Handbook of Experimental Pharmacology

Volume 284

The *Handbook of Experimental Pharmacology* is one of the most authoritative and influential book series in pharmacology. It provides critical and comprehensive discussions of the most significant areas of pharmacological research, written by leading international authorities. Each volume in the series represents the most informative and contemporary account of its subject available, making it an unrivalled reference source.

HEP is indexed in PubMed and Scopus.

Monika Schäfer-Korting • Ulrich S. Schubert
Editors

Drug Delivery and Targeting

Springer

Editors
Monika Schäfer-Korting
Pharmacology and Toxicology
Freie Universität Berlin
Berlin, Germany

Ulrich S. Schubert
Laboratory of Organic and Macromolecular Chemistry (IOMC)
Friedrich Schiller University Jena
Jena, Germany

ISSN 0171-2004 ISSN 1865-0325 (electronic)
Handbook of Experimental Pharmacology
ISBN 978-3-031-52863-7 ISBN 978-3-031-52864-4 (eBook)
https://doi.org/10.1007/978-3-031-52864-4

This Springer imprint is published by the registered company Springer Nature Switzerland AG
The registered company address is: Gewerbestrasse 11, 6330 Cham, Switzerland

Paper in this product is recyclable.

Preface

In 2010, "Drug Delivery" has been published – volume 197 of the most authoritative book series in pharmacology, the *Handbook of Experimental Pharmacology* edited by Springer, Heidelberg – now Springer Nature. The book series dates back to Dr A. Heffner and exists for about 100 years; the main focus is on essential pathological processes and the interference of active agents (drugs) with those. The volume "Drug Delivery" has broadened the view on drugs as clinical use asks for drug formulations efficiently delivering the actives to the patients and in particular to the site of disease. Facing major progress in recent *drug delivery*, the publisher has asked for a second edition, which enables to take up the enhanced understanding of cellular processes in health and disease as well as the development of agents addressing poorly accessible targets. These include genes (over)expressed in tumor cells or immunologic diseases as well as the respective proteins to name only a few. These targets challenge drug development with respect to drug delivery and targeting: drug structures sensitive to rapid degradation and with limited access to the target site ask for novel tailor-made *delivery* systems. In addition, the interference with other essential cellular pathways often induces severe adverse drug reactions, which exclude the therapeutic use. These can be overcome by *local delivery* (e.g., implantable devices for long-term treatment) and by *drug targeting,* a selective (preferential) access of the active agent to the target site, e.g. by using particulate delivery systems with targeting ligands or the target-selective activation of a prodrug.

Major improvements in drug therapy have been realized also before, e.g. by optimization of drug structures or – alternatively – the use of formulations for enhanced drug availability and adjusted periods of activity, e.g. 24 h in treatment for hypertension and hypercholesterolemia as well as several months (and beyond), e.g. in case of contraception. Now, normalization of hypercholesterolemia for weeks appears at the horizon, too. Hot topics of recent research are tumor therapies (e.g., CART therapies, anti-cancer vaccines) as well as gene therapy in hemophilia and spinal muscular atrophies among others.

Research developments in drug delivery strongly focus on design strategies using, e.g., drug carriers to overcome the general drawbacks of systemic administration. In crafting a targeted drug carrier, a crucial step is understanding the specific challenges posed by the drug, encompassing aspects such as pharmacokinetics, pharmacodynamics, on-target and off-target toxicities, and drug resistance. Beyond liposomes and lipid-based nanoparticles, various drug carriers have emerged, including polymeric nanoparticles, polymer conjugates, inorganic (silica, carbon) and metal-based nanostructures. These diverse materials can be used to physically encapsulate, adsorb, or chemically conjugate both small-molecule drugs and macromolecules. The enrichment of the drug carrier in the cell/organ/tissue of interest can be ensured through passive or active targeting by physical and/or chemical modulation of the carrier materials. Also new drug products for topical administration such as microneedle patches have broadened the application fields of this non-invasive, convenient, and easy-to-use route.

Due to the significant increases in lifetime (worldwide almost 4 years increase from 2005 to 2015), patients suffering from severe and often chronic diseases (cancer, diabetes, and neurological diseases) increase in numbers and challenge therapy and health systems worldwide. Innovative agents, nucleic acid-based drugs including gene therapy, proteins and cell therapeutics can be an answer, yet challenge delivery because of large size and very rapid degradation in vivo while their hydrophilicity is another challenge because of limited access to the target site because of lipid barriers. While healing of a disease by a single treatment is the final goal, this is reached only in rare cases, and currently limited observation periods do not allow to exclude recurrences in future life. Yet, results seen so far stimulate ongoing research.

Life expectancy and wellbeing, however, are challenged by the age-related increase in tumors and neurological diseases in particular. Moreover, the increasing world population and travelling are driving factors spreading infections in all ages. Thus, there is a major need for respective drugs as well as stable, most efficient, well-tolerated, readily adaptable, and easy-to-use vaccines allowing for comprehensive vaccination as evidenced by the success of COVID-19 vaccination and vaccine adaptation to mutants – and in the future, perhaps, to cancer as well.

In general, drugs are produced in pharmaceutical companies, each batch is checked for quality and the product is delivered via pharmacies. The current book that is divided up into four parts provides insights into the state of the art of drug development and upcoming improvements in drug formulations (Part I), visualization (Part II), and target-specific delivery (Part III). The final section (Part IV) focuses on current major challenges – formulations of critical and new agents as well as the testing and approval of drugs used in rare diseases (Advanced Therapeutic Medicinal Products, ATMPs). These drugs pose and will pose problems in production, shipping, and use – and thus significantly challenge health systems. Moreover, the low number of patients challenges or even excludes clinical testing in accordance with general standards. A further pivotal challenge lies in upscaling to cGMP-compliant production, encompassing the establishment of analytical methods and characterization standards – an aspect that has been overlooked in recent years in terms of research and investment focus.

Yet, despite the major progress obtained, most severe diseases remain which still ask for reliable drug delivery to the site of disease and preclinical and clinical testing in accordance with the highest standards should allow to retard or even inhibit aggravation as already seen in tumor therapy. These include, e.g., nonalcoholic steatohepatitis (NASH) resulting in fibrotic remodeling of the liver culminating in liver cancer as well as impaired bone regeneration in poorly healing injuries.

Taken together advanced delivery systems pave the clinical use of nucleic acids and cell therapies as underpinned by the Nobel Award for Medicine and Physiology in 2023: "The impressive flexibility and speed with which mRNA vaccines can be developed pave the way for using the new platform also for vaccines against other infectious diseases" and "may also be used to deliver therapeutic proteins and treat some cancer types." (Nobel Committee 2023)

To achieve this goal, the pharmaceutical industry attaches great importance to the development of customized delivery systems: "The effective and targeted transport of active ingredients is crucial to achieve the desired therapeutic effect. Optimized lipid nanoparticles (LNP) and new excipients are, therefore, of central importance for the further development of mRNA drugs that go beyond the available vaccines. The new handbook 'Drug Delivery and Targeting' represents an important contribution to further enhance the field." (Dr Florian Mann, Bayer AG, Pharmaceuticals, Drug Delivery Innovation, 2023)

The editors acknowledge major thanks to all the authors for their contributions. Coherence of chapters has become possible by an intense cooperation with authors of other chapters. We would also like to thank our esteemed colleague and long-standing editor of the HEP series, Dr Walter Rosenthal from Jena, for inviting and bringing together the editors of this volume. Moreover, we express our deep thanks to Dr Stephanie Schubert, Jena, for her critical view and her most efficient every-day process management. Finally, we acknowledge our thanks to Ms Susanne Dathe and Alamelu Damodharan from Springer Nature for continuous support.

We welcome any feedback to the book by the readers.

Berlin, Germany Monika Schäfer-Korting
Jena, Germany Ulrich S. Schubert

Contents

Part I

Nanoparticles and Other Advanced Technologies

Knowledge-Based Design of Multifunctional Polymeric Nanoparticles

Mira Behnke, Caroline T. Holick, Antje Vollrath, Stephanie Schubert, and Ulrich S. Schubert

Contents

Abstract

Conventional drug delivery systems (DDS) today still face several drawbacks and obstacles. High total doses of active pharmaceutical ingredients (API) are often difficult or impossible to deliver due to poor solubility of the API or undesired clearance from the body caused by strong interactions with plasma proteins. In addition, high doses lead to a high overall body burden, in particular if they cannot be delivered specifically to the target site. Therefore, modern DDS must not only be able to deliver a dose into the body, but should also overcome the hurdles mentioned above as examples. One of these promising devices are polymeric nanoparticles, which can encapsulate a wide range of APIs despite having different physicochemical properties. Most importantly, polymeric

M. Behnke · C. T. Holick · A. Vollrath · S. Schubert · U. S. Schubert (✉)
Laboratory of Organic and Macromolecular Chemistry (IOMC), Friedrich Schiller University Jena, Jena, Germany

Jena Center for Soft Matter (JCSM), Friedrich Schiller University Jena, Jena, Germany
e-mail: ulrich.schubert@uni-jena.de

M. Schäfer-Korting, U. S. Schubert (eds.), *Drug Delivery and Targeting*,
Handbook of Experimental Pharmacology 284, https://doi.org/10.1007/164_2023_649

nanoparticles are tunable to obtain tailored systems for each application. This can already be achieved via the starting material, the polymer, by incorporating, e.g., functional groups. This enables the particle properties to be influenced not only specifically in terms of their interactions with APIs, but also in terms of their general properties such as size, degradability, and surface properties. In particular, the combination of size, shape, and surface modification allows polymeric nanoparticles to be used not only as a simple drug delivery device, but also to achieve targeting. This chapter discusses to what extent polymers can be designed to form defined nanoparticles and how their properties affect their performance.

Keywords

Active pharmaceutical ingredient · Drug delivery system · Formulation method · Nanoparticle · Polymer · Targeting

Abbreviations

API	Active pharmaceutical ingredient
FDA	Food and Drug Administration
GA	Glycolic acid
HHB	Hydrophilic-hydrophobic balance
LA	Lactic acid
LCST	Lower critical solution temperature
NIR	Near-infrared
PEG	Poly(ethylene glycol)
PGA	Poly(glycolic acid)
PLA	Poly(lactic acid)
PLGA	Poly(lactic-*co*-glycolic acid)
RESS	Rapid expansion of supercritical solutions
RGD	Arginylglycylaspartic acid
ROS	Reactive oxygen species
SC-CO_2	Supercritical carbon dioxide
SLNP	Solid lipid nanoparticle
UCST	Upper critical solution temperature

1 Introduction

The term nanoparticle has been encountered in more and more contexts in recent years; in addition to medical/pharmaceutical applications, it can also be found in lifestyle products such as cosmetics or even the construction industry and the military. However, there is a lack of a sharp and, above all, uniform definition. What nanoparticles have in common is that they are objects whose longest and shortest axes differ only slightly in length, whereas there is inconsistency in dimensions. While, for example, the International Organization for Standardization (ISO) is oriented to the term "nanoscale" and, therefore, specifies the size of nanoparticles as lying between 1 and 100 nm (ISO/TR 18401:2017(en)), one finds in the many publications on the subject significantly higher orders of magnitude up to 1,000 nm, whereby in some cases the more general term "nanomaterials" is also used (Jo et al. 2015; Zielinska et al. 2020; Jeevanandam et al. 2018).

Polymeric nanoparticles are defined within this chapter as being completely polymer based (in contrast to polymer-containing nanomedicines like liposomes, solid lipid nanoparticles (SLNP), or polymer-coated metal nanoparticles) and can be classified into solid nanoparticles, micelles, nanogels, polymersomes, core shell particles, and polyplexes. Solid nanoparticles are colloidal systems, which can form nanocapsules or nanospheres. Nanocapsules have a liquid or solid core with the compound to be delivered, which is surrounded by a solid polymer shell (Zielinska et al. 2020). Nanospheres, on the other hand, do not have a shell, but consist of a dense polymer matrix (Deng et al. 2020). Hydrogel nanoparticles, or nanogels, consist of polymers with crosslinkable groups that enable a network to be formed by chemical or physical entanglement. They combine the advantages of hydrogels, such as swelling by water, and conventional nanoparticles, e.g. improved bioavailability of the cargo (Wibowo et al. 2021). Polymersomes are polymeric vesicles in which a polymeric bilayer surrounds an aqueous core. They allow the transport of hydrophilic drugs. In contrast to the similar liposomes, the formation of these particles is based on the self-assembly of amphiphilic block copolymers. If, on the other hand, a core forming polymeric particle is present, which has, e.g., a shell of lipids, cell membrane or inorganic/organic materials, one speaks of core shell nanoparticles. These combine the advantages of polymeric particles, such as stability or controllable release of active ingredients, with the biomimetic advantages of the shell. Polyplexes consist of ionic, mostly cationic, polymers, which can transport nucleic acids through electrostatic interaction and complexation and protect them from enzymatic degradation. If amphiphilic polymers are used, they can self-assemble in aqueous systems and form micellar structures (Wibowo et al. 2021; Prabhu et al. 2015). The hydrophobic part forms the inner core of the nanoparticle and embeds the drug. The hydrophilic polymer is building a shell on the outside that protects the polymer and particle from opsonization and prevents rapid detection as well as clearance by the immune system (Fam et al. 2020). This effect is known as stealth effect and is exploited for prolonged blood circulation and enhanced drug delivery efficiency (Fam et al. 2020). Nanoparticles are further divided into different categories depending on the starting material. (1) Carbon-based: They consist entirely of carbon, including fullerenes (C60), graphene, carbon nanotubes, carbon nanofibers, and carbon black; (2) Inorganic-based: Based on metal or metal oxide and semiconductors such as silicon or ceramic; (3) Lipid-based: With lipid functions; and (4) Polymer-based: The polymers can be of natural, synthetic, or semi-synthetic origin and can be biodegradable or non-biodegradable. Both lipid- and polymer-based nanoparticles are used as drug carriers (Jeevanandam et al. 2018; Sur et al. 2019; Khan et al. 2019).

The manifold diversity of polymer synthesis makes it possible to develop tailor-made polymers and their nanoparticles for the desired applications (Fig. 1).

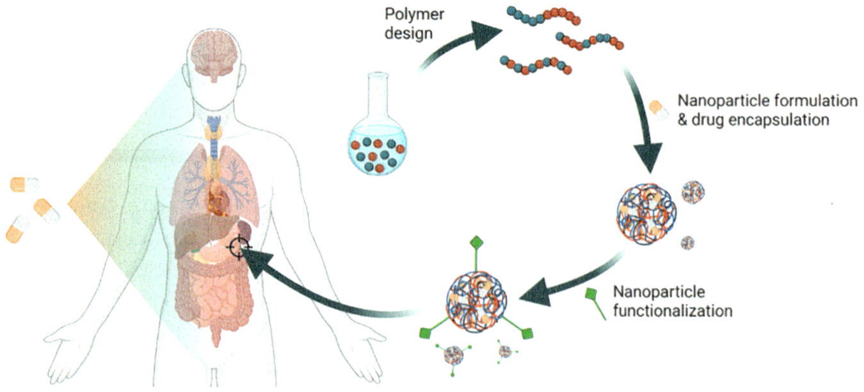

Fig. 1 Design of multifunctional polymeric nanoparticles for targeted drug delivery application

Polymer-based nanoparticles can be manufactured with different methods. For all techniques, the cargo (which can be, e.g., an active pharmaceutical ingredient (API) including proteins and genetic material for drug delivery, or a dye for diagnosis) is dissolved, attached, encapsulated, or trapped in the matrix in such a way that it is protected from unwanted degradation (Sur et al. 2019). This provides the opportunity of controlled release of the cargo as well as site-specific delivery and increased bioavailability once administered to the patient (Jo et al. 2015; Afsharzadeh et al. 2018). By utilization of polymeric nanoparticles as drug delivery vehicles it is possible to overcome even intact biological barriers such as the blood–brain barrier or blood–kidney barrier, which would not be possible for crude drugs or genes (Jo et al. 2015).

2 Polymers for Nanoparticles

Polymers are particularly well suited as carrier materials as they can be modified almost without limits. The formulated polymeric particles can be effectively adapted to the respective need in terms of size, charge, shape, hydrophilic–hydrophobic balance (HHB), softness, degradability, drug release, and targeting (Jo et al. 2015). The structure and composition of the polymer determine to a large extent not only the properties of the polymer, but also those of the subsequent nanoparticle (Fig. 2).

Polymers are molecules that consist of covalently connected single units (so-called monomers) and were introduced to the world in the early 1920s by Hermann Staudinger. They can consist of one type of monomer, in which case they are referred to as homopolymers or they may contain different monomers that are distributed randomly, alternating or block-like in the so-called copolymers (Fig. 2) (Koltzenburg et al. 2017).

Polymers can be categorized in naturally occurring and synthetically created polymers. Natural polymers derive from animal- and plant-based sources and are

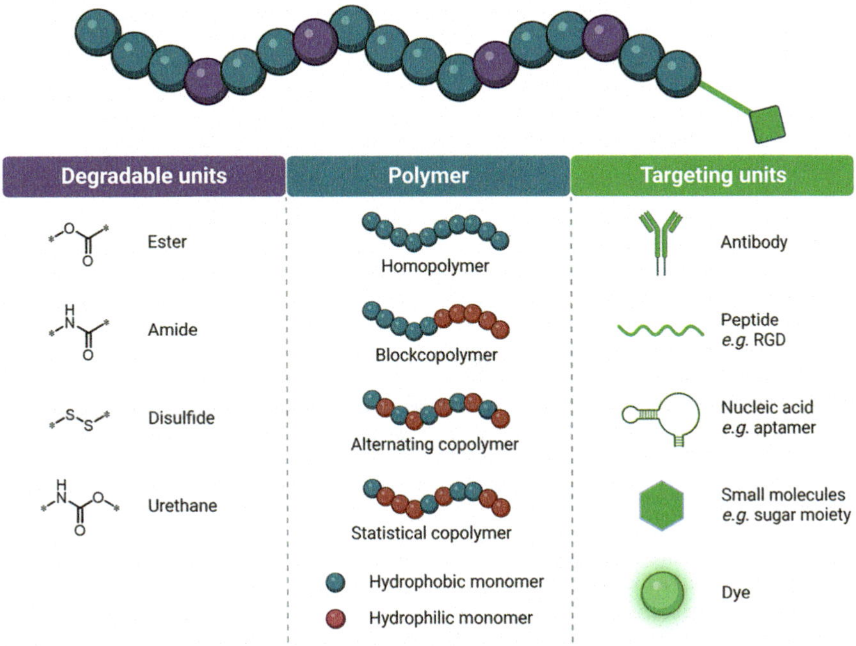

Fig. 2 Schematic representation and examples of structural units that are essential in polymer design for nanoparticle-based drug delivery approaches

often highly biocompatible and non-toxic at various concentrations. However, they are prone to high batch-to-batch variability, which might result in poor particle quality after nanoparticle formulation. Chemically modified natural polymers are usually named semi-synthetic polymers (Jarai et al. 2020). Synthetic polymers, on the other hand, are obtained by polymerizing (various) monomers, e.g., via step- or chain growth reactions, and are highly adjustable in their structure and, thus, in their properties, making them suitable for manifold applications. The step-growth reaction can be used for monomers with two functional groups, e.g., for synthesis of polyamides or polyesters. Here, oligomers are formed first, before reacting at higher conversions leading to molecules with a higher molar mass. Each molecule can act as a new monomer and has the same reactivity as the original monomer. This is in contrast to chain growth reactions, which require an active group to which the monomers can be attached to grow the chain. Typical examples are radical- and ionic polymerization reactions, and only a small fraction of the molecules are involved in the polymerization. In radical polymerization, only radical molecules can start a reaction while the rest remain unreactive. Molecules of higher molar mass can be obtained very quickly (Koltzenburg et al. 2017). Examples for various natural and synthetic polymers and their characteristics are listed in Table 1.

There are several polymers that are approved by, e.g., the Food and Drug Administration (FDA) or the European Medicines Agency (EMA) and used as

Table 1 Selection of different classes of polymers used in nanoparticles and their main characteristics

Class	Polymer	Characteristics
Natural polymers		
Polysaccharide	Hyaluronic acid[a]	Biodegradable (Jarai et al. 2020), function in tumor cell proliferation (Wong et al. 2020)
	Cellulose[a]	Low cost (Khine and Stenzel 2020)
	Chitosan[a]	Biodegradable, tunable degradation rate (Yuan et al. 2011), poor solubility (Wong et al. 2020)
Natural protein	Albumin[a]	Highly soluble, many binding sites for drugs (Wong et al. 2020)
	Collagen[a]	Biodegradable (Wong et al. 2020)
Semi-synthetic polymers		
	Acetalated dextran (AceDex)	Acid sensitive, tunable degradation kinetics (Stiepel et al. 2022)
Synthetic polymers		
Polyester	Poly(glycolic acid)[a] (PGA)	High crystallinity, biodegradable (Jarai et al. 2020; Calzoni et al. 2019)
	Poly(lactic acid)[a] (PLA)	Bioresorbability (Jarai et al. 2020; Tyler et al. 2016)
	Poly(lactic-*co*-glycolic acid)[a] (PLGA)	Tunable degradation rate (Jarai et al. 2020; Calzoni et al. 2019)
	Polycaprolactone[a] (PCL)	Slow degradation (Jarai et al. 2020)
Polyamine	Poly(ethylene imine)[a] (PEI)	Cationic nature allows formulation with negatively charged genes (polyplexes) (Jarai et al. 2020), cytotoxic at higher concentrations (Bus et al. 2017)
Polypeptide	Poly(lysine)[a]	Antimicrobial activity, cationic (may form polyplexes) (Shukla et al. 2012)
Poly(*N*-acryl-amides)	Poly(*N*-isopropylacryl-amide)[a] (PNIPAAm)	Thermoresponsive (LCST ~32°C) (Chung et al. 1999), not biocompatible for blood-contacting application (Nishimura et al. 2022)
Polyether	Polyethyleneglycol[a] (PEG)	Stealth effect, water soluble (Mohapatra et al. 2019)
	Poly(methyl methacrylate) (PMMA)	High permeability for drugs, resistant to chemical hydrolysis (Sahu et al. 2018)

[a] Legally approved polymers for medical applications

packaging materials for drug delivery applications also in nanomedicines. However, of the FDA-approved polymer-containing products, only a few, such as Genexol PM® or Nanoxel®, can be grouped under the term polymeric nanoparticles. Moreover, many polymer-based prodrugs, inactive precursors of drugs that are bioconverted (Najjar and Karaman 2019), and drug-polymer conjugates such as PEGIntron, Oncaspar, and Copaxone are on the market as well as polymer-containing nanoparticles (with polymers being only a minor part and not a structural unit) like liposomes (e.g., Doxil®, AmBisome®, Marqibo®) or solid lipid nanoparticles (SLNP, e.g., Comirnaty®, Spikevax®) (Mitchell et al. 2021; Werner et al. 2013).

2.1 Important Aspects in Polymer Design

By choosing the right polymer, characteristics such as biocompatibility, biodegradability, and hydrophobicity/hydrophilicity can be tuned to achieve better performances of the nanoparticle in vivo. In addition, polymers can be modified after polymerization to improve the targeting abilities of the nanoparticle (see Fig. 2).

Hydrophilicity/Hydrophobicity Polymers can be hydrophilic, hydrophobic, or amphiphilic as often observed for block copolymers. Depending on the type of polymer or composition of the polymers used, it is possible to obtain different nanoparticle structures. The hydrophilic-hydrophobic balance (HHB) describes the ratio of the different proportions within a polymer and determines directly the HHB of the particles. Although the HHB strongly affects the polymer aggregate morphology, this relationship is often not considered. By adjusting the amphiphilicity of the block copolymers, the dimensions of polymeric nanoparticles, such as the length of worms, can be controlled (Figg et al. 2017). Furthermore, the internal pore size of bicontinuous polymer nanospheres can also be tuned via the HHB (McKenzie et al. 2015).

When using an amphiphilic block copolymer, the hydrophilic polymer on the outside can protect the polymer or particle from nonspecific cellular uptake, molecular recognition, and protein adhesion. Specifically, opsonization, rapid detection, and clearance by the immune system (stealth effect) are prevented (Fam et al. 2020). The most prominent example of a polymer with a stealth effect is PEG. However, the so-called PEGylation of polymers and particles also entails considerable disadvantages, which is referred to as the "PEG dilemma." Due to the stimulation of anti-PEG antibodies, that are widely present in humans due to the frequent use of PEG also in cosmetics, accelerated blood clearance can prevent PEGylated particles from efficiently reaching their desired site of action resulting in lower performance (Hou et al. 2021; Nogueira et al. 2020; Knop et al. 2010).

In addition to this, anti-PEG antibodies can also lead to hypersensitivity reactions, which manifests as pseudo allergy in humans (Figg et al. 2017; Nogueira et al. 2020). Besides these disadvantages, another problem of the use of PEG is the possible formation of toxic side products during synthesis, such as 1,4-dioxane and PEG oligomers due to sequential oxidation when using PEG of lower molar masses (Knop et al. 2010). Consequently, it is important to establish PEG alternatives. Currently water-soluble polyoxazolines (Bludau et al. 2017), in particular poly(2-methyl/ethyl-2-oxazoline), poly(sarcosine) (Nogueira et al. 2020), or polyglycerol (Hauptstein et al. 2021) are in the focus of research.

Biocompatibility and Biodegradability Biocompatibility and biodegradability are two main points of interest when creating nanoparticles for biomedical application. Hereby, biocompatibility is defined as the ability of a material to elicit a specific host response and the interaction of a material with a system without a risk of toxicity or immune responses (Ghasemi-Mobarakeh et al. 2019). Consequently, the materials used must be either biocompatible, biodegradable, and the degradation products biocompatible, or they need to be completely eliminated as such before any unfavorable reaction occurs (Vauthier and Bouchemal 2009). As a consequence, biodegradability is very important, since it not only lowers the risk of large molecules but also simplifies drug release (Karlsson et al. 2018; Marin et al. 2013).

For controlled degradation and the release of APIs, different triggers can be integrated into the polymer depending on the site of action, which enable a release profile for optimal treatment. If the polymer has a hydrolysis-sensitive group, e.g., ester moieties, it can react with water and a hydrolytic degradation occurs. Enzymes such as esterases can catalyze the reaction (Marin et al. 2013). Known polymers with hydrolysable groups are polyesters, polyamides, polyurethanes, and polyanhydrides. When copolymerized with other monomers, it is possible to further adjust the degradation rate. The best-known example is PLGA, which is copolymerized from lactic acid (LA) and glycolic acid (GA). The degradability of PLGA depends on the molar ratio of LA and GA, the resulting crystallinity, and the molar mass. Amorphous regions are more prone to degradation compared to crystalline ones, which means an increase in the PGA content would lead to a decrease in degradability, since PGA reduces chain rearrangement. Increasing the number of crystalline parts also leads to a reduction of water absorption, which additionally hinders hydrolytic degradation (Elmowafy et al. 2019; Zhou and Xanthos 2008). The only exception to this is PLGA with an equal proportion of PLA and PGA. Besides the molecular order, higher molar masses result in slower degradation rates, because chain–chain crossing of the polymer backbones hinders chain cleavage (Elmowafy et al. 2019). Aside from hydrolysis, oxidation caused by reactive oxygen species (ROS) can also lead to degradation due to the formation of free radicals, e.g., in polymers such as poly(ethylene)s, poly(urethane)s, or poly(ether)s. In particular in inflamed tissues, leukocytes and macrophages produce ROS such as nitric oxide, hydrogen peroxide, and superoxide to a higher extent (Marin et al. 2013).

In addition to the previously mentioned polymer degradation options, particles can release their cargo with the help of a trigger. Such triggers can be divided into external and internal. Internal stimuli are, e.g., changes in pH value, redox potential or specific enzymes, while external ones are temperature, light, or ultrasound (Chang et al. 2021). Internal stimuli preferably occur in inflamed areas and tumors. Moreover, anaerobic metabolism is enhanced due to insufficient oxygen supply (Cheng et al. 2013). This pH change can be exploited for cargo release, e.g., by incorporating primary or tertiary amines into the polymer structure, the polymer, respectively nanoparticle, can be protonated at the slightly acidic conditions leading to dissolution of the before hydrophobic polymer and, thus, drug release (Elsabahy and Wooley 2012).

Thermoresponsive polymers usually change their solubility in water at a critical temperature, named lower or upper critical solution temperature (LCST, UCST). When a polymer becomes soluble below a certain temperature due to more prominent polymer–water interactions (hydrogen bonding) and turns insoluble above that temperature due to stronger polymer–polymer interactions (the entropic contributions are larger than the hydrogen bonds), it is called an LCST polymer. Poly(*N*-isopropylacrylamide) is a prominent example with a LCST preferably at physiological temperatures (Chung et al. 1999). UCST describes the opposite effect (Chung et al. 1999; Bordat et al. 2019). In case of LCST polymers, the change in the HHB leads to a change in the morphology of the polymer. Once the LCST is reached, the polymer chains collapse and the drug is released from the carrier (Crucho 2015; de la Rosa et al. 2016). However, using LCST polymers for drug encapsulation may be disadvantageous due to the insufficient release of hydrophobic drugs, which are miscible with the hydrophobic core above the LCST. Because of that, UCST polymeric carriers recently emerged a great potential. UCST is based on interactions as hydrogen bonding or electrostatic interactions, e.g., in poly(*N*-acryloyl glycinamide) (PNAGA). These polymers can form micelles in aqueous medium below the UCST and release the encapsulating drug fully with increasing temperature when the polymer is solubilized (Le et al. 2022).

Ultrasound represents an upcoming and promising trigger because of its non-invasive nature, application in a controlled manner, and deep tissue penetration. Ultrasound is a form of pressure waves, which are already used in the fields of diagnostic imaging, therapeutic purposes, or a combination of both. Drug release by ultrasound can be achieved in manifold ways. Most famous is the release of a drug in a thermosensitive structure. When the waves propagate into the tissue, energy will be absorbed resulting in heating, which leads to disruption of the nanostructure and the cargo is released (Entzian and Aigner 2021; Tehrani Fateh et al. 2021). In addition to the combined variant, ultrasound can also lead to drug release through mechanical effects. Continuous oscillation of the microbubbles creates shear stress that destroys the carrier, allowing the drug to be released (Tu et al. 2021).

The usage of light as external trigger generally suffers from poor tissue transparency (Wang et al. 2017). Therefore, near-infrared (NIR) light, which can penetrate deeper into tissue, is applied for the disruption of the nanoparticle with light-responsive groups. Examples are here light-cleavable polymers based on aliphatic polycarbonates that absorb light of specific wavelength leading to degradation. The light-responsive group can be incorporated in three different ways: (1) As a polymer endgroup, which leads to self-immolative reactions, (2) by photocleavable linkers as monomers in the backbone or (3) by pendant chains along the backbone, which leads to cyclization (Sun et al. 2018).

Depending on the polymer, either external or internal triggers can be used for degradation, but also in combination in the form of cycle amplification as in the case of polyurethanes. Here, external triggers cause the formation of highly reactive primary amino groups, which activate built-in triggers resulting in a release of more primary amino groups, thereby triggering the degradation of nanoparticles, which consequently results in higher sensitivity even at trace amounts of external stimuli (Tan et al. 2021).

2.2 Functional Units for Targeted Drug Delivery

The targets in the patient to which the nanoparticles should preferentially and selectively deliver the incorporated API can be addressed in two different ways: Passively and actively. Passive targeting concentrates on the nanoparticle size or circulation time, as well as on the biology of the targeted area, for instance leakiness (Attia et al. 2019). Active targeting aims to deliver the drug specifically to the envisaged site by modifying the polymer with moieties of molecular recognition (Steichen et al. 2013). This way of drug delivery is more beneficial due to less unspecific interactions between the drug and the healthy tissue resulting in a reduction in side effects (Steichen et al. 2013). For the introduction of targeting units, simple, fast, and efficient reaction conditions are required. The so-called bioconjugate chemistry uses originally occurring functionalities of the targeting ligands or slightly modified ligands bearing a reactive functional group without changing the ligand's properties and respective orthogonal groups on the polymer side (Algar 2017). Prominent examples are acylation, e.g. amidation via activation with reactive esters, aminolysis, or reactions in the sense of click chemistry (Ulbrich et al. 2016; Hermanson 2013). The latter allows to modify the polymer or particle in a well-defined matter with mild reaction conditions, high yields and without non-desired by-products (Geng et al. 2021). The term "click chemistry" stands thereby for various reactions, e.g. azide-alkyne, thiol-ene and Diels-Alder reactions and was awarded with the Nobel Prize in 2022 (Geng et al. 2021).

Targeting ligands can be coupled directly to the polymer after polymerization, preferably under homogeneous reaction conditions, or to the surface of the nanoparticle after their initial preparation, which is then a heterogeneous reaction in water. Surface post-modification includes thereby the introduction of targeting units (e.g., proteins or functional groups with different charges) as well as the attachment of hydrophilic polymers for stealth behavior. In addition to the mentioned conjugation methods, however, nonspecific interactions, e.g., adsorption of proteins, can also be used for surface modification.

In general, the analysis of the particle's surface is very challenging due to the high polymer/ligand ratio and often very low ligand concentrations (Alkilany et al. 2019). Coupling of the targeting ligand directly to the polymer is beneficial for the subsequent analysis but generally limited due to solubility and stability issues of the ligand. In addition, the ligand might not be exposed to the surface of the particles after formulation. The surface functionalization of the particle may prevent this, but other questions arise: (1) How many of the end functionalities introduced for the binding of targeting or structural units are present on the surface and available for specific binding; (2) how many targeting or structural units are bound to the surface. The latter depends not only on the number of theoretical binding possibilities but also on the properties of the ligands, i.e., their steric demand, charge, which may prevent the binding of several or even many ligands simultaneously. The stability of the particle suspension is also influenced by the modification. For example, proteins that offer several functional groups for binding to the particle surface bear the risk of cluster formation if they bind to different particles at the same time. The following section will provide an overview of typical targeting ligands.

Antibodies Antibodies belong to the most used targeting moieties such as FDA-approved rituximab (Sultan et al. 2022; Accardo et al. 2014). This targeting is characterized by high specificity and good binding affinities (Accardo et al. 2014; Carter et al. 2016). However, they are very expensive and stability problems as well as immunogenicity problems may occur if non-humanized antibodies are used (Accardo et al. 2014).

Aptamers Having high binding specificity and affinity makes aptamers to "synthetic antibodies" (Wu et al. 2015). Aptamers are short, single-stranded oligonucleotides, which show lower toxicity and lower immunogenicity (Uhl et al. 2018). The easy production with a low batch-to-batch variation combined with the beneficial properties mentioned before makes them strong candidates for specific drug delivery. However, being based on nucleic acids, aptamers face the danger of degradation in biological media (Zhao et al. 2020).

Peptides The wide variety of possible sequences also in large batch synthesis shows the potential of peptides as targeting ligands for different receptors. Despite their comparatively lower immunogenicity, the use of peptides as a target bears the disadvantage of lower target affinity and metabolic instability due to protease degradation. The latter can be solved by using specific uncoded amino acids (Accardo et al. 2014; Lu et al. 2020). The best known is the RGD (arginylglycylaspartic acid) peptide, which is renowned for its integrin affinity. Integrins are predominantly found in tumor tissues resulting in RGD frequently used for its targeting (Yoo et al. 2019).

Small Molecules Small molecules include ligands with a molar mass below 1 kDa such as dyes, sugars, and vitamins amongst others. Because of their simplicity of chemistry of conjugation and stability, these molecules belong to the first targeting ligands used (Zhao et al. 2020; Friedman et al. 2013). Most famous under this small molecule category is folic acid, a vitamin, which is used by all cells for nucleotide synthesis. Therefore, receptors for folic acid are expressed in various cells (Zhao et al. 2020). The vitamin also facilitates efficient intracellular delivery after its mediated endocytosis (Zhao et al. 2020).

Another important class are monosaccharides, for instance glucose, mannose, or galactose. These sugar moieties are known for their low toxicity, high stability, and biocompatibility (Chen et al. 2020). Since sugars can bind to lectin receptors and glucose transporter 1, which are found in many human cells, glycosylation represents a common strategy for the modification of nanoparticles. Limitations of the use of monosaccharides are the still ongoing research about the different glycosylation types and their understanding, the possible clearance of glycosylated formulations by various barriers and enzymes, and multiple targeting of several sites due to the omnipresent receptors (Chen et al. 2020).

A less popular but emerging example of small molecules as targeting ligands are dyes. Due to limitations such as poor hydrophilicity, photostability or low detection sensitivity in biological systems, only a few NIR dyes are accessible for such purposes. Polymethine (cyanine) fluorophores are, in contrast to conventional dyes, known to be cleared via specific organs, which makes them particularly interesting for organ-specific targeting (Luo et al. 2011). In the last decade, polymethine dyes were coupled to polymers and processed into nanoparticles as promising organ-selective theranostic devices (Press et al. 2014, 2017).

3 Formulation of Nanoparticles

3.1 Methods

A variety of methods are available for the preparation of nanoparticles. In general, a distinction is made between top-down and bottom-up methods. In simple terms, the top-down methods are used to break down the required nanoparticles from larger structures, while the bottom-up methods are used to assemble small structures such as atoms or molecules into the desired nanoparticles. When selecting the right method, the central question is the solubility of polymer and API. The following criteria, among others, should also be considered: Scale-up requirement, complexity, cost, yield, and, most importantly the ability to control the particle properties. In the following, the most prominent formulation techniques will be briefly introduced.

Nanoprecipitation Nanoprecipitation is a very simple method and, thus, one of the most used ones. In this approach, the polymer is dissolved in an organic solvent, the so-called "solvent" and mixed with an aqueous phase, the "non-solvent". The decisive factor here is the miscibility of solvent and non-solvent, which leads to the immediate precipitation of the polymer. The technique is not dependent on surfactants or external energy and is, thus, economically favored. Nevertheless, it has the disadvantage that is not possible to encapsulate hydrophilic drugs to a sufficient degree as the physical forces lead to the leaking of the drug outside the particle matrix (Shkodra-Pula et al. 2020).

Emulsion The polymer is dissolved in an organic solvent, which, in contrast to nanoprecipitation, must not be miscible with the aqueous phase. To produce particles, both phases need to be mixed with each other by utilizing external forces, for example by using ultrasonication, so that an emulsion is formed, which is stabilized by surfactants. The polymer-containing organic solvent forms the inner phase and the aqueous solution the outer phase. The evaporation of the organic solvent then causes the nanoparticles to harden over time. The single emulsion technique is frequently used for hydrophobic cargo, whereas the double emulsion method can be used to entrap hydrophilic cargo (Shkodra-Pula et al. 2020). For double emulsion, the cargo, e.g. genetic material or proteins in water, is first emulsified in a small volume with an excess of organic phase. To this primary emulsion, an excess of aqueous phase is added to form the water-in-oil-in-water emulsion.

Microfluidic The formulation of nanoparticles using microfluidic devices has become increasingly important in the last few years as it offers the possibility to influence the physicochemical properties of the particles more precisely. The particles can be prepared by nanoprecipitation as well as emulsion depending on the chip and materials used. In the case of chips with two inlets and one outlet, the active ingredient is often dissolved together with the polymer in the organic phase and then mixed with the aqueous phase connected to the second inlet. In contrast to conventional methods, the formulation occurs within channels in the micro scale, where the fluids are manipulated. Among others, the particle properties can be influenced by the geometry of the channels and the conditions (concentrations, flow speed, surfactants) applied during the formulation (Tian et al. 2022).

Electrospraying For electrospray formulation, the dissolved polymer and API is directed through a spray system with the aim of splitting the spray into fine-defined droplets by applying a high voltage to the nozzle. Due to the reduced surface tension effect, a so-called Taylor cone is initially formed, which then breaks into the charged droplets. These droplets can then be collected by using a grounded plate or a glass with cross-linker containing solution. Yet, shear effects in the nozzle and the thermal effects on the active ingredient are critical, which means that this technique can be only applied to a few selected APIs (Sridhar and Ramakrishna 2013).

Spray Drying Another simple method, which is also used in the food industry, is spray drying. For this approach, the liquid feed is first atomized. The droplets formed subsequently meet a hot air stream so that the solvent will be removed. The particles obtained are entrained by the air flow and can be collected. Depending on the solubility of the API and the excipients including the polymer, up to four-fluid nozzles can be used for different solvents (Wong and John 2016).

Supercritical Techniques The term "supercritical fluid technology" covers many variants such as the static supercritical fluid process (SSF), the gas antisolvent process (GAS), and the rapid expansion of supercritical solutions (RESS), but also many others. Supercritical fluids, such as supercritical carbon dioxide (SC-CO_2), can be generated under very high pressures. In particular, RESS has the potential to be a green alternative to other methods since additional purification steps are not required. In this process, the mixture of polymer and API is first supersaturated with SC-CO_2 and then expanded into a vessel under non-pressurized conditions through an appropriate small orifice. In contrast to other production methods, such as spray drying, the particles grow to the intended size and are not shattered. In particular materials with a high molar mass and polarity are often only poorly soluble in supercritical fluids and, thus, not suitable or require the use of co-solvents, which residues are also criticized (Byrappa et al. 2008).

PRINT Technology Another bottom-up method for the production of nanoparticles is the particle replication in nonwetting templates (PRINT) technology. Here, the particles are formed in precisely defined molds under the influence of heat, so that monodisperse size- and shape-specific nanoparticles can be obtained. Depending on the mold used, particles from 80 nm to a few micrometers can be produced (Perry et al. 2011).

Besides the presented methods, however, there are other less frequently used techniques such as the salting-out method and emulsion polymerization (Rao and Geckeler 2011). Usually, several methods are suitable for one polymer/API system, the exact specifications of the particles to be produced must, therefore, be determined. Depending on the type of application and the intended target, a certain size range and morphology must be complied, while also considering material, equipment, and general costs. In addition to the initial question of suitability, the scale of production must also be addressed. For example, in smaller laboratory scales nanoprecipitation may be superior due to good practicability, low equipment cost, a fast process, and the small amounts of polymer required. But in larger scales, microfluidic as a continuous manufacturing method with operator-independent results may balance these points and be superior. For all methods, the formulation of nanoparticles represents a multifactorial process. The individual variables must be carefully considered in the development of formulation protocols. Even small changes in individual variables and even more substantial in combination can significantly change the properties of the particles. Thus, the development of protocols is a time-consuming and cost-intensive process, which, however, can be accelerated by the latest developments in artificial intelligence via machine learning (Tao et al. 2021; Mekki-Berrada et al. 2021).

Another important part of the manufacturing process is the purification of the particles to make them suitable for biomedical applications. Depending on the preparation method, various impurities can occur, which can be present both in suspension and adsorbed onto the particles. In order to remove solvent residues, surfactants, salts, particle aggregates, or free API precipitates, the particles are often purified by centrifugation, filtration, or dialysis (Crucho and Barros 2017). These aspects also need to be considered when developing a good manufacturing practice (GMP) conform production of nanoparticles as medications.

3.2 Impact of Formulation Parameters on Particle Properties

Active Pharmaceutical Ingredient To be able to use nanoparticles as a delivery device, the APIs must be encapsulated in the particles or bound to their surface. The solubility of the API thereby directly influences the choice of the manufacturing method (and vice versa) and the need for further formulation components such as a co-solvent. Hydrophobic APIs can be encapsulated often straightforwardly with the already mentioned techniques since the hydrophobic core of the particles forms the perfect environment. The encapsulation of hydrophilic cargo, on the other hand, can be very challenging and often only realized with emulsion-based techniques and the utilization of surfactants or when using nanogels. During the encapsulation procedure of generally hydrophobic APIs, the API's solubility often undergoes a change whereby the metastable amorphous form is converted into a more stable, but poorly soluble, crystalline form (Crucho and Barros 2017). To prevent this conversion and to enhance the solubility of the drug, the amorphous solid dispersion technique has been established. Herein, the polymer is used to prevent the crystallization of the API (Newman and Zografi 2022). However, this requires that the interactions, e.g., van der Waals or hydrogen bonds, between API and polymer are high and that the polymeric component can dissolve the API and encapsulate a large part of it.

The API also affects the subsequent particle properties. Although its encapsulation often leads to an increase in particle size, the reverse effect can also be observed, for example when the charge of the polymer and API is opposite. This then results in denser packing within the particle, which can increase the stability of the particles, also because less active ingredient may be released unintentionally. The presence of free API can lead to instabilities and should, therefore, always be examined as part of quality control, e.g., by using microscopy techniques such as scanning electron microscopy.

Formulation Additives Depending on the preparation method and the stability of the particles during the production process and their storage, additional formulation agents, so-called additives or excipients, are required (Thakur and Gupta 2006). One of the most applied additives in formulation are surfactants, such as polysorbate, poly(vinyl alcohol) or poloxamers, which enable the production process, e.g., stabilization of dispersions in emulsion methods. Surfactants have a strong influence on the properties of the particles, in particular regarding size/size distribution, loading capacity, and surface charge which, in turn, alters the interaction of the particles with cells (Benfer and Kissel 2012). Thus, the proportion of additives can be used to deliberately affect the properties and the performance of the particles. However, a high concentration of surfactant can lead to undesirable side effects and the extent of their use is chosen carefully. There are difficulties to remove surfactants afterward as they often remain adsorbed on the surface of the particles. Depending on the toxicity of the additive, time-consuming and cost-intensive purification steps may be necessary.

In addition to surfactants, other excipients like lyoprotectants are applied in the production and storage of nanoparticles such as polyol compounds or sugars (trehalose, sucrose) (Ngamcherdtrakul et al. 2018). They are used to preserve the properties of the particles even after freeze-drying to remain the low surface roughness (Fonte et al. 2015).

4 Influence of the Nanoparticle Characteristics on Their Performance

The performance of the particle and its cargo depends on the final particle characteristics which are reflected mostly by the size, shape, charge, softness, hydrophilicity/hydrophobicity, and stability (degradability) (see Fig. 3).

Size The size of the particles represents a very crucial factor since it directly influences their physical properties, such as significant changes in surface to volume ratios (Carmignani et al. 2022; An et al. 2019). In addition, nanoparticles lose their colloidal character with increasing size since sedimentation becomes more prone above a size of about 200 nm. Besides these two aspects, the biological interaction is another very important issue that has to be pointed out. For nanoparticles that are administered systemically, for example, it must be ensured that they remain in the body for a sufficiently long time without being removed prematurely by the reticuloendothelial system. Size limitations can be caused by binding interactions, e.g., due to steric factors, special biological functions, or specific biological compartments (Betzer et al. 2017; Shilo et al. 2015). In particular for biomedical applications, toxicity and biocompatibility have to be considered – the smaller the nanoparticle, the easier the migration (Dolai et al. 2021). The renal excretion has an

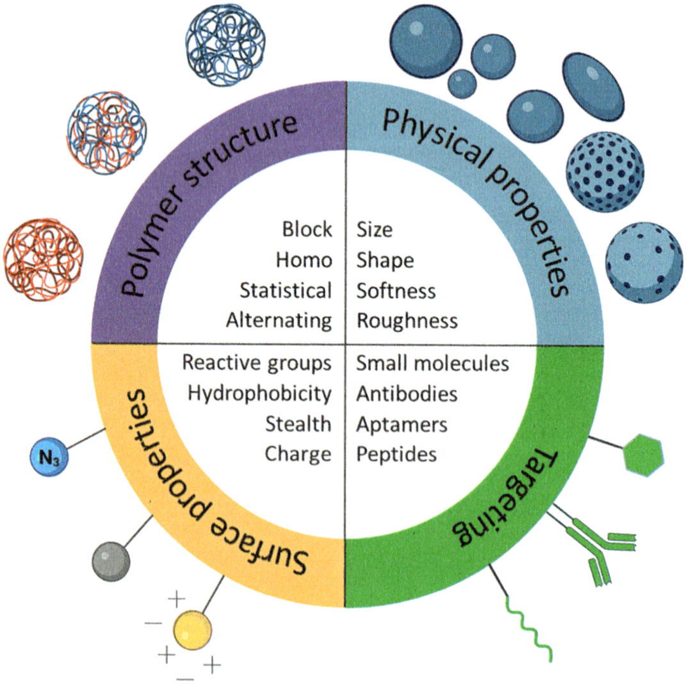

Fig. 3 Tunable structural features of polymeric nanoparticles for optimal drug delivery properties

upper cut-off limit of approx. 48 kDa, which would represent dimensions below 5.5 nm. When considering other in vivo pathways, particles up to 2,000 nm can still escape the pulmonary capillaries (Elsabahy and Wooley 2012; Choi et al. 2007; Jain and Stylianopoulos 2010; Yang et al. 2012; Zhang et al. 2021). Even on cellular level, the nanoparticle uptake mechanisms are directly correlated to the size of the particles applied. Nanoparticles below 200 nm are known to be endocytosed by many cell types, whereas micropinocytosis and phagocytosis are usually the main uptake mechanisms above 200 nm. The uptake kinetics are also influenced by the size and uptake mechanism, respectively (Vollrath et al. 2013). However, there is a lack of a consistent and generally valid statement on the specific role of particle size, as it strongly depends on the biological environment and planned application including the targeted organ, tissue, and cells (Dolai et al. 2021; Albanese et al. 2012).

Charge The surface charge (ζ-potential) decisively influences the colloidal stability of the nanoparticles and can prevent coalescence and aggregation if the repulsive forces are stronger compared to the Van der Waals attractive forces between the particles (Asem et al. 2021). The surface charge of nanoparticles is mainly determined by the underlying polymeric structure, but also by the additives used in the formulation (surfactants, etc.). Neutral- and negatively charged polymers usually result in a negative ζ-potential of the formulated particles, whereas polymers with cationic or protonable functionalities, e.g., amines, result in positively charged particles. Surfactants can render the nanoparticles neutral.

The ζ-potential of a particle influences its cellular uptake, biodistribution, and interaction with the biological environment (Jo et al. 2015). On the one hand, positively charged particles are described to offer the advantages of better imaging, gene transfer, and drug delivery, but on the other hand, often show a higher cytotoxicity (Frohlich 2012). The uptake of the particles, nevertheless, is cell-dependent. Thus, in principle, cationic particles are better internalized by non-phagocytic cells, whereas anionic nanoparticles are taken up more by phagocytic cells (Frohlich 2012). Depending on the charge of the particles, organ/tissue-specific biological distributions can occur. For example, cationic nanoparticles are more readily accumulated in the kidney compared to anionic nanoparticles (Huang et al. 2021). It can be deduced that the performance of nanoparticulate drug delivery systems also depends on their charge density and charge polarity. However, the ζ-potential can shift again in vivo to slightly negative values due to the accumulation of proteins and should, therefore, be considered when designing nanoparticles for the intended cellular uptake (Jo et al. 2015).

Shape The shape of the nanoparticles can be used to control the interaction of ligands, cellular uptake, transport, cytotoxicity, and finally their degradation (Frohlich 2012; Champion et al. 2007). For instance, a non-spherical form of the particles can lead to "cell-evading" due to an altered attachment and internalization behavior (Jo et al. 2015; Jindal 2017). Furthermore, the shape of the nanoparticles can be used to influence their circulation time. For example, filomicelles (worm-like micelles) can circulate in the blood much longer than spherical nanoparticles and, thus, have a higher chance of cellular uptake (Zhao et al. 2016). The geometry of particles also affects their cell adhesion properties, e.g., elongated or flattened particles show stronger adhesion to the cell membrane than their spherical representatives. Therefore, there is already some speculation that nanocrystals and other shapes than the classical nanospheres and nanorods could be increasingly used for medical purposes in the future (Jo et al. 2015). The shape of the particles depends mainly on two factors: (1) The material used and (2) the manufacturing method (Gardey et al. 2022). The therapeutic success of particles with different shapes may also depend on the characteristics of the patients, e.g. their blood pressure and blood compositions or tissue and blood vessel condition, which can result in the greatest therapeutic success only being possible with a combination of different nanoparticle shapes (Uhl et al. 2018). Due to the strong influence of the shape on the performance of the particles in vivo, it is considered a key factor, at least equivalent to the size, in the design of nanoparticles as drug delivery devices (Petros and DeSimone 2010).

Crystallinity As mentioned already above, the HHB value of the particles is directly dependent on the bulk polymer (Vollrath et al. 2021). While designing drug delivery vehicles, it needs to be considered that the composition of the polymer and the ratio of hydrophobic to hydrophilic areas also affects the encapsulation of the API and needs to be adapted to this, depending on whether the agent itself has a rather hydrophilic or hydrophobic character (Gad et al. 2016). An additional property that is influenced by the HHB is the crystallinity of the nanoparticles. This, in turn, influences the degradation of the particles and, thus, the release of the active ingredient as well as its cellular uptake (Bandelli et al. 2018). For instance, higher drug release rates can be obtained for polyesters at low degrees of crystallinity (Karavelidis et al. 2011).

Softness Softness describes the plasticity and malleability of the particles (Rostom and Dadmun 2020). Besides the diffusion behavior, softness also has an impact on the adhesion behavior of the particles. The particles' hardness can be controlled by the crosslinking density in case of nanogels (Rostom and Dadmun 2020). The higher the density, the harder the particle, and the diffusion movement in a linear matrix is reduced (Rostom and Dadmun 2020). For the adhesion behavior of the particles, the softer they are, the stronger is their adhesion (Yang et al. 2013). In particular in view of the use of particles as a drug delivery device, the aspect of their circulation time is crucial. Studies have shown that soft particles circulate longer in the blood than harder particles, as shown, for instance, in nanogels with lower elastic modulus (Merkel et al. 2011; Anselmo et al. 2017).

5 Future Perspective

Polymeric nanoparticles offer promising opportunities for future applications, as a variety of active substances can be administered to treat different disease conditions. They can be used not only as drug delivery devices, but also for diagnostic purposes, e.g., in cancer medicine and for combining both in the field of theranostics. It should be mentioned that polymeric nanoparticles have advantages not only as a simple drug delivery device, but also with targeting function compared to conventional dosage forms, enabling customized therapy, e.g., for cancer and infectious diseases. By lowering the applied doses due to targeted application, the strain on the organism as a whole and adverse drug reactions can be reduced. Moreover, by using polymer-based nanoformulations it is possible to make existing but not yet formulatable APIs administrable, as well as efficiently encapsulate hydrophilic or hydrophobic drugs. Another advantage is the adaptability and development speed of nanoformulations, which has been demonstrated unrivaled for Covid-19 vaccines with solid lipid nanoparticles. The use of polymeric nanoparticles as a targeted drug delivery device is advantageous over other starting materials due to more flexible customization options. Thus, the development of new polymers such as polyoxazolines enables the opportunity to respond to emerging obstacles, such as the aforementioned PEG allergy (Nogueira et al. 2020). However, despite the great potential, only a few approaches make it to market approval. Difficulties in the reproducibility and precision of production among others are reasons for this. In recent years, the numbers of clinical trials of nanomedicine have increased significantly, with few approved by the FDA. These data show that the translation of nanomedicine is difficult due to various obstacles, which are not only technical, but also industrial and economical nature. With the current pandemic and SLNPs being approved in the wake of it, an approval of new polymer-based nanoparticle formulations can be expected. In this context, it is not only important to bring the capacities of the production of pharmapolymers but also those of nanoparticles to a high-throughput level.

Acknowledgments The authors gratefully acknowledge funding by the Deutsche Forschungsgemeinschaft (DFG, SFB 1278, projects A04, C01, D01, D02 and T01, project number 316213987) and the Thüringer Aufbaubank (TAB, project "Innovative Pharmapolymers"). Images were created using BioRender.

References

Accardo A, Aloj L, Aurilio M, Morelli G, Tesauro D (2014) Receptor binding peptides for target-selective delivery of nanoparticles encapsulated drugs. Int J Nanomedicine 9:1537–1557

Afsharzadeh M, Hashemi M, Mokhtarzadeh A, Abnous K, Ramezani M (2018) Recent advances in co-delivery systems based on polymeric nanoparticle for cancer treatment. Artif Cells Nanomed Biotechnol 46:1095–1110

Albanese A, Tang PS, Chan WCW (2012) The effect of nanoparticle size, shape, and surface chemistry on biological systems. Annu Rev Biomed Eng 14:1–16

Algar WR (2017) Chemoselective and bioorthogonal ligation reactions. Wiley-VCH, pp 1–36

Alkilany AM, Zhu L, Weller H, Mews A, Parak WJ, Barz M, Feliu N (2019) Ligand density on nanoparticles: a parameter with critical impact on nanomedicine. Adv Drug Deliv Rev 143:22–36

An L, Zhang D, Zhang L, Feng G (2019) Effect of nanoparticle size on the mechanical properties of nanoparticle assemblies. Nanoscale 11:9563–9573

Anselmo AC, Prabhakarpandian B, Pant K, Mitragotri S (2017) Clinical and commercial translation of advanced polymeric nanoparticle systems: opportunities and material challenges. Transl Mater Res 4:014001

Asem H, Zheng W, Nilsson F, Zhang Y, Hedenqvist MS, Hassan M, Malmström E (2021) Functional nanocarriers for drug delivery by surface engineering of polymeric nanoparticle post-polymerization-induced self-assembly. ACS Appl Bio Mater 4:1045–1056

Attia MF, Anton N, Wallyn J, Omran Z, Vandamme TF (2019) An overview of active and passive targeting strategies to improve the nanocarriers efficiency to tumour sites. J Pharm Pharmacol 71:1185–1198

Bandelli D, Helbing C, Weber C, Seifer M, Muljajew I, Jandt KD, Schubert US (2018) Maintaining the hydrophilic hydrophobic balance of polyesters with adjustable crystallinity for tailor-made nanoparticles. Macromolecules 51:5567–5576

Benfer M, Kissel T (2012) Cellular uptake mechanism and knockdown activity of siRNA-loaded biodegradable DEAPA-PVA-g-PLGA nanoparticles. Eur J Pharm Biopharm 80:247–256

Betzer O, Shilo M, Opochinsky R, Barnoy E, Motiei M, Okun E, Yadid G, Popovtzer R (2017) The effect of nanoparticle size on the ability to cross the blood-brain barrier: an in vivo study. Nanomedicine 12:1533–1546

Bludau H, Czapar AE, Pitek AS, Shukla S, Jordan R, Steinmetz NF (2017) POxylation as an alternative stealth coating for biomedical applications. Eur Polym J 88:679–688

Bordat A, Boissenot T, Nicolas J, Tsapis N (2019) Thermoresponsive polymer nanocarriers for biomedical applications. Adv Drug Deliv Rev 138:167–192

Bus T, Englert C, Reifarth M, Borchers P, Hartlieb M, Vollrath A, Hoeppener S, Traeger A, Schubert US (2017) 3rd generation poly(ethylene imine)s for gene delivery. J Mater Chem B 5: 1258–1274

Byrappa K, Ohara S, Adschiri T (2008) Nanoparticles synthesis using supercritical fluid technology – towards biomedical applications. Adv Drug Deliv Rev 60:299–327

Calzoni E, Cesaretti A, Polchi A, Di Michele A, Tancini B, Emiliani C (2019) Biocompatible polymer nanoparticles for drug delivery applications in cancer and neurodegenerative disorder therapies. J Funct Biomater:10

Carmignani A, Battaglini M, Sinibaldi E, Marino A, Vighetto V, Cauda V, Ciofani G (2022) In vitro and ex vivo investigation of the effects of polydopamine nanoparticle size on their antioxidant and photothermal properties: implications for biomedical applications. ACS Appl Nano Mater 5:1702–1713

Carter T, Mulholland P, Chester K (2016) Antibody-targeted nanoparticles for cancer treatment. Immunotherapy 8:941–958

Champion JA, Katare YK, Mitragotri S (2007) Particle shape: a new design parameter for micro- and nanoscale drug delivery carriers. J Control Release 121:3–9

Chang D, Ma Y, Xu X, Xie J, Ju S (2021) Stimuli-responsive polymeric nanoplatforms for cancer therapy. Front Bioeng Biotechnol 9:707319

Chen F, Huang G, Huang H (2020) Sugar ligand-mediated drug delivery. Future Med Chem 12: 161–171

Cheng R, Meng F, Deng C, Klok H-A, Zhong Z (2013) Dual and multi-stimuli responsive polymeric nanoparticles for programmed site-specific drug delivery. Biomaterials 34:3647–3657

Choi HS, Liu W, Misra P, Tanaka E, Zimmer JP, Ipe BI, Bawendi MG, Frangioni JV (2007) Renal clearance of quantum dots. Nat Biotechnol 25:1165–1170

Chung JE, Yokoyama M, Yamato M, Aoyagi T, Sakurai Y, Okano T (1999) Thermo-responsive drug delivery from polymeric micelles constructed using block copolymers of poly (N-isopropylacrylamide) and poly(butylmethacrylate). J Control Release 62:115–127

Crucho CIC (2015) Stimuli-responsive polymeric nanoparticles for nanomedicine. ChemMedChem 10:24–38

Crucho CIC, Barros MT (2017) Polymeric nanoparticles: a study on the preparation variables and characterization methods. Mater Sci Eng C 80:771–784 de la Rosa VR, Woisel P, Hoogenboom R (2016) Supramolecular control over thermoresponsive polymers. Mater Today 19:44–55

Deng SY, Gigliobianco MR, Censi R, Di Martino P (2020) Polymeric nanocapsules as nanotechnological alternative for drug delivery system: current status, challenges and opportunities. Nanomaterials 10:847

Dolai J, Mandal K, Jana NR (2021) Nanoparticle size effects in biomedical applications. ACS Appl Nano Mater 4:6471–6496

Elmowafy EM, Tiboni M, Soliman ME (2019) Biocompatibility, biodegradation and biomedical applications of poly(lactic acid)/poly(lactic-co-glycolic acid) micro and nanoparticles. J Pharm Investig 49:347–380

Elsabahy M, Wooley KL (2012) Design of polymeric nanoparticles for biomedical delivery applications. Chem Soc Rev 41:2545–2561

Entzian K, Aigner A (2021) Drug delivery by ultrasound-responsive nanocarriers for cancer treatment. Pharmaceutics 13:1135

Fam SY, Chee CF, Yong CY, Ho KL, Mariatulqabtiah AR, Tan WS (2020) Stealth coating of nanoparticles in drug-delivery systems. Nanomaterials 10:787

Figg CA, Carmean RN, Bentz KC, Mukherjee S, Savin DA, Sumerlin BS (2017) Tuning hydrophobicity to program block copolymer assemblies from the inside out. Macromolecules 50:935–943

Fonte P, Araújo F, Seabra V, Reis S, van de Weert M, Sarmento B (2015) Co-encapsulation of lyoprotectants improves the stability of protein-loaded PLGA nanoparticles upon lyophilization. Int J Pharm 496:850–862

Friedman AD, Claypool SE, Liu R (2013) The smart targeting of nanoparticles. Curr Pharm Des 19: 6315–6329

Frohlich E (2012) The role of surface charge in cellular uptake and cytotoxicity of medical nanoparticles. Int J Nanomedicine 7:5577–5591

Gad A, Kydd J, Piel B, Rai P (2016) Targeting cancer using polymeric nanoparticle mediated combination chemotherapy. Int J Nanomed Nanosurg:2

Gardey E, Sobotta FH, Quickert S, Bruns T, Brendel JC, Stallmach A (2022) ROS-sensitive polymer micelles for selective degradation in primary human monocytes from patients with active IBD. Macromol Biosci 22:2100482

Geng Z, Shin JJ, Xi Y, Hawker CJ (2021) Click chemistry strategies for the accelerated synthesis of functional macromolecules. J Polym Sci A Polym Chem 59:963–1042

Ghasemi-Mobarakeh L, Kolahreez D, Ramakrishna S, Williams D (2019) Key terminology in biomaterials and biocompatibility. Curr Opin Biomed Eng 10:45–50

Hauptstein N, Pouyan P, Kehrein J, Dirauf M, Driessen MD, Raschig M, Licha K, Gottschaldt M, Schubert US, Haag R, Meinel L, Sotriffer C, Lühmann T (2021) Molecular insights into site-specific interferon-α2a bioconjugates originated from PEG, LPG, and PEtOx. Biomacromolecules 22:4521–4534

Hermanson GT (2013) Bioconjugate techniques, 3rd edn. Academic Press, Boston, pp 549–785

Hou X, Zaks T, Langer R, Dong Y (2021) Lipid nanoparticles for mRNA delivery. Nat Rev Mater 6:1078–1094

Huang Y, Wang J, Jiang K, Chung EJ (2021) Improving kidney targeting: the influence of nanoparticle physicochemical properties on kidney interactions. J Control Release 334:127–137

Jain RK, Stylianopoulos T (2010) Delivering nanomedicine to solid tumors. Nat Rev Clin Oncol 7: 653–664

Jarai BM, Kolewe EL, Stillman ZS, Raman N, Fromen CA (2020) Nanoparticles for biomedical applications. Elsevier, pp 303–324

Jeevanandam J, Barhoum A, Chan YS, Dufresne A, Danquah MK (2018) Review on nanoparticles and nanostructured materials: history, sources, toxicity and regulations. Beilstein J Nanotechnol 9:1050–1074

Jindal AB (2017) The effect of particle shape on cellular interaction and drug delivery applications of micro- and nanoparticles. Int J Pharm 532:450–465

Jo DH, Kim JH, Lee TG, Kim JH (2015) Size, surface charge, and shape determine therapeutic effects of nanoparticles on brain and retinal diseases. Nanomedicine 11:1603–1611
Karavelidis V, Karavas E, Giliopoulos D, Papadimitriou S, Bikiaris D (2011) Evaluating the effects of crystallinity in new biocompatible polyester nanocarriers on drug release behavior. Int J Nanomedicine 6:3021–3032
Karlsson J, Vaughan HJ, Green JJ (2018) Biodegradable polymeric nanoparticles for therapeutic cancer treatments. Annu Rev Chem Biomol Eng 9:105–127
Khan I, Saeed K, Khan I (2019) Nanoparticles: properties, applications and toxicities. Arab J Chem 12:908–931
Khine YY, Stenzel MH (2020) Surface modified cellulose nanomaterials: a source of non-spherical nanoparticles for drug delivery. Mater Horiz 7:1727–1758
Knop K, Hoogenboom R, Fischer D, Schubert US (2010) Poly(ethylene glycol) in drug delivery: pros and cons as well as potential alternatives. Angew Chem Int Ed 49:6288–6308
Koltzenburg S, Maskos M, Nuyken O (2017) Polymer chemistry. Springer, Berlin, pp 1–16
Le M, Huang W, Chen K-F, Lin C, Cai L, Zhang H, Jia Y-G (2022) Upper critical solution temperature polymeric drug carriers. Chem Eng J 432:134354
Lu J, Xu H, Xia J, Ma J, Xu J, Li Y, Feng J (2020) D- and unnatural amino acid substituted antimicrobial peptides with improved proteolytic resistance and their proteolytic degradation characteristics. Front Microbiol 11:563030
Luo S, Zhang E, Su Y, Cheng T, Shi C (2011) A review of NIR dyes in cancer targeting and imaging. Biomaterials 32:7127–7138
Marin E, Briceño MI, Caballero-George C (2013) Critical evaluation of biodegradable polymers used in nanodrugs. Int J Nanomedicine 8:3071–3090
McKenzie BE, Friedrich H, Wirix MJM, de Visser JF, Monaghan OR, Bomans PHH, Nudelman F, Holder SJ, Sommerdijk NAJM (2015) Controlling internal pore sizes in bicontinuous polymeric nanospheres. Angew Chem Int Ed 54:2457–2461
Mekki-Berrada F, Ren ZK, Huang T, Wong WK, Zheng F, Xie JX, Tian IPS, Jayavelu S, Mahfoud Z, Bash D, Hippalgaonkar K, Khan S, Buonassisi T, Li QX, Wang XN (2021) Two-step machine learning enables optimized nanoparticle synthesis. NPJ Comput Mater 7:55
Merkel TJ, Jones SW, Herlihy KP, Kersey FR, Shields AR, Napier M, Luft JC, Wu HL, Zamboni WC, Wang AZ, Bear JE, DeSimone JM (2011) Using mechanobiological mimicry of red blood cells to extend circulation times of hydrogel microparticles. Proc Natl Acad Sci U S A 108:586–591
Mitchell MJ, Billingsley MM, Haley RM, Wechsler ME, Peppas NA, Langer R (2021) Engineering precision nanoparticles for drug delivery. Nat Rev Drug Discov 20:101–124
Mohapatra A, Uthaman S, Park I-K (2019) Polymeric nanoparticles as a promising tool for anti-cancer therapeutics. Academic Press, pp 205–231
Najjar A, Karaman R (2019) The prodrug approach in the era of drug design. Expert Opin Drug Deliv 16:1–5
Newman A, Zografi G (2022) Considerations in the development of physically stable high drug load API-polymer amorphous solid dispersions in the glassy state. J Pharm Sci
Ngamcherdtrakul W, Sangvanich T, Reda M, Gu S, Bejan D, Yantasee W (2018) Lyophilization and stability of antibody-conjugated mesoporous silica nanoparticle with cationic polymer and PEG for siRNA delivery. Int J Nanomedicine 13:4015–4027
Nishimura S, Nishida K, Ueda T, Shiomoto S, Tanaka M (2022) Biocompatible poly(N-(-ω-acryloyloxy-n-alkyl)-2-pyrrolidone)s with widely-tunable lower critical solution temperatures (LCSTs): a promising alternative to poly(N-isopropylacrylamide). Polym Chem 13:2519–2530
Nogueira SS, Schlegel A, Maxeiner K, Weber B, Barz M, Schroer MA, Blanchet CE, Svergun DI, Ramishetti S, Peer D, Langguth P, Sahin U, Haas H (2020) Polysarcosine-functionalized lipid nanoparticles for therapeutic mRNA delivery. ACS Appl Nano Mater 3:10634–10645
Perry JL, Herlihy KP, Napier ME, DeSimone JM (2011) PRINT: a novel platform toward shape and size specific nanoparticle theranostics. Acc Chem Res 44:990–998

Petros RA, DeSimone JM (2010) Strategies in the design of nanoparticles for therapeutic applications. Nat Rev Drug Discov 9:615–627

Prabhu RH, Patravale VB, Joshi MD (2015) Polymeric nanoparticles for targeted treatment in oncology: current insights. Int J Nanomedicine 10:1001–1018

Press AT, Traeger A, Pietsch C, Mosig A, Wagner M, Clemens MG, Jbeily N, Koch N, Gottschaldt M, Bézière N, Ermolayev V, Ntziachristos V, Popp J, Kessels MM, Qualmann B, Schubert US, Bauer M (2014) Cell type-specific delivery of short interfering RNAs by dye-functionalised theranostic nanoparticles. Nat Commun 5:5565

Press AT, Butans MJ, Haider TP, Weber C, Neugebauer S, Kiehntopf M, Schubert US, Clemens MG, Bauer M, Kortgen A (2017) Fast simultaneous assessment of renal and liver function using polymethine dyes in animal models of chronic and acute organ injury. Sci Rep 7:15397

Rao JP, Geckeler KE (2011) Polymer nanoparticles: preparation techniques and size-control parameters. Prog Polym Sci 36:887–913

Rostom S, Dadmun MD (2020) The impact of nanoparticle softness on its tracer diffusion coefficient in all polymer nanocomposites. J Appl Phys 127:074303

Sahu A, Solanki P, Mitra S (2018) Curcuminoid-loaded poly(methyl methacrylate) nanoparticles for cancer therapy. Int J Nanomedicine 13:101–105

Shilo M, Sharon A, Baranes K, Motiei M, Lellouche JPM, Popovtzer R (2015) The effect of nanoparticle size on the probability to cross the blood-brain barrier: an in-vitro endothelial cell model. J Nanobiotechnol 13:19

Shkodra-Pula B, Vollrath A, Schubert US, Schubert S (2020) Colloids for nanobiotechnology. Elsevier, pp 233–252

Shukla SC, Singh A, Pandey AK, Mishra A (2012) Review on production and medical applications of ε-polylysine. Biochem Eng J 65:70–81

Sridhar R, Ramakrishna S (2013) Electrosprayed nanoparticles for drug delivery and pharmaceutical applications. Biomatter 3:24281

Steichen SD, Caldorera-Moore M, Peppas NA (2013) A review of current nanoparticle and targeting moieties for the delivery of cancer therapeutics. Eur J Pharm Sci 48:416–427

Stiepel RT, Pena ES, Ehrenzeller SA, Gallovic MD, Lifshits LM, Genito CJ, Bachelder EM, Ainslie KM (2022) A predictive mechanistic model of drug release from surface eroding polymeric nanoparticles. J Control Release 351:883–895

Sultan MH, Moni SS, Madkhali OA, Bakkari MA, Alshahrani S, Alqahtani SS, Alhakamy NA, Mohan S, Ghazwani M, Bukhary HA, Almoshari Y, Salawi A, Alshamrani M (2022) Characterization of cisplatin-loaded chitosan nanoparticles and rituximab-linked surfaces as target-specific injectable nano-formulations for combating cancer. Sci Rep 12:468

Sun J, Birnbaum W, Anderski J, Picker M-T, Mulac D, Langer K, Kuckling D (2018) Use of light-degradable aliphatic polycarbonate nanoparticles as drug carrier for photosensitizer. Biomacromolecules 19:4677–4690

Sur S, Rathore A, Dave V, Reddy KR, Chouhan RS, Sadhu V (2019) Recent developments in functionalized polymer nanoparticles for efficient drug delivery system. Nano-Struct Nano-Objects 20:100397

Tan JJ, Deng ZY, Song CZ, Xu J, Zhang YB, Yu Y, Hu JM, Liu SY (2021) Coordinating external and built-in triggers for tunable degradation of polymeric nanoparticles via cycle amplification. J Am Chem Soc 143:13738–13748

Tao HC, Wu TY, Aldeghi M, Wu TC, Aspuru-Guzik A, Kumacheva E (2021) Nanoparticle synthesis assisted by machine learning. Nat Rev Mater 6:701–716

Tehrani Fateh S, Moradi L, Kohan E, Hamblin MR, Shiralizadeh Dezfuli A (2021) Comprehensive review on ultrasound-responsive theranostic nanomaterials: mechanisms, structures and medical applications. Beilstein J Nanotechnol 12:808–862

Thakur R, Gupta RB (2006) Formation of phenytoin nanoparticles using rapid expansion of supercritical solution with solid cosolvent (RESS-SC) process. Int J Pharm 308:190–199

Tian F, Cai L, Liu C, Sun J (2022) Microfluidic technologies for nanoparticle formation. Lab Chip 22:512–529

Tu L, Liao Z, Luo Z, Wu Y-L, Herrmann A, Huo S (2021) Ultrasound-controlled drug release and drug activation for cancer therapy. Exp Dermatol 1:20210023

Tyler B, Gullotti D, Mangraviti A, Utsuki T, Brem H (2016) Polylactic acid (PLA) controlled delivery carriers for biomedical applications. Adv Drug Deliv Rev 107:163–175

Uhl CG, Gao Y, Zhou S, Liu Y (2018) The shape effect on polymer nanoparticle transport in a blood vessel. RSC Adv 8:8089–8100

Ulbrich K, Holá K, Šubr V, Bakandritsos A, Tuček J, Zbořil R (2016) Targeted drug delivery with polymers and magnetic nanoparticles: covalent and noncovalent approaches, release control, and clinical studies. Chem Rev 116:5338–5431

Vauthier C, Bouchemal K (2009) Methods for the preparation and manufacture of polymeric nanoparticles. Pharm Res 26:1025–1058

Vollrath A, Schallon A, Pietsch C, Schubert S, Nomoto T, Matsumoto Y, Kataoka K, Schubert US (2013) A toolbox of differently sized and labeled PMMA nanoparticles for cellular uptake investigations. Soft Matter 9:99–108

Vollrath A, Kretzer C, Beringer-Siemers B, Shkodra B, Czaplewska JA, Bandelli D, Stumpf S, Hoeppener S, Weber C, Werz O, Schubert US (2021) Effect of crystallinity on the properties of polycaprolactone nanoparticles containing the dual FLAP/mPEGS-1 inhibitor BRP-187. Polymers 13:2557

Wang Y, Deng Y, Luo H, Zhu A, Ke H, Yang H, Chen H (2017) Light-responsive nanoparticles for highly efficient cytoplasmic delivery of anticancer agents. ACS Nano 11:12134–12144

Werner ME, Cummings ND, Sethi M, Wang EC, Sukumar R, Moore DT, Wang AZ (2013) Preclinical evaluation of Genexol-PM, a nanoparticle formulation of paclitaxel, as a novel radiosensitizer for the treatment of non-small cell lung cancer. Int J Radiat Oncol Biol Phys 86:463–468

Wibowo D, Jorritsma SHT, Gonzaga ZJ, Evert B, Chen S, Rehm BHA (2021) Polymeric nanoparticle vaccines to combat emerging and pandemic threats. Biomaterials 268:120597

Wong TW, John P (2016) Advances in spray drying technology for nanoparticle formation. Springer, pp 329–346

Wong KH, Lu A, Chen X, Yang Z (2020) Natural ingredient-based polymeric nanoparticles for cancer treatment. Molecules 25:3620

Wu X, Chen J, Wu M, Zhao JX (2015) Aptamers: active targeting ligands for cancer diagnosis and therapy. Theranostics 5:322–344

Yang ST, Luo JB, Zhou QH, Wang HF (2012) Pharmacokinetics, metabolism and toxicity of carbon nanotubes for biomedical purposes. Theranostics 2:271–282

Yang ST, Razavizadeh BBM, Pelton R, Bruin G (2013) Nanoparticle flotation collectors-the influence of particle softness. ACS Appl Mater Interfaces 5:4836–4842

Yoo J, Park C, Yi G, Lee D, Koo H (2019) Active targeting strategies using biological ligands for nanoparticle drug delivery systems. Cancer 11:640

Yuan Y, Chesnutt BM, Haggard WO, Bumgardner JD (2011) Deacetylation of chitosan: material characterization and in vitro evaluation via albumin adsorption and pre-osteoblastic cell cultures. Materials 4:1399–1416

Zhang W, Mehta A, Tong Z, Esser L, Voelcker NH (2021) Development of polymeric nanoparticles for blood–brain barrier transfer – strategies and challenges. Adv Sci 8:2003937

Zhao H, Lin ZY, Yildirimer L, Dhinakar A, Zhao X, Wu J (2016) Polymer-based nanoparticles for protein delivery: design, strategies and applications. J Mater Chem B 4:4060–4071

Zhao Z, Ukidve A, Kim J, Mitragotri S (2020) Targeting strategies for tissue-specific drug delivery. Cell 181:151–167

Zhou Q, Xanthos M (2008) Nanoclay and crystallinity effects on the hydrolytic degradation of polylactides. Polym Degrad Stab 93:1450–1459

Zielinska A, Carreiro F, Oliveira AM, Neves A, Pires B, Venkatesh DN, Durazzo A, Lucarini M, Eder P, Silva AM, Santini A, Souto EB (2020) Polymeric nanoparticles: production, characterization, toxicology and ecotoxicology. Molecules 25:3731

Stimuli-Responsive Non-viral Nanoparticles for Gene Delivery

Liên S. Reichel and Anja Traeger

Contents

Abstract

Considering nucleic acids as the language of life and the genome as the instruction manual of cells, their targeted modulation promises great opportunities in treating and healing diseases. In addition to viral gene transfer, the overwhelming power of non-viral mRNA-based vaccines is driving the development of novel gene transporters. Thereby, various nucleic acids such as DNA (pDNA) or RNA (mRNA, siRNA, miRNA, gRNA, or ASOs) need to be delivered, requiring a transporter due to their high molar mass and negative charge in contrast to classical agents. This chapter presents the specific biological hurdles for using nucleic acids and shows how new materials can overcome these.

L. S. Reichel · A. Traeger (✉)
Institute of Organic and Macromolecular Chemistry (IOMC), Friedrich Schiller University Jena, Jena, Germany

Jena Center for Soft Matter (JCSM), Friedrich Schiller University Jena, Jena, Germany
e-mail: anja.traeger@uni-jena.de

M. Schäfer-Korting, U. S. Schubert (eds.), *Drug Delivery and Targeting*,
Handbook of Experimental Pharmacology 284, https://doi.org/10.1007/164_2023_694

Keywords

Gene delivery · Gene therapy · Lipid · Nanomedicine · Non-viral · Polymer · Vaccination

Abbreviation

ApoE	Apolipoprotein E
ASO	Antisense oligonucleotide
CART	Charge-altering releasable transporters
CMC	Critical micelle concentration
CPPs	Cell-penetrating peptides
CRISPR	Clustered regularly interspaced short palindromic repeats
DEAE	Diethylaminoethyl
DMAEA	N,N-(Dimethylamino)ethyl acrylate
DNA	Desoxyribonucleic acid
DOTAP	1,2-Dioleoyl-3-trimethylammonium-propane
dsDNA	Double-stranded desoxyribonucleic acid
DSPC	Distearoylphosphatidylcholine
FDA	Food and Drug Administration
GALA peptide	Glutamic acid-alanine-leucine-alanine repeat peptide
GalNAc	N-Acetylgalactosamin
gRNA	Guide ribonucleic acid
LDH	L-Lactatdehydrogenase
LNP	Lipid nanoparticle
miRNA	Micro-ribonucleic acid
mRNA	Messenger ribonucleic acid
PAMAM	Polyamidoamine
PAsp	Poly(aspartic acid)s
PDMAEMA	Poly[2-(dimethylamino)ethyl methacrylate]
pDNA	Plasmid desoxyribonucleic acid
PEG	Polyethylenglycol
PEI	Polyethylenimine
PIC	Polyion complex
PLL	Poly-L-lysine
PPI	Polypropyleneimine
RNA	Ribonucleic acid
s.c.	Subcutaneous
SARS-CoV-2	Severe acute respiratory syndrome coronavirus type 2
siRNA	Short interfering ribonucleic acid
SORT	Selective organ targeting
ssDNA	Single-stranded desoxyribonucleic acid
ZPP	Zwitterionic phospholipidated polymers

1 Genetic Material as Active Ingredient for Drug Delivery

Innovative clinical solutions with rapid and targeted treatments based on flexible technologies are currently highly required. Nanomedicine is considered a key technology of the twenty-first century. New therapy concepts are being tested in clinical trials, and some have already received regulatory approval (Germain et al. 2020; Afonin et al. 2020). Among the numerous applications of nanomedicine, gene transfer occupies a prominent position due to its promising and enormous potential. The beauty of nucleic acids as an active ingredient is their chemical simplicity (phosphates, sugars, a handful of nucleotides) combined with high biological variability. For their delivery, the conserved negatively charged phosphates in the backbone of RNA as well as DNA can be used for interactions with polymers or lipids. These electrostatic interactions form the basis for their interaction with carrier materials, so that small changes in the nucleotide sequence have little effect on the formulation process, but allow rapid adaptation to different indications. Although the potential is immense, genetic material also poses various challenges. It is a biopolymer with a higher molar mass (around 333 Da per nucleotide) and a strong negative charge, resulting in good water solubility. In the presence of degradation enzymes its stability is low, and free nucleic acids can trigger an immune response based on evolutionary-optimized mechanisms to protect us from viral gene manipulation (Kulkarni et al. 2021).

Although the conserved backbone is used for complexation, the physicochemical parameters of the different genetic materials influence the choice of delivery material. RNA, which needs to be delivered into the cytoplasm, is more labile to nucleases and shows higher immunogenicity than DNA. Therefore, modified nucleotides were proposed, and chemical modifications were introduced (Kulkarni et al. 2021; Cui et al. 2022). Due to the different sugar backbone, they show a higher linear charge density and rigidity than DNA (Gaspar et al. 2020). mRNA is a single-stranded nucleotide with amphiphilic character, allowing hydrophobic interactions with transport molecules. It contains several hundred nucleotides and is more flexible compared to DNA or siRNA and ssDNA (Gaspar et al. 2020). Short interfering RNA (siRNA) is a double-stranded RNA, typically 19–25 bp. There are several amphiphilic single-stranded RNA molecules that can modulate mRNA expression. Among them, antisense oligonucleotides (ASOs) are already used clinically (Fig. 1), while microRNAs (miRNAs), oligonucleotides derived from endogenous miRNAs, are still under clinical investigation.

One of the fastest developing genome editing technologies of today is the RNA-guided endonuclease class known as Cas9 from the CRISPR system. This system uses a gRNA, which is a short synthetic single RNA sequence. The required Cas9 protein, an enzyme that can modify the DNA once the gRNA recognizes the target DNA, needs to be co-delivered as pDNA, mRNA or protein, a challenge for delivery systems (Hsu et al. 2014).

DNA usually occurs as a double-stranded variant (dsDNA) representing a semi-flexible polymer with high negative charge densities. For therapeutic applications DNA is often encoded in plasmids (pDNA), containing a few thousand base pairs

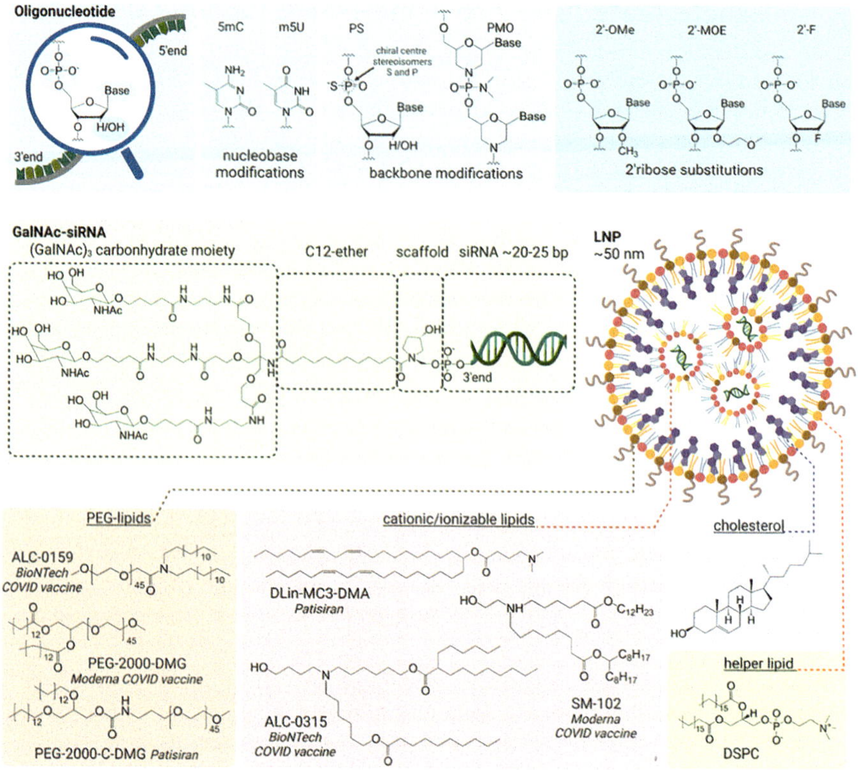

Fig. 1 Overview of approved non-viral strategies for therapeutic application of nucleic acids. Oligonucleotide: chemical modifications of backbone, sugar, or nucleobases increase their specificity, protection against degradation, circulation, and immunological properties. GalNAc-siRNA: a trivalent ligand with terminal GalNAc moieties covalently bound to siRNA, allowing hepatocyte-specific targeting of genetic material. LNP: LNPs contain multiple lipids for delivery of encapsulated siRNA or mRNA (green inside LNP)

(bp) and can thus have a molar mass of several million Da. Gene expression can be modulated by introducing pDNA into the cell nucleus. However, this additional hurdle is a major challenge, which is why only a limited number of systems have successfully entered clinical use to date. Gene therapy repairs defective genes, offering precise and potentially curative treatments for diseases without standard options.

2 Current Status of Non-viral Nanoparticle for Gene Delivery

The COVID-19 pandemic demonstrates the advantage of nucleic acids as an effective agent, enabling rapid vaccine development – including vaccines for immunotherapies of cancers. The high capacity, versatility, efficacy, safety profile, scalability, and cost-effective production process of nucleic acid vaccines facilitate the access to potent vaccines globally (Mendes et al. 2022).

However, the application of gene transfer to cure, treat, or prevent a wide range of diseases has been limited due to technical and biological obstacles. Carrier systems are required to overcome the instability, the high renal clearance, and the immune-activating potential of genetic material. For this purpose, various nanomaterials have been developed to protect nucleic acid from degradation and non-specific immune reactions and/or to transport it specifically to target tissues and cells. Nowadays, a few gene therapy products are on the market, and more than 100 clinical trials are ongoing (Halwani 2022). Clinical trials often use viral delivery systems that have been evolutionarily optimized to deliver their nucleic acids to target cells, but with biological and technical limitations, including carcinogenesis, immunogenicity, broad tropism, limited packaging potential, and difficulty of vector production. Non-viral systems have the potential to overcome many of these drawbacks. However, they have other challenges, such as limited efficacy, specificity, or biodegradability (Mintzer and Simanek 2009; Yin et al. 2014).

Figure 1 is an overview of the approved strategies for nucleic acid delivery. To name some approved non-viral delivery systems: Fomivirsen (Vitravene) is an antisense oligonucleotide (ASO) targeting specific sequences on cellular RNA and was approved in 1998 to treat cytomegalovirus infection of the retina in AIDS patients (withdrew 2002; due to more potent AIDS therapy nowadays) (Roberts et al. 2020). Mipomersen (Kynamro) is an ASO for hypercholesterolemia. Patisiran (Onpattro) is the first approved representative "first-in-class" of novel drugs based on siRNA to treat hereditary transthyretin amyloidosis in patients with stage 1 or 2 polyneuropathy (Buck et al. 2019). Moreover, Collategene, a plasmid that encodes the human hepatocyte growth factor is approved in Japan for treating patients with critical limb ischemia (Ylä-Herttuala 2019).

The approval of novel RNA-based systems has further driven advances in the development of non-viral delivery systems, such as the hepatocyte-specific *N*-acetylgalactosamine (GalNAc)-siRNA conjugates applied by s.c. injections: i) Givosiran (Givlaari) for treating acute intermittent hepatic porphyria, ii) Lumasiran (Oxlumo) for treating primary hyperoxaluria type 1, and iii) Inclisiran (Leqvio), for the treatment of hypercholesterolemia. Last but not least, further RNA-based systems are lipid-based siRNA drugs and the SARS-CoV-2 mRNA vaccines (Paunovska et al. 2022).

Beyond the intramuscularly administered SARS-CoV-2 mRNA vaccines, most approved gene therapies are locally applied or organ-targeted, e.g., to the spinal cord, eyes, or liver. A systemic administration is challenging, in particular for lipid and cationic polymer-based gene carriers. They are prone to rapid degradation, and unwanted interactions lead to, e.g., accumulation in the liver or aggregation in the bloodstream, resulting in cytotoxicity and low efficacy (Mendes et al. 2022). Systemic application without off-target accumulation by remaining organ specificity can be realized through various strategies. Active targeting can be tuned through modification of the delivery systems with different ligands to achieve ligand–receptor specific interaction. Chemical targeting can be achieved through chemical

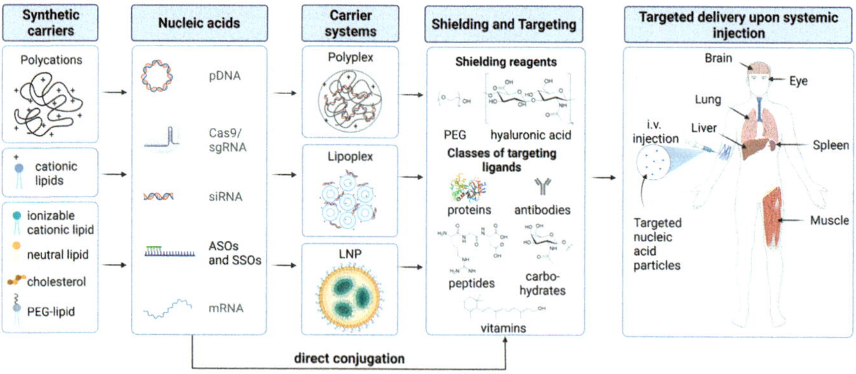

Fig. 2 Non-viral synthetic carriers and their main components, particle types as well as shielding and targeting agents for the delivery of nucleic acids to specific organ or cells upon systemic injection. According to R. C. Steffens (Steffens and Wagner 2023)

modifications to alter chemical and physiochemical properties, e.g. size and charge of LNPs and polymers, which influence their biodistribution and accumulation (Steffens and Wagner 2023). Non-viral synthetic carriers, their main components, and some of the shielding and targeting agents enable targeting extrahepatic organs, like the lung or spleen, as lymphoid organs are shown in Fig. 2. E.g. ApoE binding disorder to de-targeting the liver, inserting stealth moieties to prolong circulation time, and preventing aggregation. The biodistribution of LNPs can be changed explicitly by incorporating selective organ targeting (SORT) lipids with different chemical structures. SORT molecules can vary the pK_a value leading to interaction with specific serum proteins to form a specific protein corona with different molar masses, enriching extrahepatic organs like the lung or spleen. Incorporation of 50% of the permanent cationic DOTAP SORT lipid selectively addressed the lung (50% DOTAP SORT LNPs), incorporating 30% of anionic 18PA SORT lipid enables to target the spleen (18PA SORT LNPs) (Cao et al. 2019a). Other organ targeting strategies use FDA-approved polyester materials, particularly ionizable aminopolyesters, to optimize molar mass and charge density. Furthermore, zwitter-ionic phospholipidated polymers (ZPPs) enable systemic delivery of mRNA to the spleen and lymph nodes (Liu et al. 2021), and charge-altering releasable transporters (CARTs) are specific for splenic delivery, especially in lymphocytes (McKinlay et al. 2018). Also the reduction of off-target effect can be achieved through the use of active targeting ligands. For example, the GALA peptide mimics the hemagglutinin protein of influenza virus which can effectively transport siRNA and pDNA to the lung, and antibodies enable delivery to specific cell types (Dilliard and Siegwart 2023). Moreover, targeting specific cells within an organ can be achieved, e.g., incorporating (1) mannose moieties to shift the intrahepatic biodistribution to target liver sinusoidal endothelial cells, (2) vitamin A to target hepatic stellate cells as reservoirs for 50–80% of the vitamin A in the body, (3) siRNA-LNPs with a cyclic peptide ligand (pPB) that interacts with the platelet-derived growth factor receptor β

(Steffens and Wagner 2023). Some of the described delivery systems are currently in clinical trials, and the increasing trend in approving non-viral gene carriers highlights their importance for the future of nanomedicine.

3 Biological Hurdles for Gene Delivery

Successful delivery of nucleic acids involves several challenges, including (1) efficient packaging of genetic material, (2) bypassing clearance through off-target organs, (3) reaching the aimed tissue or desired target cell, (4) endocytosis, and (5) efficient release from the endosome, without triggering a deleterious adverse reaction (Paunovska et al. 2022). An additional challenge for in vivo applications is (6) the potential degradation by nucleases in physiological fluids, where the half-life of plasmid DNA in the blood is only about 10 min (Kawabata et al. 1995).

Thus, encapsulation or binding can protect nucleic acids and extend their circulation time. To reach the desired site of action, targeted delivery seems to be the appropriate choice, i.e., nanoparticles equipped with specific sequences that can be recognized by a specific organ, tissue, cell type, or pathogens to deliver their genetic cargo to a target site without affecting other body regions. Electrostatic repulsion between the most likely positively charged material (nucleic acid complexes with an excess of positively charged polymers or lipids) decreases the salt and protein concentrations present in the blood. This leads to colloidal instability and aggregation, resulting in, e.g., impeded transfer to the desired tissues or cells, fast clearance by macrophages and, in the worst case, triggering emboli formation (Ogris et al. 1999).

However, successful cell uptake does not necessarily correlate with successful gene expression/knock-down (Richter et al. 2020). The preferred cellular uptake pathway and frequency depend on the nanocarrier and cell type. Moreover, introducing active targeting components can positively influence cell uptake. Mainly particles and macromolecules are taken up by endocytosis. The polyelectrolyte complex of polymer and genetic material, so-called polyplexes, can be internalized for endocytosis via clathrin-dependent or independent endocytosis, caveolae-mediated endocytosis, or macropinocytosis (Bus et al. 2018). Irrespective of the route by which carriers enter the cell, filopodia, among others, promote the interaction between particles and the cell surface and the formation of intracellular vesicles (Rehman et al. 2012). Loaded vesicles can move along microtubules toward the nucleus and mature into late endosomes. They enlarge, form intraluminal vesicles, and can fuse with the lysosome to form endolysosomes. During this process, called endosomal maturation, the size, structure, intravesicular pH value (from 7.4 to 4.5), and the proteins and lipids composition of the endosomal membrane change (Fig. 3). Furthermore, the hydrolytic activity of the endolysosomes leads to a degradation of most compounds and, thus, should be avoided for successful gene transfer. Therefore, an endosomal release is considered a bottleneck for successful gene transfer.

Once the nanocarrier is locked into the endocytosis pathway, only a minority of carriers (<1–2%, two to five bursts per cell) overcome the endolysosomal barrier

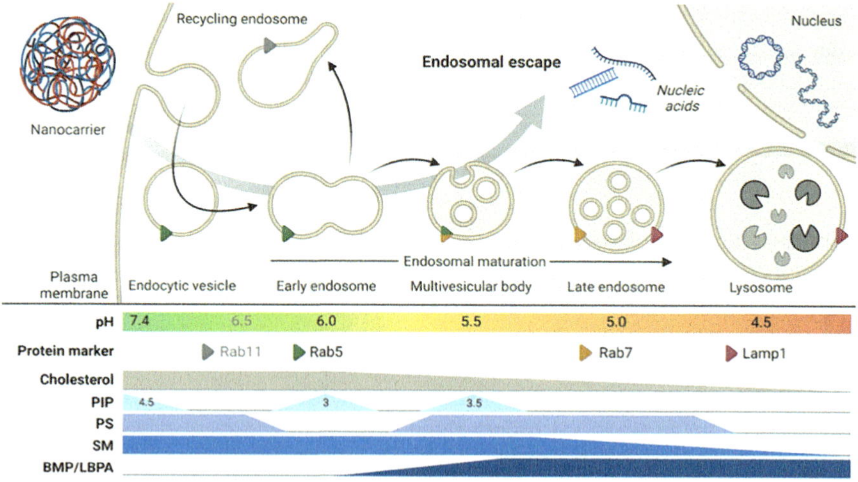

Fig. 3 Maturation of the endosome. After endocytosis, the endocytic vesicle forms the early endosome, either forming a recycling endosome or continuing through the endolysosomal pathway. In addition to membrane invagination and fusion of different vesicles, the pH value, the lipid- and the protein composition of the membrane change during endosomal maturation. *PIP* phosphoinositides (the numbers indicate the phosphate positions on the inositol ring), *PS* phosphatidylserine, *SM* sphingomyelin, *BMP/LBPA* bis(monoacylglycerol)phosphate/ lysobisphosphatidic acid. According to F. Richter et al. reprint with permission (Hausig-Punke et al. 2022)

(Rehman et al. 2013). Different hypotheses were postulated for describing the endosomal release. The most popular hypothesis is the "proton sponge effect," proposed for the frequently used polyethylenimine (PEI)-based carrier systems. The escape of the polyplex is explained by the polymer's buffer capacity that induces chloride ion influx, and osmotic imbalance leads to osmotic swelling and rupture or lysis of the endosome (Bus et al. 2018). This hypothesis is based on studies including the inhibition of acidification by bafilomycin A1 decreasing transfection, the quantification of chloride ion accumulation, and acidification within endosomes. Furthermore, modified PEI-based polymers with reduced buffer capacity revealed decreasing transfection, and the addition of the weak buffer chloroquine increased the transfection of polymers with low buffer capacity. Yet, this is contradicted by the fact that polymers without buffer capacity in the physiological range can equally transport genetic material. Calculations showed that the osmotic pressure induced by the cationic polymer's protonation is insufficient to rupture the endosomal membrane (Benjaminsen et al. 2013).

For this reason, further hypotheses have been developed, mainly dealing with a direct membrane–material interaction leading to local membrane destabilization and permeability (Bus et al. 2018), which is more comparable to the release mechanism of lipids and viral particles.

The development of new methods is an essential driver to gain new insights into cellular processes, particularly imaging techniques, but also the study of lipid bilayers, lipid vesicles, or artificial membranes. Modeling and release assays using dyes such as calcein, the LDH assay, and the red blood cell test are now well established for studying material libraries (Evans et al. 2013). In the case of lipid-based carriers, modeling their interaction with the membrane is well-advanced, which is more difficult for polymers due to their size and distribution.

4 Lipid-Based Delivery

Lipids are one of the most important and best-understood non-viral nucleic acid carriers, of which LNPs are the most exciting representatives, mainly since they were used for mRNA vaccines to fight the COVID-19 pandemic. However, even beyond that, LNPs have already been approved for siRNA application (Patisiran, see Fig. 1). Lipids exist in various classifications, with amphiphilic fats and sterols primarily applied for nanoformulation. In 1987, the term "lipofection" was introduced to describe lipid-based gene delivery (Felgner et al. 1987). Due to their amphiphilic character, lipids can form 3D structures, such as micelles, liposomes, and LNPs (Fig. 4). In this context, LNPs consist of several lipid components, e.g., approved variations contain four components; the ionizable lipid with a pH-dependent protonated amine to bind and stabilize the nucleic acids, while cholesterol, a helper lipid (e.g., DSPC), and a PEG-lipid stabilize the formulation and support the interaction with biological membranes (Fig. 1).

Several lipids have been screened to determine structure-property relationships and to optimize efficiency with a low amount of genetic material (Buck et al. 2019; Semple et al. 2010). These allowed the development of lipids with good efficacy profiles and reduced the dose required for robust in vivo effects. In addition, the optimal pK_a value, structure of the hydrophobic chains, and linker chemistry could

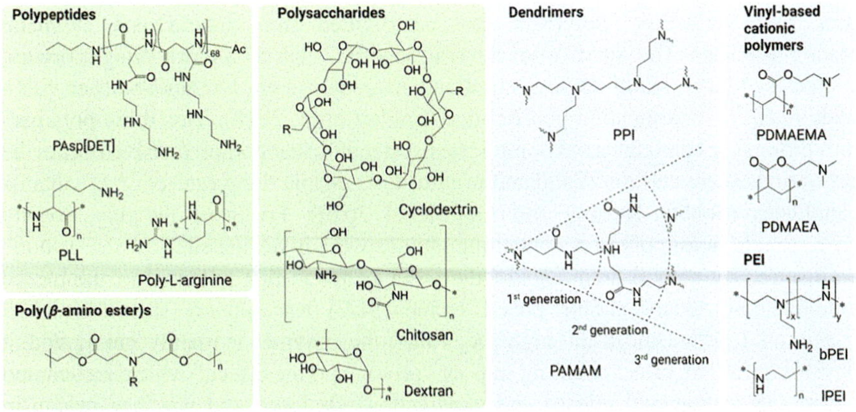

Fig. 4 Chemical structures of selected polymeric vectors commonly used for gene delivery. Biodegradable polymers are highlighted in green, and non-biodegradable polymers are highlighted in blue. * end group. R possible modification with functional amine groups

also be optimized (Zhang et al. 2021), as small changes can affect the stability, specificity, and distribution of LNPs in vivo (Paunovska et al. 2022).

The development of ionizable lipids is considered a breakthrough for the broad application of LNPs (Dolgin 2021). The original cationic lipids achieved high transfection efficiencies but caused toxic effects in cell cultures. The particles showed a short half-life in blood circulation and non-specific binding to cell surfaces. To circumvent this obstacle, the so-called ionizable lipids with a pK_a value below 7 were developed. These lipids bind to the genetic material by a pH-dependent formulation, starting with a lower pH to enable binding of the genetic material and slowly increasing to physiological pH. The formulations are neutral upon application, e.g., intravenous, intramuscular, and become charged under the acidic environment in the endosome, offering advantages for endosomal release. The protonation in the endosome offers a good interaction with the lipids of the endosomal membrane. After optimizations, ionizable lipids revealed promising results even with less genetic material, supporting their potential (Paunovska et al. 2022). Regarding the ionizable headgroup, a dimethylamino base showed high transfection efficiency (Mo et al. 2013). Conversely, substitution with sterical headgroups, e.g., diethylamino, piperazino, morpholino, or trimethylamino complicated access and increased pK_a value, exhibited lower activity (Semple et al. 2010). A pK_a value between 5.5 and 7 resulted in maximum efficiency in vivo with siRNA used in most studies (Jayaraman et al. 2012).

5 Polymer-Based Delivery Systems

So far, polymers do not play a considerable role in therapeutic gene applications, partly because they represent one of the newest technologies, and their complexity and diversity pose a challenge. Gene transfer through polymers has been intensively studied in the last decades, as they have advantages in terms of durability, production, and versatility. Polymers can be divided into natural and synthetic macromolecules. The latter offers several benefits, such as a more straightforward synthesis of large quantities, less variation between different synthesis batches, and a wide range of modification possibilities (Englert et al. 2018). This turns polymers into promising candidates but complicates systematic and comprehensive studies, as the options seem endless. Validated in-vitro tests enable the preselection of suitable candidates (Schäfer-Korting and Landsiedel 2020). For gene delivery, mainly protonizable homopolymers containing amines were investigated.

Inspired by natural amino acids, the DNA condensation potential of the biodegradable and biocompatible poly-L-lysine (PLL) was already shown in 1975 (Laemmli 1975). Due to the high pK_a value, the polymer is mainly protonated at physiological pH value, resulting in poor “proton sponge effect,” which was argued for its low endosomal release and transfection efficiency and was one reason to modify PLL, to incorporate ligands or add lysosomotropic agents (chloroquine) (Gigante et al. 2019).

PEI with a molar mass between 2 and 25 kDa was the first polycationic polymer with a high-loading density synthesized for gene delivery in 1995 (Boussif et al. 1995). It is applied in different topologies (Fig. 4). Both forms are partially protonated at physiological pH values. Due to the buffering capacity during endosomal maturation, the "proton sponge effect" was proposed for PEI (Bus et al. 2018). As a commercially available polymer, it is a prominently used control for developing novel polymer-based delivery tools for in vitro use. Its in vivo application is limited; the non-biodegradable polymer backbone induced cytotoxicity, unspecific cellular uptake, and serum interactions. Various modifications have been presented to circumvent the limitations of PEI, including PEGylation or combination with cholesterol, sugars, proteins, and the introduction of a degradable linker (Mintzer and Simanek 2009; Gigante et al. 2019).

Since then, various polymers have been developed for gene delivery. Among them, poly[2-(dimethylamino)ethyl methacrylate] (PDMAEMA) represents a well-known candidate, readily available by radical polymerizations. Controlled free radical polymerization techniques enable its synthesis with controlled molar mass, defined chain ends, compositions, and architectures (e.g., block, star, and graft polymerization) (Synatschke et al. 2011; Agarwal et al. 2012). Their easy synthesis and the presence of amines in the side chain enable more systematic investigations regarding the nature of amines or on the polymer backbone (Agarwal et al. 2012; Trützschler et al. 2018a). However, limitations in degradability and cytotoxicity restrict in vivo applications of synthetic vinyl-based cationic polymers. Thus, synthesis of multifunctional polymer structures were promoted (Trützschler et al. 2018b). Recently, the cleavable variant of DMAEMA, *N,N*-(dimethylamino)ethyl acrylate (DMAEA) gains more attention since the cationic side group can be cleaved, resulting in an anionic polymeric counterpart, also called charge-shifting polycations (Miyata et al. 2008).

In addition, complex architectures such as dendrimers can also transport genetic material, with amine-terminated polyamidoamine (PAMAM) being one of the most commonly used dendritic carriers. With each additional generation, molar mass, branching density, and toxicity increase rendering dendrimers with smaller generations more advantageous in encapsulating genetic material in the available cavities of the structures. Likewise, low-generation poly(propylene imine) (PPI) dendrimers showed the best transfection potential (Mintzer and Simanek 2009).

For potential applications, biodegradable polymers are advantageous. Chitosan is a natural linear polysaccharide valued for biodegradability and biocompatibility. It is poorly soluble in physiological envrironment but highly soluble in acidic environment or buffers since its amino groups are protonated and can form a complex with the nucleic acids. Due to its low endosomal escape capacity, further modifications of the functional groups are needed to turn chitosan into an attractive non-viral material for gene delivery (Gigante et al. 2019; Cao et al. 2019b).

Cyclodextrins are naturally occurring cyclic oligosaccharides. Its basket-shaped topology is unique, with a hydrophilic exterior and hydrophobic interior. Due to their amphiphilic character, cyclodextrins reveal high biocompatibility and permeability for biological membranes. Modifications with cationic groups and cationic polymers make them ideal for gene transfer with siRNA, respective agents are entering clinical trials (Yin et al. 2014; Cao et al. 2019b).

Dextran is likewise a biodegradable polysaccharide. Dextran reveals antithrombotic and anti-inflammatory properties, and its structure offers conjugations and modifications with hydrophobic moieties or polycations, e.g., PEI or diethylaminoethyl (DEAE). DEAE was one of the first chemical reagents used to transfer nucleic acids into cultured mammalian cells (Zarogoulidis et al. 2013).

Poly(β-amino ester)s are degradable polymers that can be synthesized in various architectures (Gao et al. 2016). These amphiphilic polymers are synthesized by conjugating amine monomers to diacrylates. They enable efficient transfection and endosomal escape and present improved biodegradability and minor cytotoxicity, as they contain biodegradable ester linkages besides cationic amines. Different polymer modifications were used to identify structure-property relationships. So far, the efficacy of the polymers appears to be due to the incorporation of hydrophobic side chains or side groups consisting of mono-alcohol or di-alcohol-containing linear amines (Anderson et al. 2003).

Furthermore, biocompatible and biodegradable peptides and proteins are promising. Besides PLL, poly(L-arginine) was applied due to its cationic charge ($pK_a > 10$) and condensation of genetic material. Mainly, modification of polymers or combination with other functionalities was described (Gigante et al. 2019; Chen et al. 2017). L-Histidine is widely used to modify polymers to enhance their endosomal activity due to the buffering capacity of charged imidazole groups (pK_a 6.0). Furthermore, cell-penetrating peptides (CPPs) were used as building blocks to tune the potential of non-viral vectors. Improved biocompatibility and excellent transfection were shown, e.g., with modified poly(aspartic acids) (PAsp), where the ethylene diamine units were located at the side chain PAsp[DET] (Miyata et al. 2008).

In recent decades, multifunctional polymeric systems have been explored. The introduction of additional functions reduces toxicity or promotes assembly into nanostructured systems and specific cellular interactions. It should not be neglected that a changed polymer architecture affects the polyplex properties, which also impacts the biological performance. Inspired by assembled virus capsids and lipid nanoparticles, hydrophobic moieties were applied. Hydrophobic interactions promote the local assembly of polymers and intensify interactions with cellular membranes, resulting in enhanced endosomal release and transfection efficiency (Rinkenauer et al. 2015). In particular, lipids or amphiphilic block copolymers with hydrophobic and hydrophilic segments can assemble into micelles, vesicles, or more complex shapes with hydrophilic and hydrophobic compartments (Fig. 5). The possible morphology can be predicted by the packing parameter p. The parameter p is influenced by the optimal area of the head group, the volume of the hydrophilic polymer chains, and the length of the hydrophilic group. A packing parameter of p below 1/3 preferentially assembles spherical micelles. For higher p-values, cylindrical micelles, vesicles, membranes, or inverse micelles can be formed (Mai and Eisenberg 2012). In particular, polymeric micelles show great potential in

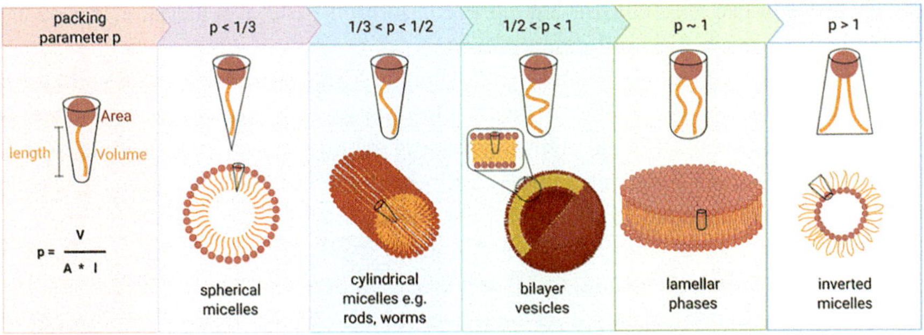

Fig. 5 Overview of nanostructure morphology as a function of the packing parameter (p) of an amphiphile (V = volume of the hydrophobic chain, A = optimal area of the hydrophilic head group, l = critical length of the alkyl chain)

nanomedicine, e.g., controlled drug distribution and release and effectively overcoming biological barriers (Cabral et al. 2018).

For human gene delivery, the stability of polymer assemblies, also known as critical micelle concentration (CMC), plays an important role. The CMC represents the concentration at which the amphiphilic polymers self-assemble into a defined nanostructure at defined pressure and temperature. Systemic (e.g., intravenous) administration may result in complex dilution below the CMC in the bloodstream. The lower concentration compared to in vitro studies may lead to reduced efficiency. One way to stabilize the micellar shape is to cross-link the micellar core (Jiang et al. 2013). Cross-linkers containing disulfide bonds stabilize the micelle architecture and can be degraded under reductive conditions inside cells.

Due to the strong electrostatic interactions between cationic polymers and nucleic acids, the core of a so-called polyion complex (PIC) micelles can be formed (Kataoka et al. 1996). Besides, the so-called micelleplexes can be formed by preformed micelles of amphiphilic polymers and subsequent complexation with genetic material. Preformed micelles offer the advantage of simultaneously introducing genetic material and hydrophobic active ingredients due to the hydrophobic compartment. Another interesting assembly for gene delivery are worm-like micellar structures, also called filamentous micelles, which have unique properties for biological applications. However, there are only few DNA delivery studies on pDNA as a template in the literature (Jiang et al. 2013; Osada et al. 2010).

6 Conclusion

Successful non-viral gene transfer involves overcoming various physicochemical and biological challenges, including stable packaging of the genetic material, targeted uptake into specific cell types, intracellular release, and transport to the site of action within cells. Thus, the gene transfer must first overcome evolutionarily optimized defense mechanisms that prevent foreign genetic material from acting inside cells to reach their full potential.

Despite many academic developments, there is a limited translation into clinics or products, known as the valley of death. One reason is that there is an enormous number of compounds, but the in vivo screening in animals is disproportionate. Only a few are tested in vivo or even adopted for industrial research. In addition, academic research is less interested in already known systems, and the industry's willingness to take risks is limited. The experimental transfer itself presents a challenge. Results are often difficult to translate from in vitro to in vivo or clinical trials, risking overlooking potential material (Paunovska et al. 2022). Better knowledge of material–cell interactions, species-specific differences, interdisciplinary understanding, standardized protocols, and reports aiming for data transparency and reproducibility is crucial. Lastly, artificial intelligence and machine-learning-based models can be applied to predict nanoparticle material properties and their pharmacodynamic and pharmacokinetic properties. Moreover, species-to-species translation and design of genetic material or carriers can be optimized for stability, efficiency, cell targeting, and therapeutic safety to promote the development of novel nanodevices, including personalized medicine.

Acknowledgment This work was supported by the Bundesministerium für Bildung und Forschung (BMBF, Germany, #13XP5034A PolyBioMik) and by the DFG-funded Collaborative Research Center PolyTarget (SFB 1278, project B01, project ID: 316213987). The authors gratefully acknowledge Dr. Stephanie Schubert for proofreading. The graphics were created with BioRender.com.

References

Afonin KA, Dobrovolskaia MA, Church G, Bathe M (2020) Opportunities, barriers, and a strategy for overcoming translational challenges to therapeutic nucleic acid nanotechnology. ACS Nano 14(8):9221–9227

Agarwal S, Zhang Y, Maji S, Greiner A (2012) PDMAEMA based gene delivery materials. Mater Today 15(9):388–393

Anderson DG, Lynn DM, Langer R (2003) Semi-automated synthesis and screening of a large library of degradable cationic polymers for gene delivery. Angew Chem Int Ed 42(27): 3153–3158

Benjaminsen RV, Mattebjerg MA, Henriksen JR, Moghimi SM, Andresen TL (2013) The possible "proton sponge" effect of polyethylenimine (PEI) does not include change in lysosomal pH. Mol Ther 21(1):149–157

Boussif O, Lezoualc'h F, Zanta MA, Mergny MD, Scherman D, Demeneix B et al (1995) A versatile vector for gene and oligonucleotide transfer into cells in culture and in vivo: polyethylenimine. Proc Natl Acad Sci U S A 92(16):7297–7301

Buck J, Grossen P, Cullis PR, Huwyler J, Witzigmann D (2019) Lipid-based DNA therapeutics: hallmarks of non-viral gene delivery. ACS Nano 13(4):3754–3782

Bus T, Traeger A, Schubert US (2018) The great escape: how cationic polyplexes overcome the endosomal barrier. J Mater Chem B 6(43):6904–6918

Cabral H, Miyata K, Osada K, Kataoka K (2018) Block copolymer micelles in nanomedicine applications. Chem Rev 118(14):6844–6892

Cao C, Zhao J, Lu M, Garvey CJ, Stenzel MH (2019a) Correlation between drug loading content and biological activity: the complexity demonstrated in paclitaxel-loaded glycopolymer micelle system. Biomacromolecules 20(4):1545–1554
Cao Y, Tan YF, Wong YS, Liew MW, Venkatraman S (2019b) Recent advances in chitosan-based carriers for gene delivery. Mar Drugs
Chen J, Guan X, Hu Y, Tian H, Chen X (2017) Peptide-based and polypeptide-based gene delivery systems. Top Curr Chem 375(2):32
Cui L, Ma R, Cai J, Guo C, Chen Z, Yao L et al (2022) RNA modifications: importance in immune cell biology and related diseases. Signal Transduct Target Ther 7(1):334
Dilliard SA, Siegwart DJ (2023) Passive, active and endogenous organ-targeted lipid and polymer nanoparticles for delivery of genetic drugs. Nat Rev Mater
Dolgin E (2021) The tangled history of mRNA vaccines. Nature 597(7876):318–324
Englert C, Brendel JC, Majdanski TC, Yildirim T, Schubert S, Gottschaldt M et al (2018) Pharmapolymers in the 21st century: synthetic polymers in drug delivery applications. Prog Polym Sci 87:107–164
Evans BC, Nelson CE, Yu SS, Beavers KR, Kim AJ, Li H et al (2013) Ex vivo red blood cell hemolysis assay for the evaluation of pH-responsive endosomolytic agents for cytosolic delivery of biomacromolecular drugs. J Vis Exp 73:e50166
Felgner PL, Gadek TR, Holm M, Roman R, Chan HW, Wenz M et al (1987) Lipofection: a highly efficient, lipid-mediated DNA-transfection procedure. Proc Natl Acad Sci U S A 84(21): 7413–7417
Gao Y, Huang J-Y, O'Keeffe Ahern J, Cutlar L, Zhou D, Lin F-H et al (2016) Highly branched poly (β-amino esters) for non-viral gene delivery: high transfection efficiency and low toxicity achieved by increasing molecular weight. Biomacromolecules 17(11):3640–3647
Gaspar R, Coelho F, Silva BFB (2020) Lipid-nucleic acid complexes: physicochemical aspects and prospects for cancer treatment. Molecules
Germain M, Caputo F, Metcalfe S, Tosi G, Spring K, Åslund AKO et al (2020) Delivering the power of nanomedicine to patients today. J Control Release 326:164–171
Gigante A, Li M, Junghänel S, Hirschhäuser C, Knauer S, Schmuck C (2019) Non-viral transfection vectors: are hybrid materials the way forward? Med Chem Commun 10(10):1692–1718
Halwani AA (2022) Development of pharmaceutical nanomedicines: from the bench to the market. Pharmaceutics 14(1)
Hausig-Punke F, Richter F, Hoernke M, Brendel JC, Traeger A (2022) Tracking the endosomal escape: a closer look at Calcein and related reporters. Macromol Biosci:2200167
Hsu PD, Lander ES, Zhang F (2014) Development and applications of CRISPR-Cas9 for genome engineering. Cell 157(6):1262–1278
Jayaraman M, Ansell SM, Mui BL, Tam YK, Chen J, Du X et al (2012) Maximizing the potency of siRNA lipid nanoparticles for hepatic gene silencing in vivo. Angew Chem Int Ed 51(34): 8529–8533
Jiang X, Qu W, Ren Y, Williford J-M, Pan D, Luijten E et al (2013) Plasmid-templated shape control of condensed DNA-polymer micelles. Adv Mater 25:227–232
Kataoka K, Togawa H, Harada A, Yasugi K, Matsumoto T, Katayose S (1996) Spontaneous formation of polyion complex micelles with narrow distribution from antisense oligonucleotide and cationic block copolymer in physiological saline. Macromolecules 29(26):8556–8557
Kawabata K, Takakura Y, Hashida M (1995) The fate of plasmid DNA after intravenous injection in mice: involvement of scavenger receptors in its hepatic uptake. Pharm Res 12(6):825–830
Kulkarni JA, Witzigmann D, Thomson SB, Chen S, Leavitt BR, Cullis PR et al (2021) The current landscape of nucleic acid therapeutics. Nat Nanotechnol 16(6):630–643
Laemmli UK (1975) Characterization of DNA condensates induced by poly(ethylene oxide) and polylysine. Proc Natl Acad Sci 72(11):4288–4292
Liu S, Wang X, Yu X, Cheng Q, Johnson LT, Chatterjee S et al (2021) Zwitterionic phospholipidation of cationic polymers facilitates systemic mRNA delivery to spleen and lymph nodes. J Am Chem Soc 143(50):21321–21330

Mai Y, Eisenberg A (2012) Self-assembly of block copolymers. Chem Soc Rev 41(18):5969–5985
McKinlay CJ, Benner NL, Haabeth OA, Waymouth RM, Wender PA (2018) Enhanced mRNA delivery into lymphocytes enabled by lipid-varied libraries of charge-altering releasable transporters. Proc Natl Acad Sci 115(26):E5859–E5E66
Mendes BB, Conniot J, Avital A, Yao D, Jiang X, Zhou X et al (2022) Nanodelivery of nucleic acids. Nat Rev Methods Primers 2(1):24
Mintzer MA, Simanek EE (2009) Nonviral vectors for gene delivery. Chem Rev 109(2):259–302
Miyata K, Oba M, Nakanishi M, Fukushima S, Yamasaki Y, Koyama H et al (2008) Polyplexes from poly(aspartamide) bearing 1,2-diaminoethane side chains induce pH-selective, endosomal membrane destabilization with amplified transfection and negligible cytotoxicity. J Am Chem Soc 130(48):16287–16294
Mo R, Sun Q, Li N, Zhang C (2013) Intracellular delivery and antitumor effects of pH-sensitive liposomes based on zwitterionic oligopeptide lipids. Biomaterials 34(11):2773–2786
Ogris M, Brunner S, Schüller S, Kircheis R, Wagner E (1999) PEGylated DNA/transferrin–PEI complexes: reduced interaction with blood components, extended circulation in blood and potential for systemic gene delivery. Gene Ther 6(4):595–605
Osada K, Oshima H, Kobayashi D, Doi M, Enoki M, Yamasaki Y et al (2010) Quantized folding of plasmid DNA condensed with block catiomer into characteristic rod structures promoting transgene efficacy. J Am Chem Soc 132(35):12343–12348
Paunovska K, Loughrey D, Dahlman JE (2022) Drug delivery systems for RNA therapeutics. Nat Rev Genet 23(5):265–280
Rehman Z, Sjollema KA, Kuipers J, Hoekstra D, Zuhorn IS (2012) Nonviral gene delivery vectors use syndecan-dependent transport mechanisms in filopodia to reach the cell surface. ACS Nano 6(8):7521–7532
Rehman ZU, Hoekstra D, Zuhorn IS (2013) Mechanism of polyplex- and lipoplex-mediated delivery of nucleic acids: real-time visualization of transient membrane destabilization without endosomal lysis. ACS Nano 7(5):3767–3777
Richter F, Martin L, Leer K, Moek E, Hausig F, Brendel JC et al (2020) Tuning of endosomal escape and gene expression by functional groups, molecular weight and transfection medium: a structure–activity relationship study. J Mater Chem B 8(23):5026–5041
Rinkenauer AC, Tauhardt L, Wendler F, Kempe K, Gottschaldt M, Traeger A et al (2015) A cationic poly(2-oxazoline) with high in vitro transfection efficiency identified by a library approach. Macromol Biosci 15(3):414–425
Roberts TC, Langer R, Wood MJA (2020) Advances in oligonucleotide drug delivery. Nat Rev Drug Discov 19(10):673–694
Schäfer-Korting MM-ES, Landsiedel R (2020) Organotypic models in drug development. Handbook of experimental pharmacology, 1st edn. Springer
Semple SC, Akinc A, Chen J, Sandhu AP, Mui BL, Cho CK et al (2010) Rational design of cationic lipids for siRNA delivery. Nat Biotechnol 28(2):172–176
Steffens RC, Wagner E (2023) Directing the way—receptor and chemical targeting strategies for nucleic acid delivery. Pharm Res 40(1):47–76
Synatschke CV, Schallon A, Jérôme V, Freitag R, Müller AHE (2011) Influence of polymer architecture and molecular weight of poly(2-(dimethylamino)ethyl methacrylate) polycations on transfection efficiency and cell viability in gene delivery. Biomacromolecules 12(12): 4247–4255
Trützschler A-K, Bus T, Reifarth M, Brendel JC, Hoeppener S, Traeger A et al (2018a) Beyond gene transfection with methacrylate-based polyplexes—the influence of the amino substitution pattern. Bioconjug Chem 29(7):2181–2194
Trützschler A-K, Bus T, Sahn M, Traeger A, Weber C, Schubert US (2018b) The power of shielding: low toxicity and high transfection performance of cationic graft copolymers containing poly(2-oxazoline) side chains. Biomacromolecules 19(7):2759–2771
Yin H, Kanasty RL, Eltoukhy AA, Vegas AJ, Dorkin JR, Anderson DG (2014) Non-viral vectors for gene-based therapy. Nat Rev Genet 15(8):541–555

Ylä-Herttuala S (2019) Gene therapy of critical limb ischemia enters clinical use. Mol Ther 27(12): 2053

Zarogoulidis P, Hohenforst-Schmidt W, Darwiche K, Krauss L, Sparopoulou D, Sakkas L et al (2013) 2-Diethylaminoethyl-dextran methyl methacrylate copolymer nonviral vector: still a long way toward the safety of aerosol gene therapy. Gene Ther 20(10):1022–1028

Zhang Y, Sun C, Wang C, Jankovic KE, Dong Y (2021) Lipids and lipid derivatives for RNA delivery. Chem Rev 121(20):12181–12277

Sustainability in Drug and Nanoparticle Processing

Dagmar Fischer

Contents

Abstract

The formulation of drugs in poly(lactic-*co*-glycolic acid) (PLGA) nanoparticles can be accomplished by various methods, with nanoprecipitation and nanoemulsion being among the most commonly used manufacturing techniques to provide access to high-quality nanomaterials with reproducible quality. Current trends turned to sustainability and green concepts leading to a re-thinking of these techniques, particularly as the conventional solvents for the dissolution of the polymer suffer from limitations like hazards for human health and natural environment. This chapter gives an overview about the different excipients used in classical nanoformulations with a special focus on the currently applied organic

D. Fischer (✉)
Division of Pharmaceutical Technology and Biopharmacy, Department of Chemistry and Pharmacy, Friedrich-Alexander-Universität Erlangen-Nürnberg, Erlangen, Germany
e-mail: dagmar.fischer@fau.de

M. Schäfer-Korting, U. S. Schubert (eds.), *Drug Delivery and Targeting*,
Handbook of Experimental Pharmacology 284, https://doi.org/10.1007/164_2023_659

solvents. As alternatives, the status quo of green, sustainable, and alternative solvents regarding their application, advantages, and limitations will be highlighted as well as the role of physicochemical solvent characteristics like water miscibility, viscosity, and vapor pressure for the selection of the formulation process, and for particle characteristics. New alternative solvents will be introduced for PLGA nanoparticle formation and compared regarding particle characteristics and biological effects as well as for in situ particle formation in a matrix consisting of nanocellulose. Conclusively, new alternative solvents are available that present a significant advancement toward the replacement of organic solvents in PLGA nanoparticle formulations.

Keywords

Drug delivery · Nanoparticles · PLGA · Polymer · Sustainability

Abbreviations

6BIGOE	6-Bromo-indirubin-3′-glycerol-oximether
BNC	Bacterial nanocellulose
CBD	Cannabidiol
DMSO	Dimethyl sulfoxide
EDTA	Ethylenediamine tetraacetic acid
EHS	Environmental, health and safety
GHS	Globally Harmonized System of Classification, Labelling and Packaging of Chemicals
ICH	International Council for Harmonization of Technical Requirements for Pharmaceuticals for Human Use
NMP	*N*-methyl-2-pyrrolidone
O/W-emulsion	Oil-water emulsion
O-phase	Organic phase
PDE	Permitted daily exposure
PEG	Polyethylene glycol
PLGA	Poly(lactic-*co*-glycolic acid)
PVA	Polyvinyl alcohol
SDS	Sodium dodecylsulfate
Tg	Glass transition temperature
TPGS	D-α-tocopherol polyethylene glycol succinate
UV	Ultraviolet
W/O/W-emulsion	Water-oil-water emulsion
W-phase	Aqueous phase

1 Introduction

The widespread use of high-throughput screening and combinatorial chemistry resulted in a large number of drugs with high potency and new targets and pathways in the body, but often insufficient bioavailability mostly due to low drug solubility, high plasma protein binding, and inefficient stability in the physiological environment. As about 60 to 70% of the newly developed drug candidates in the industrial pipeline tend to be lipophilic, controllable drug release profiles or targeted pharmacokinetics require sophisticated drug delivery systems aimed at optimizing pharmacokinetics and release characteristics (Borde et al. 2021; Ting et al. 2018).

The formulation of active substances by nanoparticle approaches has resulted in an enormous number of reports with new concepts and trends for the development and optimization of new drug carriers with varying architectures and novel carrier materials. Particularly, polymer-based nanoparticles have attracted considerable interest due to their inherent diversity of structures with readily adjustable and controllable properties. Additionally, the potential to combine therapeutics and diagnostics (theranostics), the protection of drugs, and the realization of time- and spatial-controlled specific targeting effects highlight the potential of their application (Grund et al. 2011).

The actual concepts for polymer-based drug nanoformulation technologies provide the pharmaceutical industry with strategies to solve some of the limitations associated with critical drugs and enhance their therapeutic efficiency. The preferential tasks of the recent decades were characterized by traditional nanoformulation strategies with adaption to new polymers, reduction of batch-to-batch variations, identification of critical process parameters for control and upscaling of formulation processes as well as aspects of harmonized international characterization protocols (Operti et al. 2021, 2022). However, in the last years, formulation specialists were not yet exposed to challenges that we face today in producing nanoparticles. New trends turned to sustainability and green concepts leading to a re-thinking of the current formulation techniques and excipients (Ratti 2020).

Although many natural and synthetic polymers have been described (Grund et al. 2011; Sumana et al. 2020), the present chapter is focused on poly(D,L-lactic-*co*-glycolic acid) (PLGA), a biocompatible, biodegradable, synthetic polyester polymer, widely exploited regarding the design and formulation of drug delivery systems and approved by the regulatory authorities in various applications (Makadia et al. 2011). Many different technologies have been developed to prepare particulate drug delivery systems on the basis of PLGA polymers (Ahmed 2013) to form nanospheres, i.e. solid polymer matrix systems in which the drug molecules may be chemically bound, adsorbed, dissolved, or dispersed.

In this chapter, the applicability of green concepts and sustainability for a safe and healthy environment with respect to PLGA nanoparticle formulations will be discussed. Concepts with green, sustainable, and alternative solvents as a set of principles that reduce or eliminate the use or generation of substances potentially hazardous to humans and environment, will be discussed, where the term "hazardous" includes physical (e.g., explosive, flammable), toxicological (e.g., carcinogenic, mutagenic), and global (e.g., ozone depletion, climate change) factors.

2 The Classical Way of Polymer Nanoformulation

PLGA nanoparticles can be produced from polymers with nanoemulsification and nanoprecipitation methods being among the most commonly used manufacturing techniques (Hernandez-Giottonini et al. 2020). Furthermore, the salting-out method (Türk et al. 2021), spray drying (Panda et al. 2016), supercritical liquids (Zabihi et al. 2014), electrospraying (Esmaili et al. 2018), flow focusing (Lu et al. 2016; Xu et al. 2017), and microfluidic technologies (Morikawa et al. 2018) also provided access to high-quality nanomaterials with reproducible quality (Sah et al. 2015). Particle structure and stability, particle size and polydispersity, loading efficiency, localization of the active ingredients as well as release profiles can be influenced by the formulation (Essa et al. 2020; Swider et al. 2018). In the following, two of the most important manufacturing processes for PLGA nanoparticles, the nanoprecipitation and nanoemulsification method, are briefly discussed.

Nanoprecipitation is the most simple, mild, and easy to scale up technique that is suitable for the encapsulation of hydrophobic active agents (Fig. 1) (Fessi et al. 1989). In a one-step method, an organic (O)-phase is formed by dissolution of the hydrophobic PLGA polymer and the lipophilic drug in polar, water-miscible organic solvents such as acetone, acetonitrile, dimethylformamide, dimethyl sulfoxide

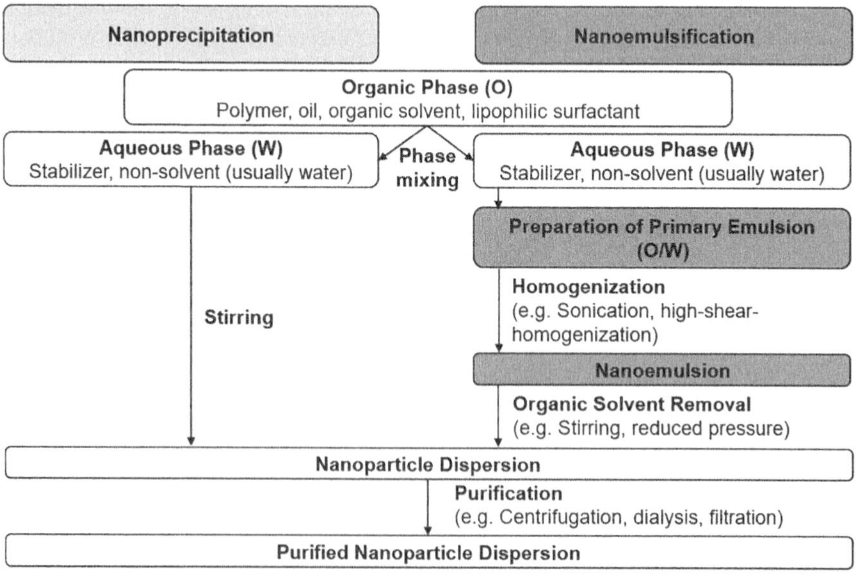

Fig. 1 A schematic overview of the process flow of both most commonly used techniques, nanoprecipitation and nanoemulsification, for the formulation of nanoparticles

(DMSO), and tetrahydrofuran (Alshamsan 2014; Beck-Broichsitter et al. 2015; Bilati et al. 2005; Huang et al. 2018). The O-phase is added dropwise by slow injection or under moderate stirring into an aqueous (W)-phase with or without one or more stabilizers (Alshamsan 2014; Shkodra-Pula et al. 2020), the latter favoring the advantage of a missing complex stabilizer removal. The organic solvent diffuses into the aqueous phase within a few milliseconds, resulting in precipitation of the polymer according to the Marangoni (nanospheres) (Galindo-Rodriguez et al. 2004; Sternling et al. 1959) or the Ouzo (nanocapsules) (Ganachaud et al. 2005; Vitale et al. 2003) effect and, therefore, particle formation. The most important experimental variables affecting the process are stirring speed, ratio of O- and W-phase, and method and rate of phase mixing (Beck-Broichsitter et al. 2010).

Alternatively, for the encapsulation of lipophilic drugs emulsification-based methods are performed requiring the formation of a nanoemulsion before particle formation (Fig. 1) (Essa et al. 2020). The hydrophobic PLGA polymer and the lipophilic active ingredient are first dissolved in an organic solvent (O-phase). Typical solvents are dichloromethane (Arafa et al. 2020) and chloroform (Panda et al. 2016), which are not miscible with water, or the partially water-miscible solvents benzyl alcohol (Konan et al. 2003), ethyl acetate (Sah et al. 2015; Ravi Kumar et al. 2004), isopropyl formate (Lee et al. 2016), and methyl ethyl ketone (Choi et al. 2002). To form an O/W-emulsion, the O-phase is added dropwise to a W-phase containing one or more stabilizers to enable emulsion formation and prevent particle aggregation. The emulsion is homogenized with a high-energy ultrasonic probe, a high-pressure homogenizer (e.g., microfluidizer), or a high-performance rotor/stator disperser (e.g., Ultra-Turrax®). Applying high-energy homogenization techniques requires the awareness of the stability of thermolabile and sensitive drugs. Depending on the solvent properties, particularly volatility and water miscibility, a classification of the emulsification methods can be made according to the type of solvent removal into emulsion-evaporation, emulsion-diffusion and emulsion-diffusion-evaporation (Pal et al. 2011). For the encapsulation of hydrophilic drugs, a double emulsion technique, preferentially for PLGA as water-oil-water (W/O/W)-emulsion, is applied where the primary emulsion is emulsified again by another phase to prepare a secondary emulsion before solvent removal (Pal et al. 2011). The characteristics of the final particles can be mainly controlled by the type of homogenization, stirring speed and time, ratio of the phases, type and concentration of the stabilizers, process temperature, and method of solvent removal.

Finally, the nanoparticles can be purified from stabilizers, non-encapsulated active ingredients and solvent residues by centrifugation (Profirio et al. 2018), ultrafiltration (Paswan et al. 2017), or dialysis (Profirio et al. 2018).

3 Excipients in PLGA Nanoformulations

3.1 Typical Components of the W-Phase

The basis for the W-phase is water that is preferred in high quality and as deionized water to avoid ions potentially affecting the emulsifier and therefore, the emulsification process. Usually, a physiological pH value is selected for the aqueous phase, but e.g. a more acidic pH value could be used for the encapsulation of acidic drugs. As an example, atorvastatin is encapsulated in PLGA nanoparticles at pH 4.0 to protonate the carboxyl group of the statin, enhance its lipophilic character, its solubility in the organic phase and in consequence, the encapsulation efficiency (Grune et al. 2021a). Unwanted changes of the pH value in the aqueous phase can be avoided by phosphate, bicarbonate, or citrate buffers. Since the presence of inorganic electrolytes may influence the stability of the emulsion, complexation and inactivation by ethylenediamine tetraacetic acid (EDTA) could be helpful (Anderson et al. 2003; Arshady 1992; Odian 2004).

One of the key excipients in the W-phase is an adequate stabilizer acting by electrostatic or steric principles. By optimized type and concentration of the stabilizer, particle sizes can be decreased, particle numbers increased, and agglomeration phenomenons decreased (Alkholief et al. 2022). In general, a low stabilizer concentration is preferred not only for economic reasons, but also due to the often observed adverse effects on physical (e.g., size, zeta potential, drug load) or biological (e.g., cell uptake) properties of the particles. E.g. 30,000–70,000 g/mol polyvinyl alcohol (PVA) (M_w values) influenced the cell uptake of PLGA nanoparticles depending on the PVA concentration used during the formulation process as it forms an interconnected network on the particle surface resulting in a modified hydrophilicity of the nanoparticles (Sahoo et al. 2002). Nonionic (e.g., Polysorbate 20, polyvinylpyrrolidone, PVA, Poloxamer), anionic (e.g., sodium dodecyl sulfate (SDS)), and cationic (e.g., cetyltrimethylammonium bromide) stabilizers are used (Sahoo et al. 2002), although nonionic stabilizers are by far the most preferred one. PVA is a commonly used stabilizer for the production of PLGA nanoparticles as well as Polysorbates, Poloxamers, and D-α-tocopherol polyethylene glycol succinate (TPGS) (Swider et al. 2018; Profirio et al. 2018; Cortés et al. 2021; Pánek et al. 2011). Nonionic stabilizers do not typically form micelles and do not lower the surface tension but seem to act by physical adsorption or chemical incorporation into the polymer particles and stabilize them via steric interference with the van der Waals attraction forces between the particles. Mechanical shear stability, freeze-thaw stability, and additional electrolyte tolerance are additional functions of the nonionic stabilizers.

To avoid hazards to health and environment, new green surfactants are now under investigation, an area which is still in its infancy for nanoformulations (Fernandez et al. 2005). The use of conventionally produced surfactants often comes along with several safety concerns, such as toxicity for microbial environment and aquatic system, soil, plants and for human and animal health. The definition of green surfactants includes bio-based amphiphilic molecules that are extracted from natural material or derived from renewable goods (Rebello et al. 2014). They can be divided into two generations: The first generation of green surfactants comprises molecules that are directly obtained by purification of plant and animal material or fully produced of renewable sources through chemical synthesis (e.g., sugar esters, saponins, alkanolamines, and alkyl polyglucosides). The second generation includes surfactants mainly produced by biological processes such as lipopeptides and glycolipids (Farias et al. 2021). Green surfactants can replace sodium dodecylsulfate as standard surfactant in nanoemulsification demonstrating the potential for SDS exchange by green alternatives (sodium lauroylsarcosinate, sodium lauroylglutamate, sodium myristoylsarcosinate) leading to comparable physico-chemical properties of the resulting polymeric nanoparticles (Baier et al. 2014).

After particle formation, the final product can optionally be supplemented with additional surfactants such as post-stabilizers to improve freeze-thaw stability or electrolyte tolerance, antioxidants, UV stabilizers, or antimicrobial preservatives to inhibit microbial growth or modifiers of rheology (Anderson et al. 2003).

3.2 The O-Phase and the Organic Solvents

Organic solvents form the basis for the organic phase in nanoformulation, acting for the dissolution of the hydrophobic polymers and lipophilic drugs. However, many of them suffer from limitations like toxicity for humans, potential environmental hazards as well as cost-intensive removal and waste disposal with a view to industrial application. According to the guideline Q3C (R8) of the International Council for Harmonization of Technical Requirements for Pharmaceuticals for Human Use (ICH) in combination with the Globally Harmonized System of Classification, Labelling and Packaging of Chemicals (GHS), organic residual solvents in drug substances, excipients, and in drug products can be categorized in three classes depending on their toxicological potential for humans (International Council for Harmonisation of Technical Requirements for Pharmaceuticals for Human Use (ICH), n.d.; Globally Harmonized System of Classification and Labelling of Chemicals (GHS), n.d.). Class I contains all "solvents to be avoided" with known or strongly suspected human carcinogenic effect as well as environmental hazards. Class II collects "solvents to be limited" such as non-genotoxic animal carcinogens or possible causative agents of other irreversible toxicity such as neurotoxicity or teratogenicity. Additionally, solvents suspected of other significant but reversible toxicities are part of class II. "Solvents with low toxic potential" to man are represented by class III where no health-based exposure limit is needed (International Council for Harmonisation of Technical Requirements for Pharmaceuticals for Human Use (ICH), n.d.). A permitted daily exposure (PDE) is set for the solvents of the different classes.

Typical examples for solvents (Table 1) applied in PLGA nanoparticle formulations (their thresholds in brackets) are class II solvents like chloroform (0.6 mg/day), acetonitrile (4.1 mg/day), *N*-methyl-3-pyrrolidone (NMP) (5.3 mg/day), dichloromethane (6 mg/day), and tetrahydrofuran (7.2 mg/day) (International

Table 1 Summary of standard organic solvents for nanoparticle preparation and their physicochemical properties including their classification according to ICH Q3C R8

Solvent	Density [g/mL]	Dyn. viscosity [mPa s]	Solubility in water [g/L]	Vapor pressure [mmHg]	ICH classification
Acetone	0.791[a]	0.32[a]	1000[b]	231[b]	III
Acetonitrile	0.787[a]	0.35[a]	>800[b]	88.80[b]	III
Chloroform	1.484[a]	0.563[a]	7.95[b]	197[b]	II
Dichloromethane	1.3255[a]	0.437[a]	0.0132[b]	435[b]	II
Dimethylacetamide	0.943[a]	0.92[b]	>100[b]	2[b]	II
Dimethyl sulfoxide	1.101[a]	2.47[a]	1000[b]	0.60[b]	III
1,4-Dioxane	1.036[a]	0.012[b]	>800[b]	38.1[b]	II
Ethyl acetate	0.9003[a]	0.423[b]	64[b]	98.4[b]	III
Methyl acetate	0.927[a]	0.364[b]	243[a]	216.2[b]	III
N-Methylpyrrolidone	1.027[b]	1.65[b]	>100[a]	0.345[b]	II
N,N-dimethyl-formamide	0.9445[b]	0.802[b]	1000[b]	3.87[b]	III
Tetrahydrofuran	0.888[a]	0.53[a]	>100[a]	162[b]	II

Taken from PubChem, except for dynam. viscosity ethyl formate (taken from Chemical & Physical Properties by Cheméo)
[a] –20°C
[b] –25°C

Council for Harmonisation of Technical Requirements for Pharmaceuticals for Human Use (ICH), n.d.). Acetone, ethyl acetate, and ethyl formate are categorized in class III with a low toxic potential for humans. Although no acute toxicity or toxicity in short-term studies could be observed for these solvents, a PDE of 50 mg/day or a maximum residual content of 0.5% was defined because studies for long-term exposure or carcinogenicity are missing (International Council for Harmonisation of Technical Requirements for Pharmaceuticals for Human Use (ICH), n.d.). However, in the last decade, aspects of sustainability including the synthesis from renewable raw materials, disposal, reusability as well as safety aspects like volatility, flash point, and hazardness for the environment have to be taken into consideration, so that the need for alternative solvents in pharmaceutical industry became one of the raising topics in polymer particle formulation.

4 Introduction of Alternative Solvents in the Nanoparticle Formulation Process: The Status Quo

Particularly the pressure for environmental protection has increased the trend toward the partial or entire substitution of the traditional, often petrochemical, organic solvents in the O-phase by green, sustainable, and alternative solvents in drug formulation. Requirements of the solvents also include low viscosity, complete or partly miscibility with water, high drug stability and solvent stability, and non-volatility (Byrne et al. 2016). For the W-phase, the situation is easy as water as basis is often overlooked as green solvent, inexpensive, widely available, not hazardous to use, and not harmful to the environment (Breslow 2010). However, two disadvantages must be taken into account for water, particularly with respect to the drying process of particles. First, a high heat of vaporization for this low molar mass molecule results in the need for high-energy impact and costs, which is relevant for industrial settings. Moreover, the removal of organic solvents enriched in water before disposal often requires extensive and cost-intensive treatments (Byrne et al. 2016).

For the new generation of solvents, the terms "green," "sustainable," and "alternative" are used. "Green" solvents in a narrower sense are biosolvents that are environmentally friendly solvents, derived from the processing of agricultural crops or waste and renewable sources such as sugars, starchy feed materials, or lignocellulosic materials (Capello et al. 2007). In a broader sense also solvents were categorized as "green" in case of (1) solvents with better environmental, health, and safety (the so-called EHS) properties, such as increased biodegradability or reduced ozone depletion potential, (2) supercritical fluids that are environmentally harmless and avoid the use of, e.g., chlorofluorocarbons, and (3) ionic liquids with a low vapor pressure and, thus, less emission to air (Capello et al. 2007). The so-called sustainable solvents are similar to green solvents, but with a view to a more holistic approach taking environmental concerns like the entire life cycle, regeneration, recycling as well as aspects of the economic development into account (Sustainability n.d.; Verband Der Chemischen Industrie n.d.; Quimidroga n.d.). "Alternative" solvents include a wider range of substances, i.e. not only the environmentally friendly solvents, but also solvents with benefits regarding health impact on humans, costs, and other elements compared to traditional solvents. Therefore, also polyethylene glycols (PEG) are considered as alternative solvents because they are non-toxic, easy to recycle, non-volatile, and hardly inflammable (Soni et al. 2020). The EHS group at Pfizer Research and Development summarized recommendations for the selection of solvents based on process and worker safety as well as environmental and regulatory considerations (Byrne et al. 2016).

To judge how green a solvent is, different frameworks were established on the basis of life cycle assessments, of the impact (toxicological, ecotoxicological, environmental, resource depletion, economic), of its production chain, its type of use, and its fate or disposal in combination with health and safety issues (Capello et al. 2007). Gu et al. (2013) defined 12 criteria to judge the solvent acceptability as shown in Table 2. However, one has to have in mind that no solvent can really meet all these requirements or can be considered as "universally" green (Winterton 2021).

One of the most common green and sustainable solvents in chemistry and pharmacy is ethyl lactate, processed from corn, with the advantages of a high boiling point, low vapor pressure, high solvency, and with respect to biological characteristics non-carcinogenicity, complete biodegradability, and easy recycling (Pereira et al. 2011). Ethyl lactate has replaced solvents such as toluene, acetone, xylene, and chlorinated solvents (Nikles et al. 2001). Another quite new example on

Table 2 List of criteria to judge for solvent acceptability as alternative solvents (according to Gu et al. (2013))

1	Technical performance according to the conventional solvents
2	Stability during handling and storage
3	High purity
4	Less or non-inflammable
5	Availability in sufficient amounts, even for long-term supply
6	Recyclability
7	Acceptable price
8	Resource and energy efficient production validated by life cycle assessment
9	Renewable sources
10	Acceptable in vitro, in vivo, and ecotoxicological profiles
11	Fully biodegradable to harmless, non-critical products
12	Conformity with regulations for transportation

the market is Cyrene™ (dihydrolevoglucosenone), a biodegradable, non-toxic (EC_{50} values >100 mg/mL in acute toxicity tests with algae, invertebrates, and fish), green and sustainable solvent, that is produced in a simple two-step synthesis from cellulose by an almost energy neutral process and is readily biodegradable to carbon dioxide and water (99% in 28 days) (Sigma-Aldrich n.d.-a). It is already successfully applied as an alternative solvent for different chemical reactions in pharmaceutical industry (Camp 2018).

Gamma-valerolactone, considered as sustainable, can be obtained from cellulose-based biomass such as wood waste by acid hydrolysis with glucose and levulinic acid as intermediates (Zhang et al. 2016). Advantages in terms of safety aspects are a high boiling point, very low vapor pressure, biodegradability, and non-toxic properties (EC_{50} values >100 mg/mL in acute toxicity tests with algae and invertebrates) (Sigma-Aldrich n.d.-b). Glycerol formal as an alternative solvent represents a mixture of a 5-membered cyclic ketal, namely 4-hydroxymethyl-1,3-dioxolane, and a 6-membered cyclic one, namely 5-hydroxy-1,3-dioxane. This glycerol-based acetal is obtained in a condensation reaction of glycerol with formaldehyde. It is a water soluble solvent with a high boiling point, low vapor pressure, and does not show an acute toxicity (LD_{50} values >2,000 mg/kg in rats, not hazardous to aquatic environment) (Carl Roth n.d.).

As summarized in Table 3, different approaches for the formulation of PLGA particles were published using alternative solvents. The methods selected for the formation and purification of PLGA particles were found to be mainly dependent on the water solubility and the vapor pressure of the alternative solvents. Emulsion processes are preferentially used in the production of particles with non-water-miscible or conditionally miscible solvents (e.g., dimethyl carbonate (Kim et al. 2018), ethyl formate (Sah 2000), methylpropionate (Lee et al. 2015), propylene carbonate (Grizić et al. 2018)). Particles with water-miscible solvents such as glycofurol (Allhenn et al. 2011), PEG (Ali et al. 2013), and isosorbide dimethyl ether (Haji Mansor et al. 2018) were formed by nanoprecipitation. Also a

Table 3 Overview of the application of alternative solvents for PLGA nano- and microparticle preparation (modified according to Grune (2022))

Solvent	Polymer	Particle size	Preparation method (solvent extraction)	Results	Reference
Carbonate esters					
Dimethyl carbonate	PLGA (75: 25)	–	Emulsion-solvent-extraction (alkaline solvent hydrolysis)	Plasticizer effect; accelerated hydrolysis improved encapsulation efficiency, reduced crystallization of drug progesterone	(Kim et al. 2018)
Propylene carbonate	PLGA (Resomer® RG 502 H, 50:50)	20–60 µm	Emulsion-solvent-extraction (alkaline solvent hydrolysis)	Plasticizing effect; reducible by alkaline hydrolysis	(Grizić et al. 2018)
Ether					
Isosorbide-dimethyl-ether	PLGA (Resomer® RG752 H, 75:25) 5 kDa PEG-25 kDa PLGA (75: 25)	200–250 nm	Phase separation (extraction)	No change of activity and structure of lysozyme and stromal cell-derived factor alpha	(Haji Mansor et al. 2018)
PEG 400	PLGA 50: 50 (Resomer® RG 504 H) PEG-PLGA (Resomer® RGP d 50155), Eudragit RL PO	80–400 nm	Nanoprecipitation (dialysis)	No change of activity after encapsulation of lysozyme and bovine serum albumin	(Ali et al. 2013)
Glycofurol	PLGA (Resomer® RG 502 H, 50:50)	100–200 µm	Emulsion-solvent-diffusion (extraction)	Controlled in vitro release over 4 h (ritonavir) to 3 weeks (Sudan III), sponge-like internal particle structure	(Allhenn et al. 2011)
Ester					
Ethyl formate	PLGA (85: 15)	93–131 µm	Emulsion-solvent-evaporation/ extraction	Compared to dichloromethane higher	(Sah 2000)

(continued)

Table 3 (continued)

Solvent	Polymer	Particle size	Preparation method (solvent extraction)	Results	Reference
			(evaporation/ extraction)	evaporation, water miscibility, lower volume of dilution phase for solvent extraction (encapsulation of progesterone)	
Methyl propionate	PLGA (75: 25)	152–440 nm	Emulsion-solvent-evaporation/ extraction (alkaline solvent hydrolysis)	Reduced process time, lower coalescence and aggregation tendency	(Lee et al. 2015)

quasi-emulsion with a viscosity increasing mixture of glycerol and PEG (1,000 g/mol) in the external aqueous W-phase was described to produce microparticles by preventing the spontaneous diffusion of the water-miscible organic solvent glycofurol (O-phase) into the aqueous phase and avoiding the formation of smaller nanoparticles (Allhenn et al. 2011).

Additionally, the removal of alternative solvent residues in the last purification step of the particle formation process depends on the type of solvent and is carried out either by extraction (e.g., glycofurol, propylene carbonate, methylpropionate (Lee et al. 2015; Grizić et al. 2018; Allhenn et al. 2011; Kim et al. 2016)), evaporation (methyl propionate (Kang et al. 2014)), or a combination of both (ethyl formate (Sah 2000)). For methyl propionate, a faster removal by evaporation than for the organic solvent ethyl acetate could be observed although both have comparable boiling points and vapor pressures (Kang et al. 2014). A special process of solvent extraction has been described for carbonate esters (methyl, dimethyl, propylene carbonate) and methyl propionate based on degradation by alkaline hydrolysis. Alternatively, methyl propionate was hydrolyzed by sodium hydroxide solution or methylamine, the latter one resulting in the formation of sponge-like particles (Lee et al. 2015; Kim et al. 2016). The removal of the residual solvent is especially important for carbonate esters and PEG as it circumvents their unwanted plasticizing effects in the final formulations (Kim et al. 2018; Grizić et al. 2018; Ali et al. 2013).

Plasticizing effects, low drug dissolving capacity, and comparably lower encapsulation efficiencies were reported as potential disadvantages of some alternative solvents. For example, the encapsulation of ibuprofen in PLGA with glycofurol as solvent showed a low encapsulation efficiency of 1.9% compared to ~63% encapsulation efficiency with dichloromethane or ethyl acetate (Allhenn et al. 2011). Vice versa, the alternative solvents offer process related advantages over the standard solvents. The aggregation tendency of the nanoparticles can be reduced during purification and after lyophilization by the use of methyl propionate compared to ethyl acetate, and the process times reduced due to the purification by alkaline hydrolysis (Lee et al. 2015). Sensitive drugs like the proteins lysozyme and albumin can be encapsulated in PLGA by nanoprecipitation using 400 g/mol PEG (PEG 400) as solvent without affecting the protein stability or activity (Ali et al. 2013). However, many unresolved questions remain that include the transferability of alternative solvents to different classes of active substances and the circumvention of the above-mentioned disadvantages such as solubility problems, plasticizing effects, low encapsulation efficiencies, or unfavorable particle sizes.

5 New PLGA Formulation Technologies for the Application of Alternative Solvents

A systematic comparison of different new methods using alternative solvents was performed in our lab (Fig. 2) using an O-phase containing PLGA (Resomer 502®) and a W-phase containing 2% PVA as stabilizer. In the best case, the standard nanoencapsulation methods with classical organic solvents can be directly transferred to the alternative solvents. The selected solvents differed in their viscosity, vapor pressure and water solubility/miscibility (Table 4). Compared to the classical organic solvent ethyl acetate, all selected alternative solvents were characterized by a lower hydrophobicity as shown by the octanol/water coefficients (Fig. 2), and a lower vapor pressure (Table 4).

The three alternative solvents with decreasing log P_{OW} values in the ranking ethyl lactate > γ-valerolactone > glycerol formal could all be formulated with similar

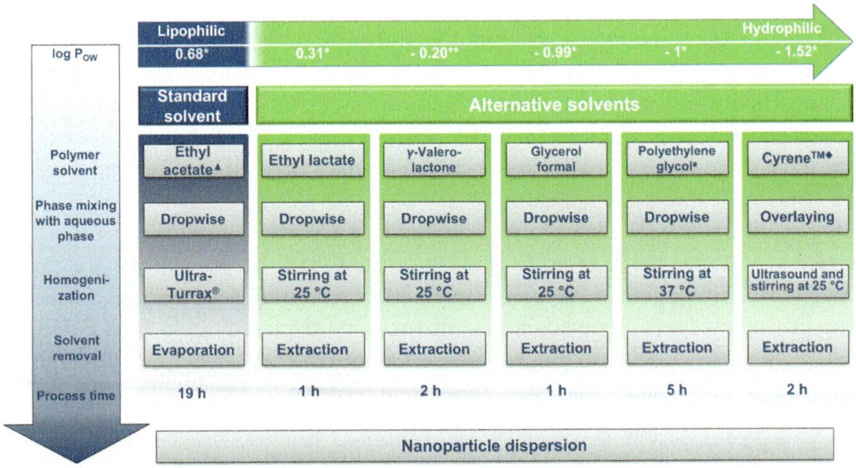

Fig. 2 Comparison of the different process steps for nanoparticle preparation using alternative solvents with varying hydrophobicity and log P_{OW} values (taken from suppliers Carl Roth and Sigma-Aldrich) in comparison to the standard nanoemulsification method with ethyl acetate as organic solvent

Table 4 Summary of organic and alternative solvents applied in the formulation of PLGA nanoparticles including their physicochemical characteristics relevant for nanoprecipitation and nanoemulsification

Functional group	Solvent	Density [g/mL]	Dyn. viscosity [mPa s]	Solubility in water [g/L]	Vapor pressure [mmHg]
Alcohol	Glycerol formal	1.219[a, #]	16[a, †]	Miscible[#]	0.23[a, #]
Carbonate ester	Dimethyl carbonate	1.07[a, **]	0.664[a, **]	138[b, **]	55.36[b, **]
	Propylene carbonate	1.2047[a, **]	2.471[b, *]	175[b, **]	0.045[b, **]
Ester	Ethyl formate	0.9168[a, **]	10.21[a, *]	88.25[b, **]	245[b, **]
	Ethyl lactate	1.03[a, **]	2.53[b, ◊]	1000[a, **]	3.75[b, **]
	Methyl propionate	0.915[b, *]	n.d.	57.8[a, *]	85.5[b, *]
	γ-Valerolactone	1.057[a, **]	2[a, *]	>100[b, **]	0.5[c, **]
Ether	Isosorbide dimethyl ether	1.15[b, *]	n.d.	2,000[a, *]	n.d.
	PEG 400	1.126[a, *]	120[a, #]	256.1[b, #]	<0.008[a, *]
	Glycofurol	1.09[a, *]	n.d.	3.420[a, *]	0.037[a, *]
Ketone	Cyrene™	1.25[a, *]	14.5[b, ⍰]	52.6[a, *]	0.21[b, *]

Taken from *Sigma-Aldrich, **PubChem, #Carl Roth, †Fisher Scientific, ◊Aparicio et al. (Aparicio et al. 2009), ⍰Salavagione et al. (2017)

[a] –20°C

[b] –25°C

[c] –28.9°C

methods. The solvents were selected due to their high water miscibility, semipolar character, and low viscosity. The polymer is dissolved in these solvents and forms nanoparticles instantaneously due to rapid solvent diffusion, when mixed dropwise or under continuous stirring with the W-phase (Pal et al. 2011). The low viscosity of the three solvents was found to be beneficial for the preparation, which can therefore be performed at room temperature.

PEG 400 was selected according to previous reports describing a precipitation process with the polymer as O-phase to encapsulate the proteins bovine serum albumin and lysozyme in PLGA (Ali et al. 2013; Eun-JungHan 2012). The underlying principle of this process is a modified solvent displacement method (Ali et al. 2013). Since PEG 400 as a semipolar solvent is miscible with water, a rapid diffusion into the W-phase takes place with precipitation of the polymer and a spontaneous formation of the nanoparticles (Pal et al. 2011). However, due to the high viscosity of the PEG 400, the nanoparticles had to be formulated at 37°C to accelerate the diffusion of PEG 400 in the W-phase and to obtain small particle sizes. This was also reported by Ali et al. who received a mixture of particles and precipitated polymer during preparations at room temperature (Ali et al. 2013). Under optimized conditions the homogenization was performed only by stirring at 650 rpm.

The most hydrophilic candidate, the dipolar aprotic solvent Cyrene™ (Murray n.d.) required a completely new procedure as standard techniques did not result in small-sized nanoparticles. The O-phase consisting of a polymer solution in Cyrene™ was carefully covered with the W-phase forming two phases. The following homogenization by ultrasonication resulted in the formation of an O/W-emulsion with an increased interfacial area. At the interface between both phases, the aprotic Cyrene™, per se not miscible with water, forms an equilibrium with its hydrate, a geminal diol by formation of two additional hydroxyl groups, which greatly increase the polarity, causing it to diffuse into the aqueous phase and precipitate the PLGA. Although several homogenization techniques with varying process parameters were investigated, the overlaying technique using Cyrene™ was found to be the best reproducible technique (Grune et al. 2021b).

As a major advantage, for all newly tested alternative solvents the number of process steps and, consequently, the process time to formulate nanoparticles could be reduced to 1–5 h depending on the type of alternative solvent. This is in contrast to the standard emulsion-diffusion-evaporation techniques using organic solvents with process times up to 19 h mainly related to the evaporation process for solvent removal. In contrast to typically used organic solvents with high vapor pressures or low boiling points, the application of alternative solvents facilitate solvent removal by the faster process of centrifugation within some hours.

As summarized in Fig. 2, which provides an overview of the process flow of all mentioned manufacturing techniques, the differences between the production methods critically depend on the type of solvent resulting in different types of phase mixing, process temperature, number of process steps, and as a result in different process times.

6 Physicochemical and Biological Characteristics of the Nanoparticles Produced with Alternative Solvents

The nanoparticle preparation techniques with the different solvents presented in the last section were evaluated and compared regarding their influence on the physicochemical characteristics of the final nanoparticles as well as their biological effects. Under optimized conditions, all formulation techniques offered the possibility to produce nanoparticles around 150–200 nm with low polydispersity (below 0.2) and monomodal size distributions. Size and morphology were confirmed by electron microscopy and atomic force microscopy showing spherical particles with smooth surfaces independent of the type of solvent (Grune et al. 2021a, b).

Ethyl acetate (nanoemulsification) and ethyl lactate (nanoprecipitation), both with lower viscosities and the highest hydrophobicity, resulted in nanoparticles with comparably high yields around 50–60% and particle sizes of about 180–200 nm and 170–180 nm, respectively, probably due to the different preparation techniques. A trend to smaller nanoparticle sizes below 180 nm could be observed for glycerol formal and PEG 400, however, for both with a lower yield compared to ethyl acetate and ethyl lactate, which could be related to different viscosities. Although PEG

400 demonstrated the highest viscosity of all alternative solvents, the increase of process temperature to 37°C accomplished the formation of small particles. The low yield might be related to the diffusion of PEG 400 into the aqueous phase, but it still has a considerable potential to solubilize PLGA (about 50%) whereby a part of the PLGA does not precipitate (Grune et al. 2021a). Although γ-valerolactone reached particle yields in the range of ethyl lactate, particles sizes were slightly larger around 200 nm. Cyrene™ was different from the other alternative solvents and formed nanoparticles with larger sizes of about 220–230 nm due to its higher hydrophilicity, formation of the geminal diols, high viscosity, and the different, layered preparation technique, as discussed above (De Bruyn et al. 2019). An influence of the solvent selection on the zeta potential of the particles around −15 to −25 mV is negligible as the surface charge was mostly dependent on the type of PLGA polymer and stabilizer used (Rietscher et al. 2016).

PLGA nanoparticle formulations with Cyrene™, ethyl lactate, and ethyl acetate exhibited similar crystallinities comparable to the pure PLGA polymer. In contrast, the use of PEG 400 resulted in plasticizing effects and a lower crystallinity of the PLGA nanoparticles with a decrease in the glass transition temperature of up to 22°C as determined by differential scanning calorimetry and Raman spectroscopy (Grune et al. 2021a). Interestingly, the particles prepared by the PEG 400 based method showed crystallinities and drug release kinetics similar to nanoparticles made of PEGylated PLGA polymer using the conventional emulsification technique (Grune et al. 2021a). Whether applied as covalent bound PEG or as solvent in the O-phase, obviously PEG incorporates between the PLGA chains, which reduces the attraction forces between the PLGA chains and lowers the glass transition temperature (Vega et al. 2012).

Regarding drug release, a biphasic diffusion-controlled release profile with a rapid drug release within the first 24 h was shown for all nanoparticle preparations (Grune et al. 2021a, b; Czapka et al. 2022). Up to 168 h no further relevant changes of the cumulative drug release could be observed. The initial burst release can be explained by the rapid hydration and diffusion of the drug adsorbed to the surface or encapsulated near the surface of the particles (Fredenberg et al. 2011). The second phase exhibits a slower diffusion of the drug through either the polymer matrix or water filled pores. However, the differences of particle crystallinity due to the different preparation methods were reflected in a modified drug release with the PEG 400 nanoparticles exhibiting a faster and higher release due to the lower crystallinity. The hydrophobicity of the selected solvent also has to be taken into consideration for the encapsulation efficiency of drugs. In a comparative study using the anti-inflammatory lipophilic indirubin derivative 6-bromo-indirubin-3′-glycerol-oximether (6BIGOE), drug loading increased in the order Cyrene™ < PEG 400 < ethyl acetate in correlation with the increasing lipophilic character of the solvent (Grune et al. 2021a, b; Czapka et al. 2022). The respective nanoparticles showed a clear anti-inflammatory effect in CD14+ monocytes after stimulation with lipopolysaccharide and were superior to the free drugs. With regard to the different preparation methods, comparable anti-inflammatory effects could be shown. Only the cell uptake of the 6BIGOE containing nanoparticles prepared by the Cyrene™

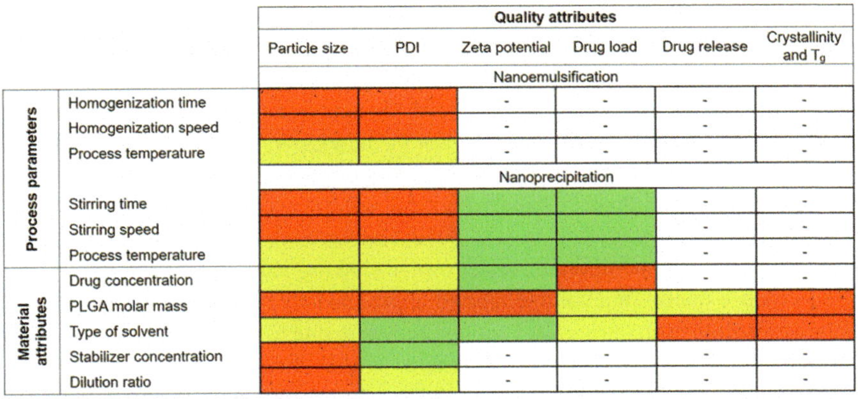

Quality attributes
Particle size
PDI
Zeta potential
Drug load
Drug release
Crystallinity and T_g
Nanoemulsification
Process parameters
Homogenization time
Homogenization speed
Process temperature
Nanoprecipitation
Stirring time
Stirring speed
Process temperature
Material attributes
Drug concentration
PLGA molar mass
Type of solvent
Stabilizer concentration
Dilution ratio

Fig. 3 Classification of the material attributes and process parameters according to their individual influence on the quality attributes (red: major, yellow: moderate, green: low)

and PEG 400 method was superior to the nanoparticles prepared by the emulsion method and needs further investigations (Czapka et al. 2022).

In a comprehensive overview as conclusion (Fig. 3), all quality attributes of the final nanoparticle preparations like particle size and polydispersity, surface charge, drug load and release, as well as crystallinity were correlated with the different process parameters and the attributes of the applied materials, to identify critical factors with major impact (Grune et al. 2021a). For methods with classical and alternative solvents, homogenization speed and time played the most crucial role for the particle size distribution, whereas the process temperature was only relevant for the higher viscous solvents to form small particles. All other attributes were less effected by the process parameters. With respect to the material attributes, PLGA molar mass, stabilizer concentration, and dilution ratio of the two phases mainly determined the particle size. Of all parameters tested, the PLGA molar mass had the most relevant impact affecting many of the quality attributes. Although the type of solvent determined the particle size and drug load, the highest influence was found for the drug release depending on the crystallinity.

7 Applicability of Alternative Solvents for In Situ Formation of Particles in Matrices

The applicability of alternative solvents for emulsion and precipitation methods raised the question whether an in situ formation of particles in complex matrices would also be feasible with alternative solvents. Therefore, the biosynthetically produced, sustainable hydrogel bacterial nanocellulose (BNC) was used as a model matrix that consists of <5% physically cross-linked cellulose binding >95% water. The material is used for a broad variety of biomedical applications including implants, wound dressings, tissue engineering, and drug delivery (Klemm et al. 2021; Pötzinger et al. 2017). The rationale for the combination of BNC and polymer particles was to introduce a lipophilic compartment within the hydrophilic matrix, enabling the homogenous incorporation and the controlled release of lipophilic drugs, which could be beneficial for long-acting active wound dressings and tissue engineering. For the dissolution of the PLGA, three different alternative solvents were selected, namely PEG 400, Cyrene™, and ethyl lactate and compared to *N*-methyl-2-pyrrolidone, a standard organic solvent typically used for the formulation of in situ implants (Kempe et al. 2010; Pandya et al. 2014). This organic phase was homogenously incorporated under orbital shaking at room temperature into the nanocellulose matrix in a volume ratio of approximately 1:15 to avoid uncontrolled polymer precipitation during the loading procedure due to the mixing with the water bound by BNC. Afterwards, the BNC matrix was shaken in an excess of ultrapure water to enable solvent exchange, to initialize particle formation by phase inversion and to ensure sufficient solvent removal (Fig. 4a) (Bellmann et al. 2023).

Due to the concentration gradient between the fluid bound by the BNC matrix and the aqueous surrounding, two diffusional movements are relevant for the polymer precipitation: (1) The diffusion of solvent molecules from the BNC matrix to the aqueous surrounding (solvent efflux) and (2) the diffusion of water from the aqueous surrounding into the BNC matrix (non-solvent influx). The concentration of the non-solvent water within the cellulose network increases over time and overcomes a critical value, leading to a separation of the polymer solution into a polymer-rich and a polymer-lean phase. With a further increase of the water concentration, the polymer-rich phase solidifies (Parent et al. 2013). Therefore, the diffusivity of the solvents turned out to be a critical factor for the phase inversion dynamics within the hydrogel matrix. Additionally, water miscibility, viscosity, molar mass, and the critical water concentration for precipitation were identified as critical parameters for the selection of solvents for this approach.

Whereas the highly viscous solvents PEG 400 and Cyrene™ were not successful for particle incorporation due to an inhomogeneous distribution in the BNC matrix, ethyl lactate and NMP demonstrated the homogenous incorporation of PLGA particles. The presence of PLGA was verified by Fourier-transform infrared spectroscopy and scanning electron microscopy and revealed the formation of spherical PLGA microparticles with diameters from 1 to 5 μm attached to the cellulose fibers. As an example, the lipophilic anti-inflammatory drug cannabidiol was encapsulated in the PLGA particles to evaluate the drug delivery capabilities of the developed formulation approach. In contrast to conventional formulation approaches for BNC matrices, particle encapsulation of the drugs led to a sustained release with linear kinetics over up to 10 days (Fig. 4b).

The performance of the systems was independent of whether NMP or ethyl lactate was used for particle formation, which demonstrated the applicability of the green solvent. When using ethyl lactate for the formulation process, every compound of the delivery system can be manufactured from sustainable resources. The ability to form polymeric particles within BNC matrices enables numerous possibilities for BNC based biomedical applications, such as drug delivery systems, active medical devices, or extracellular matrices for tissue engineering.

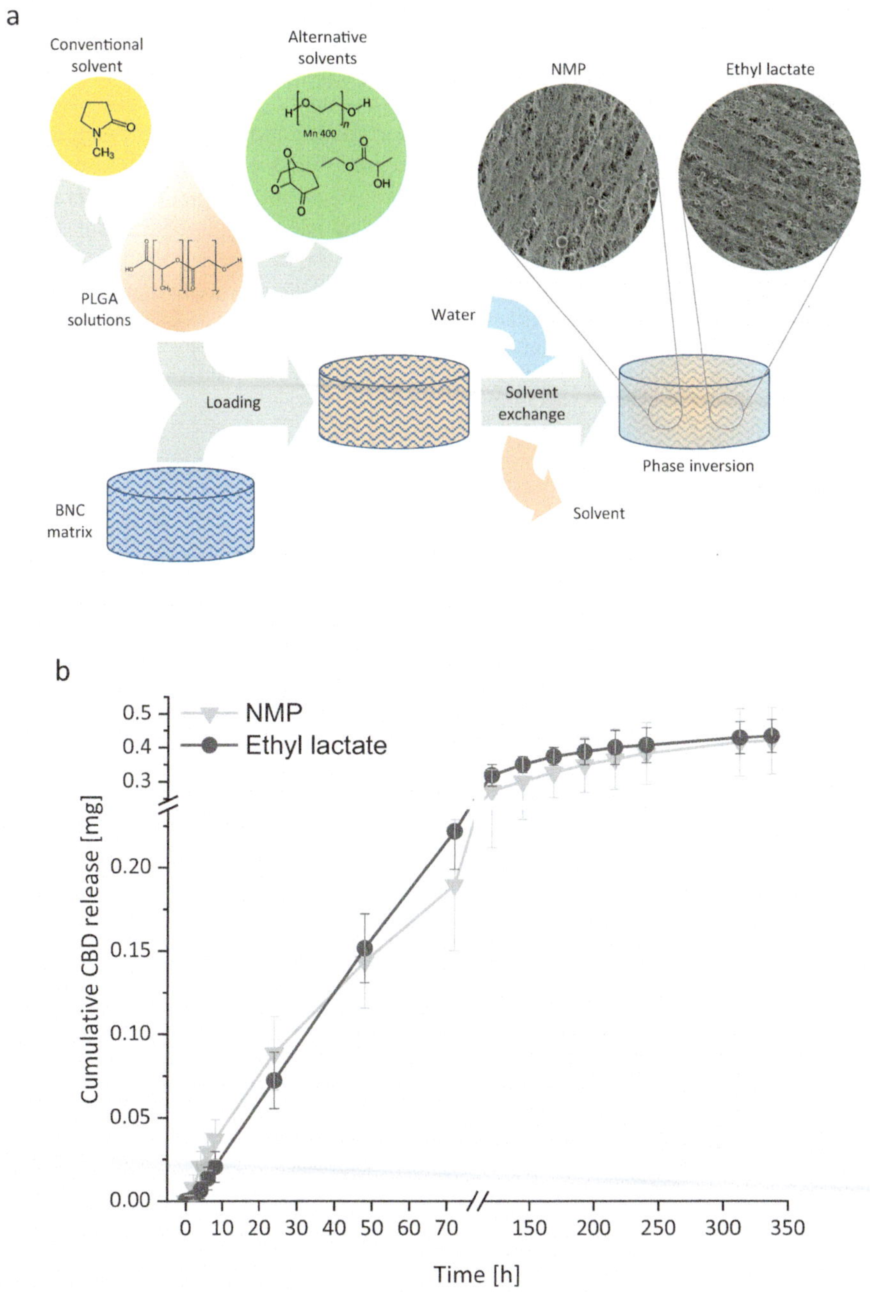

Fig. 4 (**a**) Formulation concept of the in situ particle formation in a matrix consisting of bacterial nanocellulose. (**b**) Drug release of cannabidiol (CBD) compared between particle containing nanocellulose matrices using NMP and ethyl lactate as solvents for precipitation (mean ± SD, $n = 6$)

8 Conclusion

Since the 1990s, green chemistry approaches have grown into a significant area that could provide the drug formulation technologists with a plethora of new ideas for green, sustainable, or alternative solvents to formulate nanoparticles by precipitation or emulsification. Future challenges will not only focus on the principal question how these solvents can be applied into these processes, but also on the transferability to different classes of active ingredients and the transfer into larger scales.

Acknowledgments The author would like to thank Tom Bellmann, Sandra Hübner, Christian Kroh, Alexander Weber, and Jan Westhoff for their excellent editorial support during manuscript preparation. This work was supported by the DFG-funded Collaborative Research Centre PolyTarget (SFB 1278, project number 316213987, project C02) and the Free State of Thuringia and the European Social Funds (2019 FGR 0095; nanoCARE4skin).

References

Ahmed N (2013) Polymeric drug delivery systems for encapsulating hydrophobic drugs. Drug delivery strategies for poorly water-soluble drugs, 1st edn. Wiley, pp 151–197

Ali ME et al (2013) Polyethylene glycol as an alternative polymer solvent for nanoparticle preparation. Int J Pharm 456:135–142

Alkholief M et al (2022) Effect of solvents, stabilizers and the concentration of stabilizers on the physical properties of poly(d,l-lactide-co-glycolide) nanoparticles: encapsulation, in vitro release of indomethacin and cytotoxicity against HepG2-cell. Pharmaceutics 14

Allhenn D et al (2011) Microsphere preparation using the untoxic solvent glycofurol. Pharm Res 28:563–571

Alshamsan A (2014) Nanoprecipitation is more efficient than emulsion solvent evaporation method to encapsulate Cucurbitacin I in PLGA nanoparticles. Saudi Pharm J 22:219–222

Anderson CD et al (2003) Emulsion polymerisation and latex applications. Rapra Technol

Aparicio S et al (2009) The green solvent ethyl lactate: an experimental and theoretical characterization. Green Chem 11:65–78

Arafa MG et al (2020) Chitosan-coated PLGA nanoparticles for enhanced ocular anti-inflammatory efficacy of atorvastatin calcium. Int J Nanomedicine 15:1335–1347

Arshady R (1992) Suspension, emulsion, and dispersion polymerization: a methodological survey. Colloid Polym Sci 270:717–732

Baier G et al (2014) Stabilization of nanoparticles synthesized by miniemulsion polymerization using "Green" amino-acid based surfactants. Macromolecules 337:9–17

Beck-Broichsitter M et al (2010) Preparation of nanoparticles by solvent displacement for drug delivery: a shift in the "Ouzo Region" upon drug loading. Eur J Pharm Sci 41:244–253

Beck-Broichsitter M et al (2015) Solvent selection causes remarkable shifts of the "Ouzo Region" for poly(lactide-co-glycolide) nanoparticles prepared by nanoprecipitation. Nanoscale 7:9215–9221

Bellmann T et al (2023) In situ formation of polymer microparticles in bacterial Nanocellulose using alternative and sustainable solvents to incorporate lipophilic drugs. Pharmaceutics 15:559

Bilati U et al (2005) Development of a nanoprecipitation method intended for the entrapment of hydrophilic drugs into nanoparticles. Eur J Pharm Sci 24:67–75

Borde S et al (2021) Ternary solid dispersions: classification and formulation considerations. Drug Dev Ind Pharm 47:1011–1028

Breslow R (2010) The principles of and reasons for using water as a solvent for green chemistry. Handbook of green chemistry

Byrne FP et al (2016) Tools and techniques for solvent selection: green solvent selection guides. Sustain Chem Processes 4:7

Camp JE (2018) Bio-available solvent cyrene: synthesis, derivatization, and applications. ChemSusChem 11:3048–3055

Capello C et al (2007) What is a green solvent? A comprehensive framework for the environmental assessment of solvents. Green Chem 9:927–934

Carl Roth (n.d.) Safety data sheet (SDS) glycerol formal version 2.0 de; [Available from: https://www.carlroth.com/medias/SDB-0798-DE-DE.pdf?context=bWFzdGVyfHNlY3VyaXR5RGF0YXNoZWV0c3wyNjg2NDN8YXBwbGljYXRpb24vcGRmfHNlY3VyaXR5RGF0YXNoZWV0cy9oNjUvaDBmLzkwMjcyMjczODU4ODYucGRmfDFkMGRjZDM5YTMzNmY3NGI2ZGY4MjJjNzNmZDY1YmNmMmQ4ZTAwMmY4MGE2ODhjNjg4MGFiNGVjODNmOTk3MzM. Accessed on 14 Nov 2022

Choi S-W et al (2002) Thermodynamic parameters on poly(d,l-lactide-co-glycolide) particle size in emulsification–diffusion process. Colloids Surf A Physicochem Eng Asp 201:283–289

Cortés H et al (2021) Non-ionic surfactants for stabilization of polymeric nanoparticles for biomedical uses. Materials 14:3197

Czapka A et al (2022) Drug delivery of 6-bromoindirubin-3′-glycerol-oxime ether employing poly(d,l-lactide-co-glycolide)-based nanoencapsulation techniques with sustainable solvents. J Nanobiotechnology 20:5

De Bruyn M et al (2019) Geminal diol of dihydrolevoglucosenone as a switchable hydrotrope: a continuum of green nanostructured solvents. ACS Sustain Chem Eng 7:7878–7883

Esmaili Z et al (2018) Development and characterization of electrosprayed nanoparticles for encapsulation of curcumin. J Biomed Mater Res A 106:285–292

Essa D et al (2020) The design of poly(lactide-co-glycolide) nanocarriers for medical applications. Front Bioeng Biotechnol 8:48

Eun-JungHan A-HI-J (2012) Analysis of residual solvents in polylactide-co-glycolide nanoparticles. J Pharm Investig 42:251–256

Farias CBB et al (2021) Production of green surfactants: market prospects. Electron J Biotechnol 51:28–39

Fernandez AM et al (2005) New green surfactants for emulsion polymerization. Prog Org Coat 53: 246–255

Fessi H et al (1989) Nanocapsule formation by interfacial polymer deposition following solvent displacement. Int J Pharm 55:R1–R4

Fredenberg S et al (2011) The mechanisms of drug release in poly(lactic-co-glycolic acid)-based drug delivery systems – a review. Int J Pharm 415:34–52

Galindo-Rodriguez S et al (2004) Physicochemical parameters associated with nanoparticle formation in the salting-out, emulsification-diffusion, and nanoprecipitation methods. Pharm Res 21: 1428–1439

Ganachaud F et al (2005) Nanoparticles and nanocapsules created using the ouzo effect: spontaneous emulisification as an alternative to ultrasonic and high-shear devices. ChemPhysChem 6: 209–216

Globally Harmonized System of Classification and Labelling of Chemicals (GHS) (n.d.) United Nations; [Available from: https://www.unece.org/fileadmin/DAM/trans/danger/publi/ghs/ghs_rev08/ST-SGAC10-30-Rev8e.pdf. Accessed on 14 Nov 2022]

Grizić D et al (2018) Microparticle preparation by a propylene carbonate emulsification-extraction method. Int J Pharm 544:213–221

Grund S et al (2011) Polymers in drug delivery – state of the art and future trends. Adv Eng Mater 13:B61–B87

Grune CS (2022) Verwendung von alternativen Lösungsmitteln zur Verkapselung von lipophilen Naturstoffen in polyesterbasierte Nanopartikel. Pharmaceutical Technology and Biopharmacy, Institute of Pharmacy, Friedrich Schiller University Jena, p 17

Grune C et al (2021a) Sustainable preparation of anti-inflammatory atorvastatin PLGA nanoparticles. Int J Pharm 599:120404

Grune C et al (2021b) Cyrene™ as an alternative sustainable solvent for the preparation of poly (lactic-co-glycolic acid) nanoparticles. J Pharm Sci 110:959–964
Gu Y et al (2013) Bio-based solvents: an emerging generation of fluids for the design of eco-efficient processes in catalysis and organic chemistry. Chem Soc Rev 42:9550–9570
Haji Mansor M et al (2018) Development of a non-toxic and non-denaturing formulation process for encapsulation of SDF-1α into PLGA/PEG-PLGA nanoparticles to achieve sustained release. Eur J Pharm Biopharm 125:38–50
Hernandez-Giottonini KY et al (2020) PLGA nanoparticle preparations by emulsification and nanoprecipitation techniques: effects of formulation parameters. RSC Adv 10:4218–4231
Huang W et al (2018) Tuning the size of poly(lactic-co-glycolic acid) (PLGA) nanoparticles fabricated by nanoprecipitation. Biotechnol J 13
International Council for Harmonisation of Technical Requirements for Pharmaceuticals for Human Use (ICH) (n.d.) ICH Q3C (R8) Residual solvents – scientific guideline [Available from: https://www.ema.europa.eu/en/documents/regulatory-procedural-guideline/ich-guideline-q3c-r8-impurities-guideline-residual-solvents-step-5_en.pdf; Accessed on 14 Nov 2022]
Kang J et al (2014) Applicability of non-halogenated methyl propionate to microencapsulation. J Microencapsul 31:323–332
Kempe S et al (2010) Non-invasive in vivo evaluation of in situ forming PLGA implants by benchtop magnetic resonance imaging (BT-MRI) and EPR spectroscopy. Eur J Pharm Biopharm 74:102–108
Kim Y et al (2016) Methylamine acts as excellent chemical trigger to harden emulsion droplets into spongy PLGA microspheres. RSC Adv 6:85275–85284
Kim H et al (2018) Solvent hydrolysis rate determines critical quality attributes of PLGA microspheres prepared using non-volatile green solvent. J Biomater Sci Polym Ed 29:35–56
Klemm D et al (2021) Biotech nanocellulose: a review on progress in product design and today's state of technical and medical applications. Carbohydr Polym 254:117313
Konan YN et al (2003) Preparation and characterization of sterile sub-200 nm meso-tetra (4-hydroxylphenyl)porphyrin-loaded nanoparticles for photodynamic therapy. Eur J Pharm Biopharm
Lee Y et al (2015) Chemical approach to solvent removal during nanoencapsulation: its application to preparation of PLGA nanoparticles with non-halogenated solvent. J Nanopart Res 17:453
Lee Y et al (2016) Simple emulsion technique as an innovative template for preparation of porous, spongelike poly(lactide-co-glycolide) microspheres with pore-closing capability. J Mater Sci 51:6257–6274
Lu M et al (2016) Microfluidic hydrodynamic focusing for synthesis of nanomaterials. Nano Today 11:778–792
Makadia HK et al (2011) Poly lactic-co-glycolic acid (PLGA) as biodegradable controlled drug delivery carrier. Polymers (Basel) 3:1377–1397
Morikawa Y et al (2018) The use of an efficient microfluidic mixing system for generating stabilized polymeric nanoparticles for controlled drug release. Biol Pharm Bull 41:899–907
Murray J (n.d.) CYRENE™: a new bio-based dipolar aprotic solvent; [Available from: https://communities.acs.org/t5/GCI-Nexus-Blog/CYRENE-A-New-Bio-based-Dipolar-Aprotic-Solvent/ba-p/15488. Accessed on 14 Nov 2022]
Nikles SM et al (2001) Ethyl lactate: a green solvent for magnetic tape coating. Green Chem 3:109–113
Odian G (2004) Principles of polymerization
Operti MC et al (2021) PLGA-based nanomedicines manufacturing: technologies overview and challenges in industrial scale-up. Int J Pharm 605:120807
Operti MC et al (2022) Industrial scale manufacturing and downstream processing of PLGA-based nanomedicines suitable for fully continuous operation. Pharmaceutics:14
Pal SL et al., Nanoparticle: an overview of preparation and characterization. 2011
Panda A et al (2016) Formulation and characterization of clozapine and risperidone co-entrapped spray-dried PLGA nanoparticles. Pharm Dev Technol 21:43–53

Pandya YN et al (2014) Implants and controlled released drug delivery system
Pánek J et al (2011) Polymeric nanoparticles stabilized by surfactants: kinetic studies. J Dispers Sci Technol 32:1105–1110
Parent M et al (2013) PLGA in situ implants formed by phase inversion: critical physicochemical parameters to modulate drug release. J Control Release 172:292–304
Paswan SK et al (2017) Purification of drug loaded PLGA nanoparticles prepared by emulsification solvent evaporation using stirred cell ultrafiltration technique. Pharm Res 34:2779–2786
Pereira CSM et al (2011) Ethyl lactate as a solvent: properties, applications and production processes – a review. Green Chem 13:2658–2671
Pötzinger Y et al (2017) Bacterial nanocellulose: the future of controlled drug delivery? Ther Deliv 8:753–761
Profirio D et al (2018) Formulation of functionalized PLGA nanoparticles with folic acid-conjugated chitosan for carboplatin encapsulation. Eur Polym J 108:311–321
Quimidroga (n.d.) Alternative solvents to traditional solvents. [Available from: https://www.quimidroga.com/en/2022/03/08/alternative-solvents-to-traditional-solvents/. Accessed on 14 Nov 2022]
Ratti R (2020) Industrial applications of green chemistry: status, challenges and prospects. SN Appl Sci 2:263
Ravi Kumar MN et al (2004) Preparation and characterization of cationic PLGA nanospheres as DNA carriers. Biomaterials 25:1771–1777
Rebello S et al (2014) Surfactants: toxicity, remediation and green surfactants. Environ Chem Lett 12:275–287
Rietscher R et al (2016) Impact of PEG and PEG-b-PAGE modified PLGA on nanoparticle formation, protein loading and release. Int J Pharm 500:187–195
Sah H (2000) Ethyl formate – alternative dispersed solvent useful in preparing PLGA microspheres. Int J Pharm 195:103–113
Sah E et al (2015) Recent trends in preparation of poly(lactide-co-glycolide) nanoparticles by mixing polymeric organic solution with antisolvent. J Nanomater 2015:794601
Sahoo SK et al (2002) Residual polyvinyl alcohol associated with poly (D,L-lactide-co-glycolide) nanoparticles affects their physical properties and cellular uptake. J Control Release 82:105–114
Salavagione HJ et al (2017) Identification of high performance solvents for the sustainable processing of graphene. Green Chem 19:2550–2560
Shkodra-Pula B et al (2020) Encapsulation of the dual FLAP/mPEGS-1 inhibitor BRP-187 into acetalated dextran and PLGA nanoparticles improves its cellular bioactivity. J Nanobiotechnology 18:73
Sigma-Aldrich (n.d.-a) Safety data sheet (SDS) cyrene version 6.6; [Available from: https://www.sigmaaldrich.com/DE/en/sds/sial/807796. Accessed on 15 Nov 2022]
Sigma-Aldrich (n.d.-b) Safety data sheet (SDS) γ-valerolactone version 7.0; [Available from https://www.sigmaaldrich.com/DE/de/sds/aldrich/v403. Accessed on 14 Nov 2022]
Soni J et al (2020) Polyethylene glycol: a promising approach for sustainable organic synthesis. J Mol Liq 315:113766
Sternling CV et al (1959) Interfacial turbulence: hydrodynamic instability and the Marangoni effect. AICHE J 5:514–523
Sumana M et al (2020) Biodegradable natural polymeric nanoparticles as carrier for drug delivery. Integrative nanomedicine for new therapies. Springer, pp 231–246
Sustainability (n.d.) United Nations. [Available from: https://www.un.org/en/academic-impact/sustainability. Accessed 16 Mar 2023]
Swider E et al (2018) Customizing poly(lactic-co-glycolic acid) particles for biomedical applications. Acta Biomater 73:38–51
Ting JM et al (2018) Advances in polymer design for enhancing oral drug solubility and delivery. Bioconjug Chem 29:939–952
Türk CTŞ et al (2021) Development and in-vitro evaluation of chitosan chloride decorated PLGA based polymeric nanoparticles of nimesulide. J Pharm Res 25:379–387

Vega E et al (2012) Role of Hydroxypropyl-β-cyclodextrin on freeze-dried and gamma-irradiated PLGA and PLGA-PEG Diblock copolymer nanospheres for ophthalmic Flurbiprofen delivery. Int J Nanomedicine 7:1357–1371

Verband Der Chemischen Industrie (n.d.) VCI position on chemicals strategy for sustainability: Verband Der Chemischen Industrie; [Available from: https://www.vci.de/ergaenzende-downloads/2020-11-09-vci-position-en-eu-chemicals-strategy.pdf. Accessed on 16 Mar 2023]

Vitale SA et al (2003) Liquid droplet dispersions formed by homogeneous liquid–liquid nucleation: "The Ouzo Effect". Langmuir 19:4105–4110

Winterton N (2021) The green solvent: a critical perspective. Clean Techn Environ Policy 23:2499–2522

Xu J et al (2017) Controllable microfluidic production of drug-loaded PLGA nanoparticles using partially water-miscible mixed solvent microdroplets as a precursor. Sci Rep 7:4794

Zabihi F et al (2014) High yield and high loading preparation of curcumin–PLGA nanoparticles using a modified supercritical antisolvent technique. Ind Eng Chem Res 53:6569–6574

Zhang JF et al (2016) Dihydrolevoglucosenone (Cyrene) as a green alternative to N, N-dimethylformamide (DMF) in MOF synthesis. ACS Sustain Chem Eng 4:7186

Advanced Formulation Approaches for Proteins

Corinna S. Schlosser, Gareth R. Williams, and Karolina Dziemidowicz

Contents

Abstract

Proteins and peptides are highly desirable as therapeutic agents, being highly potent and specific. However, there are myriad challenges with processing them into patient-friendly formulations: they are often unstable and have a tendency to aggregate or degrade upon storage. As a result, the vast majority of protein actives are delivered parenterally as solutions, which has a number of disadvantages in terms of cost, accessibility, and patient experience. Much work has been undertaken to develop new delivery systems for biologics, but to date this has

C. S. Schlosser · G. R. Williams (✉) · K. Dziemidowicz
UCL School of Pharmacy, University College London, London, UK
e-mail: g.williams@ucl.ac.uk

M. Schäfer-Korting, U. S. Schubert (eds.), *Drug Delivery and Targeting*,
Handbook of Experimental Pharmacology 284, https://doi.org/10.1007/164_2023_647

led to relatively few products on the market. In this chapter, we review the challenges faced when developing biologic formulations, discuss the technologies that have been explored to try to overcome these, and consider the different delivery routes that can be applied. We further present an overview of the currently marketed products and assess the likely direction of travel in the next decade.

Keywords

Biologic · Formulation · Peptide · Pharmaceutical technology · Protein

Abbreviations

API	Active pharmaceutical ingredient
COPD	Congestive obstructive pulmonary disease
EHD	Electrohydrodynamic processes
EMA	European Medicines Agency
FDA	Food and Drug Administration
HME	Hot-melt extrusion
IFN	Interferon
IV	Intravenous
MMAD	Mass median aerodynamic diameter
PEG	Polyethylene glycol
PLA	Poly(lactic acid)
PLGA	Poly(lactic-co-glycolic acid)
SC	Subcutaneous

1 Introduction

Biologics, or biological drugs, are a potent class of active pharmaceutical ingredients (APIs) that includes vaccines, cell and gene therapy, and recombinant therapeutic proteins. Currently, around 50% of the top 100 drugs are biologics, most of which are protein based (Park et al. 2022). Whilst promising therapeutically due to their high specificity and relatively low toxicity compared to small molecule drugs, proteins are notoriously difficult to deliver to the site of action. At present, the patient-preferred route of oral delivery is virtually impossible for proteins due to extremely low bioavailability (<1%) (Nie et al. 2021). This is primarily due to the acidic pH of the gastric fluids and digestive enzymes that cause the breakdown of delicate protein structures. Permeability is also a challenge. The majority of protein therapeutics are therefore given parenterally, but their short half-lives require frequent injections to maintain therapeutic efficacy. This, in turn, becomes a logistical challenge if the treatment requires administration by a healthcare professional. Moreover, the invasive nature of injections negatively affects patient adherence and pushes protein drugs further down the treatment guidelines, giving preference to cheaper orally delivered small molecule drugs.

There is therefore a strong need for novel formulation technologies aiming at prolonged and effective delivery of therapeutic proteins without the loss of their functionality. This chapter discusses techniques as well as delivery routes currently used in protein drug delivery, and gives an outlook into how the field may develop in the coming years.

2 Techniques Used in Protein Drug Delivery

Most pharmaceutical proteins suffer from poor stability during storage, transport and administration, for example due to temperature fluctuations, light exposure or agitation. To decrease the risk of protein breakdown before it is delivered to the patient, almost half of protein pharmaceuticals are formulated as solids. Typically, these are reconstituted to solutions before administration. Such solid formulations can be obtained through a variety of routes, including formulating emulsions or using microfluidics, freeze-drying, spray-drying, spray-freeze-drying and electrohydrodynamic processes (Chen et al. 2021; Moreira et al. 2021; Mu et al. 2021; Tomeh and Zhao 2020; Wang 2015).

2.1 Freeze-Drying

Freeze-drying, often referred to as lyophilisation, is the primary method of solid-state protein formulation production (Chen et al. 2021; Wang 2015). Despite long processing times and high operating costs, around 50% of the Food and Drug Administration (FDA) and European Medicines Agency (EMA)-approved biopharmaceuticals are lyophilised products (Chen et al. 2021).

In freeze-drying (Fig. 1), the liquid sample is frozen, resulting in an ice-crystal matrix which is followed by the application of a vacuum (Chen et al. 2021). Under vacuum the ice crystals directly pass from the solid state into the vapour phase (a process called sublimation), leaving an anhydrous solid product behind (Chen et al. 2021; Ishwarya et al. 2015). The latter comprises a porous material that requires reconstitution prior to administration by a healthcare professional (Muralidhara and Wong 2020). To prevent aggregation and denaturation of proteins during the freezing process, cryoprotectants such as non-reducing sugars (e.g. sucrose and trehalose), amino acids, proteins or polyols are often used (Emami et al. 2018). Lyophilisation is commonly used in the formulation of monoclonal antibodies, such as Herceptin (trastuzumab), Remicade (infliximab) or Keytruda (pembrolizumab) (Gervasi et al. 2018).

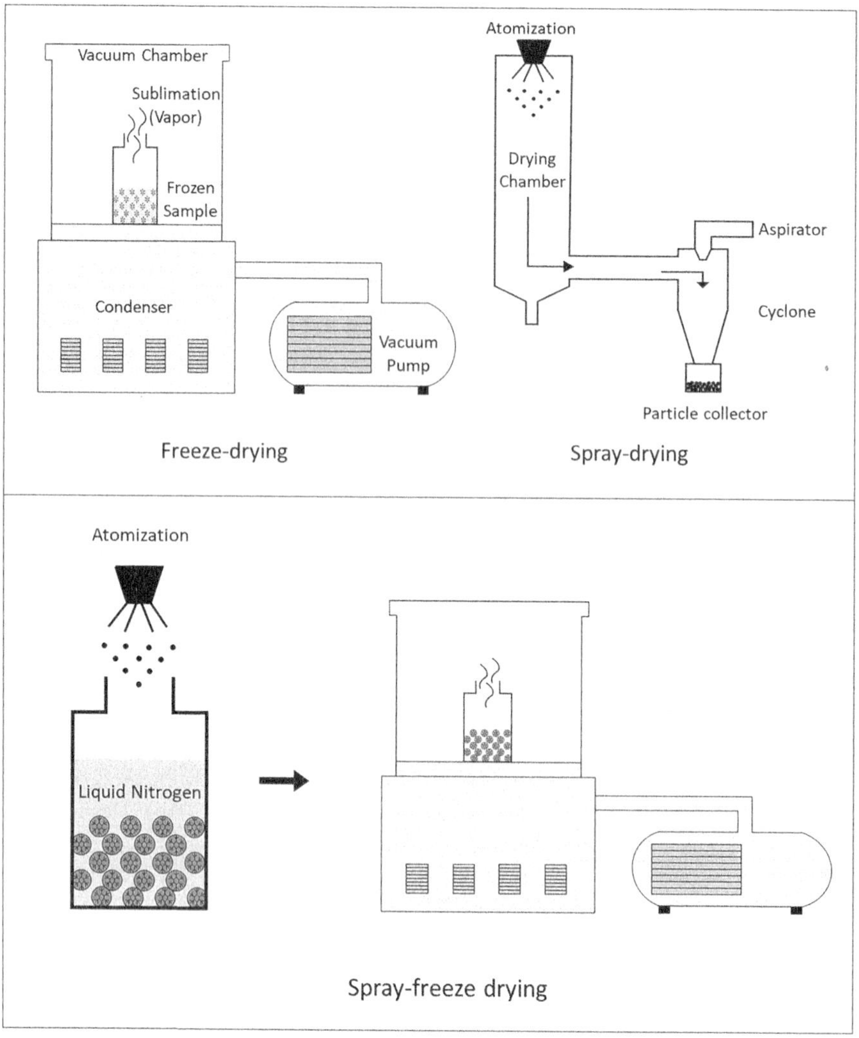

Fig. 1 A schematic image of the freeze-drying, spray-drying and spray-freeze drying set-up

2.2 Spray-Drying

Spray-drying is a scalable technology allowing large-scale production of therapeutics with high batch-to-batch reproducibility (Angkawinitwong et al. 2015). A typical spray-drying system (Fig. 1) is composed of four parts, namely an atomiser (nozzle), a drying chamber, a cyclone recovery unit and an aspirator (Chen et al. 2021; Angkawinitwong et al. 2015). A solution of the active ingredient and any excipients is atomised into fine droplets and dried by blowing over hot dry air or an inert gas (e.g. nitrogen), which leads to rapid evaporation of the solvent (Angkawinitwong et al. 2015). The aspirator attracts the dry particles towards the cyclone recovery unit to allow product collection (Angkawinitwong et al. 2015). The physical properties of the spray-dried particles are controlled by instrument settings (e.g. atomiser, feed rate, air flow, aspirator) and feedstock composition (e.g. solvent and solution concentration) (Chen et al. 2021; Angkawinitwong et al. 2015). The properties of the spray-dried particles, in particular the particle size, can thus be optimised to meet requirements for specific routes of administration (e.g. inhalation). Exubera (insulin) and Raplixa (thrombin + fibrinogen) are both examples of spray-dried products which have obtained FDA approval in 2006 and 2015 respectively (Chen et al. 2021; Geraldes et al. 2020; Arpagaus 2018; McKeage 2015).

2.3 Spray-Freeze Drying

Spray-freeze drying combines the spray-drying and freeze-drying processes. This technique is not currently adopted for manufacturing of commercial pharmaceutical products but has seen an increase in research interest for processing of thermosensitive biopharmaceutical active ingredients (Chen et al. 2021). The spray-freeze drying process (Fig. 1) first atomises the solution into droplets (spraying) that freezes upon contact with a cold liquid (e.g. liquid nitrogen) (freezing) (Chen et al. 2021; Ishwarya et al. 2015; Wanning et al. 2015; Costantino et al. 2002). The solvent then sublimes from the frozen particles under vacuum (drying) (Wanning et al. 2015; Costantino et al. 2002). The resulting particles are generally porous and possess good flowability (Ishwarya et al. 2015; Wanning et al. 2015). Optimising processing parameters and excipients used can prevent particle agglomeration and protein denaturation (Ishwarya et al. 2015). The spray-freeze drying technique is particularly attractive for pulmonary drug delivery due to the favourable aerodynamic properties of the resultant particles and has been applied to vaccines, insulin, calcitonin, teriparatide and anti-IgE monoclonal antibodies, amongst others (Wanning et al. 2015; Vishali et al. 2019; Poursina et al. 2017).

2.4 Electrohydrodynamic Processes

In recent years, electrohydrodynamic processes (EHD), which include electrospinning and electrospraying have been widely explored for the formulation of biopharmaceuticals (Li et al. 2010; Briggs and Arinzeh 2014; Chen et al. 2010; Gomez et al. 1998; Domján et al. 2020; Angkawinitwong et al. 2017; Lee et al. 2020; Lancina et al. 2017). Electrospinning and electrospraying are sister technologies and use the same basic experimental apparatus (Fig. 2), which consists of four main components: a syringe pump, a high voltage supply, a metallic needle (often described as the 'spinneret') and a collector (Williams et al. 2018). An electric field is maintained between a positively charged spinneret and the collector, which can be grounded or negatively charged. The charged liquid exiting the spinneret is

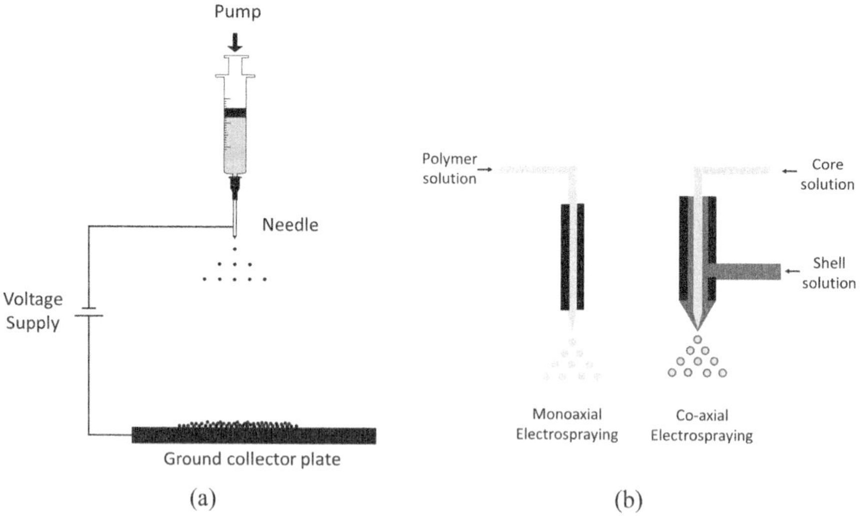

Fig. 2 Schematic image of (**a**) the electrohydrodynamic technique of electrospraying and (**b**) monoaxial and co-axial spinnerets and the resultant products

drawn and solidifies at ambient temperature under the influence of the electric field, resulting in the production of fibres (electrospinning) or particles (electrospraying) in the nano- to micrometre range (Moreira et al. 2021; Williams et al. 2018). Further, by varying processing parameters (e.g. flow rate and voltage) product features such as size, morphology, composition and release behaviour can be tailored (Moreira et al. 2021; Williams et al. 2018). Monoaxial or blend EHD is achieved from a single solution but frequently requires the use of organic solvents, which could lead to denaturation of a protein therapeutic (Onyekuru et al. 2021; Focarete and Tampieri 2018). Protection of biopharmaceuticals from organic solvents and denaturation can be achieved in a co-axial set-up where a two-needle concentric spinneret processes two separate solutions (e.g. aqueous core and organic shell) and results in core-shell materials (Onyekuru et al. 2021; Focarete and Tampieri 2018). EHD-produced nanoparticles and nanofibers for the delivery of protein therapeutics have to date mainly been evaluated at the pre-clinical stage or as proof of concept (Godakanda et al. 2022), but the technique appears to have promise.

2.5 Emulsions

Emulsions are thermodynamically unstable dispersions of two immiscible (oil and water) liquids, where one (dispersed phase) is distributed uniformly throughout the other (continuous phase) (Fig. 3) (Kakran and Antipina 2014; Taylor and Aulton 2022). Emulsions are prepared by physical fission of two immiscible liquids, achieved by high-speed mixing or acoustic cavitation. Depending on the nature of the continuous phase, emulsions can be either oil-in-water (o/w) or water-in-oil

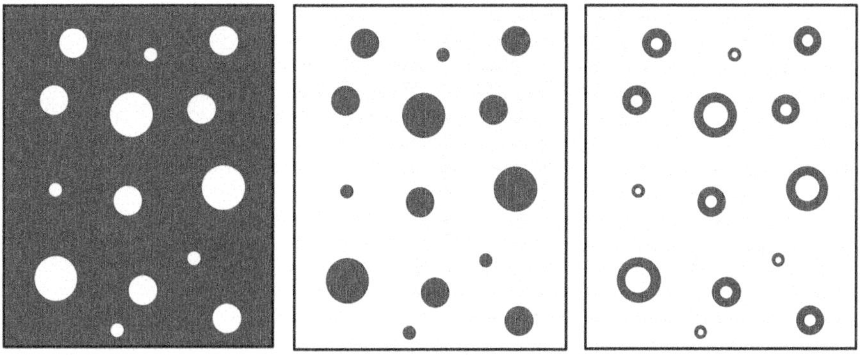

Fig. 3 The two types of single emulsion and a double emulsion (water-in-oil-in-water)

(w/o) and are stabilised by amphiphilic compounds (emulsifiers) (Kakran and Antipina 2014; Taylor and Aulton 2022). Water-in-oil emulsions allow incorporation of hydrophilic molecules, such as proteins, but there is a risk of active ingredient diffusion into the continuous phase (Iqbal et al. 2015; Jorgensen et al. 2006). For this reason, hydrophilic compounds are often formulated as double emulsions – generally water-oil-water (w/o/w) emulsions. The protein is solubilised within the inner aqueous phase which is dispersed in the oil phase forming the primary emulsion. Subsequently, this primary emulsion is dispersed into an outer aqueous phase. Emulsifiers are required at both dispersion stages and the properties of the emulsion are tailored by adapting the type and concentration of the stabiliser (Iqbal et al. 2015).

The double emulsion technique also allows preparation of polymeric particles when including a polymer into the organic phase (oil) and further evaporation of the organic solvent (Iqbal et al. 2015). A wide range of polymers have been explored for the fabrication of microparticles, however, poly(lactic-*co*-glycolic acid) (PLGA) and poly(lactic acid) (PLA) are often preferred due to their known safety profile and being FDA-approved excipients (Makadia and Siegel 2011; Tyler et al. 2016). These polymers degrade slowly via hydrolysis in vivo, releasing their drug cargo as they do so. PLA is more hydrophobic than PLGA due to the presence of a methyl side chain, which results in slower degradation and hence release (Makadia and Siegel 2011). Encapsulation within particles can prolong the half-life of otherwise unstable biomolecules, such as peptides. A notable example of this approach is Bydureon BCise, a once-weekly injectable formulation of the GLP-1 agonist exenatide licensed for type 2 diabetes, in which the peptide is encapsulated within PLGA microspheres suspended in a medium chain triglyceride vehicle (Yu et al. 2018).

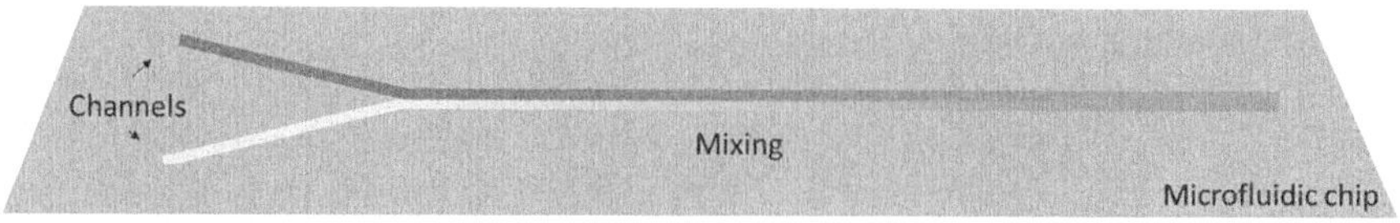

Fig. 4 Illustration of a microfluidic device composed of two channels for mixing

2.6 Microfluidics

Microfluidics allow precise and reproducible handling of nano- to picolitre volumes which, by mixing within milliseconds, results generally in monodispersed drug carriers (Tomeh and Zhao 2020; Rabiee et al. 2021; Riahi et al. 2015). Microfluidic devises are composed of micron-scaled channels, chambers, valves, pumps and mixers, which together control the flow behaviour of the fluids (Tomeh and Zhao 2020; Riahi et al. 2015; Whitesides 2006). Figure 4 shows a simple microfluidic chip containing two channels merging and thereby allowing mixing. Microfluidic devices have been employed for the production of protein loaded nanogels for controlled release, polymeric microparticles obtained by a double emulsion approach, and more generally have been used to generate lipid nanoparticles, liposomes, and micelles containing proteins such as bovine serum albumin, ovalbumin, and myoglobin (Tomeh and Zhao 2020; Bazban-Shotorbani et al. 2016; Chiesa et al. 2021; Pessi et al. 2014).

2.7 Summary of Processing Techniques

Table 1 summarises the advantages and disadvantages of the protein processing approaches described in this chapter and provides examples of products fabricated using each technique.

3 Overview of Delivery Routes

Today a range of biologics are approved as drug products, and more are expected to come on the market in the future. Table 2 presents relevant examples.

3.1 Parenteral Delivery Routes

Parenteral administration is the primary route for biologic delivery due to the poor oral bioavailability and susceptibility to degradation of these APIs (Ibeanu et al. 2020; Muralidhara and Wong 2020; Kirkby et al. 2020). Intravenous (IV) administration ensures 100% bioavailability and remains a preferred route for high-dose monoclonal antibody delivery (Ibeanu et al. 2020a; Kirkby et al. 2020). IV

Table 1 Comparison of the advantages and limitations of each processing technique

Technique	Advantages	Limitations	Clinical trials and commercial products
Freeze-drying	High recovery yields Easy process scale-up Does not require terminal sterilisation (Angkawinitwong et al. 2015)	Time and energy consuming Uneven heat transfer Vial-to-vial inhomogeneity Variable quality (Chen et al. 2021) Batch process (Ishwarya et al. 2015)	Remicade (1998), Herceptin (1998), Xolair (2003), Afrezza (2014)
Spray-drying	Achieves freely flowing powders (Ishwarya et al. 2015) Reproducibility (Chen et al. 2021) Efficiency Scalability (Chen et al. 2021; Wang 2015)	High temperature used (Chen et al. 2021) Air–water interfaces (protein denaturation) (Wang 2015) Modest yield in early work (pre-clinical) Use of solvents/surfactants (Angkawinitwong et al. 2015)	Exubera (2006)
Spray-freeze-drying	Quick freezing Highly porous particles Reduced drying times (Vishali et al. 2019)	Time and energy consuming Cost Air–water and ice–liquid interfaces (protein denaturation) (Ishwarya et al. 2015)	
Electrohydrodynamic techniques	High encapsulation efficiency (Batens et al. 2020) One-step process Ambient temperature and pressure (Etxabide et al. 2018) Low shear stress (Batens et al. 2020)	Exposure to organic solvents (Onyekuru et al. 2021; Focarete and Tampieri 2018)	Surgiclot (NCT02509208)
Emulsion approaches	Scalability (Angkawinitwong et al. 2015) Controlled release Protection from light, enzymatic degradation and oxidation (Iqbal et al. 2015)	Low encapsulation efficiencies Use of organic solvents Aqueous–organic interfaces (protein denaturation) Shear stress Sterilisation (Angkawinitwong et al. 2015) Emulsion stability (Iqbal et al. 2015)	Lupron Depot (1989) Bydureon (2012)
Microfluidics	Controlled mixing Reproducibility Low cost (Tomeh and Zhao 2020)	Production rate Scalability (Riahi et al. 2015)	

Table 2 Examples of marketed and late-stage clinical trial protein products and their route of administration

Product (API)	Indication	Clinical trial stage/year of authorisation	Route of administration
Remicade (infliximab)	Autoimmune diseases	1998	IV injection
Herceptin (trastuzumab)	Cancer	1998	IV infusion
Xolair (omalizumab)	Asthma	2003	Subcutaneous
Pegasys (PEG-INF-α-2a)	Hepatitis C	2002	Subcutaneous
Bydureon (exenatide)	Type 2 diabetes	2005	Subcutaneous
Zoladex (Goserelin acetate)	Breast and prostate cancer, endometriosis	1989	Subcutaneous
Zoma-Jet (somatropin)	Growth-hormone disorders in children	2018	Subcutaneous (jet injector)
Lupron Depot (leuprolide acetate)	Prostate cancer	1989	Intramuscular
mRNA (Covid-19) NCT05315362	Immunisation	Phase II Clinical trial	Transdermal (microneedles)
Adalimumab NCT03607903	Arthritis	Phase II Clinical trial	Transdermal (microneedles)
Insulin NCT00837512	Type I diabetes	Phase II Clinical trial	Transdermal (microneedles)
Abaloparatide NCT01674621	Osteoporosis	Phase III Clinical trial	Transdermal (microneedles)
Pulmozyme (Dornase alfa)	Cystic fibrosis	1993	Pulmonary
Exubera (insulin)	Type I and type II diabetes	2006	Pulmonary
Afrezza (insulin)	Diabetes	2014	Pulmonary
ChAdOx1 nCov-19 (NCT05007275)	Covid-19 immunisation	Stage I clinical trial	Pulmonary

administration allows for bolus injections or infusions; however, trained personnel are required for safe administration, which results in increased treatment costs (Ibeanu et al. 2020a). The invasive nature of parenteral delivery is considered one of the major drawbacks and may lead to infection, thus resulting in stricter formulation requirements and consequently further adding to costs (Shi and Li 2005; Antosova et al. 2009; Bajracharya et al. 2019; Long et al. 2020). Parenteral therapeutics must be sterile, free of pyrogen, and meet tonicity requirements (Shi and Li 2005; Akers et al. 2002). From the patient's perspective, injections are painful, and this can lead to poor treatment compliance (Antosova et al. 2009).

The use of finer needles (30G) for subcutaneous (SC) administration allows for self-administration and reduced pain upon injection (Ibeanu et al. 2020a). However, the injection volume is limited to 2 mL when given SC and this poses challenges when high doses are required for therapeutic efficacy (e.g. monoclonal antibodies) (Ibeanu et al. 2020a). Further, the bioavailability of therapeutics administered by this route is not well understood and varies between 30 and 100% (Ibeanu et al. 2020a). Neither IV and SC administration overcomes the very short half-lives of polypeptides in the blood stream, and thus require frequent dosing (Antosova et al. 2009). Sustained delivery systems favour patient adherence by reducing the injection frequency (Jorgensen et al. 2006).

Several formulation strategies have been developed to either extend the half-life of the therapeutic or prepare sustained delivery formulations releasing the therapeutic over a prolonged period and thereby reducing injection frequencies (Ibeanu et al. 2020a; Shi and Li 2005). Chemical modification of a polypeptide may increase its stability in the bloodstream (Antosova et al. 2009). One such approach is PEGylation, which refers to covalent conjugation of polyethylene glycol (PEG) to proteins (Shi and Li 2005; Jevševar et al. 2010). This results in reduced kidney filtration, proteolysis and phagocytosis, leading to an extended half-life (Shi and Li 2005). PEGylation is considered safe and is well established: the first PEGylated protein obtained FDA approval in 1990 (Jevševar et al. 2010). For example, PEGASYS consists of interferon α-2a (INF-α-2a) conjugated to a 40 kDa branched PEG moiety. It is indicated for the treatment of chronic hepatitis C (Rajender Reddy et al. 2002; EMA EMA Product Information n.d.). PEGASYS demonstrated therapeutic superiority over IFN-α-2a, particularly with regard to difficult to treat strains of the virus (Rajender Reddy et al. 2002; Drugs@FDA FDA-Approved Drugs n.d.). In addition to PEGylation, conjugation with recombinant albumin (e.g. IDELVION, FDA approval in 2016), an Fc fragment (e.g. ALPROLIX, FDA approval in 2014) or glycoPEGylation (e.g. REBINYN, FDA approval in 2017) has been successfully employed strategies for extension of recombinant factor IX half-life (Marchesini et al. 2021).

An alternative approach is the use of liposomes, small spherical vesicles which mainly consist of phospholipids, amphipathic compounds presenting both hydrophilic (head) and hydrophobic (tail) characteristics (Akbarzadeh et al. 2013). In an aqueous environment these lipids arrange themselves into a bilayer, thus forming a vesicle in which both interior and exterior are in contact with an aqueous environment (Abuwatfa et al. 2022). Liposomes have been extensively explored for cancer therapeutics, which led to the authorisation of Doxil – the first marketed liposome – in 1995 (Barenholz (Chezy) 2012). To date, two liposome-based vaccines, Epaxal and Inflexal (for hepatitis A and influenza respectively) have been approved (Bulbake et al. 2017; Kim and Jeong 2021). Both vaccines contain virus-derived protein (e.g. glycoprotein/ hemagglutinin) intercalated in the phospholipid bilayer and are therefore referred to as virosomes (Bulbake et al. 2017; Kim and Jeong 2021). Such particulate vaccines protect the antigens from enzymatic degradation and promote delivery of adjuvant/antigen to antigen presenting cells, thus promoting both a cellular and humoral immune response (Kim and Jeong 2021). The chemical composition and characteristics (e.g. size and surface charge) of liposomes influence their stability as well as their fate after administration (pharmacokinetics, biodistribution and cellular uptake). Liposomes are subjected to uptake by the

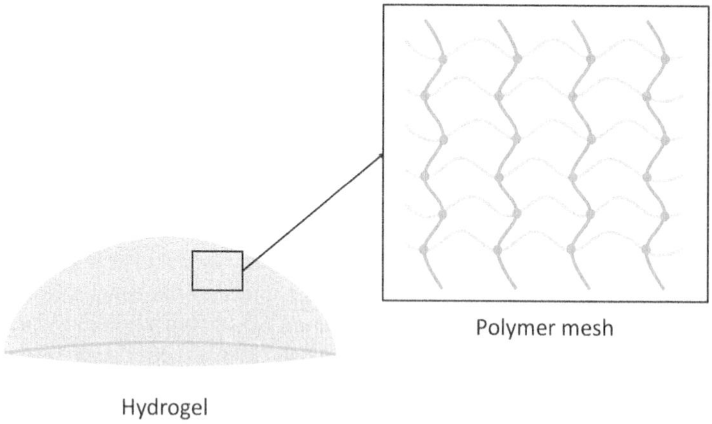

Fig. 5 Cross-linked hydrophilic polymer network forming a hydrogel

reticuloendothelial system and opsonisation, which may be overcome by incorporation of PEG. However, repeated administration of PEGylated liposomes may result in accelerated blood clearance via antibody formation against their components (Sercombe et al. 2015).

Cross-linked hydrophilic polymers forming a three-dimensional network are known as hydrogels (Fig. 5) (Li et al. 2021). The polymeric network presents pores permitting the hydrogel to retain a large amount of water, while remaining insoluble and maintaining its structure (Vermonden et al. 2012). These features make hydrogels highly suitable to accommodate high loads of peptides and proteins, creating a depot from which the therapeutic elutes (Hoare and Kohane 2008). By controlling the pore size via the density of cross-linkages, it is possible to tune the release of the active ingredient from the hydrogel matrix (Vermonden et al. 2012). Proteins generally present limited mobility within the hydrogel, which may be advantageous for maintaining their structure (Hoare and Kohane 2008). Vantas (FDA approved in 2004 for advanced prostate cancer, 50 μg/day (Food and Drug Administration Vantas Approval n.d.)) and Supprelin LA (FDA approved in 2007 for children with precocious puberty, 65 μg/day) are both implantable hydrogels delivering histrelin, a luteinising hormone-releasing hormone agonist, over 12 months.

Nano- and microparticle carriers have been extensively investigated for the sustained delivery of protein therapeutics. Many of the approved sustained-release formulations are parenterally administered polymeric microspheres (Shi and Li 2005). For example, Lupron Depot is indicated for the treatment of prostate cancer and endometriosis (Food and Drug Administration Lupron Depot Approval n.d.). The product contains leuprolide acetate loaded microspheres achieving a sustained release of the therapeutic over up to 6 months. The monthly injections contain PLGA microspheres whereas the microspheres administered every 3–6 months are PLA based (Drugs@FDA FDA-Approved Drugs n.d.).

The use of long-term release implants may be preferential if prolonged and localised drug release is required, too. An interesting example of this delivery route is Zoladex, a marketed implant containing goserelin acetate for the treatment of prostate cancer and endometriosis. Goserelin is dispersed in a matrix of PLGA through hot-melt extrusion (HME), permitting a continuous release of the therapeutic over a 12-week period (Drugs@FDA FDA-Approved Drugs n.d.). In HME, materials are melted by employing elevated temperature and high pressure. The melt subsequently passes through the extruder where mixing, grinding and particle reduction may take place before the blend is extruded through an orifice and moulded into the desired shape (Patil et al. 2016; Zheng and Pokorski 2021). This is an unusual example however, since the high process temperatures and the shear stress occurring during HME generally exclude it as a processing technique for proteins (Zheng and Pokorski 2021).

3.2 Transdermal Delivery Route

Transdermal drug delivery describes the non-invasive delivery of therapeutics through the epidermal layers of the skin, typically with the aim of the active ingredient entering the systemic circulation (Long et al. 2020). Compared to oral or parenteral administration, transdermal delivery presents advantages such as avoidance of first pass metabolism, and reductions in the pain, trauma and infection risk associated with injections (Long et al. 2020; Prausnitz and Langer 2008).

The greatest challenge of transdermal delivery is achieving drug permeation through the stratum corneum (Kirkby et al. 2020; Prausnitz and Langer 2008; Sabbagh and Kim 2022). The skin is composed of different layers, namely the epidermis, the dermis and the subcutaneous tissue. The epidermis is comprised of five anatomical layers, the outermost layer of which is the stratum corneum (Sabbagh and Kim 2022). The stratum corneum (10–15 μm thick) is composed of corneocytes embedded in a lipid domain which is mainly made up of ceramides. It is this highly hydrophobic layer that provides an excellent barrier to external substances and prevents penetration into deeper layers (Jeong et al. 2021; Kim et al. 2012). There are three different routes for passive diffusion through the skin layers – transcellular, intercellular and trans-appendageal. The intercellular route is generally the main pathway but is limited to small lipophilic drugs, given the lipophilic nature of the stratum corneum (Mathias and Hussain 2010; Benson 2006). The low penetration rate results in low dose delivery (<10 mg) and thus often limits this route to potent drugs (Kirkby et al. 2020; Mathias and Hussain 2010; Naik et al. 2000; Prausnitz 2004).

Several strategies have been developed to overcome the skin barrier and enable delivery of a wider range of therapeutics (Prausnitz and Langer 2008; Naik et al. 2000). The aim is to reversibly disrupt the stratum corneum, permitting a temporary increase in permeability (Long et al. 2020; Prausnitz and Langer 2008), while ensuring the disruption remains localised so to avoid deep tissue injury (Prausnitz and Langer 2008). Simple approaches involve formulation adaptation or drug derivatisation to obtain more lipophilic compounds. However, for highly hydrophilic molecules such as peptides and proteins more sophisticated strategies are generally required (Naik et al. 2000). Strategies facilitating transdermal delivery of macromolecules include penetration enhancers, micro/nanocarriers, microneedles, ultrasound, electroporation/iontophoresis, jet injection, thermal ablation/ microdermabrasion and ionic liquids. These have been reviewed in detail in a number of publications (Long et al. 2020; Prausnitz and Langer 2008).

Transdermal delivery of molecules enabled by physiologically acceptable electrical current (< 1.0 mA/cm^2) is known as iontophoresis (Kalia et al. 2004; Alkilani et al. 2015). The current is generated by application of a small electrical potential (<15 V) (Long et al. 2020; Kalia et al. 2004). Iontophoresis enables the transport of ionised molecules via electromigration and electroosmosis and thereby enhances their skin permeability (Long et al. 2020; Kalia et al. 2004). The amount of drug delivered may be controlled by adapting the applied current, the duration of the application and the skin surface area (Kalia et al. 2004). The first FDA-approved iontophoretic patch (LidoSite) was commercialised in 2004, delivering lidocaine for dermal anaesthesia (Alkilani et al. 2015). The delivery of peptides and small proteins (e.g. insulin, calcitonin, human parathyroid hormone, and octreotide amongst others) by iontophoresis has been assessed in numerous pre-clinical studies, and a clinical trial (NCT05444842, comparing topical insulin with insulin iontophoresis in patients with chronic diabetic foot ulcer) is expected to produce first results by the end of 2022 (Clinical Trials.Gov n.d.). It should be mentioned, however, that in ulcers the natural skin barrier is impaired, therefore facilitating drug penetration.

It is also important to state that the choice of an appropriate animal model for in vivo pre-clinical studies is paramount to allow correlation with humans. In the context of transdermal delivery, the use of rodents often results in an overestimation of permeation as the skin of these animals is abundant in hair follicles.

Jet injectors provide a needle-free alternative to injections and directly deliver liquid therapeutics to the viable epidermis and dermis using high-pressure devices (Long et al. 2020; de Wit et al. 2015). The liquid is administered at high speed (60–140 m/s), piercing a micro hole in the skin (Long et al. 2020). The liquid diffuses through the hole to a larger area of the surrounding tissue (compared with injections) (Long et al. 2020; de Wit et al. 2015; Baxter and Mitragotri 2006). Jet injectors have been extensively used since 1955, especially for vaccination against poliomyelitis, influenza and chickenpox amongst others (Baxter and Mitragotri 2006). Jet injectors are FDA-approved and clinically available for the delivery of somatropin (Tjet; used in growth-hormone deficiency) and insulin (Long et al. 2020; Alkilani et al. 2015). A clinical trial (NCT01947556) demonstrated that the use of a jet injector to administer insulin resulted in improved pharmacokinetics by increasing the rate of absorption, giving higher peak insulin levels compared with a conventional insulin pen. The ease of use, administration discomfort and safety (measured in hypoglycaemic events) of the jet injector were comparable to the conventional insulin pen (de Wit et al. 2015).

Microneedles consist of an array of multiple micro-projections (25 to 900 μm) assembled on a supporting base, allowing painless penetration of the stratum corneum while dramatically increasing the transdermal delivery of therapeutics (Kirkby et al. 2020; Long et al. 2020). Microneedles penetrate the stratum corneum and are inserted into the epidermis, sometimes even reaching the superficial dermis, forming micro-channels through which the active ingredient can penetrate (Long et al. 2020; Prausnitz 2004). Human studies have confirmed their application to be painless (Prausnitz 2004). Furthermore, compared to parenteral injections they are less likely to cause any bleeding or infections due to their small size (Long et al. 2020).

The majority of clinical research into microneedles is focused on vaccines, which has led to the FDA approval of Fluzone. Fluzone is marketed as an intradermal influenza vaccine and gained FDA authorisation in 2011 (Bragazzi et al. 2016). Intradermal vaccination has shown to lead to a greater immune response in clinical studies compared to intramuscular injections (Arnou et al. 2009; Kim et al. 2009). An example of FDA-approved hollow microneedle system is MicronJet 600, which holds three needles of 600 μm length allowing the delivery of therapeutics in liquid form (Bhatnagar et al. 2017). The system is being employed for the administration of different therapeutics (e.g. insulin, polio vaccine) in clinical studies (phase 1 to 3) (Clinical Trials.Gov n.d.).

3.3 Pulmonary Route

The delivery of drugs via the lungs has long been employed, particularly for the treatment of pulmonary conditions such as asthma or congestive obstructive pulmonary disease (COPD), but is increasingly investigated for non-invasive systemic delivery of therapeutic agents including proteins and peptides (Mathias and Hussain 2010; Uchenna Agu et al. 2001).

The respiratory tract is characterised by extensive bifurcation and generally divided into conducting regions (e.g. nasal cavity, bronchi and bronchiole) and respiratory regions (e.g. distal bronchioles and alveoli) (Uchenna Agu et al. 2001). The lungs provide not only a large surface area of approximately 75 m^2 but also a very thin alveolar epithelium (0.1 to 0.5 μm thick), providing a permeable interface with the systemic circulation and thereby allowing for rapid absorption (Bajracharya et al. 2019; Uchenna Agu et al. 2001; Angelo et al. 2009; Heida et al. 2022). Furthermore, the lungs are well perfused and thus pulmonary delivery generally results in rapid absorption of both small molecules and macromolecules (Mathias and Hussain 2010). The permeability to macromolecules makes the pulmonary route one of the most optimal routes for the uptake of biopharmaceuticals, while also being non-invasive and painless (Kirkby et al. 2020; Heida et al. 2022; Liang et al. 2020a).

Despite these advantages, there remain several barriers to effective pulmonary delivery (Bajracharya et al. 2019; Mathias and Hussain 2010; Liang et al. 2020a). One is the muco-ciliary, an important defence mechanism trapping inhaled substances – amongst those aerosolised therapeutics – in the mucus and clearing them (Houtmeyers et al. 1999). The mucus (1–10 μm) lining the lungs and the surfactant around the alveoli (0.1 to 0.2 μm) present physical barriers to pulmonary absorption of peptides and proteins (Uchenna Agu et al. 2001). Finally, degradation by proteases and peptidases or uptake by macrophages might occur, limiting the therapeutic effect (Uchenna Agu et al. 2001; Liang et al. 2020a).

For pulmonary delivery, a formulation must be aerosolised into droplets or particles of appropriate aerodynamic characteristics (Uchenna Agu et al. 2001). An inhaled therapeutic should present a narrow particle size distribution with a mass median aerodynamic diameter (MMAD) between 1 and 5 μm to obtain good distribution throughout the lungs. The first inhaled protein formulation – Exubera (insulin) – was approved in 2006 but later withdrawn due to poor sales (Al-Tabakha 2015). Various factors may have contributed to the poor sales such as the cumbersome delivery device (Al-Tabakha 2015) and challenges in determining the administered dose (Al-Tabakha 2015). The decision to discontinue Exubera resulted in most companies terminating the development of their inhaled insulin products (Al-Tabakha 2015). However, the concept of inhaled therapies for delivery of biologics was not abandoned, with ongoing clinical trials exploring administration of antibodies (e.g. anti-IL-13 – NCT02473939), interferon (e.g. Interferon-β1a – NCT03570359), interleukins (e.g. IL-2 – NCT01590069) and sialidase fusion protein (NCT01924793) (Liang et al. 2020b).

3.4 Oral Drug Delivery

Oral administration has the advantages of high patient compliance and allowing self-administration, and thus is typically preferred (Bajracharya et al. 2019). However, oral administration of biologics results in low systemic bioavailability (<1%) (Nie et al. 2021; Moreira et al. 2021). This is, on the one hand, caused by the considerable peptidase and protease activity in the gastrointestinal (GI) tract, which is the most efficient body compartment for peptide and protein metabolism (Crommelin and Sindelar 2008). Additionally, the hydrophilic nature of polypeptides as well as their high molecular weight and the presence of ionisable groups makes absorption through the intestinal epithelium challenging (Nie et al. 2021; Moreira et al. 2021).

Another great challenge for developing polypeptide therapeutics is their fast degradation and clearance. Once in the blood stream, most display short half-lives (minutes to hours) (Crommelin and Sindelar 2008; Ibeanu et al. 2020b). This is attributed to rapid renal clearance, with the kidney glomeruli having a pore size of about 8 nm and allowing the passage of peptides and many therapeutic proteins (up to the renal threshold (~60 kDa)) (Shah 2015; Zaman et al. 2019). Moreover, these agents are also susceptible to being cleared by enzymatic activity, immune cells, or eliminated by the liver (Crommelin and Sindelar 2008; Zaman et al. 2019). As a consequence, frequent administration and higher doses are typically required to maintain therapeutic concentration (Zaman et al. 2019).

Approaches to overcome these limitations include increasing drug absorption across the intestinal membrane with permeation enhancers as well as increasing stability and half-life by conjugation to a polymer (e.g. PEG) or encapsulation into polymeric particles (Antosova et al. 2009). The most successful strategy to date is the use of permeation enhancers, and two distinct formulations employing this have obtained FDA approval (Brayden and Maher 2021). Oral octreotide capsules, licensed for acromegaly treatment, contain a combination of lipophilic (polysorbate-80, glyceryl monocaprylate, glyceryl tricaprylate and glyceryl monooleate) and hydrophilic (polyvinylpyrrolidone and sodium caprylate) excipients, creating an oily suspension which transiently opens epithelial tight junctions and allows the passage of hydrophilic molecules (<10 kDa) (Brayden and Maher 2021).

Rybelsus (semaglutide) was formulated with the proprietary salcaprozate sodium (SNAC) absorption enhancers facilitating absorption across the gastric epithelia (Lewis et al. 2022; Twarog et al. 2019) and was approved by the FDA in 2019 for the treatment of diabetes. Orally administered semaglutide matches bioavailability achieved in the injectable version of the same drug, but only if administered in a fasted state. As a result, Rybelsus administration requires no food intake 1 h before and 2 h after administration, and with no more than 120 mL liquid (Food and Drug Administration Rybelsus Approval n.d.), which may potentially affect treatment adherence and patient acceptability. In pharmacokinetic studies, maximum plasma concentration was achieved 1 h post administration; however, between-subject absorption variability remains high (Berg et al. 2022).

4 Conclusions and Future Outlook

The increasing importance of proteins and peptides in modern medicine will inevitably shift the field of pharmaceutical formulation towards more innovative solutions and advanced drug delivery platforms. With biologics being considered for a wider range of therapeutic indications, such as GLP-1 peptides now routinely prescribed for obesity treatment, there is a significant commercial incentive for developing patient-friendly and affordable delivery platforms of such agents. Undoubtedly, the approval of the first oral peptide tablet in 2019 was a major advancement in the field of biomolecule drug delivery, but further formulation developments are required to increase patient acceptability and ease of administration, even in the case of orally delivered formulations.

The last 20 years have seen major progress in protein drug delivery, but the impact on patient outcomes has been relatively low so far. The existing protein formulation techniques implemented by industry suffer from multiple disadvantages, and the academic research into emerging technologies such as EHD processes or spray freeze-drying often does not reach the pre-clinical testing stage. This is likely to change in the future as major pharmaceutical companies become more open to investing in and implementing innovative solutions in their formulation development pathways. The next decade is therefore likely to see the maturation of emerging technologies towards clinical trials, as well as further enhancements of existing formulations to improve therapeutic efficacy and user experience.

References

Abuwatfa WH, Awad NS, Pitt WG, Husseini GA (2022) Thermosensitive polymers and thermo-responsive liposomal drug delivery systems. Polymers (Basel) 14:925. https://doi.org/10.3390/polym14050925

Akbarzadeh A, Rezaei-Sadabady R, Davaran S, Joo SW, Zarghami N, Hanifehpour Y, Samiei M, Kouhi M, Nejati-Koshki K (2013) Liposome: classification, preparation, and applications. Nanoscale Res Lett 8:102. https://doi.org/10.1186/1556-276X-8-102

Akers MJ, Vasudevan V, Stickelmeyer M (2002) Formulation development of protein dosage forms. In: Development and manufacture of protein pharmaceuticals. pp 47–127

Alkilani A, McCrudden MT, Donnelly R (2015) Transdermal drug delivery: innovative pharmaceutical developments based on disruption of the barrier properties of the stratum corneum. Pharmaceutics 7:438–470. https://doi.org/10.3390/pharmaceutics7040438

Al-Tabakha MM (2015) Future prospect of insulin inhalation for diabetic patients: the case of Afrezza versus Exubera. J Control Release 215:25–38. https://doi.org/10.1016/j.jconrel.2015.07.025

Angelo R, Rousseau K, Grant M, Leone-Bay A, Richardson P (2009) Technosphere® insulin: defining the role of technosphere particles at the cellular level. J Diabetes Sci Technol 3:545–554. https://doi.org/10.1177/193229680900300320

Angkawinitwong U, Sharma G, Khaw PT, Brocchini S, Williams GR (2015) Solid-state protein formulations. Ther Deliv 6:59–82. https://doi.org/10.4155/tde.14.98

Angkawinitwong U, Awwad S, Khaw PT, Brocchini S, Williams GR (2017) Electrospun formulations of bevacizumab for sustained release in the eye. Acta Biomater 64:126–136. https://doi.org/10.1016/j.actbio.2017.10.015

Antosova Z, Mackova M, Kral V, Macek T (2009) Therapeutic application of peptides and proteins: parenteral forever? Trends Biotechnol 27:628–635. https://doi.org/10.1016/j.tibtech.2009.07.009

Arnou R, Icardi G, De Decker M, Ambrozaitis A, Kazek M-P, Weber F, Van Damme P (2009) Intradermal influenza vaccine for older adults: a randomized controlled multicenter phase III study. Vaccine 27:7304–7312. https://doi.org/10.1016/j.vaccine.2009.10.033

Arpagaus C (2018) Pharmaceutical particle engineering via Nano spray drying – process parameters and application examples on the laboratory-scale. Int J Med Nano Res 5. https://doi.org/10.23937/2378-3664.1410026

Bajracharya R, Song JG, Back SY, Han H-K (2019) Recent advancements in non-invasive formulations for protein drug delivery. Comput Struct Biotechnol J 17:1290–1308. https://doi.org/10.1016/j.csbj.2019.09.004

Barenholz (Chezy) Y (2012) Doxil® – the first FDA-approved nano-drug: lessons learned. J Control Release 160:117–134. https://doi.org/10.1016/j.jconrel.2012.03.020

Batens M, Dewaele L, Massant J, Teodorescu B, Clasen C, Van den Mooter G (2020) Feasibility of electrospraying fully aqueous bovine serum albumin solutions. Eur J Pharm Biopharm 147: 102–110. https://doi.org/10.1016/j.ejpb.2019.12.011

Baxter J, Mitragotri S (2006) Needle-free liquid jet injections: mechanisms and applications. Expert Rev Med Devices 3:565–574. https://doi.org/10.1586/17434440.3.5.565

Bazban-Shotorbani S, Dashtimoghadam E, Karkhaneh A, Hasani-Sadrabadi MM, Jacob KI (2016) Microfluidic directed synthesis of alginate nanogels with tunable pore size for efficient protein delivery. Langmuir 32:4996–5003. https://doi.org/10.1021/acs.langmuir.5b04645

Benson HA (2006) Transfersomes for transdermal drug delivery. Expert Opin Drug Deliv 3:727–737. https://doi.org/10.1517/17425247.3.6.727

Berg S, Edlund H, Goundry WRF, Bergström CAS, Davies NM (2022) Considerations in the developability of peptides for oral administration when formulated together with transient permeation enhancers. Int J Pharm 628:122238. https://doi.org/10.1016/j.ijpharm.2022.122238

Bhatnagar S, Dave K, Venuganti VVK (2017) Microneedles in the clinic. J Control Release 260: 164–182. https://doi.org/10.1016/j.jconrel.2017.05.029

Bragazzi NL, Orsi A, Ansaldi F, Gasparini R, Icardi G (2016) Fluzone® intra-dermal (Intanza®/Istivac® Intra-dermal): An updated overview. Hum Vaccin Immunother 12:2616–2627. https://doi.org/10.1080/21645515.2016.1187343

Brayden DJ, Maher S (2021) Transient permeation enhancer® (TPE®) technology for oral delivery of octreotide: a technological evaluation. Expert Opin Drug Deliv 18:1501–1512. https://doi.org/10.1080/17425247.2021.1942838

Briggs T, Arinzeh TL (2014) Examining the formulation of emulsion electrospinning for improving the release of bioactive proteins from electrospun fibers. J Biomed Mater Res A 102:674–684. https://doi.org/10.1002/jbm.a.34730

Bulbake U, Doppalapudi S, Kommineni N, Khan W (2017) Liposomal formulations in clinical use: an updated review. Pharmaceutics 9:12. https://doi.org/10.3390/pharmaceutics9020012

Chen P, Sun Y, Zhu Z, Wang R, Shi X, Lin C, Ye Y (2010) A controlled release system of superoxide dismutase by electrospun fiber and its antioxidant activity in vitro. J Mater Sci Mater Med 21:609–614. https://doi.org/10.1007/s10856-009-3927-6

Chen Y, Mutukuri TT, Wilson NE, Zhou (Tony) Q (2021) Pharmaceutical protein solids: drying technology, solid-state characterization and stability. Adv Drug Deliv Rev 172:211–233. https://doi.org/10.1016/j.addr.2021.02.016

Chiesa E, Greco A, Riva F, Dorati R, Conti B, Modena T, Genta I (2021) Hyaluronic acid-based nanoparticles for protein delivery: systematic examination of microfluidic production conditions. Pharmaceutics 13:1565. https://doi.org/10.3390/pharmaceutics13101565

Clinical Trials.Gov (n.d.). https://clinicaltrials.gov/

Costantino HR, Firouzabadian L, Wu C, Carrasquillo KG, Griebenow K, Zale SE, Tracy MA (2002) Protein spray freeze drying. 2. Effect of formulation variables on particle size and stability. J Pharm Sci 91:388–395. https://doi.org/10.1002/jps.10059

Crommelin DJA, Sindelar RD (2008) Pharmaceutical biotechnology: fundamentals and applications. CRC Press

de Wit HM, Engwerda EEC, Tack CJ, de Galan BE (2015) Insulin administered by needle-free jet injection corrects marked hyperglycaemia faster in overweight or obese patients with diabetes. Diabetes Obes Metab 17:1093–1099. https://doi.org/10.1111/dom.12550

Domján J, Vass P, Hirsch E, Szabó E, Pantea E, Andersen SK, Vigh T, Verreck G, Marosi G, Nagy ZK (2020) Monoclonal antibody formulation manufactured by high-speed electrospinning. Int J Pharm 591:120042. https://doi.org/10.1016/j.ijpharm.2020.120042

Drugs@FDA FDA-Approved Drugs (n.d.). https://www.accessdata.fda.gov/scripts/cder/daf/index.cfm

EMA EMA Product Information (n.d.). https://www.ema.europa.eu/en/glossary/product-information

Emami F, Vatanara A, Park EJ, Na DH (2018) Drying technologies for the stability and bioavailability of biopharmaceuticals. Pharmaceutics 10

Etxabide A, Garrido T, Uranga J, Guerrero P, de la Caba K (2018) Extraction and incorporation of bioactives into protein formulations for food and biomedical applications. Int J Biol Macromol 120:2094–2105. https://doi.org/10.1016/j.ijbiomac.2018.09.030

Focarete ML, Tampieri A (2018) Core-shell nanostructures for drug delivery and theranostics: challenges, strategies, and prospects for novel carrier systems, 1st edn. Woodhead Publishing, Duxford

Food and Drug Administration Lupron Depot Approval (n.d.) In: https://www.accessdata.fda.gov/drugsatfda_docs/nda/98/019732s012_lupron.cfm

Food and Drug Administration Rybelsus Approval (n.d.). https://www.accessdata.fda.gov/drugsatfda_docs/nda/2019/213051Orig1s000TOC.cfm

Food and Drug Administration Vantas Approval (n.d.) In: https://www.accessdata.fda.gov/drugsatfda_docs/nda/2004/021732s000_VantasTOC.cfm

Geraldes DC, Beraldo-de-Araújo VL, Pardo BOP, Pessoa Junior A, Stephano MA, de Oliveira-Nascimento L (2020) Protein drug delivery: current dosage form profile and formulation strategies. J Drug Target 28:339–355. https://doi.org/10.1080/1061186X.2019.1669043

Gervasi V, Dall Agnol R, Cullen S, McCoy T, Vucen S, Crean A (2018) Parenteral protein formulations: an overview of approved products within the European Union. Eur J Pharm Biopharm 131:8–24. https://doi.org/10.1016/j.ejpb.2018.07.011

Godakanda VU, Dziemidowicz K, de Silva RM, de Silva KMN, Williams GR (2022) Electrospun fibers in drug delivery. In: Vaseashta A, Bölgen N (eds) Electrospun nanofibers: principles, technology and novel applications. Springer, Cham, pp 159–181

Gomez A, Bingham D, de Juan L, Tang K (1998) Production of protein nanoparticles by electrospray drying. J Aerosol Sci 29:561–574. https://doi.org/10.1016/S0021-8502(97)10031-3

Heida R, Hinrichs WL, Frijlink HW (2022) Inhaled vaccine delivery in the combat against respiratory viruses: a 2021 overview of recent developments and implications for COVID-19. Expert Rev Vaccines 21:957–974. https://doi.org/10.1080/14760584.2021.1903878

Hoare TR, Kohane DS (2008) Hydrogels in drug delivery: progress and challenges. Polymer (Guildf) 49:1993–2007. https://doi.org/10.1016/j.polymer.2008.01.027

Houtmeyers E, Gosselink R, Gayan-Ramirez G, Decramer M (1999) Regulation of mucociliary clearance in health and disease. Eur Respir J 13:1177. https://doi.org/10.1034/j.1399-3003.1999.13e39.x

Ibeanu N, Egbu R, Onyekuru L, Javaheri H, Tee Khaw P, Williams GR, Brocchini S, Awwad S (2020a) Injectables and depots to prolong drug action of proteins and peptides. Pharmaceutics 12:999. https://doi.org/10.3390/pharmaceutics12100999

Ibeanu N, Egbu R, Onyekuru L, Javaheri H, Khaw PT, Williams GR, Brocchini S, Awwad S (2020b) Injectables and depots to prolong drug action of proteins and peptides. Pharmaceutics 12:1–42

Iqbal M, Zafar N, Fessi H, Elaissari A (2015) Double emulsion solvent evaporation techniques used for drug encapsulation. Int J Pharm 496:173–190. https://doi.org/10.1016/j.ijpharm.2015.10.057

Ishwarya SP, Anandharamakrishnan C, Stapley AGF (2015) Spray-freeze-drying: a novel process for the drying of foods and bioproducts. Trends Food Sci Technol 41:161–181. https://doi.org/10.1016/j.tifs.2014.10.008

Jeong WY, Kwon M, Choi HE, Kim KS (2021) Recent advances in transdermal drug delivery systems: a review. Biomater Res 25:24. https://doi.org/10.1186/s40824-021-00226-6

Jevševar S, Kunstelj M, Porekar VG (2010) PEGylation of therapeutic proteins. Biotechnol J 5: 113–128. https://doi.org/10.1002/biot.200900218

Jorgensen L, Moeller EH, van de Weert M, Nielsen HM, Frokjaer S (2006) Preparing and evaluating delivery systems for proteins. Eur J Pharm Sci 29:174–182. https://doi.org/10.1016/j.ejps.2006.05.008

Kakran M, Antipina MN (2014) Emulsion-based techniques for encapsulation in biomedicine, food and personal care. Curr Opin Pharmacol 18:47–55. https://doi.org/10.1016/j.coph.2014.09.003

Kalia YN, Naik A, Garrison J, Guy RH (2004) Iontophoretic drug delivery. Adv Drug Deliv Rev 56:619–658. https://doi.org/10.1016/j.addr.2003.10.026

Kim E-M, Jeong H-J (2021) Liposomes: biomedical applications. Chonnam Med J 57:27. https://doi.org/10.4068/cmj.2021.57.1.27

Kim Y-C, Quan F-S, Yoo D-G, Compans RW, Kang S-M, Prausnitz MR (2009) Improved influenza vaccination in the skin using vaccine coated microneedles. Vaccine 27:6932–6938. https://doi.org/10.1016/j.vaccine.2009.08.108

Kim Y-C, Park J-H, Prausnitz MR (2012) Microneedles for drug and vaccine delivery. Adv Drug Deliv Rev 64:1547–1568. https://doi.org/10.1016/j.addr.2012.04.005

Kirkby M, Hutton ARJ, Donnelly RF (2020) Microneedle mediated transdermal delivery of protein, peptide and antibody based therapeutics: current status and future considerations. Pharm Res 37: 117. https://doi.org/10.1007/s11095-020-02844-6

Lancina MG, Shankar RK, Yang H (2017) Chitosan nanofibers for transbuccal insulin delivery. J Biomed Mater Res A 105:1252–1259. https://doi.org/10.1002/jbm.a.35984

Lee D-S, Kang DW, Choi G-W, Choi H-G, Cho H-Y (2020) Development of level A in vitro–vivo correlation for electrosprayed microspheres containing leuprolide: physicochemical, pharmacokinetic, and pharmacodynamic evaluation. Pharmaceutics 12:36. https://doi.org/10.3390/pharmaceutics12010036

Lewis AL, McEntee N, Holland J, Patel A (2022) Development and approval of rybelsus (oral semaglutide): ushering in a new era in peptide delivery. Drug Deliv Transl Res 12:1–6. https://doi.org/10.1007/s13346-021-01000-w

Li X, Su Y, Liu S, Tan L, Mo X, Ramakrishna S (2010) Encapsulation of proteins in poly(l-lactide-co-caprolactone) fibers by emulsion electrospinning. Colloids Surf B Biointerfaces 75:418–424. https://doi.org/10.1016/j.colsurfb.2009.09.014

Li Y, Yang HY, Lee DS (2021) Advances in biodegradable and injectable hydrogels for biomedical applications. J Control Release 330:151–160. https://doi.org/10.1016/j.jconrel.2020.12.008

Liang W, Pan HW, Vllasaliu D, Lam JKW (2020a) Pulmonary delivery of biological drugs. Pharmaceutics 12:1025. https://doi.org/10.3390/pharmaceutics12111025

Liang W, Pan HW, Vllasaliu D, Lam JKW (2020b) Pulmonary delivery of biological drugs. Pharmaceutics 12:1–28

Long L, Zhang J, Yang Z, Guo Y, Hu X, Wang Y (2020) Transdermal delivery of peptide and protein drugs: strategies, advantages and disadvantages. J Drug Deliv Sci Technol 60:102007. https://doi.org/10.1016/j.jddst.2020.102007

Makadia HK, Siegel SJ (2011) Poly lactic-co-glycolic acid (PLGA) as biodegradable controlled drug delivery carrier. Polymers (Basel) 3:1377–1397. https://doi.org/10.3390/polym3031377

Marchesini E, Morfini M, Valentino L (2021) Recent advances in the treatment of hemophilia: a review. Biologics 15:221–235

Mathias NR, Hussain MA (2010) Non-invasive systemic drug delivery: developability considerations for alternate routes of administration. J Pharm Sci 99:1–20. https://doi.org/10.1002/jps.21793

McKeage K (2015) Raplixa™: a review in improving surgical haemostasis. Clin Drug Investig 35:519–524. https://doi.org/10.1007/s40261-015-0307-5

Moreira A, Lawson D, Onyekuru L, Dziemidowicz K, Angkawinitwong U, Costa PF, Radacsi N, Williams GR (2021) Protein encapsulation by electrospinning and electrospraying. J Control Release 329:1172–1197. https://doi.org/10.1016/j.jconrel.2020.10.046

Mu X, Agostinacchio F, Xiang N, Pei Y, Khan Y, Guo C, Cebe P, Motta A, Kaplan DL (2021) Recent advances in 3D printing with protein-based inks. Prog Polym Sci 115:101375. https://doi.org/10.1016/j.progpolymsci.2021.101375

Muralidhara BK, Wong M (2020) Critical considerations in the formulation development of parenteral biologic drugs. Drug Discov Today 25:574–581. https://doi.org/10.1016/j.drudis.2019.12.011

Naik A, Kalia YN, Guy RH (2000) Transdermal drug delivery: overcoming the skin's barrier function. Pharm Sci Technol Today 3:318–326. https://doi.org/10.1016/S1461-5347(00)00295-9

Nie T, Wang W, Liu X, Wang Y, Li K, Song X, Zhang J, Yu L, He Z (2021) Sustained release systems for delivery of therapeutic peptide/protein. Biomacromolecules 22:2299–2324. https://doi.org/10.1021/acs.biomac.1c00160

Onyekuru LC, Moreira A, Zhang J, Angkawinitwong U, Costa PF, Brocchini S, Williams GR (2021) An investigation of alkaline phosphatase enzymatic activity after electrospinning and electrospraying. J Drug Deliv Sci Technol 64:102592. https://doi.org/10.1016/j.jddst.2021.102592

Park H, Otte A, Park K (2022) Evolution of drug delivery systems: from 1950 to 2020 and beyond. J Control Release 342:53–65. https://doi.org/10.1016/j.jconrel.2021.12.030

Patil H, Tiwari RV, Repka MA (2016) Hot-melt extrusion: from theory to application in pharmaceutical formulation. AAPS PharmSciTech 17:20–42. https://doi.org/10.1208/s12249-015-0360-7

Pessi J, Santos HA, Miroshnyk I, Yliruusi J, Weitz DA, Mirza S (2014) Microfluidics-assisted engineering of polymeric microcapsules with high encapsulation efficiency for protein drug delivery. Int J Pharm 472:82–87. https://doi.org/10.1016/j.ijpharm.2014.06.012

Poursina N, Vatanara A, Rouini MR, Gilani K, Rouholamini Najafabadi A (2017) Systemic delivery of parathyroid hormone (1–34) using spray freeze-dried inhalable particles. Pharm Dev Technol 22:733–739. https://doi.org/10.3109/10837450.2015.1125924

Prausnitz MR (2004) Microneedles for transdermal drug delivery. Adv Drug Deliv Rev 56:581–587. https://doi.org/10.1016/j.addr.2003.10.023

Prausnitz MR, Langer R (2008) Transdermal drug delivery. Nat Biotechnol 26:1261–1268. https://doi.org/10.1038/nbt.1504

Rabiee M, Namaei Ghasemnia N, Rabiee N, Bagherzadeh M (2021) Microfluidic devices and drug delivery systems. In: Biomedical applications of microfluidic devices, Elsevier, pp 153–186

Rajender Reddy K, Modi MW, Pedder S (2002) Use of peginterferon alfa-2a (40 KD) (Pegasys®) for the treatment of hepatitis C. Adv Drug Deliv Rev 54:571–586. https://doi.org/10.1016/S0169-409X(02)00028-5

Riahi R, Tamayol A, Shaegh SAM, Ghaemmaghami AM, Dokmeci MR, Khademhosseini A (2015) Microfluidics for advanced drug delivery systems. Curr Opin Chem Eng 7:101–112. https://doi.org/10.1016/j.coche.2014.12.001

Sabbagh F, Kim BS (2022) Recent advances in polymeric transdermal drug delivery systems. J Control Release 341:132–146. https://doi.org/10.1016/j.jconrel.2021.11.025

Sercombe L, Veerati T, Moheimani F, Wu SY, Sood AK, Hua S (2015) Advances and challenges of liposome assisted drug delivery. Front Pharmacol 6

Shah DK (2015) Pharmacokinetic and pharmacodynamic considerations for the next generation protein therapeutics. J Pharmacokinet Pharmacodyn 42:553–571. https://doi.org/10.1007/s10928-015-9447-8

Shi Y, Li L (2005) Current advances in sustained-release systems for parenteral drug delivery. Expert Opin Drug Deliv 2:1039–1058. https://doi.org/10.1517/17425247.2.6.1039

Taylor KMG, Aulton ME (2022) Aulton's pharmaceutics – the design and manufacture of medicines, 6th edn. Elsevier

Tomeh MA, Zhao X (2020) Recent advances in microfluidics for the preparation of drug and gene delivery systems. Mol Pharm 17:4421–4434. https://doi.org/10.1021/acs.molpharmaceut.0c00913

Twarog C, Fattah S, Heade J, Maher S, Fattal E, Brayden DJ (2019) Intestinal permeation enhancers for oral delivery of macromolecules: a comparison between salcaprozate sodium (SNAC) and sodium caprate (c10). Pharmaceutics 11

Tyler B, Gullotti D, Mangraviti A, Utsuki T, Brem H (2016) Polylactic acid (PLA) controlled delivery carriers for biomedical applications. Adv Drug Deliv Rev 107:163–175. https://doi.org/10.1016/j.addr.2016.06.018

Uchenna Agu R, Ikechukwu Ugwoke M, Armand M (2001) The lung as a route for systemic delivery of therapeutic proteins and peptides. Respir Res 2. https://doi.org/10.1186/rr58

Vermonden T, Censi R, Hennink WE (2012) Hydrogels for protein delivery. Chem Rev 112:2853–2888. https://doi.org/10.1021/cr200157d

Vishali DA, Monisha J, Sivakamasundari SK, Moses JA, Anandharamakrishnan C (2019) Spray freeze drying: emerging applications in drug delivery. J Control Release 300:93–101. https://doi.org/10.1016/j.jconrel.2019.02.044

Wang W (2015) Advanced protein formulations. Protein Sci 24:1031–1039. https://doi.org/10.1002/pro.2684

Wanning S, Süverkrüp R, Lamprecht A (2015) Pharmaceutical spray freeze drying. Int J Pharm 488:136–153. https://doi.org/10.1016/j.ijpharm.2015.04.053

Whitesides GM (2006) The origins and the future of microfluidics. Nature 442:368–373. https://doi.org/10.1038/nature05058

Williams GR, Raimi-Abraham BT, Luo CJ (2018) Nanofibres in drug delivery, 1st edn. UCL Press, London

Yu M, Benjamin MM, Srinivasan S, Morin EE, Shishatskaya EI, Schwendeman SP, Schwendeman A (2018) Battle of GLP-1 delivery technologies. Adv Drug Deliv Rev 130:113–130. https://doi.org/10.1016/j.addr.2018.07.009

Zaman R, Islam RA, Ibnat N, Othman I, Zaini A, Lee CY, Chowdhury EH (2019) Current strategies in extending half-lives of therapeutic proteins. J Control Release 301:176–189. https://doi.org/10.1016/j.jconrel.2019.02.016

Zheng Y, Pokorski JK (2021) Hot melt extrusion: an emerging manufacturing method for slow and sustained protein delivery. WIREs Nanomed Nanobiotechnol 13:e1712. https://doi.org/10.1002/wnan.1712

Microneedle and Polymeric Films: Delivery of Proteins, Peptides and Nucleic Acids

Yu Wu, Aaron R. J. Hutton, Anjali Kiran Pandya, Vandana B. Patravale, and Ryan F. Donnelly

Contents

Y. Wu · A. R. J. Hutton · R. F. Donnelly (✉)
School of Pharmacy, Queen's University Belfast, Belfast, UK
e-mail: R.Donnelly@qub.ac.uk

A. K. Pandya
School of Pharmacy, Queen's University Belfast, Belfast, UK

Department of Pharmaceutical Sciences and Technology, Institute of Chemical Technology, Nathalal Parekh Marg Matunga, Mumbai, Maharashtra, India

V. B. Patravale
Department of Pharmaceutical Sciences and Technology, Institute of Chemical Technology, Nathalal Parekh Marg Matunga, Mumbai, Maharashtra, India

M. Schäfer-Korting, U. S. Schubert (eds.), *Drug Delivery and Targeting*,
Handbook of Experimental Pharmacology 284, https://doi.org/10.1007/164_2023_653

Abstract

In the last 20 years, protein, peptide and nucleic acid-based therapies have become the fastest growing sector in the pharmaceutical industry and play a vital role in disease therapy. However, the intrinsic sensitivity and large molecular sizes of biotherapeutics limit the available routes of administration. Currently, the main administration routes of biomacromolecules, such as parenteral, oral, pulmonary, nasal, rectal and buccal routes, each have their limitations. Several non-invasive strategies have been proposed to overcome these challenges. Researchers were particularly interested in microneedles (MNs) and polymeric films because of their less invasiveness, convenience and greater potential to preserve the bioactivity of biotherapeutics. By facilitating with MNs and polymeric films, biomacromolecules could provide significant benefits to patients suffering from various diseases such as cancer, diabetes, infectious and ocular diseases. However, before these devices can be used on patients, how to upscale MN manufacture in a cost-effective and timely manner, as well as the long-term safety of MN and polymeric film applications necessitates further investigation.

Keywords

Biotherapeutics · Microneedles · Polymeric films · Transdermal drug delivery

Abbreviations

CTGF	Connective tissue growth factor
CyA	Cyclosporine A
HA	Hyaluronic acid
HIV	Human immunodeficiency virus
HPMC	Hydroxypropyl methylcellulose
LbL	Layer-by-layer
MN	Microneedle
NP	Nanoparticle
OVA	Ovalbumin
PCL	Polycaprolactone
PE	Polyelectrolyte
PVA	Polyvinyl alcohol
PVP	Polyvinylpyrrolidone
TDDS	Transdermal drug delivery system
VEGF	Vascular endothelial growth factor

1 Current Challenges of Peptides, Proteins and Nucleic Acid Delivery Strategies

Protein, peptide and nucleic acid-based therapies are now widely available and considered first-line treatments for various chronic diseases. However, due to hydrophilicity and susceptibility to enzymatic degradation, these biomolecules are predominately delivered via the parenteral route, which has several disadvantages (Singh et al. 2008). Parenteral delivery is often costly, with many injectable biotherapeutics manufactured under aseptic conditions. Furthermore, in aqueous environments, biotherapeutics are prone to chemical and physical degradation thus leading to reduced shelf life and negative effects on drug potency (Brown 2005). For this reason, protein-based therapeutics are maintained within a specific temperature range, typically 2–8°C, however, the necessity for 'cold chain' storage and correct handling is another additional expense. Hypodermic injections also induce pain, needle phobia, hypersensitivity and lipohypertrophy (Bashyal et al. 2016). This can result in reduced compliance and the need for medical supervision. Improper needle practices and disposal can also increase the risk of blood-borne pathogen transmission. Although appropriate training measures and equipment have been put in place, needle stick injuries still put a considerable burden on the healthcare service through both direct and indirect costs (Mannocci et al. 2016). As a result, needle-free delivery of proteins, peptides and nucleic acids has the potential to improve compliance, enhance safety, decrease costs and reduce pain. To this end, oral, pulmonary, nasal, rectal and buccal delivery have all been investigated, however, these present their own challenges. Thus, a less invasive route of administration with higher patient compliance is highly desirable.

2 Introduction of Microneedle System and Polymeric Film

Innovations in formulation science have been leading the biopharmaceutical industry towards significant changes, especially overcoming the pitfalls of the above-mentioned administration routes. A massive effort has been devoted to developing new approaches to enable controlled and efficient delivery of biomacromolecules at the desired site of action. Among various drug delivery systems under development, MNs and polymeric films constitute important parts of systems with potential in this direction.

2.1 Introduction of MNs

MNs are an attractive technology that bypasses the barrier of biological membranes and deliver drugs in close proximity to the target tissue, enabling higher delivery efficiency. MNs consist of micron-sized needles supported by a baseplate. The height of each needle is typically between 25 and 2,000 μm, which is long enough to penetrate biological membranes while short enough to reduce discomfort and pain caused by nerve irritation (Thakur Singh et al. 2017). Originally, MNs were developed to facilitate transdermal drug delivery as they can dramatically enhance the skin permeability of drug molecules, especially macromolecules. Based on its safety, capability to bypass hepatic first-pass metabolism, excellent ease of administration, and superb convenience and persistence among patients, transdermal drug delivery systems (TDDS) have emerged as an attractive alternative to oral or parenteral pathways. However, the biggest challenge for transdermal drug delivery is that only therapeutic molecules with molecular weight less than 1 kDa, high lipophilicity and a certain polarity can diffuse passively through skin barriers and achieve therapeutically effective doses (Mueller et al. 1858). The *stratum corneum* is the primary barrier for transdermal drug delivery, severely limiting the delivery of macromolecules. Based on the inherent characteristics of MNs, they are long enough to penetrate the *stratum corneum* and short enough to avoid damage to the dermis or nerve endings, making it painless (Moffatt et al. 2017). Thus, MNs tend to be a smart device to bypass the *stratum corneum* barrier and successfully deliver macromolecules in an efficient and minimally invasive manner.

A variety of materials such as silicon, ceramic, metal, silica glass, carbohydrate and polymers have been used to fabricate different types of MNs via various fabrication methods (Waghule et al. 2019). To date, five typical sub-groups of MNs, namely solid, coated, hollow, dissolving and hydrogel-forming MNs have been widely investigated for drug delivery. The principles of these MNs are shown in Fig. 1. The unique properties, functions, fabrication methods, pros and cons of these MNs are mentioned and discussed below.

2.1.1 Solid MNs

As shown in Fig. 1a, solid MNs work based on a 'poke and patch' strategy. Initially, MNs are inserted into the target tissue and then removed to form microchannels. Subsequently, drug-loaded reservoirs (e.g. patch, gel and solution) are applied on the poked site and drug molecules can migrate through the generated microchannels by passive diffusion (Prausnitz 2017). Various materials have been used to fabricate solid MNs, such as silicon, metals, glass and non-biodegradable and biodegradable polymers. Solid MNs made of silicon were the first MN developed for transdermal drug delivery (Henry et al. 1998). Subsequently, in 2003, McAllister fabricated metal MNs and demonstrated the ability to use metal MNs to facilitate the transdermal delivery of macromolecules (e.g. bovine serum albumin and insulin) (McAllister et al. 2003). Solid MNs can also be used in combination with iontophoresis for efficient and targeted delivery of therapeutic molecules (Wu et al. 2007; Han and Das 2013). Notably, Kaushik et al. measured the pain scale after applying the solid MNs, and the results demonstrated that compared with conventional hypodermic needles, the pain and tissue damage induced by MNs are negligible (Kaushik et al. 2001). Since they are always made of silicon and metal, solid MNs have superior mechanical properties and sharp tips, making them ready to penetrate skin barriers. Solid MNs are also simple to manufacture at low cost. Despite the many benefits offered by solid MNs, this technology still has several drawbacks that cannot be overlooked. The insertion of metal MNs has the potential to cause an irritation

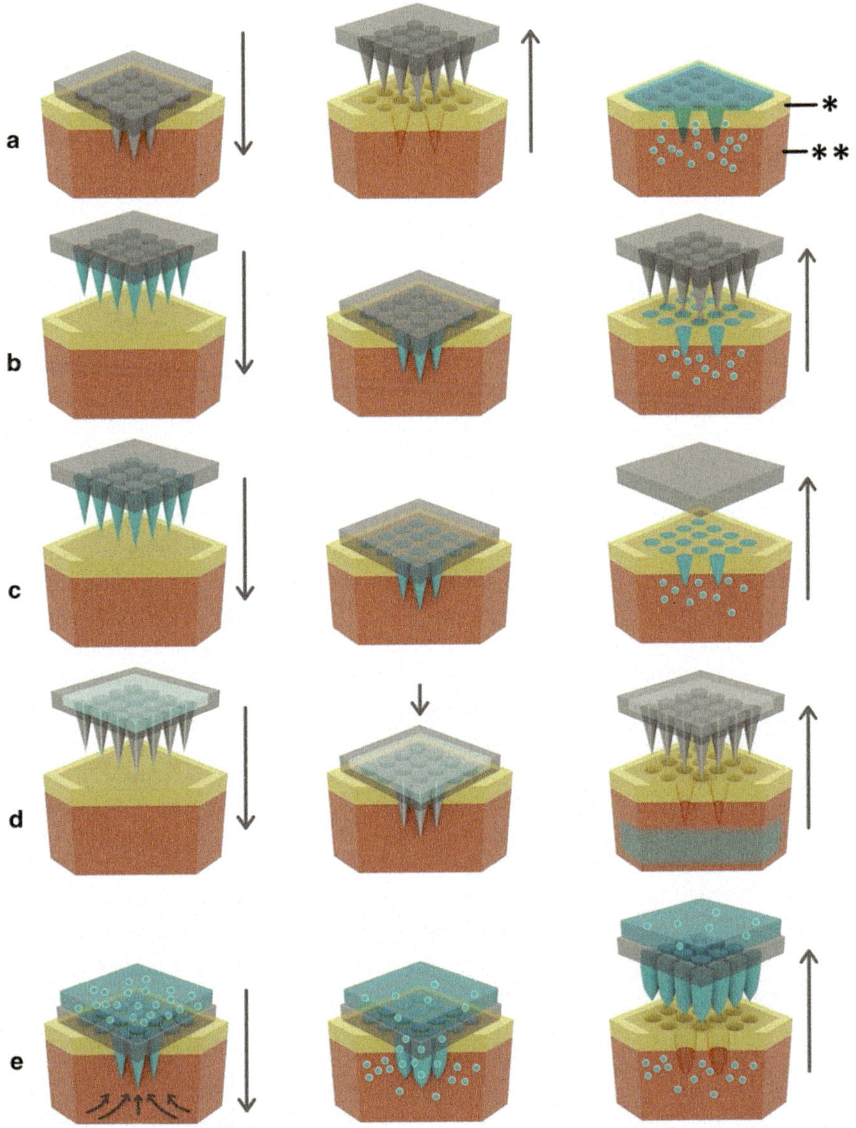

Fig. 1 Schematic representation of different types of MNs applied to the skin to achieve enhanced transdermal drug delivery, *stratum corneum, **epidermis. (**a**) Solid MNs following the 'poke and patch' strategy. (**b**) Coated MNs following the 'coat and poke' strategy. (**c**) Dissolving MNs following the 'poke and release' strategy. (**d**) Injection of drug molecules using hollow MNs. (**e**) Hydrogel-forming MNs absorb skin interstitial fluid upon application to the skin. Adapted from (Kirkby et al. 2020) with permission from Springer, Copyright [2020]

reaction and solid MNs also exhibit poor drug permeability control, as the created microchannels close quickly due to self-healing, resulting in poor delivery efficiency and reproducibility.

2.1.2 Coated MNs

Coated MNs work based on the strategy of 'coat and poke', in which drugs are pre-coated onto the shafts of the needles and then the coated MNs are inserted into the target tissue. After insertion, the drug molecules coated on solid MNs can be directly deposited and accumulated at the dosed site. Based on this principle of coated MNs, the efficacy of drug delivery largely depends on how successfully the drug layer is coated onto MNs (Gill and Prausnitz 2007a). To coat MNs, various approaches have been investigated, including dip coating, inkjet coating, immersion coating, drop coating and spray coating (Ingrole and Gill 2019). These coating methods can be mainly classified into two groups, the old group and the novel group. In the old group, therapeutic molecules were coated on the entire MN arrays, including the baseplate. As described in the first publication of coated MNs, by using the immersion coating method the entire MN was coated with medication solution (Matriano et al. 2002). However, it is challenging to deliver the drug localised in the baseplate of MNs as the baseplate will be removed prior to use and can be determined as waste (McCrudden et al. 2015). Thus, the novel methods such as dip coating and inkjet printing that can specially coat drug molecules in the MN tips without contaminating the baseplate of MNs were developed to improve delivery efficiency and reduce drug wastage (Ingrole and Gill 2019). Figure 2 summarised the potential outcomes of these two types of coating methods.

Coated MNs are a versatile delivery system that can be applied to deliver a variety of molecules, including small molecules, proteins, viruses and even microparticles (Gill and Prausnitz 2007b). However, due to the small size of the needles and the fact that drug molecules can only be coated onto the surface of the MNs, the loading capacity of coated MNs is typically quite low (Li et al. 2017). This type of MNs has been reported to have poor accuracy and reproducibility, as the sharpness of the needles will be reduced after coating, which affects insertion capability and ultimately leads to poor delivery efficiency (Jiang et al. 2007).

2.1.3 Hollow MNs

Like conventional hypodermic needles, hollow MNs have a hollow bore and also deliver drug molecules by instilling a drug solution through the inserted needle. However, hollow MNs needle sizes are significantly smaller than conventional hypodermic needles (2 mm in length, 26–30 gauge), typically ranging from 33 to 35 gauge in outer diameter and 150 μm in length (Gill et al. 2008; Gupta et al. 2011). Hollow MNs are typically made of glass, metal, polymer and silicon by various fabrication methods, such as isotropic etching, laser micromachining, deep reactive ion etching, integrated lithographic moulding technique, wet chemical etching and X-ray photolithography (Ita 2015).

Hollow MNs have attracted great attention from researchers because they are capable of offering various advantages over conventional hypodermic needles. Due

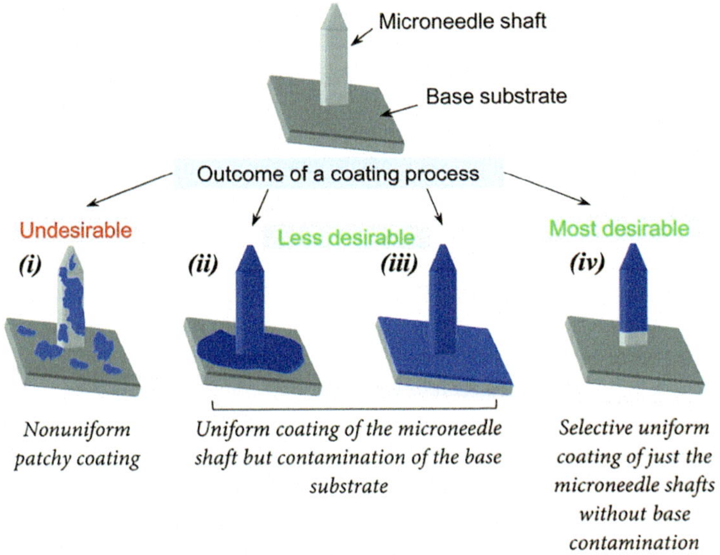

Fig. 2 Possible outcomes of a MN coating process. (i) Coating are randomly produced and do not cover the surfaces uniformly, (ii) coating cover the MN shaft but also a small region of the baseplate of the MNs, (iii) coating cover the entire MN uniformly, (iv) coating cover exclusively to the shaft of the MN without contaminating the baseplate. Adapted from (Ingrole and Gill 2019) with permission from The American Society for Pharmacology and Experimental Therapeutics, Copyright [2019]

to their much smaller dimension than traditional hypodermic needles, hollow MNs can deliver therapeutic molecules in a minimally invasive manner without posing compliance issues. After being inserted into the skin, hollow MNs directly deposit therapeutic molecules into the epidermis. Thus, it can be used to efficiently transfer a wide range of molecules, even biotherapeutics such as proteins, peptides and nucleic acids. In addition, as more therapeutic molecules can be accommodated into the empty space inside the needle, compared to solid and dissolving MNs, this form of MNs can administer large doses of drugs. The pressure inside the hollow MNs can be controlled by adjusting the dimension of the needle bore, and in turn, the infusion rate of drug solution can be modulated for rapid bolus injection or a slow infusion, as the drug solution is delivered in a pressure-driven fashion (Kaushik et al. 2001; Kim et al. 2014). In addition to administering therapeutic molecules, hollow MNs can also be used to extract interstitial fluid and blood from the body.

Although hollow MNs have been shown to be effective in facilitating drug delivery, their disadvantages cannot be ignored. Due to the materials (e.g. silicon, glass, metal) and small dimensions of hollow MNs, they are brittle and associated with the risk of blockage and breaking. Moreover, the fabrication of hollow MNs is always complicated and costly (Thakur Singh et al. 2017; Patel et al. 2011).

2.1.4 Dissolving MNs

Different from other types of MNs, the dissolving MNs are made of water-soluble polymers and are typically prepared by integrating drug molecules into biodegradable and biocompatible polymers. The administration of a dissolving MN is sought to be a straightforward patient-friendly application, similar to conventional patches by gentle thumb pressing on the skin, which can significantly reduce clinician visits (Than et al. 2018). After being inserted into the target tissue and in contact with interstitial fluid, the inserted needle-part of MNs will soften, dissolve and then release drug molecules. This smart MN design has plenty of attractive points for transdermal drug delivery. Primarily, as dissolving MNs are made of biodegradable polymers that automatically soften and disappear in the human tissue, they will not generate biohazardous sharps wastage like solid and hollow MNs. In this regard, the rate of drug release from MNs can be directly controlled by altering the composition of the polymer matrix. Dissolving MNs are self-administrable and do not need to be retrieved from the target tissue after insertion, eliminating the risk of broken MNs remaining in the dosed tissue and improving patient compliance.

A further advantage is that unlike solid, coated and hollow MNs, dissolving MNs can reliably deliver all drug molecules loaded in MNs and provide highly accurate reproducible results, as the punctured MNs dissolve completely and serve themselves as implants in the skin tissue after application.

Although dissolving MNs have a variety of advantages and are extensively applied for transdermal drug administration, this type of MN is subject to several minor constraints. Due to the small needle size and the fact that drug molecules are localised exclusively into the needle-part, dissolving MNs always have limited loading capacity (Migalska et al. 2011). Hence, until now, dissolving MNs are only suitable for the administration of highly potent drugs.

2.1.5 Hydrogel-Forming MNs

The most recent type of MNs is hydrogel-forming MNs, which are made of swellable polymers like crosslinked hydrogels. Because of the hydrophilic nature of the hydrogels, hydrogel-forming MNs easily absorb water and swell after being inserted into the skin. Based on this principle, hydrogel-forming MNs can be used for a variety of applications. Hydrogel-forming MNs can be used to administer drugs to the skin, either by incorporating therapeutic molecules into the polymeric structure during fabrication or by loading drugs into a separate reservoir and attaching it on top of the hydrogel-forming MNs (Turner et al. 2021). Additionally, hydrogel-forming MNs can also be used as a minimally invasive diagnostic method. Due to its swellable nature, upon insertion into the skin, interstitial fluid will be absorbed, which can be used as a source of biomarkers for further diagnosis.

Due to their unique structure, hydrogel-forming MNs are thought to have numerous advantages: (1) As hydrogel-forming MNs are made of nearly invisible needles attached to the base support and the insertion depth is not far enough to trigger pain receptors, minimal invasiveness is considered an inherent benefit of the hydrogel-forming MNs. (2) Unlike dissolving and coated MNs, in which drugs can be only loaded into the needle section and always result in limited drug loading, in hydrogel-forming MNs, therapeutic molecules can be loaded into a separate reservoir, thereby acquiring a higher drug loading capacity. (3) By adjusting the polymer crosslinking ratio the drug release rate can be easily tunable, which is difficult to manage in conventional forms of MNs. (4) The development of hydrogel-forming MNs can also overcome the biocompatibility issues associated with silicon or metallic MNs, which are linked to the risk of toxicity.

2.2 Introduction of Polymeric Films

Thin films were originally developed in the 1970s as an alternative to tablets and capsules for paediatric and geriatric patients with dysphagia (Bala et al. 2013). Following its initial application as a fast-dissolving oral dosage form, polymeric films have been widely used in transdermal and cosmetic applications. Polymeric films exhibit unique physio-chemical properties and advantages, such as good flexibility, drug loading capacity, rapid dissolution at the site of action, avoidance of first-pass metabolism, patient compliance and localised delivery, which contribute to improved delivery of biotherapeutics. Films have been widely used to deliver biotherapeutics via buccal, ocular, sublingual and transdermal routes. Numerous manufacturing methods used in the fabrication of films include solvent casting, hot melt extrusion, electrospinning and 3D bioprinting.

Thin films have garnered particular interest due to their compatibility with numerous natural, semi-synthetic and synthetic materials, such as silicon, silicon carbide, titanium dioxide, alumina, polymers like polyvinyl alcohol (PVA), polyvinylpyrrolidone (PVP), cellulose derivatives, chitosan, gums and alginate (Yan et al. 2009). Polyelectrolytes (PEs) based films have been highly explored for their film forming abilities driven by the ionisable surface groups, enabling fabrication of PE nano-assemblies for biomedical and healthcare applications (Díez-Pascual and Rahdar 2022). A Layer-by-Layer (LbL) approach is the simplest way to design PE-based nano-assemblies for the delivery of biomolecules, such as polypeptides, glycoproteins, glycosaminoglycans and DNA. LbL has been an appealing technique due to its ability to encompass multiple actives and multiple film layering (Park et al. 2018). Polymers have attracted attention due to their ability to undergo distinct modifications in chemical properties and mechanical strength to improve performance. These systems also offer aesthetic appeal, which is crucial in determining patient compliance.

3 Application of MNs and Polymeric Films in Facilitating Delivery of Protein, Peptide and Nucleic Acid

The bioavailability and stability of biomacromolecules delivered orally will be significantly reduced and affected by the protease enzymes in the gastrointestinal tract. Although 100% bioavailability can be achieved by delivering biomacromolecules directly into the bloodstream, long-term administration of biomacromolecules by the parenteral route also has its own drawbacks. Due to the highly invasive nature of conventional hypodermic needles, repeated parenteral administration is always associated with poor patient compliance as it may lead to needle phobia, pain and complications (e.g. phlebitis and tissue necrosis) (Morales et al. 2017). Furthermore, as biomacromolecules are always rapidly cleared from the blood, frequent administration is required to maintain therapeutic levels, which may cause systemic adverse effects. In the parenteral route, biomacromolecules are always in a liquid state and are easily denatured during long-term storage without the addition of stabilisers and under suitable conditions. To make matters worse, protein denaturation not only reduces their therapeutic activity but may also cause toxicity and immunogenicity (Truong-Le et al. 2015). Thus, a novel administration device with improved patient compliance, less invasion, improved stability of biomacromolecules and allows for rapid onset of drug action is highly desired. MNs and polymeric films have been investigated and widely applied to treat various diseases due to their ability to deliver proteins, peptides and nucleic acids in an efficient, stable and minimally invasive manner.

3.1 Miscellaneous Indications of Microneedles

MNs have been investigated to detect protein biomarkers in dermal interstitial fluids and thus diagnose infectious diseases. Ganesan et al. reported the utility of solid MNs for minimally invasive transdermal biosensing of CD4 T^{+} cell counts in blood (Ganesan et al. 2013). After the application of solid MNs, microchannels were generated and can be used to obtain blood directly from the veins. By quantifying the number of CD4 cells in the blood, HIV diagnosis can be performed in a reliable, convenient and low-cost way. Subsequently, Ganesan applied a similar device to quantify Ebola virus in blood samples, which can be used to diagnose viral haemorrhagic fever (Ganesan 2013). In this setup, biofluids were transported to the sensing chamber through microchannels and samples were quantified based on antigen–antibody reactions.

In addition to being applied for infectious disease diagnosis, MNs can also be utilised to deliver protein-based vaccines to combat infectious diseases. Due to its cost-effectiveness, treatment-effectiveness and versatility, protein-based vaccination has been recognised as a mainstream prophylaxis for infectious diseases. Compared with the conventional vaccination, which is induced by subcutaneous or intramuscular injection of vaccines and always results in poor patient compliance, a MN is simple to use, less invasive and has improved efficacy. Based on these benefits, MNs have been extensively researched as a delivery platform for protein and peptide vaccines.

Matriano et al. used various routes, including intradermal, subcutaneous and intramuscular administration to deliver the model antigen (OVA) and compared their immune responses. Results indicated that intradermal administration of OVA-coated MNs induced an immune response comparable to conventional hypodermic needles, which was 50-fold greater than subcutaneous and intramuscular administration (Matriano et al. 2002). Consistently, by using influenza vaccines as model antigens, Sean et al. (2016) and Kommareddy et al. (2012) also proved that the introduction of intradermally administered MNs could significantly improve immunogenicity of influenza antigens compared to those delivered via intramuscular injection. Furthermore, they proved that dissolving MNs also improved viral clearance as well as provided additional benefits to the patients such as being less invasive and enabling self-administration at home, saving time and money.

Based on its minimally invasive, potentially self-administrable nature, MNs have been introduced to benefit insulin administration. Solid MNs could significantly facilitate the transdermal delivery of biomacromolecules, including insulin and BSA (McAllister et al. 2003). Following the application of a 1 cm^2 patch, the concentration of insulin in the blood was thought to be sufficient to combat diabetes. Unlike solid MNs requiring multiple steps for insulin administration, Ross et al. investigated insulin coated metal MNs, which can deliver insulin in a more convenient and rapid way (Ross et al. n.d.). The utility of inkjet printing technology could coat a thin and homogenous layer on metal MNs while maintaining insulin integrity during the coating process.

Compared to the solid MNs discussed above, hollow MNs are able to provide a faster insulin onset as hollow MNs contain a hollow bore and therapeutic molecules can be delivered by pressure-driven flow. McAllister et al. developed single hollow MNs fabricated from glass. As proved in diabetic rats, hollow MNs can effectively decrease blood glucose levels within 5 h post-dosing (McAllister et al. 2003). To further speed up insulin onset, Roxhed et al. developed a hybrid system of hollow MNs and electronically controlled liquid dispensers, as shown in Fig. 3. After a 3-h dosing period, the plasma concentration of insulin applied by electrically driven active administration was fivefold greater than in the passive administration group, resulting in a significant reduction in blood glucose level (Roxhed et al. 2008).

Due to their favourable biocompatibility, biodegradability and simple manufacturing method, dissolving MNs have been extensively investigated for insulin delivery. The ability of HA-based dissolving MNs to deliver insulin was evaluated in diabetic rats and compared to subcutaneous injection using conventional hypodermic needles. Results indicated that insulin administered using dissolving MNs could efficiently get access to the systemic circulation and generate comparable efficacy to subcutaneous injection in decreasing blood glucose levels (Liu et al. 2012).

Courtenay et al. investigated dissolving and hydrogel-forming MNs to deliver bevacizumab, a recombinant monoclonal antibody that has been approved by the FDA to treat various cancers. By quantifying the serum and tissue concentrations of bevacizumab, the MNs were demonstrated to be capable of providing sustained drug delivery to systemic and lymph circulation. Thus, the developed MNs could potentially provide a novel transdermal delivery platform to deliver biomacromolecules to treat cancer (Courtenay et al. 2018). Furthermore, Wang et al. utilised dissolving MNs fabricated from silk protein, a natural biopolymer with excellent biocompatibility and controllable degradability, to deliver multiple drugs, including bevacizumab, temozolomide and thrombin to treat glioblastoma. According to the

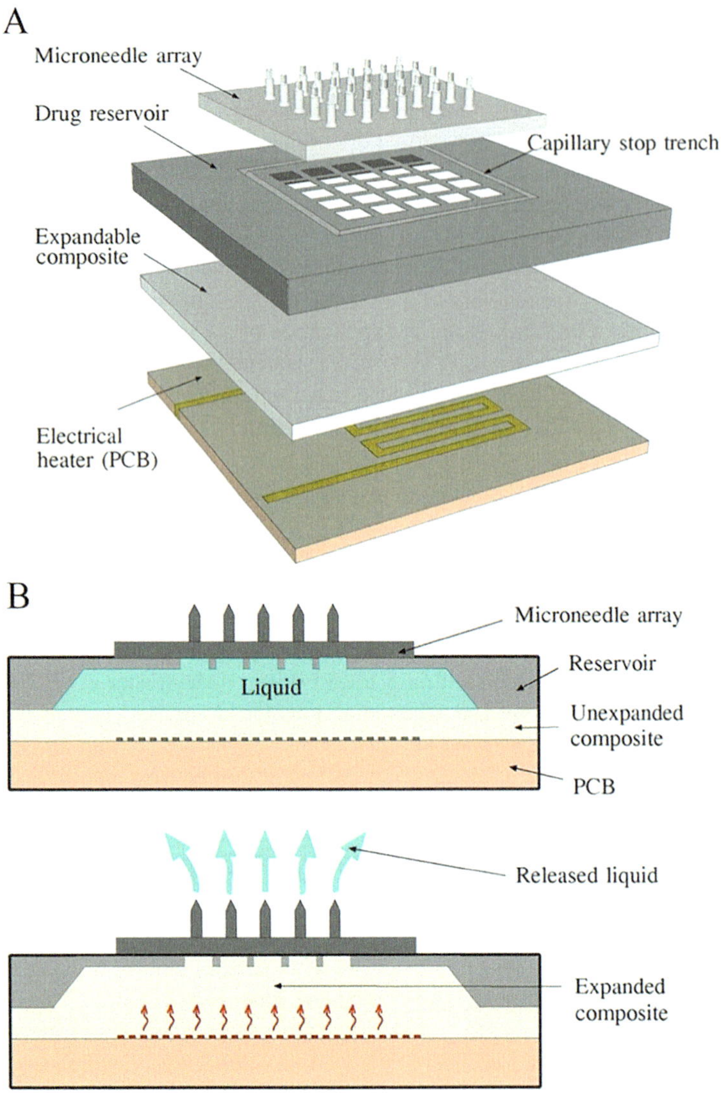

Fig. 3 Schematic representation of (**a**) the exploded view and (**b**) the principle of operation of the MN-based transdermal patch. Adapted from (Roxhed et al. 2008) with permission from IEEE, Copyright [2008]

findings in tumour-bearing mice, multidrug-loaded silk protein MNs could significantly reduce the tumour volume and improve the survival rate in mice when compared with conventional intravenous injection. Thus, the MNs developed here are considered a promising pathway to deliver biomacromolecules for the treatment of glioblastoma with improved efficiency and less toxicity (Wang et al. 2022).

Apart from directly killing tumour cells, MNs can also exert anti-tumour effects via immunotherapy, in which therapeutic cancer vaccines can be used to activate the body's immune system to attack cancer cells. Zaric et al. used dissolving MNs to deliver antigen-encapsulated nanoparticles (NPs) specifically to skin dendritic cells, resulting in a robust antigen-specific T-cell immune response. The model antigen (OVA) was encapsulated in PLGA NPs to prolong the retention time and sustain vaccine release in the skin. After dissolving MNs are inserted and dissolved in the skin, NPs can be generated, thereby bypassing the barrier of the skin stratum corneum and facilitating the delivery of biomacromolecules. The results indicate that the hybrid system of OVA-loaded PLGA NPs and dissolving MNs can not only prolong the retention of antigens in the skin but also maintain antigen stability in MNs, thereby acquiring long-term safe and efficient therapy. Furthermore, in vivo studies in mice proved that this hybrid system could induce a significant level of antigen-specific cellular immunity, resulting in efficient tumour clearance (Zaric et al. 2013).

To bypass the barriers of the eye and efficiently deliver biomacromolecules to the back of the eye, Wu et al. developed dissolving MNs made of biodegradable and biocompatible polymers (PVA and PVP) to deliver the model protein (OVA). In this investigation, a hybrid system of NPs and dissolving MNs was developed to sustain the release of the protein. As shown in ex vivo studies, compared to the conventional administration routes (i.e. eye drops and gel), the dissolving MNs could significantly improve protein delivery efficiency to the back of the eye. Thus, the developed dissolving MNs were believed to be a promising device for posterior segment delivery of biomacromolecules (Wu et al. 2021).

GhavamiNejad et al. reported a smart use of MNs for hypoglycaemia relief. In this study, a composite MN patch with hypoglycaemia-triggered release property was fabricated from photo-crosslinked MeHA with embedded multifunctional microgels, which could trigger the release of glucagon at low glucose levels, thereby treating hypoglycaemia (GhavamiNejad et al. 2019).

Chi et al. developed dissolving MNs composed of chitosan and VEGF to promote wound healing. The temperature-sensitive hydrogel was used to encapsulate VEGF in the micropores of chitosan MNs, which means that the release of the VEGF can be controlled by temperature. As the inflammation response at the wound sites can increase the temperature, the smart release of VEGF can be achieved. Both in vitro and in vivo studies demonstrated the superior ability of MNs to promote collagen deposition, angiogenesis and inflammatory inhibition. Based on these positive results, MNs possess great potential to renew wound healing therapies (Chi et al. 2020).

3.2 Miscellaneous Indications of Polymeric Films

Due to their convenience, biocompatibility and non-invasiveness, polymeric films have been developed for vaccine delivery. Anandhakumar and Raichur proposed a multilayer multifunctional film platform composed of polyelectrolyte-silver nanocomposites for remotely activated delivery of biotherapeutics. Alternate adsorption of poly(allylamine hydrochloride) and dextran sulphate was undertaken on a glass substrate followed by silver nanoparticles. Ciprofloxacin hydrochloride and bovine serum albumin were immobilised within the polymeric network of the polyelectrolyte multilayer film. The release of the antibacterial agents was triggered using ultrasonication and laser light, resulting in substantial antibacterial activity against *Staphylococcus aureus* (Anandhakumar and Raichur 2013).

Polymeric films have also been widely investigated as non-invasive delivery systems for insulin to treat diabetes in a patient-acceptable manner. For example, insulin-encapsulated NPs made of PEG-*b*-PLA copolymer were embedded into chitosan films for buccal delivery (Giovino et al. 2013). It was observed that the films enabled a 1.8-fold enhancement in insulin permeation via the EpiOral™ buccal tissue construct in comparison to insulin solution (Giovino et al. 2013). Moreover, polymeric films composed of cationic polymethacrylate derivative are called ERL, alone and in combination with hydroxypropyl methylcellulose (HPMC) were explored for buccal delivery of insulin-encapsulated NPs (Morales et al. 2014). ERL films were found to have better film properties and resulted in higher insulin permeation across human buccal mucosa over insulin loaded to HPMC films as well as insulin solution. Another investigation in buccal delivery of insulin comprised of a flexible bilayer film, in which the first layer consisted of a drug containing mucoadhesive layer made from chitosan-ethylenediaminetetraacetic acid hydrogel and the second layer was impermeable ethyl cellulose. The mucoadhesive transbuccal film formulation showed 17% higher insulin bioavailability and a considerable hypoglycaemic effect compared to subcutaneously injected insulin (Cui et al. 2009).

Moreover, polymeric films have also been investigated for local and systemic delivery of anti-tumour agents. Ceron Jayme et al. constructed a DNA-based polymeric film loaded with chlorine aluminum phthalocyanine (AlClPc) for photodynamic therapy in mucosal cancer (Ceron Jayme et al. 2020). The cell viability of oral squamous cell carcinoma cells was effectively reduced by more than 30% following administration through the polymeric film, indicating the great potential of polymeric films for localised treatment of cancer. Systemic release of anticancer drugs from multilayer nanofilms was demonstrated by Cho et al. The authors designed nanofilms to control drug release by changing the DNA structure. They synthesised unique 3D DNA origami structures with hairpin, X and Y shapes to deliver the model anticancer drug doxorubicin (Cho et al. 2014). The multilayer films were prepared using an LbL approach and consisted of positively charged poly-L-Lysine paired with negatively charged DNA molecules. In this experiment, it was found that the structure of this multilayer film not only controlled the drug release but also stabilised the structure of the biotherapeutics and maintained their activity even in the presence of protein-rich serum. This system also demonstrated promise in the development of DNA-engineered nanosurfaces for controlled biotherapeutics release (Cho et al. 2014).

Polymeric films have also been used to alleviate eye diseases. Cyclosporine A (CyA)-loaded mucoadhesive chitosan films were developed to inhibit interleukin-2 secretion in concanavalin A activated Jurkat T cells, thereby treating ocular inflammatory diseases (Hermans et al. 2014). The chitosan film system was presented as a promising long-acting mucoadhesive delivery vehicle for CyA. Furthermore, sustained delivery of ranibizumab within the vitreous cavity using a twin biodegradable nanoporous polycaprolactone (PCL) thin film-based device has also been studied for the treatment of retinal neovascularisation (Lance et al. 2016). The device showed a release of up to 12 weeks in vivo with good tolerance and no immune response, making it a potential ocular delivery platform for biotherapeutics.

Castleberry et al. reported a nanolayered siRNA delivery platform for silencing the connective tissue growth factor (CTGF), a key mediator of TGFβ pro-fibrotic response in wound healing (Castleberry et al. 2016). In this study, nanolayer films were applied to sutures for burn scar management and tested in a rat model of scarring caused by third-degree burns. The results indicated that the introduction of polymeric films could sustain the release of siRNA for more than 5 days, resulting in effective scar prevention.

4 Conclusion and Future Prospects

To improve patient compliance, minimally invasive administration of peptides, proteins and nucleic acids has been an area of particular interest in recent times. Yet, current delivery options for these biomolecules remain limited, with proteins and nucleic acids typically restricted to the traditional hypodermic needle and syringe. Recently, alternative drug delivery approaches for peptides, proteins and nucleic acids using both thin films and MNs have garnered particular attention. For instance, both start-up and established pharmaceutical companies are striving to design a wide range of therapeutic thin films for the delivery of biotherapeutics via oral, sublingual, buccal, ocular, as well as transdermal routes. Although challenges pertaining to formulation optimisation for large-scale manufacturing persist, thin films seem to be gaining in popularity amongst patients. Transdermal delivery using MNs also provides a convenient, minimally invasive, patient-friendly route of drug administration. By overcoming the formidable barrier posed by the skin's outermost layer, the *stratum corneum*, MNs have been shown to be effective in the delivery of peptides, proteins and nucleic acids across the skin without the need for a conventional needle and syringe. Notably, MNs have captured the attention of investors in recent times, with the World Economic Forum listing MNs as one of the Top Ten Emerging Technologies in 2020. This proves that there is a real desire to move away from the traditional syringe and needle, offering a minimally invasive alternative. Nevertheless, upscale manufacturing of MN technology has proven to be particularly challenging. At present, a number of key regulatory questions need to be addressed such as assurance of delivery, sterility, long-term stability and dosing accuracy. Importantly, both academics and industrial partners have been trying to resolve these regulatory concerns. For instance, recent work has investigated the use of primary packaging in maintaining MN stability, developed viable feedback mechanisms to confirm skin insertion, examined the effect of multiple skin application and assessed the impact of different sterilisation methods on MNs. Therefore, continued collaboration among academics, industrial partners and shareholders will certainly bring both thin films and MNs for biotherapeutic administration ever closer to the market.

References

Anandhakumar S, Raichur AM (2013) Polyelectrolyte/silver nanocomposite multilayer films as multifunctional thin film platforms for remote activated protein and drug delivery. Acta Biomater 9:8864–8874. https://doi.org/10.1016/j.actbio.2013.06.012

Bala R, Khanna S, Pawar P, Arora S (2013) Orally dissolving strips: a new approach to oral drug delivery system. Int J Pharm Investig 3:67. https://doi.org/10.4103/2230-973x.114897

Bashyal S, Noh G, Keum T, Choi YW, Lee S (2016) Cell penetrating peptides as an innovative approach for drug delivery; then, present and the future. J Pharm Investig 46:205–220. https://doi.org/10.1007/s40005-016-0253-0

Brown LR (2005) Commercial challenges of protein drug delivery. Expert Opin Drug Deliv 2:29–42. https://doi.org/10.1517/17425247.2.1.29

Castleberry SA, Golberg A, Sharkh MA, Khan S, Almquist BD, Austen WG, Yarmush ML, Hammond PT (2016) Nanolayered siRNA delivery platforms for local silencing of CTGF reduce cutaneous scar contraction in third-degree burns. Biomaterials 95:22–34. https://doi.org/10.1016/j.biomaterials.2016.04.007

Ceron Jayme C, Ferreira Pires A, Tedesco AC (2020) Development of DNA polymer films as a drug delivery system for the treatment of oral cancer. Drug Deliv Transl Res 10:1612–1625. https://doi.org/10.1007/s13346-020-00801-9

Chi J, Zhang X, Chen C, Shao C, Zhao Y, Wang Y (2020) Antibacterial and angiogenic chitosan microneedle array patch for promoting wound healing. Bioact Mater 5:253–259. https://doi.org/10.1016/j.bioactmat.2020.02.004

Cho Y, Lee JB, Hong J (2014) Controlled release of an anti-cancer drug from DNA structured nanofilms. Sci Rep 4. https://doi.org/10.1038/srep04078

Courtenay AJ, McCrudden MTC, McAvoy KJ, McCarthy HO, Donnelly RF (2018) Microneedle-mediated transdermal delivery of bevacizumab. Mol Pharm 15:3545–3556. https://doi.org/10.1021/acs.molpharmaceut.8b00544

Cui F, He C, He M, Tang C, Yin L, Qian F, Yin C (2009) Preparation and evaluation of chitosan-ethylenediaminetetraacetic acid hydrogel films for the mucoadhesive transbuccal delivery of insulin. J Biomed Mater Res A 89:1063–1071. https://doi.org/10.1002/jbm.a.32071

Díez-Pascual AM, Rahdar A (2022) LbL nano-assemblies: a versatile tool for biomedical and healthcare applications. Nanomaterials 12. https://doi.org/10.3390/nano12060949

Ganesan AV (2013) A novel MEMS based immunosensor for Ebola virus detection. ASME Int Mech Eng Congr Expo Proc 7 B:1–5. https://doi.org/10.1115/IMECE2013-66025

Ganesan AV, Kishore Kumar D, Banerjee A, Swaminathan S (2013) MEMS based microfluidic system for HIV detection. Proc IEEE Conf Nanotechnol:557–560. https://doi.org/10.1109/NANO.2013.6721005

GhavamiNejad A, Li J, Lu B, Zhou L, Lam L, Giacca A, Wu XY (2019) Glucose-responsive composite microneedle patch for hypoglycemia-triggered delivery of native glucagon. Adv Mater 31:1–7. https://doi.org/10.1002/adma.201901051

Gill HS, Prausnitz MR (2007a) Coated microneedles for transdermal delivery. J Control Release. https://doi.org/10.1016/j.jconrel.2006.10.017

Gill HS, Prausnitz MR (2007b) Coating formulations for microneedles. Pharm Res 24:1369–1380. https://doi.org/10.1007/s11095-007-9286-4

Gill HS, Denson DD, Burris BA, Prausnitz MR (2008) Effect of microneedle design on pain in human volunteers. Clin J Pain. https://doi.org/10.1097/AJP.0b013e31816778f9

Giovino C, Ayensu I, Tetteh J, Boateng JS (2013) An integrated buccal delivery system combining chitosan films impregnated with peptide loaded PEG-b-PLA nanoparticles. Colloids Surf B Biointerfaces 112:9–15. https://doi.org/10.1016/j.colsurfb.2013.07.019

Gupta J, Felner EI, Prausnitz MR (2011) Rapid pharmacokinetics of intradermal insulin administered using microneedles in type 1 diabetes subjects. Diabetes Technol Ther. https://doi.org/10.1089/dia.2010.0204

Han T, Das DB (2013) Permeability enhancement for transdermal delivery of large molecule using low-frequency sonophoresis combined with microneedles. J Pharm Sci 102:3614–3622. https://doi.org/10.1002/jps.23662

Henry S, McAllister DV, Allen MG, Prausnitz MR (1998) Microfabricated microneedles: a novel approach to transdermal drug delivery. J Pharm Sci. https://doi.org/10.1021/js980042+

Hermans K, Van Den Plas D, Kerimova S, Carleer R, Adriaensens P, Weyenberg W, Ludwig A (2014) Development and characterization of mucoadhesive chitosan films for ophthalmic delivery of cyclosporine A. Int J Pharm 472:10–19. https://doi.org/10.1016/j.ijpharm.2014.06.017

Ingrole RSJ, Gill HS (2019) Microneedle coating methods: a review with a perspective. J Pharmacol Exp Ther 370:555–569. https://doi.org/10.1124/jpet.119.258707

Ita K (2015) Transdermal delivery of drugs with microneedles – potential and challenges. Pharmaceutics 7(3):90–105. https://doi.org/10.3390/pharmaceutics7030090

Jiang J, Gill HS, Ghate D, McCarey BE, Patel SR, Edelhauser HF, Prausnitz MR (2007) Coated microneedles for drug delivery to the eye. Invest Ophthalmol Vis Sci 48:4038–4043. https://doi.org/10.1167/iovs.07-0066

Kaushik S, Hord AH, Denson DD, McAllister DV, Smitra S, Allen MG, Prausnitz MR (2001) Lack of pain associated with microfabricated microneedles. Anesth Analg:502–504. https://doi.org/10.1097/00000539-200102000-00041

Kim YC, Grossniklaus HE, Edelhauser HF, Prausnitz MR (2014) Intrastromal delivery of bevacizumab using microneedles to treat corneal neovascularization. Invest Ophthalmol Vis Sci. https://doi.org/10.1167/iovs.14-15257

Kirkby M, Hutton ARJ, Donnelly RF (2020) Microneedle mediated transdermal delivery of protein, peptide and antibody based therapeutics: current status and future considerations. Pharm Res 37:1–18. https://doi.org/10.1007/s11095-020-02844-6

Kommareddy S, Baudner BC, Oh S, Kwon SY, Singh M, O'Hagan DT (2012) Dissolvable microneedle patches for the delivery of cell-culture-derived influenza vaccine antigens. J Pharm Sci 101:1021–1027. https://doi.org/10.1002/jps.23019

Lance KD, Desai TA, Bernards DA, Ciaccio NA, Good SD, Mendes TS, Kudisch MAX, Chan E, Ishikiriyama M, Bhisitkul RB (2016) In vivo and in vitro sustained release of ranibizumab from a nanoporous thin-film device. Drug Deliv. Transl, Res

Li J, Zeng M, Shan H, Tong C (2017) Microneedle patches as drug and vaccine delivery platform. Curr Med Chem. https://doi.org/10.2174/0929867324666170526124053

Liu S, Jin M, Quan Y, Kamiyama F, Katsumi H (2012) The development and characteristics of novel microneedle arrays fabricated from hyaluronic acid , and their application in the transdermal delivery of insulin. J Control Release 161:933–941. https://doi.org/10.1016/j.jconrel.2012.05.030

Mannocci A, De Carli G, Di Bari V, Saulle R, Unim B, Nicolotti N, Carbonari L, Puro V, La Torre G (2016) How much do needlestick injuries cost? A systematic review of the economic evaluations of needlestick and sharps injuries among healthcare personnel. Infect Control Hosp Epidemiol 37:635–646. https://doi.org/10.1017/ice.2016.48

Matriano JA, Cormier M, Johnson J, Young WA, Buttery M, Nyam K, Daddona PE (2002) Macroflux® microprojection array patch technology: a new and efficient approach for intracutaneous immunization. Pharm Res 19:63–70. https://doi.org/10.1023/A:1013607400040

McAllister DV, Wang PM, Davis SP, Park JH, Canatella PJ, Allen MG, Prausnitz MR (2003) Microfabricated needles for transdermal delivery of macromolecules and nanoparticles: fabrication methods and transport studies. Proc Natl Acad Sci U S A 100:13755–13760. https://doi.org/10.1073/pnas.2331316100

McCrudden MTC, Torrisi BM, Al-Zahrani S, McCrudden CM, Zaric M, Scott CJ, Kissenpfennig A, McCarthy HO, Donnelly RF (2015) Laser-engineered dissolving microneedle arrays for protein delivery: potential for enhanced intradermal vaccination. J Pharm Pharmacol 67:409–425. https://doi.org/10.1111/jphp.12248

Migalska K, Morrow DIJ, Garland MJ, Thakur R, Woolfson AD, Donnelly RF (2011) Laser-engineered dissolving microneedle arrays for transdermal macromolecular drug delivery. Pharm Res 28:1919–1930. https://doi.org/10.1007/s11095-011-0419-4

Moffatt K, Wang Y, Raj Singh TR, Donnelly RF (2017) Microneedles for enhanced transdermal and intraocular drug delivery. Curr Opin Pharmacol 36:14–21. https://doi.org/10.1016/j.coph.2017.07.007

Morales JO, Huang S, Williams RO, McConville JT (2014) Films loaded with insulin-coated nanoparticles (ICNP) as potential platforms for peptide buccal delivery. Colloids Surf B Biointerfaces 122:38–45. https://doi.org/10.1016/j.colsurfb.2014.05.025

Morales JO, Fathe KR, Brunaugh A, Ferrati S, Li S, Montenegro-Nicolini M, Mousavikhamene Z, McConville JT, Prausnitz MR, Smyth HDC (2017) Challenges and future prospects for the delivery of biologics: oral mucosal, pulmonary, and transdermal routes. AAPS J 19:652–668. https://doi.org/10.1208/s12248-017-0054-z

Mueller J, Oliveira JSL, Barker R, Trapp M, Schroeter A, Brezesinski G, Neubert RHH (1858) The effect of urea and taurine as hydrophilic penetration enhancers on stratum corneum lipid models. Biochim Biophys Acta Biomembr 2016:2006–2018. https://doi.org/10.1016/j.bbamem.2016.05.010

Park S, Han U, Choi D, Hong J (2018) Layer-by-layer assembled polymeric thin films as prospective drug delivery carriers: design and applications. Biomater Res 22. https://doi.org/10.1186/s40824-018-0139-5

Patel SR, Lin ASP, Edelhauser HF, Prausnitz MR (2011) Suprachoroidal drug delivery to the back of the eye using hollow microneedles. Pharm Res 28:166–176. https://doi.org/10.1007/s11095-010-0271-y

Prausnitz MR (2017) Engineering microneedle patches for vaccination and drug delivery to skin. Annu Rev Chem Biomol Eng 8:177–200. https://doi.org/10.1146/annurev-chembioeng-060816-101514

Ross S, Scoutaris N, Lamprou D, Douroumis D (n.d.) Inkjet printing of insulin microneedles for transdermal delivery 44

Roxhed N, Samel B, Nordquist L, Griss P, Stemme G (2008) Painless drug delivery through microneedle-based transdermal patches featuring active infusion. IEEE Trans Biomed Eng 55: 1063–1071. https://doi.org/10.1109/TBME.2007.906492

Sean MRP, Sullivan P, Koutsonanos DG, del Pilar M, Martin J-WL, Zarnitsyn V, Murthy N, Compans RW, Skountzou I (2016) Dissolving polymer microneedle patches for influenza vaccination. Physiol Behav 176:139–148. https://doi.org/10.1038/nm.2182.Dissolving

Singh R, Singh S, Lillard JW (2008) Past, present, and future technologies for oral delivery of therapeutic proteins. J Pharm Sci 97:2497–2523. https://doi.org/10.1002/jps.21183

Thakur Singh RR, Tekko I, McAvoy K, McMillan H, Jones D, Donnelly RF (2017) Minimally invasive microneedles for ocular drug delivery, expert opin. Drug Deliv 14:525–537. https://doi.org/10.1080/17425247.2016.1218460

Than A, Liu C, Chang H, Duong PK, Cheung CMG, Xu C, Wang X, Chen P (2018) Self-implantable double-layered micro-drug-reservoirs for efficient and controlled ocular drug delivery. Nat Commun 9:1–12. https://doi.org/10.1038/s41467-018-06981-w

Truong-Le V, Lovalenti PM, Abdul-Fattah AM (2015) Stabilization challenges and formulation strategies associated with oral biologic drug delivery systems. Adv Drug Deliv Rev 93:95–108. https://doi.org/10.1016/j.addr.2015.08.001

Turner JG, White LR, Estrela P, Leese HS (2021) Hydrogel-forming microneedles: current advancements and future trends. Macromol Biosci 21. https://doi.org/10.1002/mabi.202000307

Waghule T, Singhvi G, Dubey SK, Pandey MM, Gupta G, Singh M, Dua K (2019) Microneedles: a smart approach and increasing potential for transdermal drug delivery system. Biomed Pharmacother 109:1249–1258. https://doi.org/10.1016/j.biopha.2018.10.078

Wang Z, Yang Z, Jiang J, Shi Z, Mao Y, Qin N, Tao TH (2022) Silk microneedle patch capable of on-demand multidrug delivery to the brain for glioblastoma treatment. Adv Mater 34. https://doi.org/10.1002/adma.202106606

Wu XM, Todo H, Sugibayashi K (2007) Enhancement of skin permeation of high molecular compounds by a combination of microneedle pretreatment and iontophoresis. J Control Release 118:189–195. https://doi.org/10.1016/j.jconrel.2006.12.017

Wu Y, Vora LK, Wang Y, Adrianto MF, Tekko IA, Waite D, Donnelly RF, Thakur RRS (2021) Long-acting nanoparticle-loaded bilayer microneedles for protein delivery to the posterior segment of the eye. Eur J Pharm Biopharm 165:306–318. https://doi.org/10.1016/j.ejpb.2021.05.022

Yan W, Hsiao VKS, Zheng YB, Shariff YM, Gao T, Huang TJ (2009) Towards nanoporous polymer thin film-based drug delivery systems. Thin Solid Films 517:1794–1798. https://doi.org/10.1016/j.tsf.2008.09.080

Zaric M, Lyubomska O, Touzelet O, Poux C, Al-Zahrani S, Fay F, Wallace L, Terhorst D, Malissen B, Henri S, Power UF, Scott CJ, Donnelly RF, Kissenpfennig A (2013) Skin dendritic cell targeting via microneedle arrays laden with antigen-encapsulated poly-D, l-lactide-co-glycolide nanoparticles induces efficient antitumor and antiviral immune responses. ACS Nano. https://doi.org/10.1021/nn304235j

Advances in Vaccine Adjuvants: Nanomaterials and Small Molecules

Bingbing Sun, Min Li, Zhiying Yao, Ge Yu, and Yubin Ma

Contents

Abstract

Adjuvants have been extensively and essentially formulated in subunits and certain inactivated vaccines for enhancing and prolonging protective immunity against infections and diseases. According to the types of infectious diseases and the required immunity, adjuvants with various acting mechanisms have been designed and applied in human vaccines. In this chapter, we introduce the advances in vaccine adjuvants based on nanomaterials and small molecules. By reviewing the immune mechanisms induced by adjuvants with different characteristics, we aim to establish structure–activity relationships between the physicochemical properties of adjuvants and their immunostimulating capability

B. Sun (✉) · M. Li · Z. Yao · G. Yu · Y. Ma
State Key Laboratory of Fine Chemicals, School of Chemical Engineering and Frontiers Science Center for Smart Materials Oriented Chemical Engineering, Dalian University of Technology, Dalian, China
e-mail: bingbingsun@dlut.edu.cn

M. Schäfer-Korting, U. S. Schubert (eds.), *Drug Delivery and Targeting*,
Handbook of Experimental Pharmacology 284, https://doi.org/10.1007/164_2023_652

for the development of adjuvants for more effective preventative and therapeutic vaccines.

Keywords

Adjuvant · Aluminum · Physicochemical property · STING agonist · Structure–activity relationship · Toll-like receptor agonist

Abbreviations

AAHPs	Amorphous aluminum hydroxyphosphate nanoparticles
AAHS	Amorphous aluminum hydroxyphosphate sulfate
AlOOH	Aluminum oxyhydroxide
APC	Antigen presenting cell
CD	Cluster of differentiation
CpG	Cytosine-phosphodiester-guanine
DC	Dendritic cell
FDA	Food and Drug Administration
HAP	Hydroxyapatite
HBsAg	Hepatitis B surface antigen
HIV	Human immunodeficiency virus
HPV	Human papillomavirus
IFN-γ	Interferon-γ
IgG	Immunoglobulin G
IL	Interleukin
LNPs	Lipid nanoparticles
LPS	Lipopolysaccharide
mRNA	Messenger ribonucleic acids
NLRP3	NOD-like receptor thermal protein domain associated protein 3
NR	Nanorice
ODNs	Oligodeoxynucleotides
OVA	Ovalbumin
Poly(I:C)	Polyriboinosinic acid-polyribocytidylic acid
RBD	Receptor-binding domain
SARS-CoV-2	Severe acute respiratory syndrome coronavirus 2
STING	Stimulator of interferon genes
Th1	Type 1 T helper
Th2	Type 2 T helper
TLR	Toll-like receptor
TNF-α	Tumor necrosis factor-α
VLPs	Virus-like particles
WHO	World Health Organization

1 Introduction

Prophylactic vaccination is the most powerful tool for the prevention and further control of pandemic of infectious diseases. WHO statistics show that with the increase of the coverage rate of preventive vaccination year by year, the global cases of infectious diseases, e.g., measles, diphtheria, pertussis, tetanus, rubella, etc., are decreasing (Immunization Dashboard n.d.). Depending on the types of antigens, various vaccine platforms have been developed, including antigen protein-based vaccines such as traditional inactivated and attenuated live vaccines, subunit vaccines and virus-like particle vaccines, as well as genetic material-based vaccines, e.g., DNA vaccines, mRNA vaccines, and viral vector vaccines (Dai and Gao 2021). Among these, pure antigen-based vaccines such as subunit and recombinant protein vaccines exhibit higher safety records; however, their immunogenicity has been compromised (Pollet et al. 2021). In order to improve the immunogenicity of antigens and save antigens, adjuvants are required to be formulated in vaccines. With decades of studies and applications, various adjuvants such as aluminum salt-based adjuvants, oil-in-water adjuvants, Toll-like receptor (TLR) agonists, etc., have been formulated in approved human vaccines (Shi et al. 2019). Additionally, adjuvants with more potent adjuvanticity have been examined extensively in pre-clinical or clinical studies (Sun and Xia 2016). In this review, we aim to introduce recent advances in vaccine adjuvants, including nanomaterials and small molecules. Moreover, we discuss structure–activity relationships (SARs) between the characteristics of adjuvants and their adjuvanticity, which would facilitate the rational design of more robust vaccine adjuvants.

2 Nanomaterials as Adjuvants

2.1 Aluminum-Based Adjuvants

Aluminum salts are the most commonly used human vaccine adjuvants with the longest history (Gregorio et al. 2008). Since potassium aluminum sulfate was reported to enhance the immunogenicity of diphtheria vaccines (Glenny 1930), aluminum salts have been utilized in human vaccines such as hepatitis B, tetanus, and diphtheria, etc. Up to now, 25 aluminum salt-containing human vaccines have been authorized by FDA (Shi et al. 2019).

Currently, three kinds of aluminum salts are used as adjuvants for licensed human vaccines (Shi et al. 2019). Aluminum hydroxide adjuvants form needle-like nanoparticles and are characterized as aluminum oxyhydroxide (AlOOH) (Sun and Xia 2016). Aluminum phosphate adjuvants are determined as amorphous aluminum hydroxyphosphate, $Al(OH)_m(PO_4)_n$ (Liang et al. 2021), forming a network of platy nanoparticles. Amorphous aluminum hydroxyphosphate sulfate (AAHS; $Al(OH)_x(PO_4)_y(SO_4)_z$) forms nanomeshes (Caulfield et al. 2007). In addition to the morphology, the surface charge is another important difference due to the different chemical compositions of the various aluminum salts. Aluminum hydroxide carries positive charges, aluminum phosphate has the opposite charges, and AAHS adjuvant is almost electrically neutral in physiological conditions (HogenEsch et al. 2018).

Aluminum salts can trigger Type 2 T helper (Th2)-biased immunity with no or minimum Type 1 T helper (Th1)-mediated immune responses. However, the poorly controlled physicochemical characteristics of aluminum salts hinder detailed mechanistic studies determining their immunological effects (Sun et al. 2013). A library of AlOOH nanoparticles with different shapes, crystalline properties, and hydroxyl contents was prepared to evaluate the effect of these properties on their capability to activate the NOD-like receptor thermal protein domain associated protein 3 (NLRP3) inflammasome and further antigen-specific immune responses. The in vitro study showed that AlOOH nanorods with higher hydroxyl content and lower crystallinity efficiently activate the NLRP3 inflammasome and stimulate IL-1β secretion. In the in vivo *ovalbumin (OVA)* model, AlOOH nanorods with higher hydroxyl content elicited higher OVA-specific IgG_1 titers. AlOOH nanoparticles (about 112 nm) and microparticles (about 9.3 μm) were established for comparing the effect of particle size of AlOOH on their immunostimulating capability (Li et al. 2014). Nano-sized particles triggered a stronger and more durable antigen-specific immune response in *OVA* and *Bacillus anthracis antigen* models, which was partially attributed to enhanced antigen adsorption, improved antigen uptake, and stronger NLRP3 inflammasome activation (Ruwona et al. 2016). Furthermore, a library of engineered aluminum oxyhydroxide nanorods with well-defined aspect ratios (the ratios of the length to the diameter of materials) was designed (Fig. 1) (Liang et al. 2022). Higher aspect ratio (51 ± 14), lower surface free energy (SFE $= 32$ mJ/m^2), and more hydrophobic surface led to stronger membrane depolarization, antigen uptake, and antigen presenting cell (APC) maturation. By utilizing *hepatitis B surface antigen (HBsAg) virus-like particles (VLPs)* and *severe acute respiratory syndrome coronavirus 2 (SARS-CoV-2) receptor-binding domain (RBD)*, in vivo studies showed that higher aspect ratio mediated stronger humoral immunity with improved dendritic cell (DC) maturation and antigen trafficking into lymph nodes (LNs). It is suggested that the role of aspect ratio is critical for the modulation of adjuvanticity of AlOOH nanorods. Furthermore, a variety of AlOOH nanorods with controlled surface modification served to evaluate the effect of surface properties on the inflammatory response and immunogenicity potentiation (Sun et al. 2017). NH_2-modified AlOOH nanorods exhibited stronger capability to promote NLRP3 inflammasome activation compared with pristine and SO_3H-modified AlOOH nanorods. The in vivo study demonstrated that cationic surface modification (-NH_2) enhanced the adjuvanticity of AlOOH nanorods in *OVA antigen* model, suggesting the critical role of surface properties on the reasonable design of AlOOH adjuvants. Additionally, various amorphous aluminum hydroxyphosphate nanoparticles (AAHPs) exhibiting well-controlled surface charges were engineered to explore the interaction mechanism between AAHPs and immune cells (Fig. 2) (Liang et al. 2021). Positive charges mediated higher cell membrane perturbation, inflammatory responses, and further the immune activation compared with the negatively-charged or neutral nanoparticles. By using *Staphylococcus aureus* (*S. aureus*) recombinant proteins (*manganese ion transport*

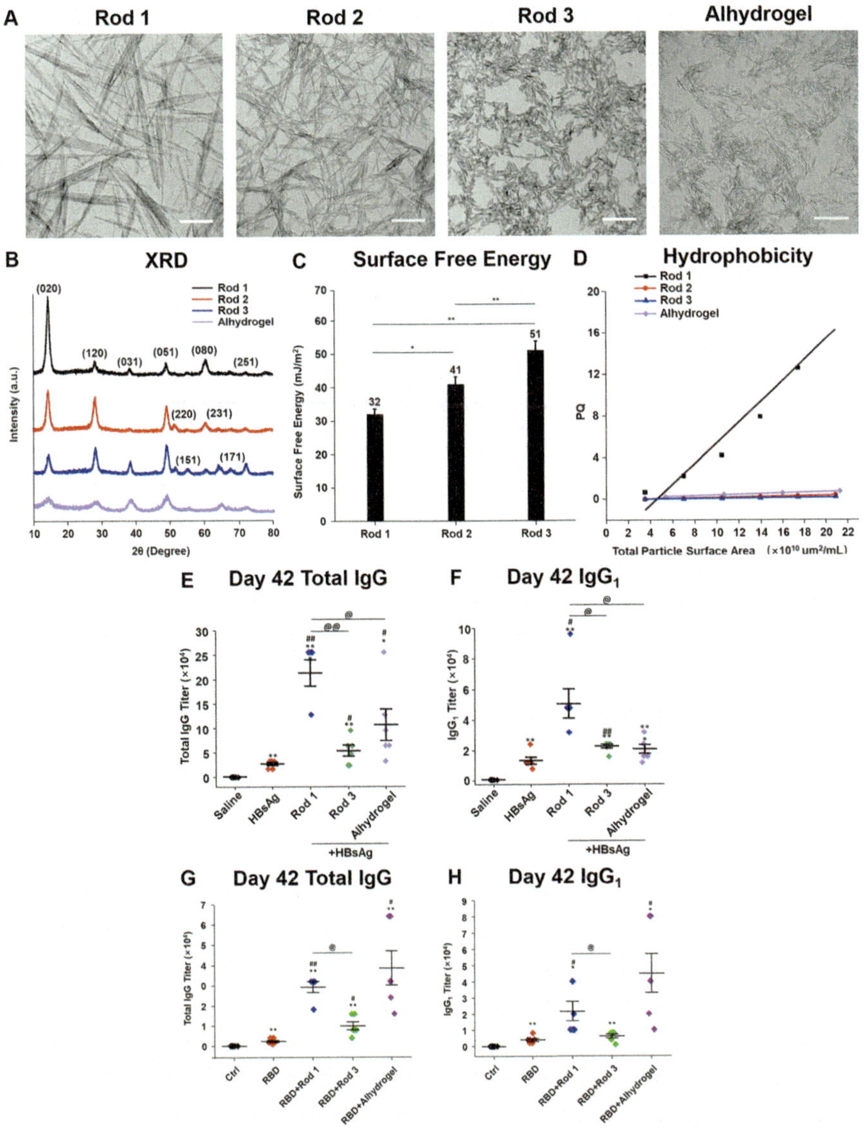

Fig. 1 The HBsAg- or RBD-specific antibody productions mediated by the physicochemical properties of engineered AlOOH nanorods. (**a**) Representative morphologies of AlOOH nanorods. The scale bar is 100 nm. (**b**) XRD spectra and (**c**) surface free energies. (**d**) Relative hydrophobicity of AlOOH nanorods. Serum HBsAg-specific (**e**) total IgG and (**f**) IgG_1 titers, and RBD-specific (**g**) total IgG and (**h**) IgG_1 titers (Liang et al. 2022) (with permission)

protein C (MntC) and *mutant staphylococcal enterotoxin B (mSEB)*), AAHP nanoadjuvant with positive charges elicited potent and durable humoral immunity, which provided the most effective protection against *S. aureus* challenge. In

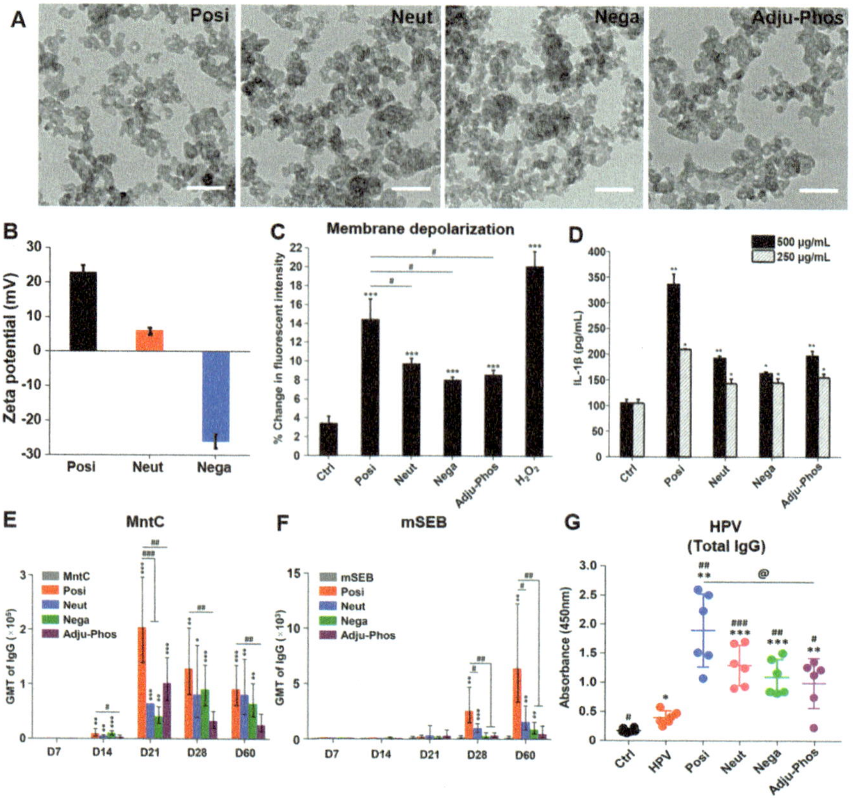

Fig. 2 The immune responses mediated by the surface charge of engineered amorphous aluminum hydroxyphosphate nanoparticles (AAHPs). The antigen models are *manganese ion transport protein C (MntC)*, *mutant staphylococcal enterotoxin B (mSEB)*, and *human papillomavirus (HPV)* antigens. (**a**) The morphologies of AAHPs with various surface charges. The scale bar is 100 nm. (**b**) Zeta potentials of AAHPs. (**c**) Membrane depolarization induced by AAHPs (250 μg/mL) in bone marrow-derived macrophages (BMDMs) for 1 h. H_2O_2 was used as a control. (**d**) IL-1β production induced by AAHPs in BMDMs for 48 h. Serum (**e**) MntC- and (**f**) mSEB-specific total IgG titers. (**g**) Serum HPV-specific total IgG production. Ctrl, saline, Posi, AAHP with positive charge, Neut, AAHP with neutral charge, Nega, AAHP with negative charge, Adju-Phos, commercial aluminum phosphate adjuvant (Liang et al. 2021) (with permission)

addition, positively-charged AAHP nanoparticles also promoted antigen-specific antibody production in the *human papillomavirus (HPV) type 18 VLP* model. Altogether, these studies suggested that the physicochemical properties of aluminum salts modulate the interaction at the nano-bio interface and determine their adjuvanticity.

Regarding the poor Th1-type immune responses, stable nanoparticles (nanoalum) were developed from commercial adjuvant Alhydrogel by using poly(acrylic acid) (PAA) polymer as a stabilizing agent to determine the effect of size and aggregate state of AlOOH on the adjuvanticity (Orr et al. 2019). In a *recombinant tuberculosis*

(TB) vaccine antigen (ID93) model, the PAA-stabilized nanoalum (PAA:nanoalum) elicited improved Th1-type immune responses including higher secretions of IFN-γ and TNF-α from $CD4^+$ T cells as well as ID93-specific IgG_{2c} titers. The in vivo results in *recombinant influenza hemagglutinin (rHA)*-immunized C57BL/6 mice demonstrated that the nanoalum provided potent immunogenicity and enhanced protective efficacy against lethal influenza compared with microparticle Alhydrogel. Therefore, engineering aluminum salt-based nanoadjuvants with well-controlled physicochemical properties facilitate the design of efficient adjuvant for human vaccines.

The depot effect, enhanced antigen presentation by APCs, NLRP3 inflammasome activation, stimulation of $CD4^+$ T cells, perturbation of DC membrane, and complement activation, have been proposed as immune-enhancing mechanisms of aluminum adjuvants. Both of them are related to the adsorption of antigens on the adjuvant, and it is believed that a large number of antigens adsorbed on aluminum adjuvants are more conducive to the exertion of immune effects (Sun and Xia 2016). WHO has required that at least 80% of antigens be adsorbed on aluminum adjuvants in *diphtheria and tetanus toxoid vaccines* (Clapp et al. 2011). Thus, the adsorption behavior of antigens on adjuvants has become a key factor that must be considered to exert the immune effect of vaccines.

The adsorption of antigens by adjuvants can be achieved through various physical or chemical effects such as electrostatic interaction, hydrophobic interaction, ligand exchange, etc. (Al-Shakhshir et al. 1995). Electrostatic interaction is a common one that occurs when adjuvants and antigens carry opposite charges. The charges of adjuvant and antigen can be determined by their isoelectric points (pI). The pI of aluminum hydroxide adjuvant and aluminum phosphate adjuvant are about 11.0 and 5.0, respectively (Al-Shakhshir et al. 1994). Therefore, at neutral pH (pH = 7.4), positively-charged aluminum hydroxide adjuvant preferentially adsorbs antigens with pI less than 7.4 and negatively-charged aluminum phosphate adjuvant preferentially adsorbs antigens with pI greater than 7.4 (Al-Shakhshir et al. 1995). The ligand exchange is the strongest interaction between aluminum adjuvants and antigens. Since phosphate binds aluminum more strongly than hydroxyl groups, phosphate can replace hydroxyl groups on the adjuvant surface to form an inner sphere surface complex with aluminum (Iyer et al. 2003). The interaction between phospholipids in *hepatitis B antigens* and aluminum adjuvants has been shown to be ligand exchange (Hansen et al. 2009). Hydrophobic interaction is the tendency of nonpolar or partially nonpolar chains, molecules, or particles to aggregate when they are immersed in water (Oss 1995). Although most of the hydrophobic residues are buried inside the proteins, there are still some hydrophobic residues on the protein surface, which may interact with adjuvants (Al-Shakhshir et al. 1995).

Regarding these different interaction mechanisms, there are many factors that affect the interaction between antigens and adjuvants, including the physicochemical properties of antigens and adjuvants, buffer compositions, etc. To enhance immunogenicity, many studies have focused on modifying antigens to modulate interactions. The *human immunodeficiency virus (HIV) envelope antigens* were modified with short peptide immunogens composed of repeated phosphoserine (pSer) residues, which promoted the binding to aluminum hydroxide through ligand exchange, and further slowed down the elimination of immunogen in the body to promote humoral immunity (Moyer et al. 2020). *RBD immunogen of SARS-CoV-2* was modified with free cysteine by pSer peptide, which effectively promoted binding to alum and delayed antigen clearance, resulting in significant germinal center responses and neutralizing antibody titers in mice (Rodrigues et al. 2021). Phosphate treatment of AlOOH adjuvants attenuated ligand exchange with *HBsAg* and *HIV 1 gp140 antigens*, reducing antigen adsorption strength and resulting in a stronger immune response (Hansen et al. 2009, 2011).

In recent years, nanomaterials have been extensively utilized as vaccine adjuvants and can achieve optimal immunogenicity by engineering their physicochemical properties (Liang et al. 2022). Similarly, the well-controlled properties of engineered nanomaterials are also suitable for screening vaccine formulations in a systematic fashion. AlOOH nanorods were engineered to establish adsorption isotherms with *HBsAg*, *RBD*, *bovine serum albumin (BSA)* and *OVA* (Yu et al. 2022). The adsorptive capacity of the antigen was related to the specific surface area of AlOOH, and the adsorptive strength was related to the surface hydroxyl content. In addition, higher surface hydroxyl content is more likely to cause destabilization of the absorbed antigen. A series of self-assembled rice-like AlOOH nanoparticles (nanorices, NRs) with low surface free energy (SFE) was engineered to improve the suspension stability of vaccine formulations (Fig. 3) (Bi et al. 2022). After

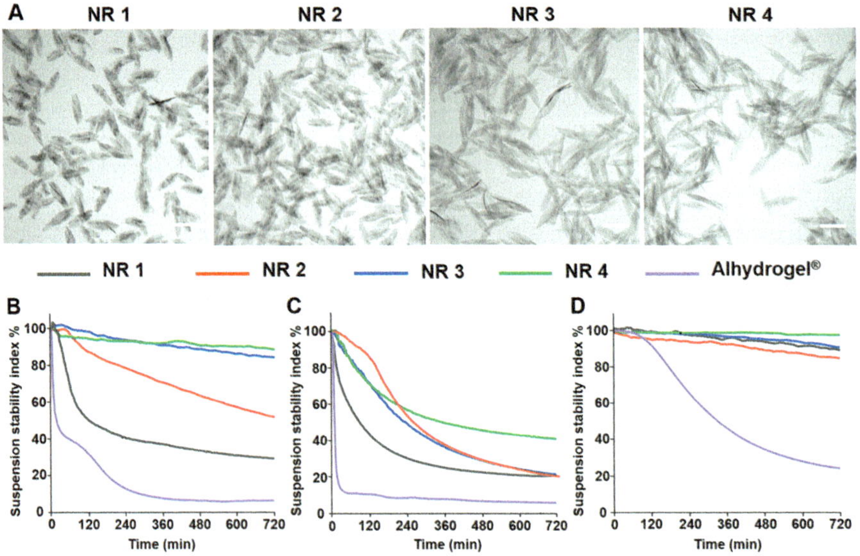

Fig. 3 The morphologies and suspension stability indexes of AlOOH nanorices (NRs). (**a**) Morphologies of NRs. The scale bar is 500 nm. Suspension stability indexes of (**b**) NR-HBsAg VLP, (**c**) NR-HPV VLP, and (**d**) NR-BSA complexes in 30 mM of NaCl within 12 h were determined by aggregation analysis via UV-vis absorption spectroscopy (Bi et al. 2022) (with permission)

adsorbing *HBsAg VLPs*, *HPV VLPs* and *BSA*, complexes of NRs and antigens showed higher stability compared to Alhydrogel-antigen complexes.

2.2 Other Inorganic Nanomaterials

Due to the lack of cellular immune response induced by alum-based nanoadjuvants, inorganic nanomaterials with efficient adjuvanticity, e.g., calcium phosphate, silica-based nanoparticles, and metal-based nanomaterials, have been studied as adjuvant candidates (Lin et al. 2017; Yang et al. 2017a; Wang et al. 2021a).

Calcium phosphate had been formulated in the *diphtheria-tetanus-pertussis vaccines* in France (Lin et al. 2017). Compared with alum-based adjuvants, calcium phosphate triggers more balanced humoral and cellular immune responses (Zhang et al. 2021a). Hydroxyapatite (HAP) is the most stable form of calcium phosphate with higher immunostimulation potentials (Lange et al. 2009). HAP nanoparticles with a diameter of 100–400 nm induced higher levels of *OVA*-specific IgG titer than smaller and larger ones (Hayashi et al. 2016). Small needle-shaped nanoparticles induced a stronger inflammatory response compared with larger-sized spherical HAP particles (Lebre et al. 2017). In addition, a variety of HAP nanospheres and nanorods were prepared to systematically study the relationship between aspect ratio of HAP and immunity (Fig. 4) (Zhang et al. 2021a). HAP nanorods with higher aspect ratio (19 ± 7) mediated higher antibody productions, IFN-γ release, and CD107α expression on CD8$^+$ T cells in the *HBsAg* model. A higher aspect ratio induced stronger cell membrane depolarization and cellular uptake, enhanced the release of cathepsin B and the production of mitochondrial reactive oxygen species, and promoted the inflammatory response. Moreover, higher aspect ratio of HAP nanorods enhanced antigen persistence and immune cell recruitments. In addition, the doping of active ingredients is regarded as a potential way to enhance adjuvanticity of HAP nanoparticles. Si-doped HAP nanorods with different Si/P molar ratios were prepared. Si doping (incorporation of Si elements into HAP nanorods during synthesis process) induced enhanced antigen delivery in LNs and further promoted Th1- and Th2-type immune responses in the *OVA* model (Wang et al. 2019).

As biocompatible and biodegradable nanomaterials, silica-based nanoparticles have been clinically used for drug delivery in the treatment of cardiovascular diseases and cancers (Janjua et al. 2021). In addition, due to their potentials to enhance immune responses, silica nanomaterials are potential candidates of both adjuvants and vaccine delivery vehicles (Yang et al. 2017a; Sun et al. 2015). The immunity induced by silica nanomaterials is determined by the physicochemical properties such as size, shape, surface charge, hydrophobicity, surface modification, etc. (Li et al. 2019; Hong et al. 2020).

Recently, a series of 80-nm mesoporous silica nanoparticles (MSNs) with various pore sizes were developed to explore the influence of pore size of MSNs on the immunogenicity of silica-adjuvanted vaccines (Hong et al. 2020). Larger pores elicited higher cross-presentation of *OVA* antigens and promoted lymph node

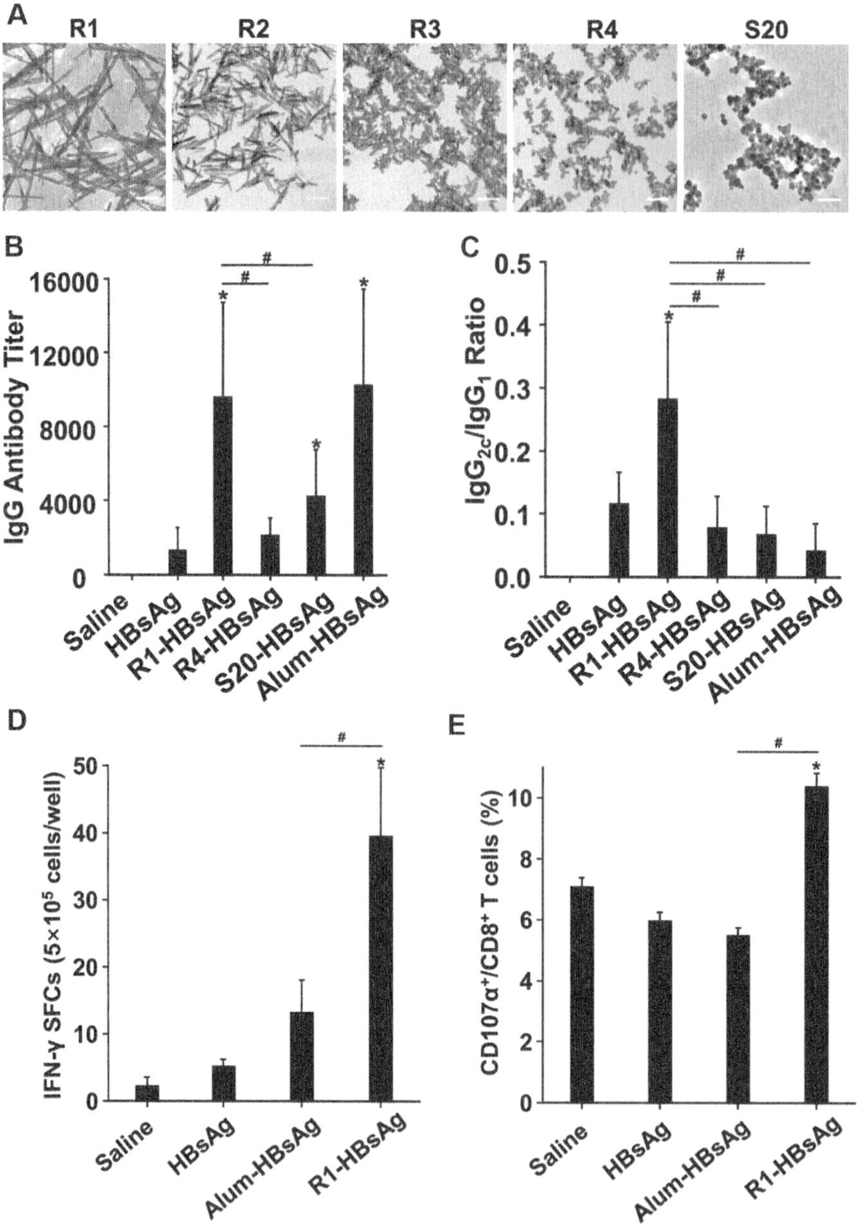

Fig. 4 The HBsAg-specific humoral and cellular immunity induced by HAP nanoparticles with various aspect ratios. (**a**) Morphologies of HAP nanorods. The scale bar is 150 nm. (**b**) Serum HBsAg-specific total IgG titer. (**c**) IgG_{2c}/IgG_1 ratio of treated mice. (**d**) Statistic figures of IFN-γ spot-forming cells (SFCs). (**e**) CD107α expression on $CD8^+$ T cells (Zhang et al. 2021a) (with permission)

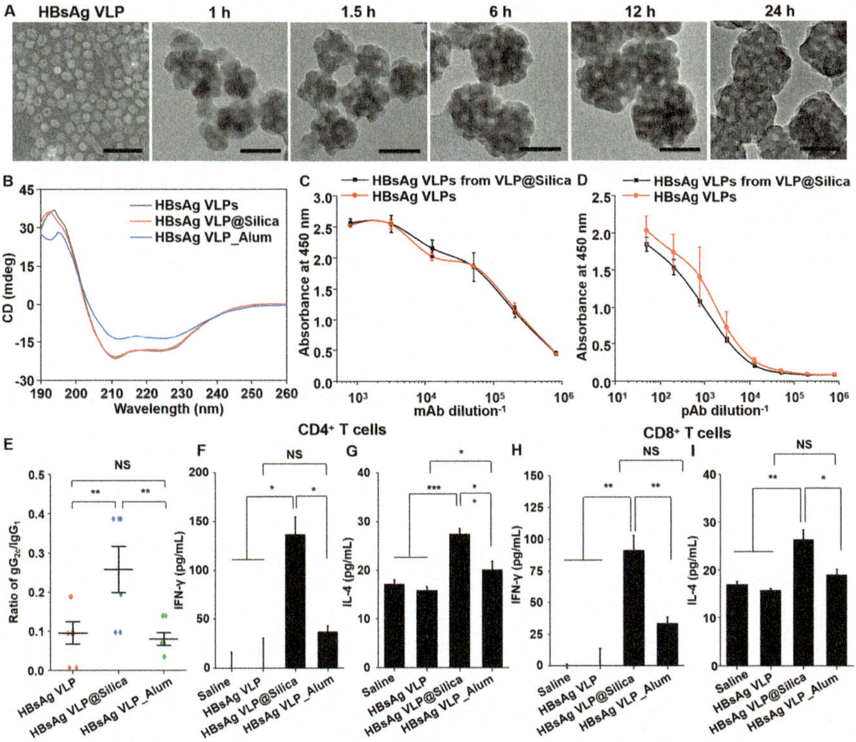

Fig. 5 Raspberry-like VLP@Silica vaccine templated with HBsAg VLPs enhances humoral and cellular immunity. (**a**) The synthesis dynamics of HBsAg VLP@Silica nanoparticles. The scale bar is 100 nm. (**b**) The circular dichromatic spectra of HBsAg VLP@Silica, HBsAg VLP_Alum and HBsAg VLPs. The affinity of (**c**) monoclonal antibody (mAb) and (**d**) polyclonal antibody (pAb) for eluted HBsAg VLPs from VLP@Silica. (**e**) The ratios of HBsAg-specific IgG_{2c} to IgG_1. The productions of (**f, h**) IFN-γ and (**g, i**) IL-4 by HBsAg-stimulated (**f, g**) $CD4^+$ and (**h, i**) $CD8^+$ T cells (Li et al. 2022) (with permission)

targeting and immune activation. *HBsAg VLPs* and *HPV 18 VLPs* served as biotemplates to prepare raspberry-like self-assembling silica-adjuvanted nanovaccines (VLP@Silica) for inducing balanced humoral and cellular immunities compared with alum-adjuvanted vaccines (Fig. 5) (Li et al. 2022). Both HBsAg VLP@Silica and HPV VLP@Silica improved antigen-specific antibody titer levels and T cell-mediated immunity in vivo. Lysosomal escape and cytosolic delivery of antigens, Th1- and Th2-type cytokine productions in bone marrow-derived dendritic cells (BMDCs) were induced and APC activation and migration into LNs were promoted compared with alum group. $-NH_2$ and $-C_{18}$ groups were modified on the surface of mesoporous silica nanorods (MSNRs) for evaluating the effect of silica surface groups on their adjuvanticity (Yang et al. 2017a). MSNRs modified with hydrophobic $-C_{18}$ induced the most efficient antigen uptake and endosomal-lysosomal escape, and elicited highest IFN-γ secretion and antibody release in

OVA-immunized mice. Moreover, bare MSNRs and MSNR-NH_2 showed Th2-biased (humoral) immune responses, while MSNR-C_{18} exhibited Th1-biased immune responses, suggesting the profound effect of surface functional groups of nanoadjuvants on the immune responses. In addition, binuclear aluminum complex was used to modify dendritic mesoporous silica nanoparticles (DMSNs) to form aluminosilicate (AS) materials (Yang et al. 2020). The modification of high-density ^{VI}Al-OH enhanced endosome escape and cellular immunity of AS in the *OVA* model. In addition, ^{VI}Al-OH-modified AS with positive charges promoted antigen loading, minimized aggregation, and improved cellular uptake.

Additionally, many other inorganic nanomaterials, e.g., Mn, Zn, Au, and Ag-based nanomaterials, etc., have been studied as adjuvants (Sun and Xia 2016; Wang et al. 2021a; Roy et al. 2014). A colloidal manganese salt (MnJ) was prepared as an immune potentiator to induce humoral and cellular immune responses (Zhang et al. 2021b). Further mechanistic study demonstrated that Mn^{2+} enhanced uptake and presentation of antigens, and further formed germinal center with activation of both NLRP3 and cGAS-STING pathways. Cubic manganese oxide nanoparticles with negative charges were formulated as adjuvants into *SARS-CoV-2 RBD*-based nanovaccines to induce humoral and cellular immunity (Wang et al. 2021a). RBD antigen and manganese oxide adjuvant were efficiently co-delivered into LNs, which promoted cellular uptake and immune cell activations. In mice model, the vaccine enhanced neutralizing of the pseudovirus and live coronavirus infection compared to alum-adjuvanted RBD vaccine.

2.3 Organic Nanofibers

In recent studies, also nanofibers have been shown to promote antigen presentation, activate the $CD8^+$ T cells response, and trigger humoral and cellular immune responses (Rudra et al. 2018). A series of nanofibers based on *Q11 peptides (epitope-bearing peptides of OVA)* with various surface charges were synthesized to investigate the effect of surface property on their immunogenicity (Wen et al. 2016). Positive surface charges provided by residues of amine acids promoted the uptake of nanofibers by APCs in vitro and maintained their ability to raise T cell and B cell immune responses in vivo. Negatively-charged surface of Q11 nanofibers prevented antigen-specific antibody production and T cell-mediated immunity in vivo, suggesting the requirement of avoiding excessive negative charges in peptide nanofiber-based vaccine design. Nanofibers based on flagellin proteins from *Bacillus subtilis* with different aspect ratios (the ratios of the length to the diameter of nanofibers) were prepared (Cote-Cyr et al. 2022). Flagellin ring-like nanofibers with low aspect ratio (around 1) were efficiently internalized by APCs and significantly stimulated TLR5, which promoted innate and adaptive immunities. In intranasal immunized mice, flagellin nanofibers carrying *antigen peptides from influenza A virus* enhanced antibody responses and immune protection against the lethal infection, illustrating the potential of flagellin nanofibers as antigen carriers. In addition, a series of flagella nanofibers with controlled lengths was prepared to explore length-dependent immune stimulating potentials (Fu et al. 2022). Intranasal administration of shorter nanofiber-adjuvanted *HPV* vaccines induced enhanced cellular responses to significantly inhibit tumor growth and increase survival rates in a cervical cancer model. Thus, the design of nanofiber-based adjuvants with specific properties can facilitate the enhancement of the immunogenicity of vaccines for disease prevention and treatment (O'Neill et al. 2021).

2.4 Pickering Emulsions

Pickering emulsions are emulsions stabilized by solid nano- or micro-particles accumulating at the interface between oil and water phases (Yang et al. 2017b). In comparison to traditional surfactant-stabilized emulsion adjuvants, Pickering emulsions have higher stability against coalescence, thus they are potential adjuvants and vaccine carriers. Various solid nanoparticles with good biocompatibility and adjuvanticity, e.g., alum, hydroxyapatite, silica and chitosan, etc., are used as stabilizers to improve the immunostimulating activity of Pickering emulsions and induce robust immune responses (Yang et al. 2017b). Recently, a PLGA particle-stabilized Pickering emulsion adjuvant system (PPAS) with high pliability, lateral mobility, biosafety and antigen-loading capabilities was developed to enhance immunity of vaccines (Xia et al. 2018). Pliable PPAS loading *OVA* enhanced antigen uptake and lysosome escape in vitro and promoted cell recruitment, activation of APCs, and migration into LNs in vivo. PPAS-adjuvanted OVA vaccine induced enhanced humoral and cellular immunities. When challenged with an intranasal lethal dose of influenza A virus (50 times of half lethal dose), PPAS-adjuvanted *influenza A hemagglutinin (HA)* vaccination increased the survival rate of mice. An alum-stabilized Pickering emulsion (PAPE) for improved T cell-mediated immune responses adsorbs numerous *SARS-CoV-2 RBD* antigens and promotes DC uptake and cross-presentation of RBD (Peng et al. 2020). As a result, PAPE adjuvant elicited enhanced antibody titer and IFN-γ-secreting T cells compared to the alum-adjuvanted group, suggesting more robust humoral and cellular immunities induced by PAPE adjuvanted vaccine.

3 Small Molecules as Adjuvants

3.1 TLR Agonists

Toll-like receptors (TLRs) are one of the pathogen recognition receptors (PRRs) stimulated by pathogen-associated molecular patterns including pathogen-specific carbohydrates, lipoproteins, or nucleic acids (Scheiermann and Klinman 2014). TLR activation mediates and maintains innate and adaptive immune responses, as well as memory immunity (Schmidlin et al. 2009). Thus, TLR agonists have been studied extensively as adjuvant candidates to induce protective immunity against infections and diseases.

Cytosine-phosphodiester-guanine (CpG) oligodeoxynucleotides (ODNs) are short single-stranded DNA molecules, which possess a phosphorothioate backbone and unmethylated CpG motifs (Scheiermann and Klinman 2014). They are recognized by TLR9 expressed in the endo-lysosomal compartments of immune cells such as B cells and APCs to induce pro-inflammatory cytokine production and robust immunostimulation (Shi et al. 2019). As efficient adjuvants, CpG ODNs trigger strong humoral and cellular immunities, supported by enhanced antibody titers and cytotoxic T lymphocyte generation (Shi et al. 2019). Clinical studies revealed that the inclusion of CpG ODN in *HBsAg* vaccination elicited more rapid and higher protective antibody titers in comparison to alum (Campbell 2017). Moreover, CpG ODNs induced improved Th1-type immune responses compared with Th2-biased immune responses mediated by traditional aluminum salt-based adjuvants (Klinman 2004). The *anthrax* vaccine adjuvanted by CpG ODN elicited significantly improved and accelerated systemic protection (Klinman et al. 2007). In 2017, CpG ODN 1018-containing *hepatitis B* vaccine, HEPLISAV-B, was approved by FDA (Campbell 2017). Additionally, CpG ODNs with Th1-biased immunity were used to re-direct Th2-biased immunity induced by other adjuvants including aluminum adjuvant and Freund's incomplete adjuvant (Weeratna et al. 2000). For example, the *diphtheria-tetanus-pertussis (DTP)* vaccine adjuvanted with alum (DTP-alum) promotes Th2-type responses (Sugai et al. 2005). In contrast, the inclusion of CpG ODN in this vaccine (DTP-alum/ODN) generated a shift toward balanced Th1/Th2 immune responses. Recently, CpG ODNs encapsulated by lipid nanoparticles (LNPs) were prepared to enhance immune responses (Shirai et al. 2019). LNPs carrying CpG ODNs (LNP-CpGs) induced mouse DC activation with higher cytokine productions including IL-12 and IFN-α. In mice immunized by *influenza A virus split vaccines (SV)*, LNP-CpGs promoted T cell-mediated immunity and induced enhanced SV-specific and heterologous-virus-strain-specific IgG_{2c} responses compared with CpG ODN and alum groups. Additionally, SV plus LNP-CpGs enhanced protective immune responses against homologous, heterologous, and heterosubtypic stain challenges, suggesting more robust and broad immune protection against influenza virus.

Moreover, due to the ability to trigger strong cellular responses, CpG ODNs are utilized as adjuvants in therapeutic vaccines. ODNs with class C unmethylated CpG (CpG-C) motifs enhance immunity against the chronic infection of *Hepatitis B virus (HBV)* (Zhao et al. 2022). Anti-HBV vaccine adjuvanted by CpG-C ODN promoted DC maturation and overcame immune tolerance as well as T cell exhaustion. The vaccine induced enhanced and long-lasting hepatic HBV-specific cellular immunity with improved cellular proliferation and IFN-γ production, suggesting a promising candidate for chronic hepatitis B therapeutic vaccine.

Polyriboinosinic acid-polyribocytidylic acid, Poly(I:C), is artificial double-stranded RNA (Martins et al. 2015). After binding with TLR3, Poly(I:C) activates transcription factors such as nuclear factor-κB (NF-κB) and interferon regulatory factor 3 (IRF3), and induces the transcription of cytokines, e.g., INF-α, INF-β, IL-12 and IL-6. Poly(I:C) can be also recognized by intracellular melanoma differentiation-associated protein 5 (MDA-5) and retinoic acid-inducible gene I

(RIG-I) to mediate the transcriptions of type I IFNs and proinflammatory cytokines. Thus, Poly(I:C) has been a potent adjuvant candidate for vaccine formulations. However, rapid degradation and systemic toxicities of Poly(I:C) prevent clinical use (Hafner et al. 2013). Establishment of suitable delivery systems such as emulsions, cationic liposomes, solid nanoparticles, and microspheres for carrying Poly(I:C) adjuvant is a promising strategy to protect antigens and adjuvants, efficiently deliver them to APCs and induce enhanced innate and adaptive immune responses (Gale et al. 2019).

3'-O-deacylated monophosphoryl lipid A (MPL) is a chemically modified lipopolysaccharide, which has a similar immunostimulatory activity to lipopolysaccharide (LPS) and greatly reduced toxicity (Wang et al. 2020a). Recognized by TLR4, MPL activates APCs and B cells and further sensitizes naive T cells, suggesting the capability to induce Th1- and Th2-type immunities (Becker et al. 2000). Moreover, MPL mediates antigen-specific immune responses by promoting the migration and maturation of DCs. In combination with other immunostimulants, a higher protective efficiency against infections is proved (Ulrich and Myers 1995). AS04 is a combination adjuvant composed of alum and MPL. It has been formulated in *human Papillomavirus bivalent vaccine*, CERVARIX, in 2009 (Cervarix n.d.). In addition, AS01b, a liposome-based formulation with MPL and QS-21 (an immunostimulatory saponin), was formulated in an FDA-approved *recombinant zoster vaccine*, Shingrix, in 2017 (Shi et al. 2019), triggering strong and persistent humoral and cellular immune responses (Vandepapeliere et al. 2008).

3.2 mRNA

Messenger ribonucleic acids (mRNA) are single-stranded RNA molecules (Kwon et al. 2022), which are recognized by various PRRs including TLR3, TLR7, and TLR8 to induce potent immunostimulation (Heil et al. 2004; Kariko et al. 2004). However, the poor stability of mRNA molecules in solution and in vivo decreases the efficiency of mRNA-based vaccines. Delivery systems, e.g., lipid nanoparticles (LNPs), polymers, peptides, virus-like replicon particles and emulsions, reduce mRNA degradation and trigger effective humoral and cellular immunities (Pardi et al. 2015; Wang et al. 2021b). Due to the dual roles of transiently encoding immunogenic antigens and self-adjuvant of mRNA molecules, mRNA vaccines stabilized and delivered by LNPs have enabled the approval of COVID-19 vaccines containing mRNAs encoding *SARS-CoV-2* (Moderna COVID-19 Vaccines n.d.; Pfizer-BioNTech COVID-19 Vaccines n.d.).

3.3 STING Agonists

Stimulator of interferon genes (STING) is an important protein in innate immunity, which is activated directly by cyclic dinucleotides (CDNs) as a PRR at endoplasmic reticulum (ER) to trigger Th1-type immune responses (Herck et al. 2021). Thus, the

CDN-based STING agonists including cyclic dimeric guanosine monophosphate (c-di-GMP), cyclic dimeric adenosine monophosphate (c-di-AMP), and 2′,3′-cyclic guanosine monophosphate-adenosine monophosphate (cGAMP) are widely studied as vaccine adjuvants (Herck et al. 2021). Recently, pulmonary surfactant (PS)-biomimetic liposomes encapsulating cGAMP (PS-cGAMP) were formulated as adjuvants in intranasal vaccines (Wang et al. 2020b), which transiently mediated strong innate immunity in lung. PS-cGAMP-adjuvanted *influenza* vaccines elicited robust humoral and cellular immunity in vivo. In H1N1 vaccine-immunized C57BL/6 mice, PS-cGAMP elicited cross-protection against heterosubtypic viruses including H3N2, H5N1, and H7N9 for more than half a year. Capsid-like hollow polymeric nanoparticles loading *MERS-CoV RBD* antigens and STING agonists c-di-GMP (RBD-NP(cdGMP)) were synthesized to elicit safe and effective immunity against MERS-CoV (Lin et al. 2019). The in vitro and in vivo studies showed that the viromimetic particles RBD-NP(cdGMP) promoted cellular uptake of antigens and STING agonists and further delivery into LNs. In immunized mice, RBD-specific humoral and cellular immunities were enhanced and prolonged. In a MERS-CoV-permissive transgenic mouse model, MERS-CoV vaccine induced protective immunity against MERS-CoV challenges. In addition to cyclic dinucleotides, some non-nucleotide small molecule alternatives, e.g., 5,6-dimethylxanthenone-4-acetic acid, 10-carboxymethyl-9-acridanone, and diamidobenzimidazole, are studied as STING agonists to induce enhanced and prolonged immune responses (Herck et al. 2021).

4 Conclusion

Current research will promote the establishment of structure–activity relationships between adjuvant properties and their adjuvanticity, enhance our understanding of the action mechanisms of adjuvants, and further facilitate the design of ideal engineered nanoadjuvants to improve the efficacy of vaccines. These new adjuvant candidates are expected to promote the next generation of adjuvanted vaccines. Thus, the structure–activity relationships of adjuvants and the immunogenicity, stability and biosafety of vaccines will facilitate the development of more effective preventative and therapeutic vaccines.

Acknowledgments This work was supported by the National Natural Science Foundation of China (U22A20455), National Key Research and Development Program of China (2022YFC2304305), Dalian Science and Technology Innovation Fund (2020JJ25CY015), and Fundamental Research Funds for the Central Universities (DUT21ZD216, DUT22LAB601, and DUT22QN225).

References

Al-Shakhshir R, Regnier F, White JL et al (1994) Effect of protein adsorption on the surface charge characteristics of aluminium-containing adjuvants. Vaccine 12:472–474

Al-Shakhshir RH, Regnier FE, White JL et al (1995) Contribution of electrostatic and hydrophobic interactions to the adsorption of proteins by aluminium-containing adjuvants. Vaccine 13:41–44
Becker GD, Moulin V, Pajak B et al (2000) The adjuvant monophosphoryl lipid A increases the function of antigen-presenting cells. Int Immunol 12:807–815
Bi S, Li M, Liang Z et al (2022) Self-assembled aluminum oxyhydroxide nanorices with superior suspension stability for vaccine adjuvant. J Colloid Interface Sci 627:238–246
Campbell JD (2017) Development of the CpG adjuvant 1018: a case study. Methods Mol Biol 1494:15–27
Caulfield MJ, Shi L, Wang S et al (2007) Effect of alternative aluminum adjuvants on the absorption and immunogenicity of HPV16 L1 VLPs in mice. Hum Vaccin 3:139–145
Cervarix (n.d.). https://www.fda.gov/vaccines-blood-biologics/vaccines/cervarix. Accessed 14 Oct 2022
Clapp T, Siebert P, Chen D et al (2011) Vaccines with aluminum-containing adjuvants: optimizing vaccine efficacy and thermal stability. J Pharm Sci 100:388–401
Cote-Cyr M, Zottig X, Gauthier L et al (2022) Self-assembly of flagellin into immunostimulatory ring-like nanostructures as an antigen delivery system. ACS Biomater Sci Eng 8:694–707
Dai L, Gao GF (2021) Viral targets for vaccines against COVID-19. Nat Rev Immunol 21:73–82
Fu D, Wang M, Yang T et al (2022) Self-assembled flagella protein nanofibers induce enhanced mucosal immunity. Biomaterials 288:121733
Gale EC, Roth GA, Smith AAA et al (2019) A nanoparticle platform for improved potency, stability, and adjuvanticity of poly(I:C). Adv Ther 3
Glenny AT (1930) Insoluble precipitates in diphtheria and tetanus immunization. Br Med J 2:244–245
Gregorio ED, Tritto E, Rappuoli R (2008) Alum adjuvanticity: unraveling a century old mystery. Eur J Immunol 38:2068–2071
Hafner AM, Corthesy B, Merkle HP (2013) Particulate formulations for the delivery of poly(I:C) as vaccine adjuvant. Adv Drug Deliv Rev 65:1386–1399
Hansen B, Belfast M, Soung G et al (2009) Effect of the strength of adsorption of hepatitis B surface antigen to aluminum hydroxide adjuvant on the immune response. Vaccine 27:888–892
Hansen B, Malyala P, Singh M et al (2011) Effect of the strength of adsorption of HIV 1 SF162dV2gp140 to aluminum-containing adjuvants on the immune response. J Pharm Sci 100:3245–3250
Hayashi M, Aoshi T, Kogai Y et al (2016) Optimization of physiological properties of hydroxyapatite as a vaccine adjuvant. Vaccine 34:306–312
Heil F, Hemmi H, Hochrein H et al (2004) Species-specific recognition of single-stranded RNA via toll-like receptor 7 and 8. Science 303:1526–1529
Herck SV, Feng B, Tang L (2021) Delivery of STING agonists for adjuvanting subunit vaccines. Adv Drug Deliv Rev 179:114020
HogenEsch H, O'Hagan DT, Fox CB (2018) Optimizing the utilization of aluminum adjuvants in vaccines: you might just get what you want. NPJ Vaccines 3:51
Hong X, Zhong X, Du G et al (2020) The pore size of mesoporous silica nanoparticles regulates their antigen delivery efficiency. Sci Adv 6:eaaz4462
Immunization Dashboard (n.d.). https://immunizationdata.who.int/. Accessed 14 Oct 2022
Iyer S, HogenEsch H, Hem SL (2003) Effect of the degree of phosphate substitution in aluminum hydroxide adjuvant on the adsorption of phosphorylated proteins. Pharm Dev Technol 8:81–86
Janjua TI, Cao Y, Yu C et al (2021) Clinical translation of silica nanoparticles. Nat Rev Mater 6: 1072–1074
Kariko K, Ni H, Capodici J et al (2004) mRNA is an endogenous ligand for toll-like receptor 3. J Biol Chem 279:12542–12550
Klinman DM (2004) Immunotherapeutic uses of CpG oligodeoxynucleotides. Nat Rev Immunol 4: 249–258
Klinman DM, Currie D, Lee G et al (2007) Systemic but not mucosal immunity induced by AVA prevents inhalational anthrax. Microbes Infect 9:1478–1483

Kwon S, Kwon M, Im S et al (2022) mRNA vaccines: the most recent clinical applications of synthetic mRNA. Arch Pharm Res 45:245–262

Lange T, Schilling AF, Peters F et al (2009) Proinflammatory and osteoclastogenic effects of beta-tricalciumphosphate and hydroxyapatite particles on human mononuclear cells in vitro. Biomaterials 30:5312–5318

Lebre F, Sridharan R, Sawkins MJ et al (2017) The shape and size of hydroxyapatite particles dictate inflammatory responses following implantation. Sci Rep 7:2922

Li X, Aldayel AM, Cui Z (2014) Aluminum hydroxide nanoparticles show a stronger vaccine adjuvant activity than traditional aluminum hydroxide microparticles. J Control Release 173: 148–157

Li M, Cheng F, Xue C et al (2019) Surface modification of Stober silica nanoparticles with controlled moiety densities determines their cytotoxicity profiles in macrophages. Langmuir 35:14688–14695

Li M, Liang Z, Chen C et al (2022) Virus-like particle-templated silica-adjuvanted nanovaccines with enhanced humoral and cellular immunity. ACS Nano 16:10482–10495

Liang Z, Yang Y, Yu G et al (2021) Engineering aluminum hydroxyphosphate nanoparticles with well-controlled surface property to enhance humoral immune responses as vaccine adjuvants. Biomaterials 275:120960

Liang Z, Wang X, Yu G et al (2022) Mechanistic understanding of the aspect ratio-dependent adjuvanticity of engineered aluminum oxyhydroxide nanorods in prophylactic vaccines. Nano Today 43:101445

Lin Y, Wang X, Huang X et al (2017) Calcium phosphate nanoparticles as a new generation vaccine adjuvant. Expert Rev Vaccines 16:895–906

Lin LC, Huang CY, Yao BY et al (2019) Viromimetic STING agonist-loaded hollow polymeric nanoparticles for safe and effective vaccination against middle east respiratory syndrome coronavirus. Adv Funct Mater 29:1807616

Martins KA, Bavari S, Salazar AM (2015) Vaccine adjuvant uses of poly-IC and derivatives. Expert Rev Vaccines 14:447–459

Moderna COVID-19 Vaccines (n.d.). https://www.fda.gov/emergency-preparedness-and-response/coronavirus-disease-2019-covid-19/moderna-covid-19-vaccines. Accessed 14 Oct 2022

Moyer TJ, Kato Y, Abraham W et al (2020) Engineered immunogen binding to alum adjuvant enhances humoral immunity. Nat Med 26:430–440

O'Neill CL, Shrimali PC, Clapacs ZP et al (2021) Peptide-based supramolecular vaccine systems. Acta Biomater 133:153–167

Orr MT, Khandhar AP, Seydoux E et al (2019) Reprogramming the adjuvant properties of aluminum oxyhydroxide with nanoparticle technology. NPJ Vaccines 4:1

Oss CJV (1995) Hydrophobic, hydrophilic and other interactions in epitope-paratope binding. Mol Immunol 32:199–211

Pardi N, Tuyishime S, Muramatsu H et al (2015) Expression kinetics of nucleoside-modified mRNA delivered in lipid nanoparticles to mice by various routes. J Control Release 217:345–351

Peng S, Cao F, Xia Y et al (2020) Particulate alum via Pickering emulsion for an enhanced COVID-19 vaccine adjuvant. Adv Mater 32:e2004210

Pfizer-BioNTech COVID-19 Vaccines (n.d.). https://www.fda.gov/emergency-preparedness-and-response/coronavirus-disease-2019-covid-19/pfizer-biontech-covid-19-vaccines. Accessed 14 Oct 2022

Pollet J, Chen WH, Strych U (2021) Recombinant protein vaccines, a proven approach against coronavirus pandemics. Adv Drug Deliv Rev 170:71–82

Rodrigues KA, Rodriguez-Aponte SA, Dalvie NC et al (2021) Phosphate-mediated coanchoring of RBD immunogens and molecular adjuvants to alum potentiates humoral immunity against SARS-CoV-2. Sci Adv 7

Roy R, Kumar S, Verma AK et al (2014) Zinc oxide nanoparticles provide an adjuvant effect to ovalbumin via a Th2 response in Balb/c mice. Int Immunol 26:159–172

Rudra JS, Banasik BN, Milligan GN (2018) A combined carrier-adjuvant system of peptide nanofibers and toll-like receptor agonists potentiates robust CD8+ T cell responses. Vaccine 36:438–441

Ruwona TB, Xu H, Li X et al (2016) Toward understanding the mechanism underlying the strong adjuvant activity of aluminum salt nanoparticles. Vaccine 34:3059–3067

Scheiermann J, Klinman DM (2014) Clinical evaluation of CpG oligonucleotides as adjuvants for vaccines targeting infectious diseases and cancer. Vaccine 32:6377–6389

Schmidlin H, Diehl SA, Blom B (2009) New insights into the regulation of human B-cell differentiation. Trends Immunol 30:277–285

Shi S, Zhu H, Xia X et al (2019) Vaccine adjuvants: understanding the structure and mechanism of adjuvanticity. Vaccine 37:3167–3178

Shirai S, Shibuya M, Kawai A et al (2019) Lipid nanoparticles potentiate CpG-oligodeoxynucleotide-based vaccine for influenza virus. Front Immunol 10:3018

Sugai T, Mori M, Nakazawa M et al (2005) A CpG-containing oligodeoxynucleotide as an efficient adjuvant counterbalancing the Th1/Th2 immune response in diphtheria-tetanus-pertussis vaccine. Vaccine 23:5450–5456

Sun B, Xia T (2016) Nanomaterial-based vaccine adjuvants. J Mater Chem B 4:5496–5509

Sun B, Ji Z, Liao YP et al (2013) Engineering an effective immune adjuvant by designed control of shape and crystallinity of aluminum oxyhydroxide nanoparticles. ACS Nano 7:10834–10849

Sun B, Pokhrel S, Dunphy DR et al (2015) Reduction of acute inflammatory effects of fumed silica nanoparticles in the lung by adjusting silanol display through calcination and metal doping. ACS Nano 9:9357–9372

Sun B, Ji Z, Liao YP et al (2017) Enhanced immune adjuvant activity of aluminum oxyhydroxide nanorods through cationic surface functionalization. ACS Appl Mater Interfaces 9:21697–21705

Ulrich JT, Myers KR (1995) Monopbospboryl lipid a as an adjuvant, vol 6. Springer, Boston

Vandepapeliere P, Horsmans Y, Moris P et al (2008) Vaccine adjuvant systems containing monophosphoryl lipid A and QS21 induce strong and persistent humoral and T cell responses against hepatitis B surface antigen in healthy adult volunteers. Vaccine 26:1375–1386

Wang X, Ihara S, Li X et al (2019) Si-doping increases the adjuvant activity of hydroxyapatite nanorods. Colloids Surf B Biointerfaces 174:300–307

Wang YQ, Bazin-Lee H, Evans JT et al (2020a) MPL adjuvant contains competitive antagonists of human TLR4. Front Immunol 11:577823

Wang J, Li P, Yu Y et al (2020b) Pulmonary surfactant-biomimetic nanoparticles potentiate heterosubtypic influenza immunity. Science 367

Wang Y, Xie Y, Luo J et al (2021a) Engineering a self-navigated MnARK nanovaccine for inducing potent protective immunity against novel coronavirus. Nano Today 38:101139

Wang Y, Zhang Z, Luo J et al (2021b) mRNA vaccine: a potential therapeutic strategy. Mol Cancer 20:33

Weeratna RD, McCluskie MJ, Xu Y et al (2000) CpG DNA induces stronger immune responses with less toxicity than other adjuvants. Vaccine 18:1755–1762

Wen Y, Waltman A, Han H et al (2016) Switching the immunogenicity of peptide assemblies using surface properties. ACS Nano 10:9274–9286

Xia Y, Wu J, Wei W et al (2018) Exploiting the pliability and lateral mobility of Pickering emulsion for enhanced vaccination. Nat Mater 17:187–194

Yang Y, Jambhrunkar M, Abbaraju PL et al (2017a) Understanding the effect of surface chemistry of mesoporous silica nanorods on their vaccine adjuvant potency. Adv Healthc Mater 6

Yang Y, Fang Z, Chen X et al (2017b) An overview of Pickering emulsions: solid-particle materials, classification, morphology, and applications. Front Pharmacol 8:287

Yang Y, Tang J, Song H et al (2020) Dendritic mesoporous silica nanoparticle adjuvants modified with binuclear aluminum complex: coordination chemistry dictates adjuvanticity. Angew Chem Int Ed Engl 59:19610–19617

Yu G, Liang Z, Yu Z et al (2022) Engineering the hydroxyl content on aluminum oxyhydroxide nanorod for elucidating the antigen adsorption behavior. NPJ Vaccines 7:62
Zhang L, Liang Z, Chen C et al (2021a) Engineered hydroxyapatite nanoadjuvants with controlled shape and aspect ratios reveal their immunomodulatory potentials. ACS Appl Mater Interfaces 13:59662–59672
Zhang R, Wang C, Guan Y et al (2021b) Manganese salts function as potent adjuvants. Cell Mol Immunol 18:1222–1234
Zhao H, Han Q, Yang A et al (2022) CpG-C ODN M362 as an immunoadjuvant for HBV therapeutic vaccine reverses the systemic tolerance against HBV. Int J Biol Sci 18:154–165

Biodegradable Long-Acting Injectables: Platform Technology and Industrial Challenges

Marieta Duvnjak, Alessia Villois, and Farshad Ramazani

Contents

Abstract

Long-acting injectables have been used to benefit patients with chronic diseases. So far, several biodegradable long-acting platform technologies including drug-loaded polymeric microparticles, implants (preformed and in situ forming), oil-based solutions, and aqueous suspension have been established. In this chapter, we summarize all the marketed technology platforms and discuss their challenges regarding development including but not limited to controlling drug release, particle size, stability, sterilization, scale-up manufacturing, etc. Finally, we discuss important criteria to consider for the successful development of long-acting injectables.

Marieta Duvnjak and Farshad Ramazani contributed equally to this work.

M. Duvnjak · A. Villois · F. Ramazani (✉)
Technical Research and Development, Novartis Pharma AG, Basel, Switzerland
e-mail: farshad.ramazani@novartis.com

M. Schäfer-Korting, U. S. Schubert (eds.), *Drug Delivery and Targeting*,
Handbook of Experimental Pharmacology 284, https://doi.org/10.1007/164_2023_651

Keywords

Controlled release · Extended release · Long-acting injectables · Microcrystal suspensions · Microspheres · Oil solution · PLGA microparticles · Preformed and in situ forming implants · Sustained release

Abbreviations

DCM	Dichloromethane
DLS	Dynamic light scattering
EE	Encapsulation efficiency
GDO	Glycerol dioleate
IR	Immediate release
ISFI	In situ forming implants
kGy	Kilogray
LA	Long acting
LAI	Long-acting injectables
MPs	Microparticles
Mw	Molecular weight
NMP	N-methyl-2-pyrrolidone
PCPP-SA	Poly[1,3-bis(carboxyphenoxy) propane-co-sebacic-acid]
PLGA	Poly(lactic-*co*-glycolic acid)
POE	Poly(orthoester) polymers
PVA	Polyvinyl alcohol
S/O/W	Solid-in-oil-in-water
SE/PS	Solvent extraction/phase separation
USP	United state pharmacopeia
$W_1/O/W_2$	Water-in-oil-in-water

1 Introduction

Oral is the most common and convenient route of drug administration. However, there are several limitations in that some active ingredients cannot be delivered via the oral route including among others absorption, enzymatic or acid degradation, and liver first pass effect. For such drugs parenteral delivery via intramuscular, intravenous, subcutaneous routes, etc. is an alternative. Parenteral drugs can be categorized as immediate release (IR) or long-acting (LA). LA formulations release their drugs in a controlled manner from a few days to a few months or even a year. For the treatments of chronic diseases that require frequent injection, long-acting injectables (LAI) can improve patient adherence and consequently result in effective therapy

(Bassand et al. 2022). In addition to the conventional systemic administration of LAI, there is a trend toward local drug delivery using LAIs. In this approach, the LAI is injected directly in or close to the targeted tissue resulting in efficient drug concentration in the local site of action while minimizing drug concentration in off-targeted tissues. For example, local drug delivery using LAI is used for the treatment of osteoarthritis (intraarticular injection), several cancer types (intratumorally injection or implantation), and multiple diseases that impact the posterior segment of the eye (intraocular injection) (Mansoor et al. 2009; Ramazani et al. 2016b; Kraus et al. 2018; Koh et al. 2022).

2 Platform Technologies

Marketed LAI platform technologies are categorized as polymeric and non-polymeric systems. Polymeric LAI consists of microparticles and implants (pre-formed/in situ forming). Non-polymeric LAI are drug nano/micro-crystal suspensions and oily solution of lipophilic drugs.

2.1 Polymeric Systems

In the following paragraphs, polymers that have been used in preparing LAI-marketed products are discussed. These polymers are poly(lactic-*co*-glycolic acid), polyanhydride, and poly(orthoester) polymers.

Poly(lactic-*co*-glycolic acid) (PLGA) is the most widely used polymer for LAI products development (Park et al. 2019). More than 90% of polymer-based LAI-marketed products are based on PLGA. It is an aliphatic polyester that is synthesized by ring-opening polymerization of lactic and glycolic acid monomers. PLGA is commercially available with different molecular weights, copolymer compositions, chemical structures (branched or linear), and end group (acid terminated or ester terminated) which translates in different degradation times (Makadia and Siegel 2011). In the body, PLGA is degrading via hydrolytic and enzymatic pathways. PLGA with higher content of glycolic acid degrades faster than PLGA with higher lactic acid. Glycolic acid is more hydrophilic than lactic acid which increases the water-absorbing capacity of the copolymer. Water can initiate the hydrolysis of polyester chains. Moreover, lactic ester bonds are less prone to hydrolysis than glycolic ester bonds because of the steric hindrance of methyl groups. Besides lactic to glycolic acid ratio, copolymer end group (ester or acid terminated) has an impact on the overall degradation of PLGA. It has been shown that particles prepared by an acid-terminated PLGA degrade faster as compared to an ester-terminated copolymer (Samadi et al. 2013).

Polifeprosan 20 is a random copolymer of (poly[1,3-bis(carboxyphenoxy) propane-co-sebacic-acid, 20:80] [PCPP-SA]) (McGirt et al. 2009; Wolinsky et al. 2012). This polymer is used as a matrix for local delivery of Carmustine (Gliadel® wafers) for the treatment of glioblastoma (Refer to Chap. Envisaging the future). The polymer fully degrades/eliminates in vivo for about 8 weeks. Eighty percent of SA liberated from the matrix in about 7 days, without a notable change in water-insoluble CPP copolymer, degradation starts after a lag phase of around 9 days (Domb et al. 1995). As a result of degradation, about 60% of the CPP was released from the implants over a 3-week anhydride connection between CPP-CPP diacids degrades slower than anhydride link between CPP-SA or SA-SA diacids most likely due to hydrophobicity of CPP and the steadiness of these anhydride bonds.

Poly(orthoester) polymers (POE) are another class of biodegradable polymers that have been used for controlled drug delivery. POE-IV is the most advanced polymer in this group that have a versatile erosion control rate and good biocompatibility which makes it suitable for LAI development (Heller et al. 2002). Unlike PLGA which degrades via bulk erosion, POE-IV degrades by surface erosion which is advantageous to bulk erosion as there is no accumulation of acidic degraded short polymer/monomers in the core of the particle/implant. This polymer is suitable for pH-sensitive drugs (Pandey et al. 2019). Sustol® is an in situ forming gel based on triethylene glycol POE and polyethylene glycol loaded with Granisetron for control of vomiting after chemotherapy. This polymer may open a new avenue for the future development of LAI alongside PLGA.

Apart from biodegradable polymers, a combination of endogenous polar lipids is used for in situ forming LAI ("Liquid Crystal" or FluidCrystal® technology). FluidCrystal® is based on lecithin (SPC 100) and glycerol dioleate (GDO) that are mixed with drug and dissolved in ethanol and propylene glycol (Kamali et al. 2022).

2.1.1 PLGA Microparticles

Microencapsulation refers to the manufacturing of polymer-based particles with desirable size (1–1,000 μm) where pharmaceuticals are entrapped in a polymer matrix, if the drug is dispersed or dissolved in the polymer matrix it is called microspheres but if the drug is encapsulated in the core of the particle encircled by a polymer shell, it is called microcapsules. In the following sections, we summarize the manufacturing methods of PLGA MPs.

Manufacture Processes of PLGA Microparticles

Emulsion Solvent Evaporation Methods Lipophilic drugs can be dissolved in a volatile organic solvent such as dichloromethane (DCM) along with PLGA. This organic phase is emulsified with a water phase containing emulsifiers such as polyvinyl alcohol (PVA) under shear mixing. After the formation of a stable emulsion, the organic solvent is extracted from the oily droplets into the water phase and then evaporated by elevated temperature under N_2 flow. Thereby microdroplets turn into solidified microparticles which are collected, washed several times with water and vacuum dried. The bulk microparticles are terminally sterilized if aseptic manufacturing is not used. The suspension in a vehicle containing emulsifier and osmolarity-enhancing agent is ready for use. For water-soluble drugs a water-in-oil-in-water ($W_1/O/W_2$) method can be used. In this case, the drug is dissolved in W_1 and entrapped in the organic phase (PLGA and organic solvent); this inner emulsion is then emulsified with W_2 containing water and emulsifier to form $W_1/O/W_2$. The rest of the manufacturing process is like O/W emulsion that is explained above (Ramazani et al. 2015).

Emulsification of water-soluble drugs in PLGA microparticles can be compromised by low encapsulation efficiency due to drug flux into the external water phase during emulsification and hardening of microparticles (Ramazani et al. 2016a). Water-in-oil-in-oil ($W/O_1/O_2$) has been used as an alternative for $W_1/O/W_2$ method. In this approach, the drug is dissolved in water and mixed with PLGA solution in an organic solvent. This primary emulsion is emulsified again using a non-mixable organic oil contain emulsifier (e.g., cotton oil/lecithin). The organic solvent from O_1 phase is extracted into O_2 phase which leads to the coacervation of the polymer (Park et al. 2019).

In some cases, if the drug is neither soluble in water nor in the organic solvent for microparticle manufacture, the drug can be loaded into PLGA microparticles by solid-in-oil-in-water (S/O/W) method. In this method, the micronized drug needs to be homogeneously distributed in the organic phase before emulsification. High drug loading can be achieved by this method as compared to $W_1/O/W_2$ and O/W methods. However, micronization has its own limitation, e.g., change of drug crystallinity due to jet milling (common method of micronization), controlling foreign visible particles and endotoxin as the micronized drugs cannot be sterile filtered anymore.

Spray Drying Method In this method, water insoluble drugs can be dissolved/ dispersed in an organic solution of PLGA; water-soluble drugs can be dissolved in water and added to PLGA solution and spray dried using an appropriate nozzle with different diameters and inlet/outlet temperature. Spray drying often results in high encapsulation efficiency (EE) as no water phase is used in this method (Arrighi et al. 2019). Spray drying is a simple and scalable method for microparticle manufacture. However, its drawback is high manufacturing temperature which is a limitation for sensitive drugs and drugs that can interact with PLGA, e.g., by acylation. Moreover, the batch size cannot be scaled down to milligram amount and the yield is often low in small scale which limits the use in the initial phase of drug development.

Spinning Disk Method This method is used for triamcinolone acetonide microparticle manufacture for intra-articular administration in osteoarthritis (Zilretta®). It comprises an annular spinning disk with a flat inclined surface, connected to a stirrer motor. In the middle of the disk there is a reservoir, in which the active ingredient is dispersed in the organic solvent containing biodegradable polymer. A temperature control system is available for both reservoir and the disk, to achieve controlled solvent evaporation. By applying centrifugal force, the suspension is moved from the reservoir toward the peripheral part of the disk, becoming more and more viscous because of solvent evaporation. Once the solvent is evaporated the drug-loaded MPs are solidified.

Characterization of Polymeric Microparticles

Proper analytical characterization is a key for the successful development, manufacturing, and commercialization of polymeric systems. Physicochemical properties of MPs are determined by the manufacturing process and product components (type of polymer, molecular weight, composition, and end-termination), including drug and other excipients (Park et al. 2019). Particle size and distribution, morphology, surface charge, and porosity of particles are quality parameters influencing product handling, stability, and drug release behavior. Small particles <10 μm release their payload in a brief time and they can be taken by immune systems. Large particles >200 μm may clog the needle and cause injectability issues. Particles and formulation characteristics (size, shape, density, concentration in the vehicle for injection and viscosity) are crucial factors impacting syringeability/injectability of PLGA MPs (Chitnis et al. 2019). Large particles with high density can sediment in the syringe immediately and cause needle clogging. In addition, bridging effect of polydisperse MPs during injection can cause needle clogging and injection failure. Above mentioned manufacturing methods normally produce polydisperse MPs. New manufacturing technologies such as microfluidics (Yonet-Tanyeri et al. 2022), membrane sieving (Kazazi-Hyseni et al. 2014), and printing technology (Wang et al. 2022) produce MPs with narrow size distribution and much better injectability. They hold a great promise for the future manufacture of PLGA MPs. Morphology, porosity, and particle size are usually evaluated by microscopy (optic, scanning electron, confocal, atomic force) with the addition of light laser diffraction and dynamic light scattering (DLS) for the size and surface charge of MPs.

Low drug loading capacity which is often <25% (w/w) is another limitation of MPs. This is particularly important for low-potent drugs. This limits the maximum dose of administration.

Drug quantification techniques are usually chosen based on drug properties, in most of the cases liquid chromatography (HPLC, UPLC), spectrophotometric method (UV–vis) and fluorometric assay or ELISA test in the case of biological molecules. Prior to analysis, extraction of the drug from the polymer matrix is needed.

Drug release from MPs can be tailored by MPs size, percent of drug loading (drug/polymer ratio), surface porosity, polymer (compositions, molecular weight (Mw), end group) (Otte et al. 2021). For example, smaller particle size, higher drug loading and surface porosity as well as polymer with low Mw and lower ratio of lactic to glycolic acid and acid-terminated polymer often results in faster drug release. The drug is dispersed in the polymer matrix, either molecularly or as small particles. For solid dispersion, the drug release is controlled by polymer degradation but if the encapsulated drug is molecularly dispersed, drug release is controlled by diffusion. However, there is always a combination of both diffusion and degradation that releases the drug (Fredenberg et al. 2011). Burst release is drug release within the first 24h after injection, mainly driven by the drug located close to the MP surface. Initial burst release may cause extremely high and toxic peak plasma values. Therefore, proper methods for in vitro evaluation of burst and drug release are most essential for the characterization of delivery systems; different methodologies can be utilized to evaluate drug release, such as United States Pharmacopeia (USP) apparatus II and continuous flow methods, dialysis, and sample-and-separate approach. For method development, key product attributes and mechanisms that influence release must be understood (Kim et al. 2021).

Aseptic manufacturing of PLGA MPs increases the production costs, particularly for drug products in early development phase. Moreover, terminal sterilization is the preferred choice by health authorities also for PLGA MPs as it is lethal to all microorganisms (Reinhold et al. 2012). Terminal sterilization can be performed by ethylene oxide gas, steam, dry heat, and irradiations (electron beam, X-ray, and γ-irradiation). For terminal sterilization of PLGA MPs γ-irradiation and x-ray irradiation can be used. Gamma irradiation is a commonly used method for PLGA MPs, though, it may damage the product by accelerating the degradation of PLGA and generating free radical and may crosslink the polymer chain. Though, the impact of standard dose of gamma irradiation (i.e., 25 kGy) on PLGA Mw reduction is often negligible. Nonetheless, some drug molecules particularly with reactive groups may react with PLGA under terminal sterilization or they may degrade due to energy and heat generated by gamma; thus, it is of immense importance to investigate the impact of gamma irradiation on drug product in the early stage of development. As an alternative to gamma irradiation, X-ray is faster than gamma and has the same efficiency in the elimination of microorganisms (Bittner et al. 1999; Bushell et al. 2005).

2.1.2 Implants (Preformed and In Situ Forming Implants)

Biodegradable implants like MPs are polymer-based systems that can extend the release of drugs in the body. Implants are categorized into preformed (or classical) and in situ forming implants.

Manufacturing Processes of Implants

The preformed implants are solid rods prepared by melt extrusion with a length of 10–35 mm and 1–3 mm diameter (Parent et al. 2013; Stewart et al. 2018). For temperature-sensitive drugs, melt extrusion is not an ideal method of manufacturing. Novel technologies such as printing may overcome the limitation of conventional methods for manufacturing implants with desirable shapes and sizes. One of the limitations of implants like microparticles is their low drug loading, most often <50%. Preformed implants are either injected or administered by surgical insertion. For biodegradable implants no surgical operation is needed to remove them at the end of the therapy. Depending on the size of the implants and their applicator, local pain and discomfort are reported by patients.

The limitations of preformed implants and MPs led to the development of in situ forming implants (ISFI). They are liquid or semisolid composed of drug and polymer that undergo hardening/gelation at the injection site formed by, e.g., sol-to-gel alteration initiated by physiological pH and or temperature, phase separation induced by solvent extraction, or polymer cross-linking (induced by photo-irradiation, enzymes, or ions). Moreover, organo-gelling can form implants by lyotropic liquid crystals self-assembly in an aqueous medium or thermo-sensitive hydrogels (Agarwal and Rupenthal 2013). Solvent extraction/phase separation (SE/PS) is the most common method (Vaishya et al. 2015). Atrigel® is based on PLGA dissolved in

N-methyl-2-pyrrolidone (NMP) solvent and the drug can be either dissolved or dispersed in the polymer solution. After injection, the NMP is extracted from the sol and distributed into surrounding tissues leading to the formation of solid implants loaded with drug. The drug release is like preformed implants but may have higher burst release due to organic solvent extraction. As compared to preformed implants and MPs, in situ forming implants are much simpler and do not need a complex manufacturing process and scale-up. However, NMP or other organic solvents that are used for this approach may cause local toxicity (Thakur et al. 2014). Another in situ forming gel that recently entered the market is based on FluidCrystal® technology developed by Camurus®. This system contains several lipids and a drug dissolved in ethanol and propylene glycol. Upon contact with tissue fluids, the solution transforms into a crystalline gel, which encapsulates the drug. As with Atrigel® the release mechanism is based on the degradation and dissociation of the lipid gel. Details related to the manufacturing and characterization of this type of implants have been recently reviewed (Wilkinson et al. 2022).

Characterization of Implants

In addition to technical considerations applicable to all polymer systems (Bode et al. 2019a), it is beneficial to understand depo formation and in vivo conditions influencing in-situ forming systems. For example, volume, pH, and composition of interstitial fluids at the site of injection impact the final shape and pores of the formed depot. These aspects can be simulated in vitro (Bode et al. 2019b; Li et al. 2021) and can be evaluated as described in Sect. 2.1.1.2. The same applies to preformed implants. Determination of drug loading and loading efficiency of preformed implants is like microparticles, described in Sect. 2.1.1.2. For in situ systems, drug content is determined in solution and after depot formation, also capturing the amount lost as part of burst release.

Since all biodegradable marketed implants are based on polyester polymers, their drug release can be tuned by implant size and shape, polymer composition, and surface porosity. For preformed implants, burst release is like MPs, while in situ forming systems usually exhibit higher burst release driven by solvent exchange during depo formation. This step is also critical for the development of in vitro release method (Suh et al. 2021). Evaluation of drug release is based on the same approaches as described for PLGA MPs.

Like PLGA MPs, if aseptic manufacturing is not applied, terminal sterilization using gamma irradiation is the common method for preformed implants.

2.2 Non-polymeric Systems

2.2.1 Oil-Based Solutions

Oil-based solutions of highly lipophilic (pro)drugs are another established class of LAI. The vehicle is often one of the vegetable oils like sesame, fractionated coconut, arachis or castor oil, and benzyl alcohol as cosolvent.

Manufacturing Processes of Oil-Based Solutions

Unlike manufacturing MPs, which involves extensive process development and scale-up, the manufacturing of oil-based formulation is remarkably simple. Drug is mixed, dissolved in the oil vehicle, filtered through a sterilized 0.2 μm, and filled into vials in a clean room (Weng Larsen and Larsen 2009).

Oil viscosity plays a key role in the formulation as highly viscose oils have injectability issues and low viscose oils release the drug extremely fast. Benzyl alcohol is a co-solvent in the formulation that increases the solubility of the (pro)-drug in the oil and improves injectability by reducing oil viscosity (Hines et al. 2013). Most of the active ingredients of oily solutions are engineered prodrugs based on fatty acid esters (decanoate, caproate, or enanthate) with increasing lipophilicity and solubility in the oil formulation. In addition, higher lipophilicity enhances their partitioning in the fatty tissues which works like a second depot for controlling drug release (Salem and Najib 2012). Therefore, the systemic availability of the active agents can be tuned by several approaches (Kalicharan et al. 2016).

Several oily formulations have entered the market, but a recent trend in clinical trials shows a decreasing number because of difficulties in controlling drug release necessity of drug functional groups for converting them to lipophilic prodrugs, injection pain, etc. (Sartorius et al. 2010).

Characterization of Oil-Based Solutions

Being solutions, physicochemical characterization of this type of delivery system is simple. Drug release from depos is driven by partitioning coefficient of the drug between oil and interstitial fluid. Methodologies used to evaluate it are mostly employing a "holder" for oil solution, usually a dialysis membrane fitted in conventional apparatus (Probst et al. 2017).

2.2.2 Aqueous Suspension (Micro/Nano Drug Crystals)

Crystal suspension formulation is the preferred choice when the drug needs to be administered in a concentration above its solubility in the injection medium and it has the advantage of avoiding the complexity often associated with polymeric micro/nanoparticles, gels, or implants. For such a formulation, the drug needs to be poorly soluble in the injection medium; otherwise, the release is typically too fast (Li et al. 2022).

Manufacturing Processes of Crystal Suspensions

Crystallization is a bottom-up approach to obtaining drug suspensions. It consists of a separation process in which crystals are generated starting from a liquid, gas, or amorphous solid. The supersaturation, equal to the ratio of the drug concentration and the drug equilibrium concentration, is the driving force of the process. Crystallization is composed of the following molecular steps: nucleation (primary and secondary), crystal growth, aggregation, and breakage (Orehek et al. 2021). The crystal shape and size distribution can be controlled by factors such as seed concentration, temperature, supersaturation, cooling rate, and chemical composition of the medium. The presence of polymorphs and amorphous material as a function of process conditions must be characterized and the polymorph of interest for development must be purified from the other forms.

If necessary, the crystal size can be further reduced after the crystallization process by milling the drug substance to achieve the desired crystal size distribution. Fluid energy milling and ball milling are employed to produce microcrystals in the dry state, while wet media milling, high-pressure homogenization, and cryogenic milling are used to produce nanocrystals (Loh et al. 2015). Fluid energy milling employs a compressed air stream at high velocity. Once the crystals enter the air stream, their size is reduced by the effect of crystal-crystal collision and friction. Ball milling is a technique in which the drug crystals are loaded in a vessel, together with balls or rods that can be made of various materials (ceramic, zirconia, chrome steel, etc.). Afterward, the rotation of the vessel causes the crystals to break because of friction forces and impact with the balls or rods. Wet media milling, commonly employed to produce nanocrystals, is using a similar configuration to ball milling, with the difference that the crystals and balls/rods are loaded in a liquid medium. The presence of the liquid helps in lubricating and coating the crystals, as well as reducing their adhesion to the vessel walls. However, balls/beads can be subjected to erosion, therefore potentially leading to contamination of the product (Peltonen and Hirvonen 2010). Several erosion-resistant materials can be employed such as suitable polymers or ceramics to minimize the risk of foreign matter contamination in drug products (Loh et al. 2015).

High-pressure homogenization is employed to produce nanocrystals by forcing the material through a thin gap using a piston for multiple cycles. Typical process parameters are velocities around 500 m/s and pressures of 1,000–1,500 bar. It usually requires a pre-micronization step to avoid clogging the gap. Compared to wet media milling, high-pressure homogenization is much less susceptible to material erosion and subsequent drug contamination (Loh et al. 2015). The Nanopure® variation of high-pressure homogenization is suitable for drugs susceptible to hydrolysis, thanks to the use of non-aqueous media (oil, poly(ethylene glycol), etc.), and it may be used for thermolabile drugs as well (Möschwitzer and Müller 2006).

Cryogenic milling consists of shock-freezing the material in liquid nitrogen before milling or carrying out the milling process in cryogenic conditions. This technique eases size reduction by rendering the material brittle and it is especially suitable for thermolabile drugs (Ye and Schoenung 2004).

A challenge related to suspensions is given by the limited possibility to use sterile filtration because of the size of microbes and foreign particles being in the range of drug crystals, therefore limiting the separation possibilities. For microbial contamination, alternative approaches exist, such as terminal sterilization (autoclaving or irradiation) or aseptic processing. However, aseptic processing should be the last choice, as it needs a strong justification to be accepted by the health authorities and it is not cost-effective, especially in the early development stages. For foreign particles control, a polishing filtration may be implemented to remove particles that are sufficiently larger than the drug crystals. Additionally, the source of foreign particle contamination must be identified in the process and countermeasures must be adopted.

Moreover, a choice must be made whether the product should be stored as a suspension, for instance in a pre-filled syringe, or if it must be lyophilized and then reconstituted just before administration. The first option may be preferred for simplicity, to reduce the processing steps and to ease the administration of the drug, for instance if home use is intended. In that case, the choice of crystal size affects the colloidal stability of the suspension during storage. The larger the crystals, the higher the propensity to precipitate (Stokes 2009). Instead, smaller crystals typically have a higher tendency to agglomerate; therefore, suitable stabilizers must be utilized. As an alternative, lyophilization may be a solution if the suspension tends to be physically unstable (because of precipitation, agglomeration, or flocculation) or to increase the shelf life of the product.

Characterization of Aqueous Suspensions

Physicochemical Properties Nanosuspensions have typical particle sizes between 100 and 1,000 nm, while aqueous microsuspensions can have range between 1 and 1,000 μm, although usually not going above 50 μm because of formulation injectability (Nguyen et al. 2022).

Like polymeric systems, particle size and distribution, morphology and surface properties of particles are quality parameters influencing product handling, stability, drug release behavior and host immune response and similar techniques as described in Sect. 2.1.1.2 are being utilized.

Drug Release of Nano-/Microcrystals The drug release from suspensions of drugs with low water solubility is limited and driven by the rate of dissolution from the crystal to the surrounding fluid crystal shape and size affect the release. Regarding crystal size, theoretically nanocrystals should be characterized by a faster release compared to microcrystals because the surface-to-volume ratio is higher. However, the higher surface of nanocrystals also renders them thermodynamically more unstable, therefore triggering agglomeration, which reduces the surface through which the drug can diffuse. In case that formulation is developed as flocculated suspension, administration procedure and conditions can have an impact on the flocculation state and, consequently, drug bioavailability (Smith et al. 2021). Additionally, the choice of crystal size affects the systemic and local distribution of the drug. In fact, after local administration, nanocrystals are more likely to undergo systemic circulation because of their permeation through body membranes. However, the local environment in vivo is also likely to affect the drug release with complex mechanisms, such as lymph node uptake, granuloma foreign body reaction, phagocytosis, and the enzymatic degradation of prodrugs (Darville et al. 2014, 2016; Mulay et al. 2020). Recent reviews are indicating that in addition to particle size, dose level, formulation composition, drug substance lipophilicity have a significant effect on the final in vivo performance of the product. In addition, gender, body mass index, and immune response are major contributors from the host side (Nguyen et al. 2022).

In vitro release approaches discussed in PLGA MPs section also applies to release characterization of drug crystalline suspensions.

2.3 Other Technologies

Few other LAI have been developed and marketed for example, Ligand Evolution to Active Pharmaceuticals (LEAP) technology, which is based on electrostatic interaction between anionic polymers with cationic drugs. For example, anionic polymer of sodium carmellose and cationic abarelix acetate, which is developed as LAI. Another LAI technology for peptide formulation is peptide self-assembly technology. In certain concentrations, some peptides undergo self-assembly to form nanotubes. Somatuline® Depot is marketed based on peptide self-assembly (Nkanga et al. 2020).

3 Important Criteria for Development of Long-Acting Drug Products

Table 1 summarizes important criteria for the development of LAIs from drug substance, drug product, and administration prospective. To enable low administration frequency drug substance needs to be highly potent with low plasma clearance. The first step in drug design is to understand the duration and extent of target engagement that is needed for efficacy (Bhattachar et al. 2017). It is important to design a drug molecule suitable for formulating in one of the established LAI such as PLGA MPs, implants, crystal suspension, or oil-based formulations. Small molecule drugs have a lot of opportunities to tailor their physicochemical properties. For example, rigid structures such as aromatic rings can be introduced to drug molecules and decrease their water solubility (Ritchie and Macdonald 2009). Moreover, as mentioned earlier coupling of fatty acid chain with varied sizes can increase drug lipophilicity. The size of drug molecules can also play a key role in drug release from the depot, e.g., large molecules diffuse slowly, and smaller molecules can diffuse out of their delivery system to the environment much faster. Not only low water solubility but also high solubility in organic solvents which are used for drug product

Table 1 Summary of important criteria for development of long-acting injectables

	Criteria for LAI development
Drug substance	• Potency • Physiochemically stability • Low water solubility
Drug products (formulation)	• Drug loading vs. volume of injection • Drug release vs. therapeutic dose • Scalability of the manufacturing process • Stability upon terminal sterilization otherwise use aseptic manufacturing • Long shelf-life of drug product ideally at room temperature or refrigerator (e.g., >2 years)
Administration	• Good injectability and syringeability • Biocompatibility especially local tolerability

formulation, e.g., dichloromethane and ethyl acetate for PLGA MPs is desired. A large therapeutic window is desirable to enable dosing without either toxicity, due to fast drug release, or no effect, due to slow drug release, as drug release from depot can vary with regards to patient age, gender, stage of disease, etc. Other parameters, which are important in the early development of formulation, are the physicochemical stability of the drug candidate as most often harsh conditions are involved during the drug product formulation, e.g., elevated temperature, drug dissolution in organic/ aqueous media, milling, terminal sterilization, etc.

Regarding the formulation, it is important to have a high drug loading to enable sustained drug release for an extended time. High drug loading can minimize the administration dose and decrease the volume of injection as the volume of injection is extremely limited for some tissues. For example, it is not possible to inject >5 mL intramascular or >2 mL subcutaneous as it may damage the local tissues. High drug loading can increase the burst release. For example, most of marketed PLGA formulations have drug loading <30% meaning >70% of the formulation contains PLGA. This formulation will be suspended in a vehicle for injection, which further decreases the administrable dose. In general, as summarized in Table 2, crystal suspension and oily formulation have higher drug loading as compared to polymeric systems. However, there are plenty of options to tailor drug release from polymeric systems as compared to limited options of tailoring drug release from non-polymeric systems.

As compared to IR formulations, LAI development is much more complex, time-consuming, and consequently expensive. For example, the development of particulate systems involves comprehensive process development to enable scale up from lab via pilot to manufacturing plant (Table 2). In this regard, early investment in scalable equipment and analytical tools to enable successful scale-up is vital. Further, molecular dynamics simulation can be utilized to minimize the number of experiments, get a better insight in the drug-polymer interactions, polymer degradation, and drug release performance from LAI (Kotla et al. 2022). In addition, simulation can be used for better estimation of scale-up factors.

Efficient collaboration between formulation scientists and manufacturing scientists is the key to success. Another unique challenge for solid long-acting parenteral is controlling foreign particles and endotoxin level as they cannot be sterile filtered such as solutions. Prior to manufacturing, it is necessary to wash all the equipment with various washing agents to remove any foreign particles and endotoxins. All the equipment pieces and moving joints need to be monitored for shedding any particles.

Aseptic manufacturing using filtration is possible for oily solution or in situ forming gel but for other systems terminal sterilization is more common. Therefore, they need to be stable upon terminal sterilization which makes it more challenging for sensitive drug candidates.

Conventionally, LAI are used for systemic administration using intramuscular or subcutaneous injection. However, nowadays novel routes of administration are investigated in both clinical and preclinical studies (Manna et al. 2021; Sun et al. 2021; Koh et al. 2022). There is a trend toward local administration of LAI ensuring

Table 2 Strengths and weaknesses of established LAI delivery systems

Formulation	Strength	Weakness
PLGA-based MPs	• Drug release can be modulated (e.g., from weeks to months) • In principle it is possible to load both hydrophilic and hydrophobic drugs • Smooth and soft surface → low risk of mechanical tissue irritation	• Gamma sterilization or aseptic production is required • Development is not simple and rather expensive • High drug loading is challenging, > 50% of formulation is polymer • Difficult to scale up
Preformed implants	• Drug release can be modulated to some extent • In principle it is possible to load both hydrophilic and hydrophobic drugs	• Gamma sterilization or aseptic production is required • Not simple and rather expensive • Invasive application (in some cases surgical procedures are required) • High drug loading is challenging > 50% of formulation is polymer
In situ forming implants	• Drug release can be modulated to some extent • Simple and cost-effective preparation methods • Filtration sterilization • Easy scale up	• Limitation for using organic solvents • Limited options for tailoring drug release • High drug loading is challenging > 50% of formulation is polymer
Non-PLGA based systems	• Polymers such as poly(orthoester)s that degrades via surface erosion → acid degradation is not accumulating in the delivery systems → compatible with acid-sensitive drugs	• Gamma sterilization or aseptic production is required • Not simple and rather expensive • Only few marketed products → limited knowledge available about versatility of these polymers
Crystal suspensions	• Simple and cost-effective preparation methods • Highest drug-loaded carrier system → allowing high drug dosing per volume	• Rough particle surface → high risk of mechanical tissue irritation • Micronization is required • Gamma, heat sterilization, or aseptic manufacturing is required • Limited options for tailoring drug release, e.g., by particle size tuning • Long-term stability issues especially with nanocrystals
Oil-based formulations	• Simple and cost-effective preparation methods • Filtration sterilization • Easy scale up	• Not possible for many drug molecules to form prodrug (only hydrophobic drug with functional groups) • Limited options for tailoring drug release • Injection-related pain

Table adopted with permission from (Nkanga et al. 2020)

high drug concentration at the site of action and low systemic drug exposure. Yet, it brings novel challenges for the development of these delivery systems. For example, local tolerability issues, injection volume and challenging pharmacokinetics evaluation (Bassand et al. 2022).

4 Conclusion

Long-acting injectables are used to improve patient adherence and treatment outcomes. Developability of LAI depends on the design of potent and stable drug substance, understanding the challenges regarding the development of a drug product (such as drug loading, drug release rate, shelf life, scale-up manufacture), and administration (injectability, local tolerability, and in vivo faith of the formulation). Knowing the strength and weakness of already established platform technologies such as PLGA MPs, implants, oily solution, and crystal suspensions can minimize the effort for selecting the best formulation approach for a new molecule.

References

Agarwal P, Rupenthal ID (2013) Injectable implants for the sustained release of protein and peptide drugs. Drug Discov Today 18:337–349. https://doi.org/10.1016/J.DRUDIS.2013.01.013

Arrighi A, Marquette S, Peerboom C et al (2019) Development of PLGA microparticles with high immunoglobulin G-loaded levels and sustained-release properties obtained by spray-drying a water-in-oil emulsion. Int J Pharm 566:291–298. https://doi.org/10.1016/J.IJPHARM.2019.05.070

Bassand C, Villois A, Gianola L et al (2022) Smart design of patient-centric long-acting products: from preclinical to marketed pipeline trends and opportunities. Expert Opin Drug Deliv. https://doi.org/10.1080/17425247.2022.2106213/SUPPL_FILE/IEDD_A_2106213_SM6391.XLSX

Bhattachar SN, Morrison JS, Mudra DR, Bender Editors DM (2017) Translating molecules into medicines. Springer

Bittner B, Mäder K, Kroll C et al (1999) Tetracycline-HCl-loaded poly(dl-lactide-co-glycolide) microspheres prepared by a spray drying technique: influence of γ-irradiation on radical formation and polymer degradation. J Control Release 59:23–32. https://doi.org/10.1016/S0168-3659(98)00170-9

Bode C, Kranz H, Kruszka A et al (2019a) In-situ forming PLGA implants: how additives affect swelling and drug release. J Drug Deliv Sci Technol 53:101180. https://doi.org/10.1016/J.JDDST.2019.101180

Bode C, Kranz H, Siepmann F, Siepmann J (2019b) Coloring of PLGA implants to better understand the underlying drug release mechanisms. Int J Pharm 569:118563. https://doi.org/10.1016/J.IJPHARM.2019.118563

Bushell JA, Claybourn M, Williams HE, Murphy DM (2005) An EPR and ENDOR study of γ- and β-radiation sterilization in poly (lactide-co-glycolide) polymers and microspheres. J Control Release 110:49–57. https://doi.org/10.1016/J.JCONREL.2005.09.009

Chitnis GD, Verma MKS, Lamazouade J et al (2019) A resistance-sensing mechanical injector for the precise delivery of liquids to target tissue. Nat Biomed Eng 3(8):621–631. https://doi.org/10.1038/s41551-019-0350-2

Darville N, Van Heerden M, Vynckier A et al (2014) Intramuscular administration of paliperidone palmitate extended-release injectable microsuspension induces a subclinical inflammatory reaction modulating the pharmacokinetics in rats. J Pharm Sci 103:2072–2087. https://doi.org/10.1002/JPS.24014

Darville N, Van Heerden M, Erkens T et al (2016) Modeling the time course of the tissue responses to intramuscular long-acting paliperidone palmitate nano-/microcrystals and polystyrene microspheres in the rat. Toxicol Pathol 44:189–210. https://doi.org/10.1177/0192623315618291/ASSET/IMAGES/LARGE/10.1177_0192623315618291-FIG2.JPEG

Domb AJ, Rock M, Perkin C et al (1995) Excretion of a radiolabelled anticancer biodegradable polymeric implant from the rabbit brain. Biomaterials 16:1069–1072. https://doi.org/10.1016/0142-9612(95)98902-Q

Fredenberg S, Wahlgren M, Reslow M, Axelsson A (2011) The mechanisms of drug release in poly (lactic-co-glycolic acid)-based drug delivery systems – a review. Int J Pharm 415:34–52. https://doi.org/10.1016/J.IJPHARM.2011.05.049

Heller J, Barr J, Ng SY et al (2002) Poly(ortho esters): synthesis, characterization, properties and uses. Adv Drug Deliv Rev 54:1015–1039. https://doi.org/10.1016/S0169-409X(02)00055-8

Hines M, Lyseng-Williamson KA, Deeks ED (2013) 17 α-hydroxyprogesterone caproate (Makena®): a guide to its use in the prevention of preterm birth. Clin Drug Investig 33:223–227. https://doi.org/10.1007/S40261-013-0060-6

Kalicharan RW, Schot P, Vromans H (2016) Fundamental understanding of drug absorption from a parenteral oil depot. Eur J Pharm Sci 83:19–27. https://doi.org/10.1016/J.EJPS.2015.12.011

Kamali H, Karimi M, Abbaspour M et al (2022) Comparison of lipid liquid crystal formulation and vivitrol® for sustained release of naltrexone: in vitro evaluation and pharmacokinetics in rats. Int J Pharm 611:121275. https://doi.org/10.1016/J.IJPHARM.2021.121275

Kazazi-Hyseni F, Landin M, Lathuile A et al (2014) Computer modeling assisted design of monodisperse PLGA microspheres with controlled porosity affords zero order release of an encapsulated macromolecule for 3 months. Pharm Res 31:2844–2856. https://doi.org/10.1007/S11095-014-1381-8/TABLES/2

Kim Y, Park EJ, Kim TW, Na DH (2021) Recent progress in drug release testing methods of biopolymeric particulate system. Pharmaceutics 13:1313. https://doi.org/10.3390/PHARMACEUTICS13081313

Koh E, Freedman BR, Ramazani F et al (2022) Controlled delivery of corticosteroids using tunable tough adhesives. Adv Healthc Mater:2201000. https://doi.org/10.1002/ADHM.202201000

Kotla NG, Pandey A, Kumar YV et al (2022) Polyester-based long acting injectables: advancements in molecular dynamics simulation and technological insights. Drug Discov Today:103463. https://doi.org/10.1016/J.DRUDIS.2022.103463

Kraus VB, Conaghan PG, Aazami HA et al (2018) Synovial and systemic pharmacokinetics (PK) of triamcinolone acetonide (TA) following intra-articular (IA) injection of an extended-release microsphere-based formulation (FX006) or standard crystalline suspension in patients with knee osteoarthritis (OA). Osteoarthr Cartil 26:34–42. https://doi.org/10.1016/J.JOCA.2017.10.003

Li Z, Mu H, Weng Larsen S et al (2021) An in vitro gel-based system for characterizing and predicting the long-term performance of PLGA in situ forming implants. Int J Pharm 609:121183. https://doi.org/10.1016/J.IJPHARM.2021.121183

Li M, Reichert P, Narasimhan C et al (2022) Investigating crystalline protein suspension formulations of pembrolizumab from MAS NMR spectroscopy. Mol Pharm 19:936–952. https://doi.org/10.1021/ACS.MOLPHARMACEUT.1C00915/ASSET/IMAGES/LARGE/MP1C00915_0008.JPEG

Loh ZH, Samanta AK, Sia Heng PW (2015) Overview of milling techniques for improving the solubility of poorly water-soluble drugs. Asian J Pharm Sci 10:255–274. https://doi.org/10.1016/J.AJPS.2014.12.006

Makadia HK, Siegel SJ (2011) Poly lactic-co-glycolic acid (PLGA) as biodegradable controlled drug delivery carrier. Polymers (Basel) 3:1377. https://doi.org/10.3390/POLYM3031377

Manna S, Donnell AM, Faraj RQC et al (2021) Pharmacokinetics and toxicity evaluation of a PLGA and chitosan-based micro-implant for sustained release of methotrexate in rabbit vitreous. Pharmaceutics 13:1227. https://doi.org/10.3390/PHARMACEUTICS13081227

Mansoor S, Kuppermann BD, Kenney MC (2009) Intraocular sustained-release delivery systems for triamcinolone acetonide. Pharm Res 26:770–784. https://doi.org/10.1007/S11095-008-9812-Z/FIGURES/5

McGirt MJ, Than KD, Weingart JD et al (2009) Gliadel (BCNU) wafer plus concomitant temozolomide therapy after primary resection of glioblastoma multiforme. J Neurosurg 110:583–588. https://doi.org/10.3171/2008.5.17557

Möschwitzer J, Müller RH (2006) New method for the effective production of ultrafine drug nanocrystals. J Nanosci Nanotechnol 6:3145–3153. https://doi.org/10.1166/JNN.2006.480
Mulay SR, Steiger S, Shi C, Anders HJ (2020) A guide to crystal-related and nano- or microparticle-related tissue responses. FEBS J 287:818–832. https://doi.org/10.1111/FEBS.15174
Nguyen VTT, Darville N, Vermeulen A (2022) Pharmacokinetics of long-acting aqueous nano-/microsuspensions after intramuscular administration in different animal species and humans – a review. AAPS J 25:4. https://doi.org/10.1208/S12248-022-00771-5/TABLES/1
Nkanga CI, Fisch A, Rad-Malekshahi M et al (2020) Clinically established biodegradable long acting injectables: an industry perspective. Adv Drug Deliv Rev 167:19–46. https://doi.org/10.1016/J.ADDR.2020.11.008
Orehek J, Teslić D, Likozar B (2021) Continuous crystallization processes in pharmaceutical manufacturing: a review. Org Process Res Dev 25:16–42. https://doi.org/10.1021/ACS.OPRD.0C00398/ASSET/IMAGES/LARGE/OP0C00398_0008.JPEG
Otte A, Damen F, Goergen C, Park K (2021) Coupling the in vivo performance to the in vitro characterization of PLGA microparticles. Int J Pharm 604:120738. https://doi.org/10.1016/J.IJPHARM.2021.120738
Pandey SP, Shukla T, Dhote VK et al (2019) Use of polymers in controlled release of active agents. Basic Fundamentals Drug Deliv:113–172. https://doi.org/10.1016/B978-0-12-817909-3.00004-2
Parent M, Nouvel C, Koerber M et al (2013) PLGA in situ implants formed by phase inversion: critical physicochemical parameters to modulate drug release. J Control Release 172:292–304. https://doi.org/10.1016/J.JCONREL.2013.08.024
Park K, Skidmore S, Hadar J et al (2019) Injectable, long-acting PLGA formulations: analyzing PLGA and understanding microparticle formation. J Control Release 304:125–134. https://doi.org/10.1016/J.JCONREL.2019.05.003
Peltonen L, Hirvonen J (2010) Pharmaceutical nanocrystals by nanomilling: critical process parameters, particle fracturing and stabilization methods. J Pharm Pharmacol 62:1569–1579. https://doi.org/10.1111/J.2042-7158.2010.01022.X
Probst M, Schmidt M, Tietz K et al (2017) In vitro dissolution testing of parenteral aqueous solutions and oily suspensions of paracetamol and prednisolone. Int J Pharm 532:519–527. https://doi.org/10.1016/J.IJPHARM.2017.09.052
Ramazani F, Chen W, Van Nostrum CF et al (2015) Formulation and characterization of microspheres loaded with imatinib for sustained delivery. Int J Pharm 482:123–130. https://doi.org/10.1016/J.IJPHARM.2015.01.043
Ramazani F, Chen W, Van Nostrum CF et al (2016a) Strategies for encapsulation of small hydrophilic and amphiphilic drugs in PLGA microspheres: state-of-the-art and challenges. Int J Pharm 499:358–367. https://doi.org/10.1016/J.IJPHARM.2016.01.020
Ramazani F, Van Nostrum CF, Storm G et al (2016b) Locoregional cancer therapy using polymer-based drug depots. Drug Discov Today 21:640–647. https://doi.org/10.1016/J.DRUDIS.2016.02.014
Reinhold SE, Desai KGH, Zhang L et al (2012) Self-healing microencapsulation of biomacromolecules without organic solvents. Angew Chem Int Ed 51:10800–10803. https://doi.org/10.1002/ANIE.201206387
Ritchie TJ, Macdonald SJF (2009) The impact of aromatic ring count on compound developability – are too many aromatic rings a liability in drug design? Drug Discov Today 14:1011–1020. https://doi.org/10.1016/J.DRUDIS.2009.07.014
Salem II, Najib NM (2012) Pharmacokinetics of betamethasone after single-dose intramuscular administration of betamethasone phosphate and betamethasone acetate to healthy subjects. Clin Ther 34:214–220. https://doi.org/10.1016/J.CLINTHERA.2011.11.022
Samadi N, Abbadessa A, Di Stefano A et al (2013) The effect of lauryl capping group on protein release and degradation of poly(d,l-lactic-co-glycolic acid) particles. J Control Release 172:436–443. https://doi.org/10.1016/J.JCONREL.2013.05.034
Sartorius G, Fennell C, Spasevska S et al (2010) Factors influencing time course of pain after depot oil intramuscular injection of testosterone undecanoate. Asian J Androl 12:227. https://doi.org/10.1038/AJA.2010.1

Smith WC, Bae J, Zhang Y et al (2021) Impact of particle flocculation on the dissolution and bioavailability of injectable suspensions. Int J Pharm 604:120767. https://doi.org/10.1016/J.IJPHARM.2021.120767

Stewart SA, Domínguez-Robles J, Donnelly RF, Larrañeta E (2018) Implantable polymeric drug delivery devices: classification, manufacture, materials, and clinical applications. Polymers 10: 1379. https://doi.org/10.3390/POLYM10121379

Stokes GG (2009) On the effect of the internal friction of fluids on the motion of pendulums. Math Phys Papers:1–10. https://doi.org/10.1017/CBO9780511702266.002

Suh MS, Kastellorizios M, Tipnis N et al (2021) Effect of implant formation on drug release kinetics of in situ forming implants. Int J Pharm 592:120105. https://doi.org/10.1016/J.IJPHARM.2020.120105

Sun YJ, Lin CH, Wu MR et al (2021) An intravitreal implant injection method for sustained drug delivery into mouse eyes. Cell Rep Methods 1:100125. https://doi.org/10.1016/J.CRMETH.2021.100125

Thakur RRS, McMillan HL, Jones DS (2014) Solvent induced phase inversion-based in situ forming controlled release drug delivery implants. J Control Release 176:8–23. https://doi.org/10.1016/J.JCONREL.2013.12.020

Vaishya R, Khurana V, Patel S, Mitra AK (2015) Long-term delivery of protein therapeutics. Expert Opin Drug Deliv 12(3):415–440. https://doi.org/10.1517/17425247.2015.961420

Wang J, Heshmati Aghda N, Jiang J et al (2022) 3D bioprinted microparticles: optimizing loading efficiency using advanced DoE technique and machine learning modeling. Int J Pharm 628: 122302. https://doi.org/10.1016/J.IJPHARM.2022.122302

Weng Larsen S, Larsen C (2009) Critical factors influencing the in vivo performance of long-acting lipophilic solutions-impact on in vitro release method design. AAPS J 11:762–770. https://doi.org/10.1208/S12248-009-9153-9/FIGURES/4

Wilkinson J, Ajulo D, Tamburrini V et al (2022) Lipid based intramuscular long-acting injectables: current state of the art. Eur J Pharm Sci 178:106253. https://doi.org/10.1016/J.EJPS.2022.106253

Wolinsky JB, Colson YL, Grinstaff MW (2012) Local drug delivery strategies for cancer treatment: gels, nanoparticles, polymeric films, rods, and wafers. J Control Release 159:14–26. https://doi.org/10.1016/J.JCONREL.2011.11.031

Ye J, Schoenung JM (2004) Technical cost modeling for the mechanical milling at cryogenic temperature (cryomilling). Adv Eng Mater 6:656–664. https://doi.org/10.1002/ADEM.200400074

Yonet-Tanyeri N, Amer M, Balmert SC et al (2022) Microfluidic systems for manufacturing of microparticle-based drug-delivery systems: design, construction, and operation. ACS Biomater Sci Eng 8:2864–2877. https://doi.org/10.1021/ACSBIOMATERIALS.2C00066/ASSET/IMAGES/LARGE/AB2C00066_0008.JPEG

Part II

Visualization Technologies

Visualization of Nanocarriers and Drugs in Cells and Tissue

Ulrike Alexiev and Eckart Rühl

Contents

Abstract

In this chapter, the visualization of nanocarriers and drugs in cells and tissue is reviewed. This topic is tightly connected to modern drug delivery, which relies on nanoscopic drug formulation approaches and the ability to probe nanoparticulate systems selectively in cells and tissue using advanced spectroscopic and microscopic techniques. We first give an overview of the breadth of this research field.

U. Alexiev (✉)
Fachbereich Physik, Freie Universität Berlin, Berlin, Germany
e-mail: ulrike.alexiev@fu-berlin.de

E. Rühl (✉)
Physikalische Chemie, Freie Universität Berlin, Berlin, Germany
e-mail: ruehl@zedat.fu-berlin.de

M. Schäfer-Korting, U. S. Schubert (eds.), *Drug Delivery and Targeting*,
Handbook of Experimental Pharmacology 284, https://doi.org/10.1007/164_2023_684

Then, we mainly focus on topical drug delivery to the skin and discuss selected visualization techniques from spectromicroscopy, such as scanning transmission X-ray microscopy and fluorescence lifetime imaging. These techniques rely on the sensitive and quantitative detection of the topically applied drug delivery systems and active substances, either by exploiting their molecular properties or by introducing environmentally sensitive probes that facilitate their detection.

Keywords

Fluorescence lifetime imaging · Label-free and label-based detection methods · Multimodal imaging methods · Nanocarrier-drug monitoring · Nanomaterials · Spectromicroscopy · X-ray microscopy

Acronyms

ADC	Analog-to-digital converter
CARS	Coherent anti-Stokes Raman scattering
CFD	Constant-fraction discriminator
CMS-ICC	ICC-tagged core-multishell nanocarriers
Cy3	Cyanine-3
D/DE	Dermis
DL	Dual label
EDX	Energy-dispersive X-ray emission
EPR	Electron paramagnetic resonance
FITC	Fluorescein isothiocyanate
FLIM	Fluorescence lifetime imaging microscopy
FRET	Fluorescence resonance energy transfer
HEC	Hydroxyethyl cellulose
ICC	Indocarbocyanine
MALDI	Matrix-assisted laser desorption ionization
MG-FITC	FITC-tagged tecto-dendrimer
NC	Nanocarrier
NIR	Near-infrared
NMR	Nuclear magnetic resonance
OPO	Optical parametric oscillator
PAM	Photoacoustic microscopy
PCA	Principal component analysis
PEEM	Photoemission electron microscopy
ppt	Parts per trillion
SC	Stratum corneum
SCC-25	Human tongue carcinoma cell line
SEM	Scanning electron microscopy
SIMS	Secondary ion mass spectrometry
SRS	Stimulated Raman scattering
s-SNOM	Scattering-scanning near-field optical microscopy
STXM	Scanning transmission X-ray microscopy
TAC	Time-to-amplitude converter

TCSPC	Time-correlated single photon counting
TEM	Transmission electron microscopy
TERS	Tip-enhanced Raman spectroscopy
TEWL	Transepidermal water loss
TIRFM	Total internal reflection fluorescence microscopy
TOF	Time-of-flight
TXM	Transmission X-ray microscopy
UV	Ultraviolet
VE	Viable epidermis

1 Introduction

Drug delivery to specific tissues is key for an appropriate dose at the target site in appropriate times. This often requires the development of novel drug delivery systems making use of nanochemistry and novel nanomaterials. These nanoparticulate drug delivery systems are envisioned not only to diminish adverse effects but also to increase the local exposure such that the therapeutic efficacy is increased compared to standard formulation (Gupta et al. 2012; Sahu et al. 2020).

Nanoparticulate drug delivery systems may include lipid-, protein-, and polymer-based nanoparticles, liposomes, as well as inorganic nanocarriers and delivery systems (Kurniasih et al. 2015; Patra et al. 2018). A large variety of such drug delivery systems have been described and tested within the last decades (Gregoire et al. 2020; Pena et al. 2020; Zheng et al. 2019). The emerging field of nanomedicine exploits these nanostructures for therapeutic as well as theranostic purposes (Ober et al. 2019; Ruman et al. 2020). One of the first nanoparticulate systems to be used in cancer therapy belongs to lipidic systems (Working and Dayan 1996), which include liposomes and lipid nanoparticles (Tenchov et al. 2021). Recently, lipid nanoparticles were successfully used in mRNA vaccines for the treatment of COVID19, effectively protecting and transporting mRNA to cells (Emergency Use Authorization (Eua) of the Pfizer-Biontech Covid-19 Vaccine to Prevent Coronavirus Disease 2019).

To determine the potential of these nanoparticulate drug delivery systems, various in vitro and in vivo techniques have been applied (Vogt et al. 2016). In the case of topical drug delivery for curing skin diseases, the aim is to bring the drug across the skin barrier to the site of action, where it is needed for therapeutic success (Vogt et al. 2016; Jeong et al. 2021). There, cytotoxicity, uptake, and binding efficacy to selected cells or the in vivo therapeutic potential to target tissues and cells has been evaluated (Alnasif et al. 2014; Brodwolf et al. 2020; Pischon et al. 2017).

Monitoring the distribution of drug delivery systems in cells, tissues, organs, or entire organisms as well as the drug release in vitro and in vivo is of paramount and irreplaceable importance for the development of drug delivery concepts and systems that accurately locate in diseased tissues and enable the release of the appropriate drug amount. Equally important is the monitoring of therapy success and thus the improvement of the therapeutic efficacy. Optimization of drug delivery strategies

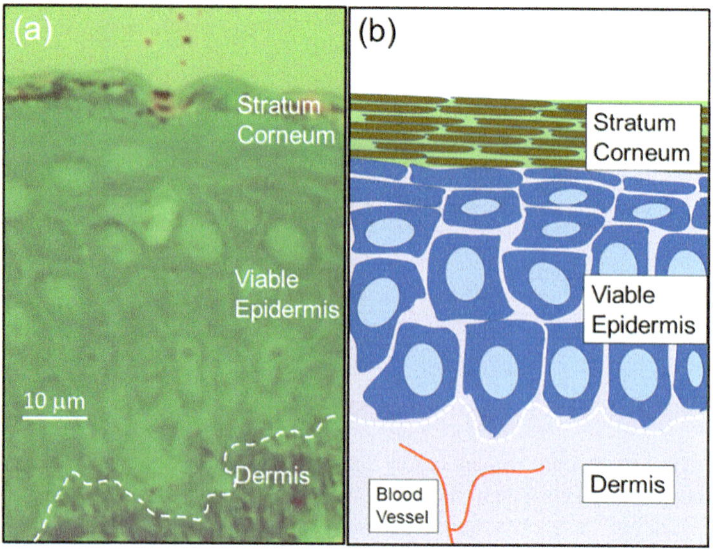

Fig. 1 Vertical section of the top layers of human skin: (**a**) optical micrograph and (**b**) cartoon. The stratum corneum consists of corneocytes separated by lipids, the viable epidermis consists mostly of keratinocytes and to a lesser extent of dendritic immune cells. The white dashed line in (**a**) and (**b**) marks the basal membrane

calls for quantitative visualization of drug penetration pathways and local drug concentrations. Visualization techniques provided by spectromicroscopy play a major role in determining spatial distributions and concentrations of the molecules of interest leading to the therapeutic capacity of novel drug delivery systems.

Here, we aim to give a brief overview on important techniques and their applications that are used for probing drugs and nanoparticles spatially resolved in biological matter with chemical specificity by methods of spectromicroscopy. Possible biological targets in the field of nanomedicine, however, are too wide for the scope of this chapter. Therefore, we consider for the sake of simplicity that the biological samples are cell monolayers, and 3D-skin models, or a skin section to be characterized with respect to the spatial distribution of nanocarriers, drugs, or drug formulations. These biological samples can be investigated by probing a variety of different physical or chemical properties, yielding qualitative and quantitative information.

As a specific example we will focus on the topical application of drug delivery systems aiming at a (epi-)dermal, follicular, or transdermal delivery. The challenge for topical drug delivery to skin is to overcome the skin barriers, the stratum corneum in particular (Vogt et al. 2016). Fig. 1 shows an optical micrograph and a cartoon of the top skin layers, representing essential barriers for topical drug delivery. The top layer of skin is the stratum corneum, which consists for intact skin of about 20 layers of thin corneocytes, where the thickness of each corneocyte is ca. 1 μm. Corneocytes are separated by thin lipid lamellae of ca. 100 nm thickness consisting of several lipid layers with repeat distances of 13 nm and 6 nm, respectively (van Smeden and Bouwstra 2016; Gorzelanny et al. 2020). The stratum corneum lipids consist of ceramides, cholesterol, fatty acids, and fatty acid esters (Candi et al. 2005). The corneocytes are connected by corneodesmosomes and tight junction remnants (Gorzelanny et al. 2020). The genesis of the stratum corneum from keratinocytes and the formation of the cornified envelope with covalently bound long-chain ω-hydroxy ceramides has been reviewed before (Candi et al. 2005). As a result, this top skin layer represents essentially a mechanical, but also a diffusion barrier for low- and high-molecular-weight species (Schulz et al. 2017), where one would expect that lipophilic drugs can be transported via the lipids. In addition, there is a size dependence for the penetration of molecular species limited to <500 Da, which is known as the 500 Da rule (Bos and Meinardi 2000), that has recently been questioned (Döge et al. 2018; Frombach et al. 2019; Volz et al. 2015). Moreover, the stratum corneum lipids lower the transepidermal water loss (TEWL). Several more barriers exist in the skin, i.e., in the stratum granulosum, between the stratum corneum and the viable epidermis, where the tight junctions are located, and below the viable epidermis where the basement membrane separates the viable epidermis from the dermis (Brandner 2016). In the former barrier, the tight junctions, specifically claudins and other plaque proteins block the penetration of high-molecular-weight drugs as well as charge-selective processes, so that the passage of ions is also reduced (Gorzelanny et al. 2020). The basement membrane consists of laminins, collagens, and proteoglycans. Besides, hair follicles and glands are located in the skin that also provide barriers (Gorzelanny et al. 2020). The difference to the above-described barriers is that the residence time of topically applied drugs or formulations is extended if entering a hair follicle (Döge et al. 2018; Frombach et al. 2019), whereas the outward flux from glands limits their penetration.

A variety of experimental techniques of low spatial resolution are known for investigating skin penetration of substances. Macroscopic information on skin is obtained from the TEWL measurements by gathering the relative humidity and temperature at the skin surface (Alexander et al. 2018). Electrical measurements consider the resistance and impedance of skin (Gorzelanny et al. 2020). Similarly, classical analytical approaches relying, e.g., on chromatography, spectroscopy (e.g., infrared, Raman), or optical microscopy (Volz et al. 2017) have either no or limited spatial resolution.

However, for obtaining a molecular understanding on nanocarrier/drug penetration and the response of tissue spatially resolved approaches are required that reach ultimately the molecular level. A variety of microscopic, spectroscopic, and structural methods can be used for monitoring and visualization of nanocarriers and drugs/drug release in cells and tissue. These methods, with a focus on high-resolution spectromicroscopies, are the topic of the next section, followed by a detailed description of few selected techniques and results demonstrating the present state-of-the-art.

2 Methodology

2.1 Overview on Spectromicroscopy Techniques

Different selected spectromicroscopy techniques for the study on biological matter with emphasis on cells and skin are schematically compiled in Fig. 2. This figure is organized as follows: A sample containing a drug or a drug nanocarrier is to be probed in biological surroundings. Here, the physical processes that are preferably suitable for their detection and quantification of these species are highlighted. These can be: (1) the absorption of electromagnetic radiation; (2) the emission of fluorescence photons; (3) scattering and reflection of radiation; (4) ionization leading to photoemission, i.e., the emission of electrons by ionizing radiation and similar probes or ions produced by ionization processes; (5) the decay of radioactive probes; and (6) there are photothermal and acoustic responses of matter.

These physical processes are best studied by spectroscopic techniques whose spatial resolution is realized by means of spectromicroscopy. The spatial resolution should be as high as possible to obtain not only macroscopic scales probed by spectroscopy but also microscopic or nanoscopic dimensions. These dimensions are required to connect observations from spectromicroscopy with a molecular understanding. The aim is to get beyond the Abbe diffraction limit of optical microscopy that is found at ~$\lambda/2$, where λ is the wavelength of the radiation.

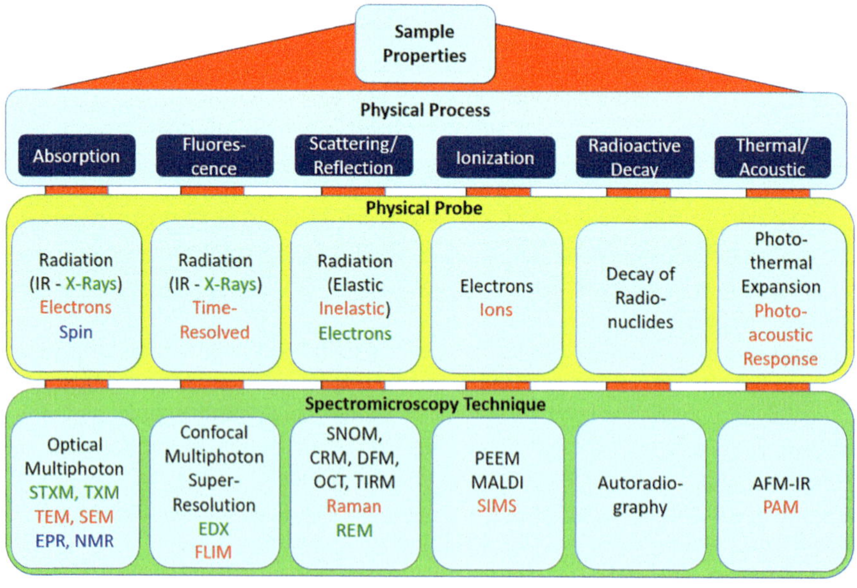

Fig. 2 Overiew on selected experimental techniques that are suitable for probing drug delivery to the skin by spectromicroscopy. Corresponding physical probes and spectromicroscopic techniques are colored alike to visualize their connection. See text for further details

As the variety of such techniques is extremely wide, it remains impossible to cover them all. It appears to be the most useful to give here a brief overview that is guided by Fig. 2. Generally, we can distinguish spectromicroscopy techniques requiring labels (sensor molecules) for selective and sensitive probing and label-free techniques. For the former, this can be fluorophore-tagged drugs or nanocarriers, fluorescent drugs, or drug mimetics. This labeling approach is often used along with fluorescence detection and appears to be simple, efficient, and appealing due to high sensitivity of fluorescence detection reaching down to single molecule detection (Volz et al. 2015). On the other hand, often highly potent drugs are not fluorescent and may change their efficacy and transport properties, if labeled by dyes. The alternative is the use of label-free techniques where the intrinsic properties of the drug or formulation are used to probe their local concentration (Graf and Rühl 2019). This ensures that non-fluorescent potent drugs or drug formulations are directly probed via their intrinsic molecular properties. However, there might be the drawback that these approaches tend to be less sensitive than those relying, e.g., on fluorescence or other sensitive labels. The use of either technique depends of course on the scientific questions and the availability of instruments to be applied to solve the scientific problems under study.

Figure 2 indicates that a variety of different physical processes can be induced by the interactions of electromagnetic radiation in different wavelength regimes, or by the impact of particles impinging on the sample of interest. Let us focus on those processes that have been used in the past to probe properties of biological matter. First, electromagnetic radiation can be absorbed by the sample. Chemical selectivity comes from the tunability of the radiation source so that distinct molecular excitations can be probed. Often, tunable photon sources including discharge lamps, lasers, or synchrotron radiation are used for absorption studies. Such radiation probes characteristic changes in optical density in one-photon transitions that are distinct for the substances of interest compared to the biological background matrix. Intense lasers are mostly available in the infrared, visible, and ultraviolet regimes, which may even allow for multiphoton absorption (Kirejev et al. 2012), a technique that can also be coupled with fluorescence microscopy (Sheppard 2020). It is even suitable for in vivo studies and may yield three-dimensional sample and target information from tomography (Koehler et al. 2011). Multiphoton absorption is of high sensitivity and selectivity, especially if resonant intermediate states of the probed species are involved or fluorescence photons are detected instead of simple absorption.

X-ray microscopy is another powerful approach in spectromicroscopy relying on absorption. Briefly, tunable X-rays have the advantage of element- and site-selective absorption and show a distinct chemical selectivity, which is advantageous for probing drugs in biological matter along with high spatial resolution, reaching below 10 nm in the soft X-ray regime (Shapiro et al. 2020). One can distinguish between scanning transmission X-ray microscopy (STXM) and transmission X-ray microscopy (TXM) (Guttmann and Bittencourt 2015). The difference between both techniques is that in STXM the sample is scanned and the transmitted photons are detected, which generates the micrograph. In TXM the sample is imaged by a zone plate on the detector for generating the micrograph. This is a similar imaging technique compared to the widely used electron microscopy, which employs fast electrons instead of photons that are either transmitted or scattered by the sample. Specifically, in transmission electron microscopy (TEM) the transmitted electrons are imaged on the detector by electron lenses probing the spatial distribution of electron density of the sample and may reach atomic resolution. The spatial resolution is superior compared to X-ray microscopy. However, there are some drawbacks, such as that thinner samples must be used for transmission electron microscopy and wet samples cannot be investigated due to the vacuum requirements of TEM. The alternative to TEM is scanning electron microscopy (SEM) where the sample is scanned across the electron beam and the transmitted or scattered electrons are detected. Chemical sensitivity can be reached from a combination with X-ray fluorescence analysis (energy-dispersive X-ray spectroscopy, EDX) (Scimeca et al. 2018). Other techniques relying on absorption processes are the resonance methods related to electron paramagnetic resonance (EPR) and nuclear magnetic resonance (NMR). These rely on resonance transitions of the Zeeman-split levels in magnetic fields due to unpaired electrons or nuclear levels, respectively. The spatial resolution is of the order of micrometers for both methods (Lee et al. 2001; Shin et al. 2011) and is still not comparable to that of optical microscopy (Sersa 2021). Fluorescence is the result of radiative de-excitation following the absorption of radiation. Often, fluorescent dyes are used as model drugs or they can be coupled to nanocarriers transporting the drugs across biological barriers (Rajes et al. 2021). Then, the fluorescent agent can be used to probe the localization or the time-dependent character of the drug/nanocarrier systems in biological samples, e.g., to monitor the drug release. Confocal microscopy or multiphoton fluorescence microscopy is limited in spatial resolution to the Abbe diffraction limit. Super-resolution fluorescence based-techniques permit substantially higher spatial resolution (Leung and Chou 2011; Valli and Sanderson 2021). Fluorescence photons can also be emitted in the X-ray regime from heavy elements following electron impact in electron microscopy, which is called energy-dispersive X-ray spectroscopy (EDX) introduced above (Mirakovski et al. 2022). Time-resolved fluorescence is a sensitive probe of the local environment of the emitting species, thus fluorescence lifetime imaging is another sensitive approach in spectromicroscopy (Alexiev et al. 2017; Boreham et al. 2017a), which is described in more detail below. If the incident radiation is inelastically scattered by the target, this opens the wide regime of Raman-based spectromicroscopy techniques, which were successfully applied to probe drugs in biological matter including skin in a label-free fashion (Zhang et al. 2007; Mao et al. 2012; Zhang et al. 2020). This approach works also for in vivo studies (Lademann et al. 2009). Besides conventional Raman techniques used for spectroscopy and spectromicroscopy, there are also advanced Raman-based approaches. This includes coherent anti-Stokes Raman scattering (CARS) (Evans et al. 2005; Fu et al. 2012), a four-wave mixing process leading to enhanced sensitivity compared to conventional Raman techniques. Stimulated Raman scattering (SRS) (Freudiger et al. 2008; Lu et al. 2015; Klossek et al. 2017; Wanjiku et al. 2019) is another, somewhat simpler to handle technique, where a tunable and a fixed wavelength infrared source is merged leading to time-correlated excitation and stimulated emission processes. This technique is by at least three orders of magnitude more sensitive than spontaneous Raman scattering. However, Raman techniques are limited in spatial resolution, which is due to the use of infrared radiation and the diffraction limit. This can be avoided by tip-enhanced Raman techniques (TERS), yielding substantially higher spatial resolution provided by the atomic-force microscopy tip along with chemical contrast provided by Raman scattering (Ashtikar et al. 2017). Besides TERS, there are other atomic-force microscopy-based techniques in spectromicroscopy. Scattering-type optical near-field microscopy (s-SNOM) is one spectromicroscopy technique that makes use of the near-field below a sharp tip of an atomic-force microscopy (Fu et al. 2012). If coupled to a tunable radiation source, one reaches spatial resolution in the nanometer regime (Kästner et al. 2018). Different tunable radiation sources in the infrared and far-infrared have been used along with s-SNOM, which includes CO- and CO_2-lasers (Keilmann et al. 2009), optical parametric oscillators (OPO) (Wirth et al. 2021), difference frequency generation of laser radiation (Hegenbarth et al. 2014), quantum cascade lasers (Schnell et al. 2020; Kanevche et al. 2021), synchrotron radiation (Kästner et al. 2018), and free electron lasers (Kuschewski et al. 2016). Especially, quantum cascade lasers have turned out to be the most convenient and intense sources for s-SNOM studies.

Ionization techniques also play a role in analyzing biological samples. The emission of electrons due to the impact of ionizing radiation (photoemission) is one sensitive probe that is exploited for spectromicroscopy by emitting electrons from the valence shell or core levels (inner-shell photoionization). However, photoelectron microscopy (PEEM) requires investigation of the sample in a high vacuum environment, which differs from most of the above-mentioned techniques that can be used at ambient conditions. There are, however, examples of applying PEEM for studying biological samples (Frazer et al. 2002, 2004). Besides detection of the emitted electrons one can also detect ions that are formed upon photoionization. One commonly used approach is matrix-assisted laser desorption (MALDI) (Caprioli et al. 1997), where an intense laser beam is impinging on the surface of the sample containing the analyte that is often probed by time-of-flight mass spectrometry (MALDI-TOF). This requires the addition of a matrix prior to the analysis while allowing for studies on biological samples (Noun et al. 2022). Commercial instruments have a low spatial resolution (>50 μm), but research efforts on proteins and lipids indicate that a spatial resolution of 5 μm can be reached (Zavalin et al. 2012, 2014), with the perspective to reach even the sub-micron range (Niehaus et al. 2019; Ma and Fernandez 2022). Certainly, this range of spatial resolution of typically 10–50 μm is substantially lower than that of electron microscopy techniques, often reaching atomic resolution, where solely the electron density of the sample is probed. Furthermore, there are secondary ion mass spectrometry (SIMS) techniques relying on ion detection. Ion beams with kinetic energies of the order of 10 keV are used for producing cations and anions without the need of labeling (Noun et al. 2022). These are probed as a function of location allowing for probing the spatial distribution of the secondary ions. The spatial resolution is for nano-SIMS ca. ≥ 50 nm with a sensitivity in the parts per trillion (ppt)-range

(Gregoire et al. 2020). The radioactive decay of unstable nuclides is also exploited for spatially resolved studies. Radiolabeled drugs or nanoparticles can be sensitively and selectively probed by autoradiography films, gamma counters, microimagers, or phosphoimager plates. This approach has the advantage that even entire organisms can be investigated, but the spatial resolution is limited to macroscopic scales of the order of 1 mm (Stojanov et al. 2012). Combination with optical microscopy allows for probing subcellular details (Gröger et al. 2013). Photothermal expansion is an atomic-force microscopy-based technique that probes locally on the nanoscale the thermal expansion of a sample irradiated by a pulsed infrared laser beam (Dazzi and Prater 2017). It is known that the photothermal expansion is proportional to the absorption of the sample, which allows for quantitative studies. The exponential drop in photothermal expansion after the photon pulse, e.g., emerging from a quantum cascade laser (Rajes et al. 2021), is sensitively probed by atomic-force microscopy, where the sensitivity of the approach depends on the transition moment of the absorption process. Suitable radiation sources used for such instruments have been pulsed OPOs and more recently quantum cascade lasers (Rajes et al. 2021; Mathurin et al. 2022). Photoacoustic microscopy (PAM) relies on the detection of ultrasound, which is generated as a response of optical absorption. It is suitable for probing, e.g., particles in biological matter with high temporal and spatial resolution (Lemaster and Jokerst 2017). This allows for probing cell organelles as well as organs (Xia et al. 2014; Wang and Hu 2012). Important for biological samples is the substantially higher penetration depth than optical microscopy, reaching several centimeters.

2.2 Selected Techniques in Spectromicroscopy

2.2.1 Scanning Transmission X-Ray Microscopy (STXM)

Scanning transmission X-ray microscopy is a technique that allows for performing spectromicroscopy studies and has been used for a variety of samples irradiated by tunable soft X-rays (Lawrence et al. 2016). It relies essentially on tunable synchrotron radiation as a light source permitting element- and site-selective excitation. Alternatively, laser plasma sources have been used, as well (Legall et al. 2012). This selective capability of primary excitation has been extensively exploited for spectroscopic investigations (Stöhr 1992). The other crucial ingredient is tight focusing of the X-rays by a Fresnel zone plate along with an order-sorting aperture. The samples under study are then placed into the focus of the zone plate, while the sample is scanned in x- and y-direction. The transmitted photons are detected by either a photomultiplier tube or a diode. The use of an absorption experiment allows for quantification by the Beer-Lambert law, which relies on the attenuation of the sample according to $\ln(I/I_0) = -\sigma \cdot c \cdot d$, where I_0 is the intensity of the incident radiation, I is the intensity of the transmitted radiation, the ratio $\ln(I_0/I)$ is often called optical density, σ is the absorption cross section, c is the concentration of the species under study, and d is the absorption path length, which is equivalent to the thickness of the sample. The thickness of the sample needs to be adjusted so that sufficient absorption occurs and still photons are transmitted to the detector. Typical values of d are of the order of 300 nm for biological samples probed by soft X-rays (Yamamoto et al. 2015). In inner-shell excitation of deeply bound electrons, typically 1 s electrons of light elements in the second row of the periodic table, such as carbon, nitrogen, or oxygen, can be excited for biologically relevant species by soft X-rays in the photon energy regime between 280 and 560 eV, corresponding to wavelengths between ~4.4 and 2.2 nm. The chemically important part concerns the distinct near-edge features, where core electrons are excited into unoccupied orbitals of the absorber (Stöhr 1992). This can provide chemical selectivity, which is due to characteristic chemical shifts of the near-edge resonances (Stöhr 1992). The other important part is the continuum cross section σ_{cont}, which follows above the absorption energy of the near-edge features (Henke et al. 1993). It is easy to quantify by $\sigma_{cont} = (A/N_A) \cdot \mu$. A corresponds to the sum of weights of the atomic constituents, μ is the tabulated and energy-dependent mass absorption coefficient, and N_A is Avogadro's number. This means that one can easily derive absolute cross sections along with the Beer-Lambert law yielding the absolute quantity of absorbers in the sample. This is often desirable for determining the efficiency of drug uptake into tissue, e.g., skin with intact or damaged barriers (Yamamoto et al. 2017). The experimental strategy for data acquisition is to take at least an X-ray micrograph of the sample at a photon energy where the species of interest absorbs and another one, where it does not absorb. This yields along with the Beer-Lambert law an image of chemical contrast of the sample of interest. In biological samples such pairs of photon energies have been used for determining the location of topically applied drug formulations in fixed skin samples (Yamamoto et al. 2015). In reality, this approach has its limitations, for the following reasons: (1) the biological matrix may give rise to cross-sensitivities, which may lead to not unique results that are uncovered after the experiments are finished (Yamamoto et al. 2015); (2) other pairs of photon energies may be desirable to investigate, but this can only be done during the access to the scanning transmission X-ray microscope. Specifically, the available beam time at synchrotron radiation facilities is limited, which requires to use the scarce time prudently; (3) energy scales in soft X-rays may slightly change with time, due to, e.g., the beam position in the storage ring, which requires to verify that the energy scale has not changed during the experiments. As a result, it has turned out to be more efficient to rely on hyperspectral imaging, where the full spectroscopic information is contained in each pixel of the X-ray micrographs (Germer et al. 2021). Then, the analysis can be done at any time after the data acquisition is terminated and is not limited to a few selected photon energies. In addition, such full data set can also be evaluated by other approaches, such as singular value decomposition along with reliable reference spectra of the species of interest (Germer et al. 2021; Koprinarov et al. 2002). This approach solves the overdetermined linear set of equations, where the unknown concentrations of the species of interest need to be determined by minimizing the residual error. The results can be compared to those determined by Beer-Lambert law (Germer et al. 2021). However, singular value decomposition is certainly favored, if there are not distinct chemical shifts in absorption energies found for identifying the species of interest in the biological matrix. Then, the full near-edge spectra appear to yield more reliable results from singular value decomposition (Germer et al. 2021), which can also be compared to other approaches, such as principal component analysis (PCA) or cluster analysis. The latter methods are contained, e.g., in standard data evaluation packages, such as MANTiS (Lerotic et al. 2014).

2.2.2 Fluorescence Techniques in Biological Matter

From the physical perspective, in vitro and in vivo fluorescence imaging relies on the excitation of the "object," i.e., the target cells or tissue together with the drug or nanocarrier, by illumination with an ultraviolet (UV) to near-infrared (NIR) light source depending on the spectral properties of the used fluorophore, the imaging agent. The photons, which excite the fluorophore, travel through the tissue layers. The emitted radiation from the excited fluorophore is shifted to higher wavelengths, corresponding to a spectral "red-shift," and requires selecting the appropriate wavelength region for the detection of the emitted photons, i.e., the detection of the fluorescence (Fig. 3(a)). The more red-shifted the excitation wavelength, the higher is the penetration depth into the tissue (Fig. 3(b)). The excitation light is partially reflected, scattered, and absorbed by endogenous fluorophores (autofluorescence) in the tissues (Fig. 3(c)) (Weissleder and Ntziachristos 2003). This affects the depth resolution, sensitivity of the fluorescence signal, and may lead to artifacts due to tissue autofluorescence. Fortunately, in the NIR wavelength region a low absorption window exists that reduces autofluorescence (Fig. 3(c)).

This explains the quest for NIR-fluorescent proteins, frequently used in optogenetics as well as in biomedical research (Nagano et al. 2022). Synthetic dyes, as often employed as imaging agents for visualization of nanocarriers and drugs, are readily available in the red and NIR region. Most of the fluorescence methods and systems currently applied in basic research and preclinical development are based on planar epi-illumination (Volz et al. 2017). These epi-illumination microscopes are simple to operate but lack depth resolution and suffer from signal non-linearities. Confocal laser-scanning microscopes provide a solution to achieve increased lateral as well as horizontal resolution (Amos and White 2003).

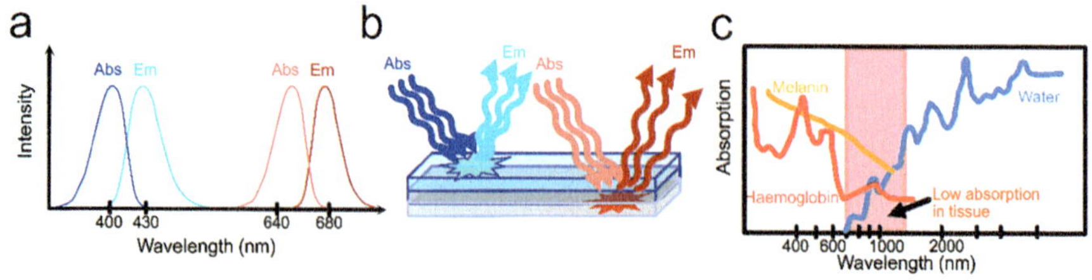

Fig. 3 (**a**) Absorption (Abs) and emission (Em) spectra of two dyes absorbing in the UV (blue) and in the red wavelength regime, (**b**) Schematic of penetration depth dependence on excitation light, (**c**) Absorption spectra of autofluorescent molecules in tissue. The NIR window devoid of autofluorescence is depicted

Usually, fluorescence intensity is linearly proportional to fluorophore concentration. However, fluorescence is highly sensitive to its environment. This may lead to fluorescence quenching (Volz et al. 2017) and obscures the intensity – concentration correlation. On the other hand, one can make use of quenching mechanisms, such as the fluorescence resonance energy transfer (FRET), where a donor dye can be fully quenched at the expense of the fluorescence of an acceptor dye. Employing judiciously placed donor and acceptor dyes, drug release can be monitored by this principle using the "turn-on" fluorescence from dequenching after drug release (Kaeokhamloed et al. 2022; Krüger et al. 2014). Other fluorophores, such as seminaphtharhodafluor or indocarbocyanine (ICC/Cy3) dyes, are sensitive to pH (Richter et al. 2015) or viscosity (Ober et al. 2019), which means that the fluorescence quantum yield of those fluorophores directly depends on the proton concentration in the environment or on the surrounding viscosity, respectively. In particular, the changes in fluorescence lifetime, i.e., the time an excited fluorophore spends in the excited state, offer insights into the microenvironment of the fluorophore.

Besides pH and viscosity, this also includes polarity, biomolecular interactions, and the presence of reactive oxygen species (Balke et al. 2018; Boreham et al. 2016; Borst and Visser 2010; Hirvonen et al. 2020; Kirchberg et al. 2011; Gronbach et al. 2020). Sect. 2.2.3 covers in more detail time-resolved fluorescence-based imaging, also called Fluorescence Lifetime Imaging Microscopy (FLIM). Single molecule/super-resolution fluorescence microscopy, most often in the flavor of total internal reflection fluorescence microscopy (TIRFM), allows, amongst other aspects, the characterization of drug delivery systems in terms of their size, shape, surface, encapsulation efficiency, as well as their interaction with cellular components and target structures, which are of importance for drug delivery efficiency (Döge et al. 2018; Volz et al. 2015; Okay 2020). Molecular parameters like drug loading, distribution, or leakage of the drug are also important parameters, e.g., for lipidic nanocarriers. Figure 4 visualizes drug loading in nanostructured lipid carriers (NLC) that depends on the formation of nanostructures within the lipid matrix (Boreham et al. 2017b; Wolf et al. 2023).

The so-called visit maps obtained from the single molecule tracks of the encapsulated fluorescent agents directly visualize the hot spots of drug distribution within the nanoparticle (Fig. 4(d–g)) (Boreham et al. 2017b). In this example, a spherical oily nanocompartment is formed, in which the drug is homogeneously distributed (Fig. 4(b, c)). A tracking free single molecule analysis (Wolf et al. 2023) revealed two distinct diffusive subpopulations with nanocompartment sizes of about 70 nm and 120 nm, which equals about 10% and 50% of the total volume of a single NLC, respectively. The third subpopulation equals the size of the nanoparticle (Fig. 4(a)), thereby indicating that part of the encapsulated agent is reaching the border of the NLC for drug release.

2.2.3 Fluorescence Lifetime Imaging (FLIM)

The fluorescence lifetime τ is the average time an exited electron remains in the excited state before relaxing to the ground state via photon emission. The

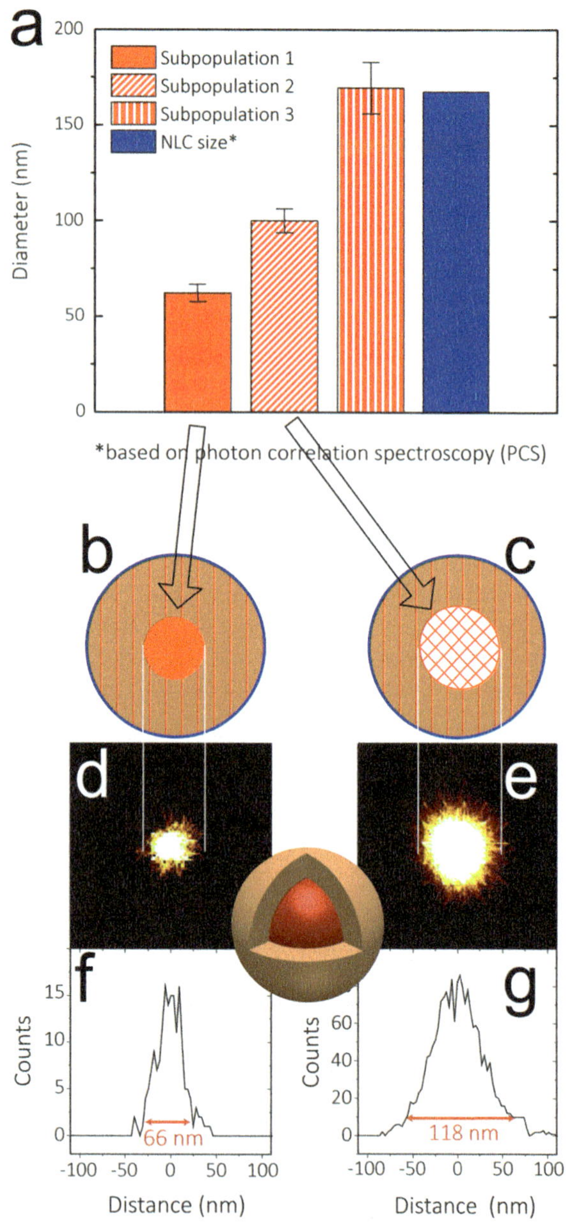

Fig. 4 Drug loading capacity in nanostructured lipid carriers (NLC) as revealed by single molecule TIRFM. (**a**) Subpopulations of drug diffusion in the NLC are compared with NLC size; (**d**–**g**) Visit maps of drug distribution within the NLC that are schematically presented in (**b**, **c**). This figure was adapted with permission from European Journal of Pharmaceutics and Biopharmaceutics, Vol. 110, by A. Boreham et al. "*Determination of nanostructures and drug distribution in lipid nanoparticles by single molecule microscopy,*" pages: 31–38, Copyright Elsevier (2017) (Boreham et al. 2017b)

fluorescence lifetime τ is dependent on the rate of photon emission k_r and the rate of the non-radiative decay processes k_{nr} with $\tau = (k_r + k_{nr})^{-1}$. For most fluorophores, the fluorescence lifetime is of the order of 100 ps to several nanoseconds. Thus, short-pulse lasers, such as Ti:sapphire lasers with pulse lengths up to 1.5 ps, supercontinuum white light lasers, or pulsed diode lasers (~ 50–200 ps pulse length), are required to excite the fluorophores (Hirvonen and Suhling 2020; Volz et al. 2018).

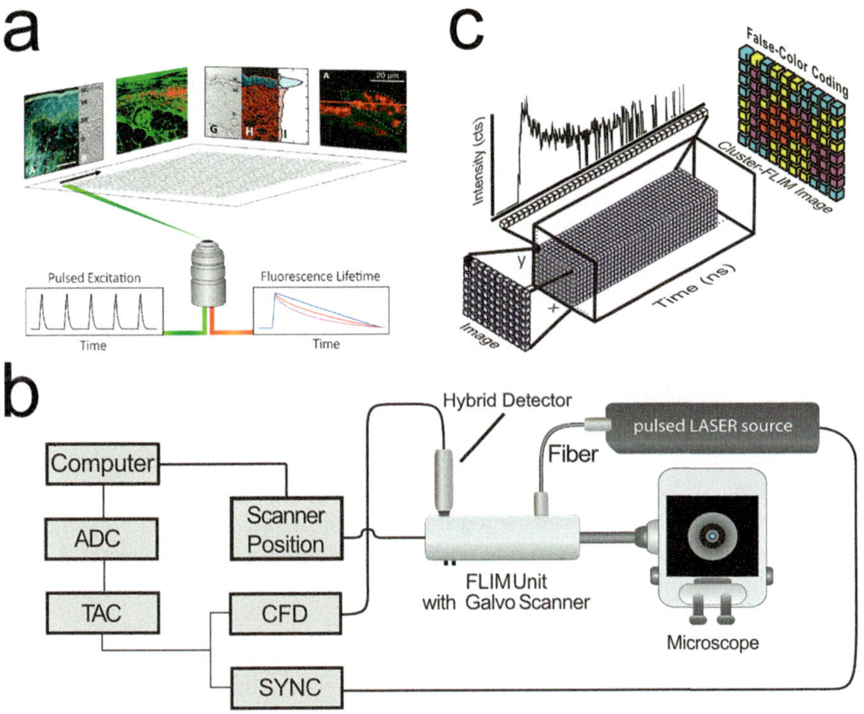

Fig. 5 (**a**) FLIM principle with picosecond laser excitation and pixelwise detection of the fluorescence lifetime curve. Pixels are color-coded with respect to the lifetime value; (**b**) Instrumentation of a typical TCSPC-based FLIM setup. Electronics (constant-fraction discriminator (CFD), time-to-amplitude converter (TAC), and analog-to-digital converter (ADC)) allow to process the captured photons, yielding the fluorescence lifetime curve in each individual pixel as shown in (**c**)

As the fluorescence quantum yield Φ is proportional to the fluorescence lifetime, $\Phi = k_r/(k_r + k_{nr})$, time-resolved fluorescence spectroscopy (fluorescence lifetime measurements) can distinguish between quenching effects, which affect the lifetime except for ground-state quenching (Volz et al. 2017), and concentration changes, which affect the intensity, i.e., the area under the fluorescence lifetime curve (see Fig. 5(c)) (Alexiev and Farrens 2014). The fluorescence lifetime can be obtained from an exponential fit with a model function to the recorded fluorescence decay curve $I(t)$ (Fig. 5(c)). Time-resolved fluorescence spectromicroscopy is named fluorescence lifetime imaging microscopy (FLIM) or in short FLI. Most FLIM setups operate in the time-domain, i.e., directly measuring the fluorescence lifetime with about 20–35 ps time resolution using time-correlated single photon counting (TCSPC) in a laser-scanning confocal microscope (Fig. 5(b)) (Alexiev et al. 2017; Poudel et al. 2020; Becker 2021). These techniques are well-suited for the study of tissue sections and live cells (monolayers, organoids) with spatial resolution down to the diffraction limit (Gronbach et al. 2020). To obtain a tomographic image deep into tissue multiphoton fluorescence techniques are required (Brodwolf et al. 2020; König 2020; Ustione and Piston 2011). Imaging of whole organisms, e.g., animals in preclinical research, requires in vivo imaging systems that combine 2D- and 3D-optical tomography (Bloch et al. 2005; Liu et al. 2019). Two-photon scanning FLIM enables this tomographic feature with lifetime resolution and a lateral resolution down to the diffraction limit (Brodwolf et al. 2020).

The drawback of FLIM in live cell or tissue imaging is that long exposure times are required to obtain a sufficient signal-to-noise ratio in each single pixel (Fig. 5(c)). For short exposure times, that are not harmful to the cells, the obtained individual lifetime curves have low photon statistics, i.e., they are quite noisy. This reduces the information content from a single fluorescence decay curve. In most cases, two decay components can be recovered.

Better statistics can be obtained at the cost of spatial resolution. Binning, i.e., the analysis of a cluster of pixels as a single pixel (e.g., a binning of 3 × 3 pixels into one pixel) where all photons are summed up to one fluorescence decay curve, increases the signal-to-noise ratio. On the analysis side, global fitting and fast lifetime fitting routines (e.g., Jo et al. (2005); Le Marois et al. (2017)) increase the certainty of the fit results. A graphically based technique, the phasor approach, is also highly successful but limited in the number of extracted fluorescence lifetime components (Digman et al. 2008). Nowadays, machine learning/deep learning algorithms facilitate and increase the certainty of lifetime extraction and fitting in FLIM (Smith et al. 2019; Mannam et al. 2020).

To meet the need of automated, fast, and fit-free fluorescence lifetime imaging required in preclinical and clinical settings, the Cluster-FLIM technique was developed that enables assumption-free extraction of the fluorescence lifetime curves with unprecedented accuracy and precision (Brodwolf et al. 2020). Cluster-FLIM uses multivariate cluster analysis techniques, without the need of any a-priori information, such as reference lifetime curves, to extract the different lifetime signatures of the various fluorescent species in the samples. Up to seven different fluorescent species with lifetime curves containing multiple decay components can be extracted. To discriminate the fluorescence lifetime signatures of five different fluorescence species Cluster-FLIM requires only 170, respectively, 90 counts per pixel to obtain 95% sensitivity (hit rate) and 95% specificity (correct rejection rate). This fit-free Cluster-FLIM technique also allows us to distinguish unequivocally between autofluorescence and target fluorescence.

3 Selected Results and Discussion

3.1 Depth Profiles of Topical Drug Delivery and Barrier Disruptions Probed by STXM

Depth profiles of drugs have been determined by scanning transmission X-ray microscopy (Wanjiku et al. 2019; Yamamoto et al. 2015, 2016; 2017, 2019; Germer et al. 2021). A prerequisite for determining such depth profiles is to measure the X-ray absorption spectra of the drug and the skin sample, as was done in earlier work for the topically applied glucocorticoid dexamethasone (Yamamoto et al. 2015, 2017). This lipophilic drug ($C_{22}H_{29}FO_5$) has a molecular weight of 392.464 g/

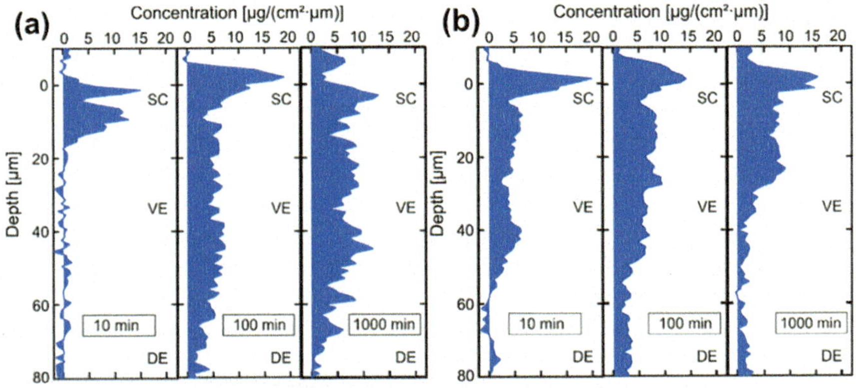

Fig. 6 (**a**) Depth profiles of dexamethasone in intact human skin obtained from scanning transmission X-ray microscopy as a function of penetration time at 10 min, 100 min, and 1,000 min, respectively; (**b**) depth profiles of dexamethasone in tape-stripped human skin obtained from scanning X-ray microscopy as a function of penetration time at 10 min, 100 min, and 1,000 min, respectively. *SC* stratum corneum, *VE* viable epidermis, *DE* dermis. See text for further details. This figure was taken with permission from European Journal of Pharmaceutics and Biopharmaceutics, Vol. 118, by K. Yamamoto et al. "*Influence of the Skin Barrier on the Penetration of Topically-Applied Dexamethasone probed by Soft X-ray Spectromicroscopy,*" pages: 30–37, Copyright Elsevier (2017) (Yamamoto et al. 2017)

mol. Its log *P*-value is 1.83 (Alvarez Núñez and Yalkowsky 1997), which means that the partitioning between an octanol and a water phase is ~67.6 times higher in the octanol phase than in the aqueous phase. This implies that one expects that the drug is found in the lipid lamellae between the corneocytes in intact stratum corneum rather than inside the corneocytes. Due to the molecular weight below 500 Da one expects that this drug is readily transported into deeper skin layers (Bos and Meinardi 2000). This is in full agreement with earlier findings as dexamethasone is used in dermatology for the treatment of inflammatory skin diseases and the mechanism of action is well-known (Ahluwalia 1998). Earlier, the depth distribution of topically applied dexamethasone was not precisely known, but it was expected that the drug forms a depot in the stratum corneum as the most lipophilic part of skin (Paturi et al. 2010). This expectation was subsequently verified by initial low spatial resolution scanning transmission X-ray microscopy (STXM) studies (Yamamoto et al. 2015). Note that the human samples studied ex vivo were taken in accordance with the Declaration of Helsinki guidelines. Skin samples were fixed in EPON resin after the treatment to become durable for later studies by STXM. They were cut into slices with a thickness of ~350 nm (see Yamamoto et al. (2017) for further details). This thickness is required for having sufficient transmission of the tunable X-rays in the wavelength range of ~2.34 nm. The STXM studies made use of two-photon energies in the O 1 s-excitation regime, where dexamethasone was element- and site-selectively excited.

Figure 6(a) shows as a specific example the result of systematic work, where the penetration time of the dexamethasone formulated in HEC gel (1.5% with a total drug dose of 600 μg/cm^2) has been systematically varied (Yamamoto et al. 2017). Three time points are shown: 10, 100, and 1,000 min. The vertical profiles of the drug concentration indicated in absolute concentrations of μg/(cm^2 μm) are derived from two-dimensional maps of the drug distribution by integrating at each depth level at pixel sizes of 100 nm, where the zero point in depth is set to the skin surface.

The resulting depth profiles with a depth resolution reduced to 1 μm indicate that label-free detection of dexamethasone yields depth profiles with absolute concentrations that show a clear temporal evolution. The stratum corneum acts as a drug reservoir and in the dermis no enhanced drug concentrations are observed. These results indicate that the stratum corneum is the major barrier for drug penetration, whereas the tight junctions at the top of the viable epidermis, i.e., the stratum granulosum, and basement membrane separating the viable epidermis from the dermis are no major barriers for dexamethasone penetration.

Figure 6(b) shows a similar sequence of results, but instead of intact human skin the samples were tape-stripped 30 times prior to topical drug exposure with the same formulation containing dexamethasone in HEC gel, as used for intact skin (Yamamoto et al. 2017). This means that the top barrier of the stratum corneum is mechanically thinned and weakened. The depth profiles indicate an about 10 times faster penetration of the drug than through intact skin.

Figure 7(a) shows a high-resolution micrograph of the stratum corneum of a skin sample that was exposed for 10 min to the dexamethasone/HEC gel formulation (Yamamoto et al. 2017). The pixel size was 50 nm and the false color image corresponds to blue color for high drug concentration, whereas low concentration is indicated by red color. Red color corresponds to optically thinner regions, which are assigned to lipids. Only, if these regions are filled with an optically thicker species, i.e., the drug dexamethasone, then there is a change in optical density. Note that the chemical contrast of dexamethasone was obtained as outlined above. The skin surface is on the right-hand side, where the outer corneocyte layers are loose and separated from each other compared to the compact regions in the lower stratum corneum. It is evident that the regions of blue color are narrow and not uniformly distributed. This implies that there is a gradient in local drug concentration, rather than some regions that are well connected to the skin surface, where the drug is leaking to deeper regions. All regions containing blue color, i.e., high drug concentration, are oriented parallel to the skin surface and have a width of ca. 100–350 nm. The distance between regions of low drug concentration is compatible with the thickness of corneocytes. This result appears to be consistent with a drug penetration path along the lipid layers separating the corneocytes. Note that no drug is found between the lipid lamellae, suggesting that dexamethasone does not penetrate efficiently corneocytes.

Figure 7(b) shows in greater detail a region that was arbitrarily chosen, where the drug penetration profile is determined vertically to the lipid lamellae, i.e., vertically to the skin surface (see arrow in Fig. 7(a)). The intensity of the local drug concentration (dashed line connecting the data points (black dots) in Fig. 7(b)) is well presented by a Gaussian profile (full line in Fig. 7(b)). This line shape is expected to occur, provided that the limited spatial resolution of the instrument, with contributions from the zone plate and X-ray monochromator, dominates the shape

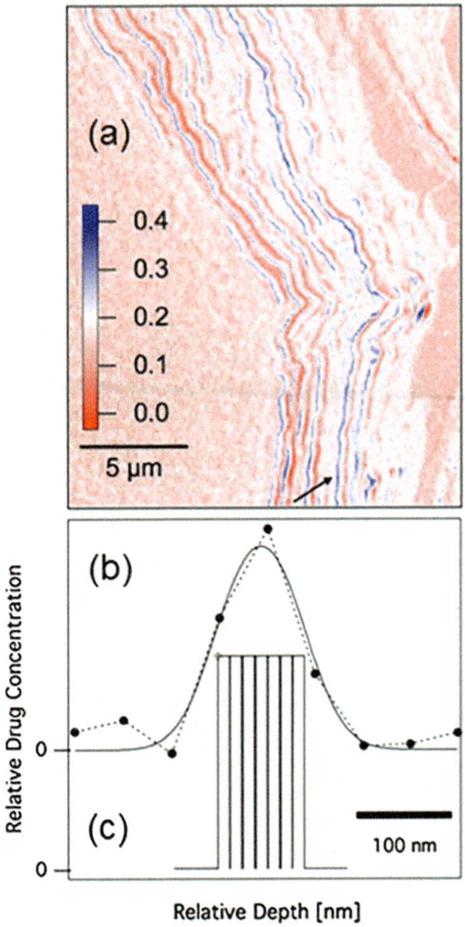

Fig. 7 (**a**) Local concentration of dexamethasone in the stratum corneum (color scale: optical density if dexamethasone is probed at 530.1 eV and 528.0 eV, respectively). The arrow corresponds to the region shown in (**b**); (**b**) Profile of local dexamethasone concentration (black dots and dashed line) and a fit with a Gaussian function leading to a rectangular profile (**c**), see text for further details. This figure was taken with permission from European Journal of Pharmaceutics and Biopharmaceutics, Vol. 118, by K. Yamamoto et al. "*Influence of the Skin Barrier on the Penetration of Topically-Applied Dexamethasone probed by Soft X-ray Spectromicroscopy,*" pages 30–37, Copyright Elsevier (2017) (Yamamoto et al. 2017)

in drug distribution. Then, one can determine the intrinsic distribution of the drug in this region.

A de-convolution with a Gaussian of 70 ± 5 nm leads to a rectangular profile of 91 nm width. This profile agrees with seven layers of lipids of 13 nm width. Such widths in lipid lamellae follow from earlier work of Bouwstra and coworkers (Bouwstra et al. 2003). There, 13 nm wide structures were identified in stratum corneum lipids, which appears to be consistent with the local drug distribution, assuming that all lipid lamellae are equally filled with the drug, as indicated in Fig. 7 (c). This result shows that STXM can provide details in local drug distributions in nanoscopic dimensions.

Barrier disruptions can be induced mechanically, as pointed out above for tape-stripping. In addition, there are also chemical ways, besides inflammatory skin diseases, to induce barrier disruptions. This was successfully done by exposing human skin to the serine protease trypsin, mostly for simulating skin inflammations (Germer et al. 2021; Frombach et al. 2018). The following example of studies shows

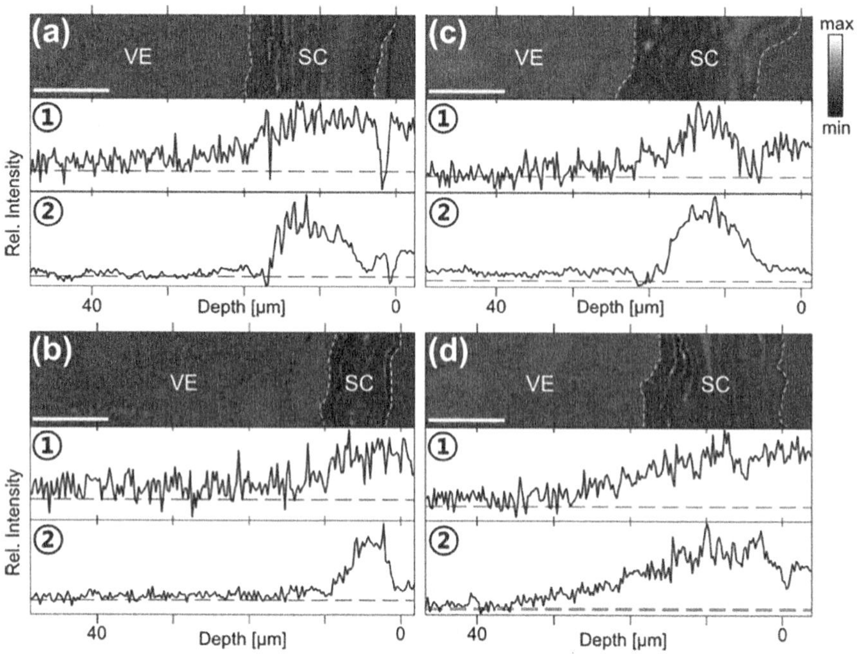

Fig. 8 Role of skin barrier damage by the serine protease trypsin. A rapamycin formulation in HEC gel was topically applied for 24 h after initial skin treatment with trypsin for (**a**) 2 h, (**b**) 4 h, (**c**) 8 h, and (**d**) 16 h, respectively. The top of each plot shows an X-ray micrograph taken at 532.0 eV. Below two different data reduction approaches are presented, showing the depth distribution of rapamycin: ① use of two-photon energies (531.1 and 530.7 eV) for selective probing of rapamycin according to the Beer-Lambert law and ② is the result of a singular value decomposition. *VE* viable epidermis, *SC* stratum corneum. The dashed white lines in the micrographs indicate the borders of the stratum corneum, the black dashed lines in the drug distribution profiles indicate the background level, scale bar: 10 µm. This figure was taken with permission from ACS Omega, Vol. 6, by G. Germer et al. "*Improved Skin Permeability after Topical Treatment with Serine Protease: Probing the Penetration of Rapamycin by Scanning Transmission X-Ray Microscopy*," pages: 12213–12222, Copyright American Chemical Society (2021) (Germer et al. 2021)

that the drug rapamycin can only penetrate human skin, if the skin is initially treated with trypsin, as probed by scanning transmission X-ray microscopy (Germer et al. 2021). Skin samples that did not undergo this treatment prior to topical application of rapamycin gave no evidence for drug penetration, even if the drug was dissolved in ethanol (Germer et al. 2021), a well-known penetration enhancer (Bommannan et al. 1991). This is in agreement with the 500 Da rule, indicating that the drug rapamycin (molecular weight: ~914 Da) cannot penetrate intact human skin (Bos and Meinardi 2000).

However, if the skin is initially treated with trypsin for variable time periods reaching from 2 to 16 h, then the drug is observed in the top skin layers (stratum corneum and viable epidermis) (Germer et al. 2021). These systematic studies are shown in Fig. 8. There, two different approaches in data evaluation are compared:

(1) using the Beer-Lambert law and (2) singular value decomposition, as outlined above. The systematic studies indicate that damage of the skin barrier is efficient already after 2 h, as reported before (Germer et al. 2021). Then, rapamycin can penetrate the stratum corneum.

The top of each section in Fig. 8 shows an X-ray micrograph of the investigated skin region covering the stratum corneum and the viable epidermis. The rapamycin distribution yields according to both data reduction approaches, i.e., Beer-Lambert law (labeled ①) and singular value decomposition (labeled ②) similar results. The drug is not localized in the lipid lamellae, as one would expect for drug penetration of a lipophilic drug, as shown for dexamethasone in Fig. 7. Rather, there is uptake into the corneocytes, so that the stratum corneum cells act as a drug reservoir. Evidently, the treatment with serine protease damages the cornified envelopes, which consist of various proteins, among them are structural proteins as loricrin, involucrin, and trichohyalin (Candi et al. 2005). Hydrolysis at the serine moieties in these proteins makes the cornified envelopes leaky, so that rapamycin can efficiently penetrate corneocytes. This situation remains similar for exposure times by trypsin for 4 and 8 h. At 16 h there is clear evidence for rapamycin in the viable epidermis, implying that the damage of the tight junction barrier by serine protease requires time. If this barrier is damaged, then topically applied rapamycin can also penetrate the viable parts of skin. These findings were further verified by high spatial resolution studies on the stratum corneum, which indicated that rapamycin is barely found in the lipids of the stratum corneum, rather than inside the corneocytes (Germer et al. 2021).

3.2 The Role of Drug Formulations Probed by STXM

Drug formulations are the key to optimize drug delivery (Mitragotri et al. 2014; Nastiti et al. 2017; Benson et al. 2019). Nanoscopic systems have been explored during the last decades, which include a variety of liposomes, micelles, and nanoparticles of different materials and architectures (Mitchell et al. 2021). Among them are core-multishell nanocarriers of dendritic polyglycerol architecture with a polar core, a non-polar shell, and an outer hydrophobic shell (see Fig. 9(a)) (Kurniasih et al. 2015).

These nanocarriers with typical molecular weights $<10^5$ Da can be filled with drugs up to a few percent of their mass, while they have diameters <10 nm and can readily be taken up by skin into the stratum corneum (Yamamoto et al. 2016). This is visualized for the example of dexamethasone (see Fig. 9(b)), which is expected to be incorporated by the non-polar shell of the nanocarriers. The question whether nanocarriers facilitate drug penetration or show a different localization in the skin matrix has been investigated by STXM, as a label-free approach to probe both the drug and the nanocarriers topically applied to human skin ex vivo (Yamamoto et al. 2016). Fig. 9(c–e) shows the spatial distribution of CMS-nanocarriers distributed after 10, 100, and 1,000 min exposure time in the stratum corneum. They were selectively probed in the O 1 s-excitation regime by evaluating changes in optical

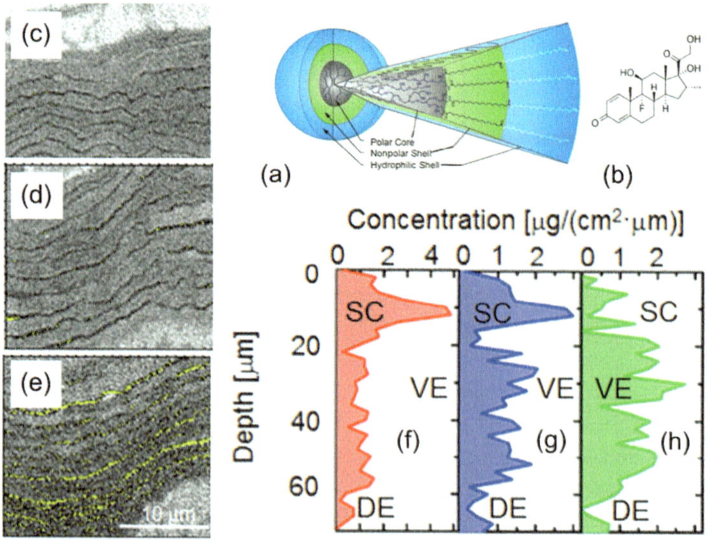

Fig. 9 Label-free detection of CMS-nanocarriers (**a**) and dexamethasone (**b**) by STXM; (**c**)–(**e**) localization of the nanocarriers in the stratum corneum, indicated by yellow color after 10 min (**c**), 100 min (**d**), and 1,000 min (**e**), respectively; vertical drug penetration profiles: 4 h penetration of dexamethasone dissolved in ethanol (**f**), 16 h penetration of dexamethasone in HEC gel (**g**), 16 h of penetration of dexamethasone-loaded nanocarriers (**h**), respectively. This material was taken with permission from Journal of Conrolled Relase, Vol. 242, by K. Yamamoto et al. *"Core-Multishell Nanocarriers: Transport and Release of Dexamethasone probed by Soft X-ray Spectromicroscopy,"* pages: 64–70, Copyright Elsevier (2016) (Yamamoto et al. 2016)

density at 531.4 eV and 535.9 eV, respectively. There, only nanocarriers gain absorption, whereas fixed skin shows no change in optical density (Yamamoto et al. 2016). After 10 min and 100 min, hardly any nanocarriers can be observed in the stratum corneum. This suggests that penetration of these dexamethasone-carrying CMS-nanoparticles is slow. The drug loading is found to be 5%, as determined by X-ray absorption. However, after 1,000 min, CMS-nanocarriers were only found in the lipid lamellae between the corneocytes (Fig. 9(e)). In the lower part of the stratum corneum this localization is less evident, which might point to enzymatic decomposition of the nanocarriers and drug release. There is no evidence for the observation of nanoscopic core-multishell nanocarriers in the viable epidermis, which points to an intact tight junction barrier that cannot be overcome by nanocarriers.

The drug penetration profiles of dexamethasone topically applied in different formulations are shown in Fig. 9(f–h). Absolute drug concentrations are derived from X-ray absorption studies. The drug penetration profiles observed after 4 h for an ethanolic dexamethasone solution (Fig. 9(f)) and dexamethasone formulated in HEC gel that penetrated for 16 h (Fig. 9(g)) are equivalent to each other: Both formulations show the highest drug concentration in the stratum corneum, acting as a reservoir, as the results shown in Fig. 6. A significantly different drug distribution is observed for core-multishell nanocarriers (Fig. 9(h)). They transport the drug efficiently through the stratum corneum so that this top skin layer is not acting as a drug reservoir. Enhanced drug concentration is rather found in the viable epidermis. This implies that nanocarriers increase the local drug concentration in the viable skin layers, where it is needed for therapeutic success, e.g., in atopic dermatitis. This also means that the drug is not lost during the passage through the stratum corneum, and the drug gets released from nanocarriers in the lower stratum corneum above the tight junctions, which cannot be passed by the nanocarriers. This explains the high local drug concentration in the viable epidermis and underscores the importance of nanocarriers for controlled drug delivery into the viable skin. A first therapeutic use of these dendritic nanocarriers in animals has been reported recently (Böhm et al. 2020).

3.3 Depth Profiles of Topical Nanocarrier-Based Drug Delivery Probed by FLIM

The versatile use of nanoparticles as drug delivery systems as well as diagnostic agents calls for sophisticated methods to observe, visualize, and quantify the drug and nanoparticles in skin tissue. The high-resolution micrographs obtained from STXM, as described in the previous section, are one example. STXM, however, is highly demanding with respect to instrumentation and experimenter skills. As another example, FLIM bioimaging will be described in this section since this technique becomes more and more available. FLIM plays an increasingly important role in revealing drug delivery and active penetration into tissue (Alexiev et al. 2017; Boreham et al. 2017a; Bloch et al. 2005) as well as in medical diagnosis (Balke et al. 2018), particularly due to the environmental sensitivity of the fluorescence lifetime.

An important requirement for fluorescence-based imaging techniques is the discrimination between autofluorescence and target fluorescence, e.g., from fluorescently-tagged nanocarriers or drugs, in the image. The Cluster-FLIM technique (see Sect. 2.2.3) allows us to distinguish unequivocally between autofluorescence and target fluorescence, as shown in the example of FITC-labeled tecto-dendrimer skin penetration (Fig. 10) (Volz et al. 2017).

Figure 11 shows the penetration of CMS-nanocarriers as visualized by Cluster-FLIM. The CMS-nanocarriers are tagged in the core by the environmentally sensitive ICC dye, yielding CMS–ICC (see Fig. 9(a)). Fluorescence tagging at the nanocarrier core diminishes possible (negative) interactions of the dye with the surrounding environment of the nanocarrier. On the other hand, steric restriction of dye mobility by the nanocarrier branches, e.g., due to interactions in the tissue, increases fluorescence quantum yield and fluorescence lifetime as clearly seen in Fig. 11(d) (Alnasif et al. 2014). The obvious differences in the fluorescence lifetime curves of ICC alone and of CMS–ICC nanocarriers, both in aqueous solution (Fig. 11(d)) and in the stratum corneum of normal skin (Fig. 11(e)) implicate a stable dye-tag and ensure that the signals observed in the stratum corneum and viable

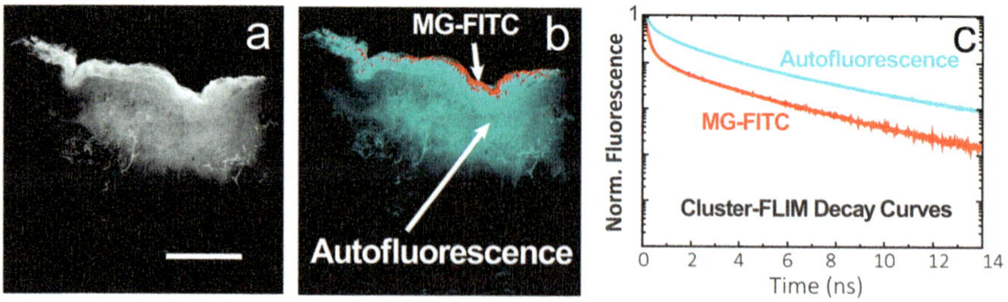

Fig. 10 Intensity-based image of a cryo-section of ex vivo skin vs. target fluorescence discrimination using Cluster-FLIM (obtained from (Volz et al. 2017)). (**a**) Intensity-based image of topically applied drug/nanocarrier (FITC-labeled tecto-dendrimer (MG-FITC) nanocarrier); (**b**) Cluster-FLIM analysis discriminates the autofluorescence lifetime (cyan) from the nanocarrier fluorescence lifetime (red). Lifetime curves are shown in (**c**). Scale bar: 200 μm. SC: stratum corneum, VE: viable epidermis. This figure was adapted with permission from Annals of the New York Academy of Science, Vol. 1,405, by P. Volz et al. "*Pitfalls in using fluorescence tagging of nanomaterials: tecto-dendrimers in skin tissue as investigated by Cluster-FLIM*," pages: 202–214, Copyright The New York Academy of Science (2017) (Volz et al. 2017)

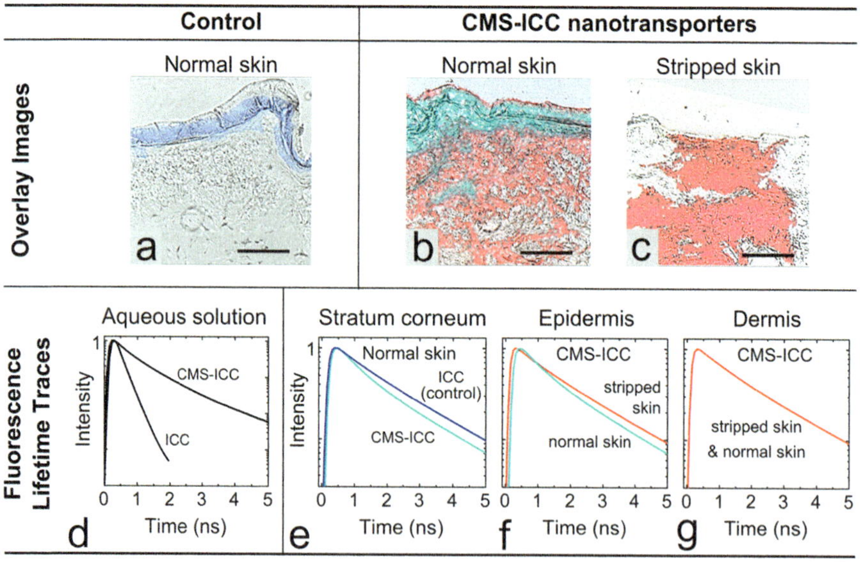

Fig. 11 FLIM-detection of ICC-tag alone (**a**) and ICC-tagged core-multishell nanocarriers (CMS-ICC) (**b**) in normal and in taped-stripped (**c**) skin cryosections, (**d**) Fluorescence lifetime curves of CMS–ICC nanocarriers and ICC in aqueous solution. The fluorescence lifetime curves (**e**–**g**) are shown in the same colors as used in the corresponding overlay images (**a**–**c**). Scale bar: 100 μm. This figure was taken with permission from Journal of Controlled Release, Vol. 185, by N. Alnasif et al. *"Penetration of normal, damaged and diseased skin — An in vitro study on dendritic core–multishell nano-transporters,"* pages: 45–50, Copyright Elsevier (2014) (Alnasif et al. 2014)

skin layers of normal and tape-stripped skin after 24 h incubation (Fig. 11(b, c)) are due to the fluorescent nanocarriers.

Note, penetration through intact stratum corneum (cyan colored areas, Fig. 11(b, e, f)) resulted in distinct differences of the CMS–ICC fluorescence lifetime curve in the stratum corneum or deeper skin layers (red colored areas, Fig. 11(b, c, f, g)). We conclude that these changes in the fluorescence lifetime curve of ICC covalently bound to CMS-nanocarriers indicate striking interactions of the nanocarriers with the lipids and/or proteins of the stratum corneum. These interactions differ from those experienced by the nanocarriers in deeper skin layers of both normal and skin barrier disrupted (tape-stripped) skin (Fig. 11(b, c)). The morphological changes to the CMS-ICC, as revealed by the fluorescence during passage through the stratum corneum are gradually reversible with further penetration into the dermis, indicating a reversible interaction with the constituents of the stratum corneum. This interpretation is supported by the results with tape-stripped skin where the stratum corneum specific changes to the fluorescence lifetime (Fig. 11(b)), cyan) are absent (Fig. 11 (c)).

Comparing the results from the FLIM experiments (Fig. 11) with those from STXM (Figs. 7 and 9(c–e)), it is evident that the latter is superior to FLIM in detecting both, the drug and nanocarrier in a single lamella of the stratum corneum with a spatial resolution in the nanometer regime. On the other hand, the environmental sensitivity of the ICC-tag enables visualization of differential and reversible interactions of the nanocarriers with the stratum corneum that vanishes upon further penetration. Since nanocarrier penetration beyond the stratum corneum was not observed in STXM experiments but in FLIM, we compare the FLIM results from two different polymer-based nanocarriers, CMS-ICC and tecto-dendrimers (MG-FITC) (Fig. 12) to obtain further insights. The penetration profile of CMS-ICC in normal skin (Fig. 12) highlights the two different environments of the CMS-ICC in the stratum corneum and in the deeper skin layers, respectively, and the decreasing core-multishell nanocarrier concentration from the photon counts. We conclude that the high sensitivity of Cluster-FLIM detects minute amounts of penetrating particles by their interactions with the environment. These interactions are probed by the ICC-tag due to its sensitivity to steric friction. Penetration, however, beyond the tight junctions was not seen for tecto-dendrimer nanocarriers (Fig. 12(d, e)) (Volz et al. 2017). This tight junction penetration barrier was visualized by immunofluorescence staining of the tight junction protein claudin-1. Claudin-1 was detected up to the stratum granulosum (Fig. 12(e)) using multi-color Cluster-FLIM for simultaneous visualization of antibodies and nanocarriers (Volz et al. 2018).

Thus, depending on the nanocarrier type, differential penetration into deeper skin layers was observed, indicating further mechanisms for drug delivery and locally enhanced drug concentrations in viable skin. Key features of beneficial nanocarrier effects for enhanced penetration are not only related to the nanocarrier size ("500 Da rule") (Bos and Meinardi 2000), but are also attributed to various physicochemical characteristics, such as rigidity, flexibility, hydrophobicity, and charge of the nanocarriers (Boreham et al. 2014, 2017b; Gupta et al. 2013). To simultaneously

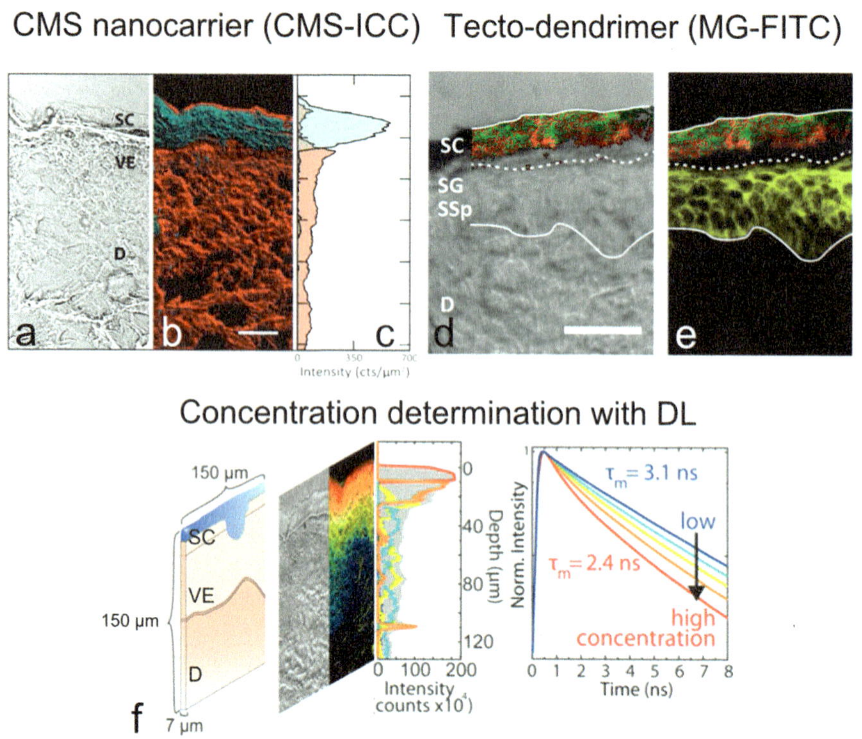

Fig. 12 (**a**–**c**) Penetration profile of CMS-ICC (**c**) from FLIM micrographs (**b**) after topical application on intact ex vivo human skin. Corresponding bright field image (**a**). Cluster-FLIM signature of CMS-ICC in cyan and red. (**d**, **e**) FLIM micrograph of tecto-dendrimer penetration in ex vivo human skin. Cluster-FLIM signature of MG-FITC in red and green, immunofluorescence staining of claudin-1 in yellow (**e**) (Volz et al. 2017). (**f**) Concentration-sensitive FLIM signature of a dual label (DL), comprising a fluorescence and EPR label. The different concentrations in the tissue section are colored according to the lifetime signatures shown at the right (Dong et al. 2021). *SC* stratum corneum, *VE* viable epidermis, *D* dermis. Figure (**a**–**c**) was adapted with permission from the Journal of Controlled Release, Vol. 185, by A. Vogt et al. *"Nanocarriers for drug delivery into and through the skin - Do existing technologies match clinical challenges?"* pages: 3–15, Copyright Elsevier (2016) (Vogt et al. 2016). Figure (**d**, **e**) was taken with permission from the Annals of the New York Academy of Science, Vol. 1,405, by P. Volz et al. "*Pitfalls in using fluorescence tagging of nanomaterials: tecto-dendrimers in skin tissue as investigated by Cluster-FLIM*," pages: 202–214, Copyright The New York Academy of Science (2017) (Volz et al. 2017). Figure (**f**) was adapted with permission from Angewandte Chemie, Vol. 1,405, by P. Dong et al. "*A Dual Fluorescence–Spin Label Probe for Visualization and Quantification of Target Molecules in Tissue by Multiplexed FLIM–EPR Spectroscopy*," pages: 14938–14,944, Copyright Angewandte Chemie Int. Ed. (2021) (Dong et al. 2021)

visualize and directly quantify the nanocarriers or drug in biological tissue, a dual label (DL) compound comprising a highly fluorescent dye together with an EPR spin probe, which also renders the fluorescence lifetime to be concentration sensitive, was developed (Dong et al. 2021). FLIM-based concentration sensitivity was estimated

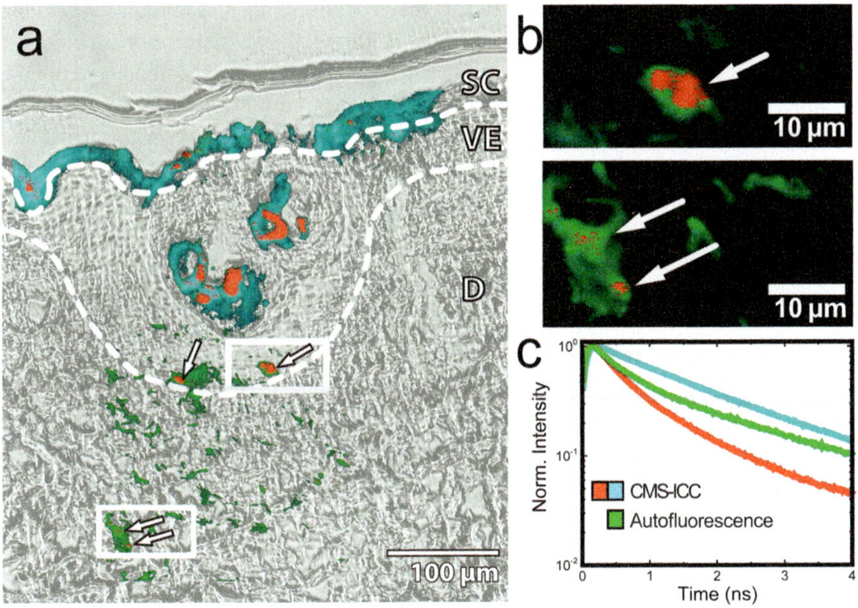

Fig. 13 Penetration profile of CMS-ICC nanocarrier from FLIM micrographs in intact ex vivo human skin. Cluster-FLIM-bright-field overlay of CMS-ICC penetration (**a**). Colored regions (according to the fluorescence lifetime signatures in (**c**)) indicate the localization of CMS-ICC. (**b**) Zoom into regions of (**a**) as indicated by white rectangles. (**c**) Fluorescence lifetime signatures. *SC* stratum corneum, *VE* viable epidermis, *D* dermis. Figure was taken with permission from Journal of Controlled Release, Vol. 299, by J. Frombach et al. "*Core-multishell nanocarriers enhance drug penetration and reach keratinocytes and antigen-presenting cells in intact human skin,*" pages: 138–148, Copyright Elsevier (2019) (Frombach et al. 2019)

down to 10 μg/cm^3 tissue from the dual label sensor in human skin cryo-section volume element (Fig. 12(f)). The dual label can easily be coupled to the drug or nanocarrier of choice, enabling in vivo and in vitro applications and paves the way for studies with unprecedented qualitative visualization ranging from fundamental biological investigations to preclinical drug research (Dong et al. 2021). Further studies should investigate the clinical relevance of this research.

Another mechanism to enhance drug delivery into skin via nanocarrier transport is through the usage of skin appendages and possible contributions from immune cells (Frombach et al. 2019). Fig. 13 shows excised full-thickness human skin with special focus on hair follicles for penetration and release of core-multishell nanocarrier encapsulated dexamethasone (Frombach et al. 2019). A global cluster analysis of CMS-ICC treated (16 h) and untreated reference skin (Fig. 13(a, b)) reveals three distinct fluorescence lifetime clusters (Fig. 13(c)). A clear-cut discrimination between the autofluorescence lifetime signature (green) and CMS-ICC (cyan, red) fluorescence lifetime signatures was found. The fast fluorescence decay signature (red) was found in the center of hair follicles and occasionally in small spots in the viable epidermis and dermis (Fig. 13(a, b)). Thus, the micrographs indicate that core-multishell nanocarriers can reach the viable tissue. Accumulation of the nanocarriers within the hair follicle may facilitate this translocation. Since the CMS-nanocarriers enrich in the entire stratum corneum reservoir, contact and uptake in upper keratinocytes as well as dendritic cells may be feasible. Moreover, recent findings implicate an increased role of skin-resident epidermal Langerhans cells and their immunofunction in the development of chronic, inflammatory skin diseases like psoriasis (Tanaka et al. 2022; Zhang et al. 2022).

The density of dendritic cells is lower than that of keratinocytes (Cruchley et al. 1994), so that it is not contradictory to other work (Yamamoto et al. 2016), where no penetration of core-multishell nanocarriers was observed in the investigated skin sections (see Fig. 9). Indeed, it was postulated that the extensive dendrite meshwork, their position around hair follicle orifices, and their capacity to modulate tight junctions facilitate a preferential uptake of CMS-nanocarriers by Langerhans cells within the skin. This newly identified aspect of CMS-nanocarrier penetration underscores the potential of CMS-nanocarrier for dermatotherapy, particularly in inflammatory skin diseases (Frombach et al. 2019).

3.4 Skin Models and Cellular Fate of Nanocarriers Visualized by FLIM

To verify that and how CMS-nanocarriers are taken up by keratinocytes, 2D cell cultures of primary keratinocytes were subjected to Cluster-FLIM analysis (Brodwolf et al. 2020). Correlation of Cluster-FLIM results to classical pharmacological uptake pathway analysis reveals that the cellular interactions of CMS-ICC, i.e., the cellular interactome of the nanocarrier sensed by the ICC(Cy3)-tag due to its sensitivity to steric friction (see Fig. 14), can directly be translated into endocytosis pathways and intracellular fate (Fig. 14). Ideally, the interactome obtained from Cluster-FLIM represents all interactions along the uptake pathway into the cell. For CMS-nanocarriers an caveolae/lipid raft mediated uptake pathway was revealed (Pelkmans and Helenius 2002). The fluorescence lifetime signatures of the different interactions shown in Fig. 14 correspond to fast initial interactions with membrane scavenger receptors (cyan), to interactions with components of lipid rafts/caveolae (yellow), and to lysosomal interactions (red), respectively.

Eventually, the nanocarriers accumulate in lysosomes with a time constant of 107 ± 9 min. The fluorescence lifetime signatures of the different interactions (Fig. 14) are colored in cyan (fast initial interaction by membrane scavenger receptor), yellow (interactions with components of lipid rafts/caveolae), and red (lysosomal interaction), respectively. The capability of Cluster-FLIM to unravel cellular pathways solely based on the interactome analysis lays the foundation for fast and automated decision making in drug and drug delivery system development using Cluster-FLIM (Brodwolf et al. 2020). A schematic of the workflow of automated interactome assessment in high-content screening is presented in Fig. 15. While for normal keratinocytes the endolysosomal pathway was identified for core-multishell nanocarriers, transformed keratinocytes (squamous cell

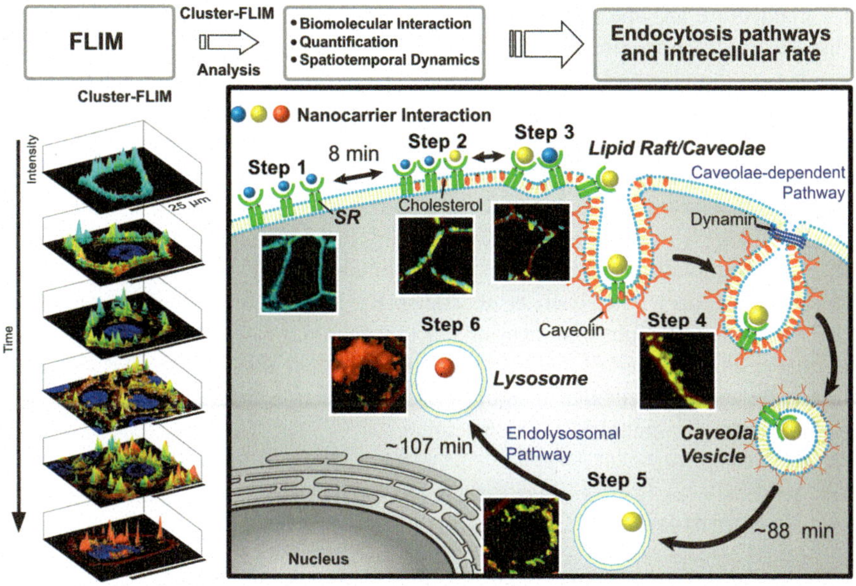

Fig. 14 Endocytosis pathway (right) of CMS-nanocarriers in primary human keratinocytes from the dynamic interaction of CMS-ICC in normal keratinocytes (left). The intracellular CMS-nanocarrier interactome is visualized by the different fluorescence lifetime signatures (cyan, yellow, red). This figure was adapted with permission from Theranostics, Vol. 299, by R. Brodwolf et al. "*Faster, sharper, more precise: Automated Cluster-FLIM in preclinical testing directly identifies the intracellular fate of theranostic in live cells and tissue,*" pages: 6322–6336, Copyright Ivyspring International Publisher (2020) (Brodwolf et al. 2020)

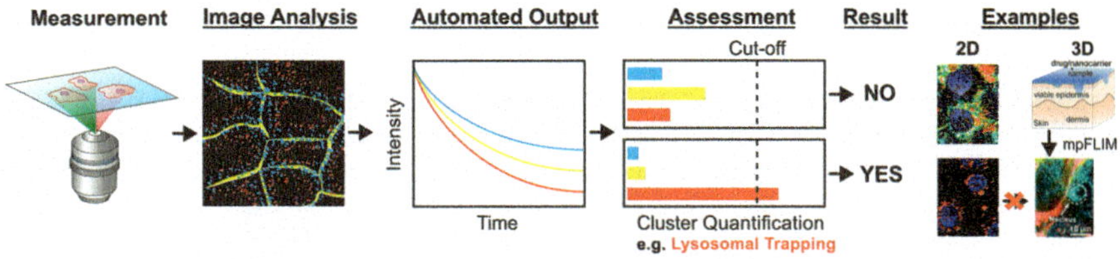

Fig. 15 Workflow of automated cellular nanocarrier interactome assessment using Cluster-FLIM in 2D- and 3D-skin models. This figure was adapted with permission (Brodwolf et al. 2020)

carcinoma, cell line SCC-25) take up nanocarriers via a different route (Fig. 15) and no lysosomal trapping (Schmitt et al. 2019) was identified. Thus, automated Cluster-FLIM analysis shows the capability to replace the visual evaluation of FLIM images, thereby fulfilling an essential requirement for high-content screening and reduction of analysis time.

As current preclinical models still have low power to predict treatment efficacy, especially in oncology (Wong et al. 2019), and monolayers of human cells lack, e.g., the architecture and the microenvironment of tumor tissue, 3D-multi-layered skin (disease) models reflecting more closely skin morphology and microenvironment are mandatory (Gronbach et al. 2020). In the example of core-multishell nanocarriers, the intracellular fate markedly differed between 2D-cell cultures and the 3D-tissue model (Fig. 15), emphasizing the need for qualified preclinical methods in drug development (Brodwolf et al. 2020; Schäfer-Korting and Zoschke 2021). This information was received as a direct outcome from the workflow of automated Cluster-FLIM, which can be transferred to any cell type and molecule of interest. Here, an example is the application of cetuximab to a 3D-multi-layered head and neck cancer model (Gronbach et al. 2020). By further combining the automated FLIM readout with bioinformatics and machine learning tools, Cluster-FLIM should become an essential part of high-content screening along the drug discovery pipeline to provide an unprecedented insight in target prediction, interaction, and pathway profiling from the spatial FLIM interactome.

4 Summary and Conclusions

Spectromicroscopy has developed during the last decades to a powerful approach for probing the penetration of drugs and drug formulations in biological matter. This review outlines the highly dynamic development of this field during the last decades and presents the enormous breadth of experimental methods and related data evaluation approaches with emphasis on STXM and FLIM. These methods are selected for being representative for spectromicroscopy methods relying, on the one hand, on sensitive fluorescence labels and, on the other hand, on label-free approaches. Key for these spectromicroscopy approaches is to use molecular properties of actives and nanoscopic drug carriers for deriving a qualitative and quantitative understanding for drug delivery processes on a molecular scale.

Acknowledgments Financial support by the German Research Foundation (DFG, a.o. SFB 1112 and SFB 1449 project ID 431232613, and RU 420/12-1) and Freie Universität Berlin is gratefully acknowledged. Beam time for STXM studies at the UVSOR III synchrotron facility (Institute for Molecular Science, Okazaku, Japan) and BESSY II (Helmholtz Zentrum Berlin, Germany) is also gratefully acknowledged.

References

Ahluwalia A (1998) Topical glucocorticoids and the skin-mechanisms of action: an update. Mediators Inflamm 7:183–193

Alexander H, Brown S, Danby S, Flohr C (2018) Research techniques made simple: transepidermal water loss measurement as a research tool. J Investig Dermatol 138:2295–2300

Alexiev U, Farrens DL (2014) Fluorescence spectroscopy of rhodopsins: insights and approaches. BBA-Bioenergetics 1837:694–709

Alexiev U, Volz P, Boreham A, Brodwolf R (2017) Time-resolved fluorescence microscopy (FLIM) as an analytical tool in skin nanomedicine. Eur J Pharm Biopharm 116:111–124

Alnasif N, Zoschke C, Fleige E, Brodwolf R, Boreham A, Rühl E, Eckl KM, Merk HF, Hennies HC, Alexiev U, Haag R, Küchler S, Schäfer-Korting M (2014) Penetration of normal, damaged and diseased skin - an in vitro study on dendritic core-multishell nanotransporters. J Control Release 185:45–50

Alvarez Núñez FA, Yalkowsky SH (1997) Correlation between log P and ClogP for some steroids. J Pharm Sci 86:1187–1189

Amos WB, White JG (2003) How the confocal laser scanning microscope entered biological research. Biol Cell 95:335–342

Ashtikar M, Langelüddecke L, Fahr A, Deckert V (2017) Tip-enhanced Raman scattering for tracking of invasomes in the stratum corneum. BBA-Gen Subjects 1861:2630–2639

Balke J, Volz P, Neumann F, Brodwolf R, Wolf A, Pischon H, Radbruch M, Mundhenk L, Gruber AD, Ma N, Alexiev U (2018) Visualizing oxidative cellular stress induced by nanoparticles in the subcytotoxic range using fluorescence lifetime imaging. Small 14:1800310

Becker W (2021) The bh TCSPC handbook (9th edition). Becker and Hickl GmbH. Available on https://www.becker-hickl.com/literature/documents/flim/the-bh-tcspc-handbook/

Benson HAE, Grice JE, Mohammed Y, Namjoshi S, Roberts MS (2019) Topical and transdermal drug delivery: from simple potions to smart technologies. Curr Drug Deliv 16:444–460

Bloch S, Lesage F, McIntosh L, Gandjbakhche A, Liang KX, Achilefu S (2005) Whole-body fluorescence lifetime imaging of a tumor-targeted near-infrared molecular probe in mice. J Biomed Opt 10:054003

Böhm D, Moré S, Moré M, Kloner L, Volkmann M, Haag R, Kohn B (2020) Nanocarrier in veterinary medicine – a pilot study for the treatment of feline hyperthyroidism with a nanocarrier based thiamazole ointment. Schweiz Arch Tierheilkd 162:223–234

Bommannan D, Potts RO, Guy RH (1991) Examination of the effect of ethanol on human stratum corneum in vivo using infrared spectroscopy. J Control Release 16:299–304

Boreham A, Pfaff M, Fleige E, Haag R, Alexiev U (2014) Nanodynamics of dendritic core-multishell nanocarriers. Langmuir 30:1686–1695

Boreham A, Pikkemaat J, Volz P, Brodwolf R, Kuehne C, Licha K, Haag R, Dernedde J, Alexiev U (2016) Detecting and quantifying biomolecular interactions of a dendritic polyglycerol sulfate nanoparticle using fluorescence lifetime measurements. Molecules 21:22

Boreham A, Brodwolf R, Walker K, Haag R, Alexiev U (2017a) Time-resolved fluorescence spectroscopy and fluorescence lifetime imaging microscopy for characterization of dendritic polymer nanoparticles and applications in nanomedicine. Molecules 22:17

Boreham A, Volz P, Peters D, Keck CM, Alexiev U (2017b) Determination of nanostructures and drug distribution in lipid nanoparticles by single molecule microscopy. Eur J Pharm Biopharm 110:31–38

Borst JW, Visser A (2010) Fluorescence lifetime imaging microscopy in life sciences. Meas Sci Technol 21:102002

Bos JD, Meinardi MMHM (2000) The 500 Dalton rule for the skin penetration of chemical compounds and drugs. Exp Dermatol 9:165–169

Bouwstra JA, Honeywell-Nguyen PL, Gooris GS, Ponec M (2003) Structure of the skin barrier and its modulation by vesicular formulations. Prog Lipid Res 42:1–36

Brandner JM (2016) Importance of tight junctions in relation to skin barrier function. Curr Probl Dermatol 49:27–37

Brodwolf R, Volz-Rakebrand P, Stellmacher J, Wolff C, Unbehauen M, Haag R, Schäfer-Korting M, Zoschke C, Alexiev U (2020) Faster, sharper, more precise: automated cluster-FLIM in preclinical testing directly identifies the intracellular fate of theranostics in live cells and tissue. Theranostics 10:6322–6336

Candi E, Schmidt R, Melino G (2005) The cornified envelope: a model of cell death in the skin. Nat Rev Mol Cell Biol 6:328–340

Caprioli RM, Farmer TB, Gile J (1997) Molecular imaging of biological samples: localization of peptides and proteins using MALDI-TOF MS. Anal Chem 69:4751–4760

Cruchley AT, Williams DM, Farthing PM, Speight PM, Lesch CA, Squier CA (1994) Langerhans cell density in normal human oral mucosa and skin: relationship to age, smoking and alcohol consumption. J Oral Pathol Med 23:55–59
Dazzi A, Prater CB (2017) AFM-IR: technology and applications in nanoscale infrared spectroscopy and chemical imaging. Chem Rev 117:5146–5173
Digman MA, Caiolfa VR, Zamai M, Gratton E (2008) The phasor approach to fluorescence lifetime imaging analysis. Biophys J 94:L14–L16
Döge N, Hadam S, Volz P, Wolf A, Schönborn KH, Blume-Peytavi U, Alexiev U, Vogt A (2018) Identification of polystyrene nanoparticle penetration across intact skin barrier as rare event at sites of focal particle aggregations. J Biophotonics 11:e201700169
Dong P, Stellmacher J, Bouchet LM, Nieke M, Kumar A, Osorio-Blanco ER, Nagel G, Lohan SB, Teutloff C, Patzelt A, Schäfer-Korting M, Calderon M, Meinke MC, Alexiev U (2021) A dual fluorescence-spin label probe for visualization and quantification of target molecules in tissue by multiplexed FLIM-EPR spectroscopy. Angew Chem Int Ed Engl 60:14938–14944
Emergency Use Authorization (Eua) of the Pfizer-Biontech Covid-19 Vaccine to Prevent Coronavirus Disease (2019) (COVID-19) in individuals 16 years of age and older. https://www.fda.gov/media/144414/download. Accessed 28 Nov 2022
Evans CL, Potma EO, Puoris'haag M, Cote D, Lin CP, Xie XS (2005) Chemical imaging of tissue in vivo with video-rate coherent anti-stokes Raman scattering microscopy. Proc Natl Acad Sci U S A 102:16807–16812
Frazer B, Gilbert B, De Stasio G (2002) X-ray absorption microscopy of aqueous samples. Rev Sci Instrum 73:1373–1375
Frazer BH, Girasole M, Wiese LM, Franz T, De Stasio G (2004) Spectromicro scope for the photoelectron imaging of nanostructures with X-rays (SPHINX): performance in biology, medicine and geology. Ultramicroscopy 99:87–94
Freudiger CW, Min W, Saar BG, Lu S, Holtom GR, He CW, Tsai JC, Kang JX, Xie XS (2008) Label-free biomedical imaging with high sensitivity by stimulated Raman scattering microscopy. Science 322:1857–1861
Frombach J, Lohan SB, Lemm D, Gruner P, Hasler J, Ahlberg S, Blume-Peytavi U, Unbehauen M, Haag R, Meinke MC, Vogt A (2018) Protease-mediated inflammation: an in vitro human keratinocyte-based screening tool for anti-inflammatory drug nanocarrier systems. Z Phys Chem 232:919–933
Frombach J, Unbehauen M, Kurniasih IN, Schumacher F, Volz P, Hadam S, Rancan F, Blume-Peytavi U, Kleuser B, Haag R, Alexiev U, Vogt A (2019) Core-multishell nanocarriers enhance drug penetration and reach keratinocytes and antigen-presenting cells in intact human skin. J Control Release 299:138–148
Fu D, Lu FK, Zhang X, Freudiger C, Pernik DR, Holtom G, Xie XS (2012) Quantitative chemical imaging with multiplex stimulated Raman scattering microscopy. J Am Chem Soc 134:3623–3626
Germer G, Ohigashi T, Yuzawa H, Kosugi N, Flesch R, Rancan F, Vogt A, Rühl E (2021) Improved skin permeability after topical treatment with serine protease: probing the penetration of rapamycin by scanning transmission X-ray microscopy. ACS Omega 6:12213–12222
Gorzelanny C, Mess C, Schneider SW, Huck V, Brandner JM (2020) Skin barriers in dermal drug delivery: which barriers have to be overcome and how can we measure them? Pharmaceutics 12: 684
Graf C, Rühl E (2019) Imaging techniques for probing nanoparticles in cells and skin. In: Gehr P, Zellner R (eds) Biological responses to nanoscale particles: molecular and cellular aspects and methodological approaches. Springer, Cham, pp 213–239
Gregoire S, Luengo GS, Hallegot P, Pena AM, Chen XQ, Bornschlogl T, Chan KF, Pence I, Obeidy P, Feizpour A, Jeong S, Evans CL (2020) Imaging and quantifying drug delivery in skin - part 1: autoradiography and mass spectrometry imaging. Adv Drug Deliv Rev 153:137–146
Gröger D, Paulus F, Licha K, Welker P, Weinhart M, Holzhausen C, Mundhenk L, Gruber AD, Abram U, Haag R (2013) Synthesis and biological evaluation of radio and dye labeled amino

functionalized dendritic polyglycerol sulfates as multivalent anti-inflammatory compounds. Bioconjug Chem 24:1507–1514
Gronbach L, Wolff C, Klinghammer K, Stellmacher J, Jurmeister P, Alexiev U, Schäfer-Korting M, Tinhofer I, Keilholz U, Zoschke C (2020) A multilayered epithelial mucosa model of head neck squamous cell carcinoma for analysis of tumor-microenvironment interactions and drug development. Biomaterials 258:120277
Gupta M, Agrawal U, Vyas SP (2012) Nanocarrier-based topical drug delivery for the treatment of skin diseases. Expert Opin Drug Deliv 9:783–804
Gupta S, Bansal R, Gupta S, Jindal N, Jindal A (2013) Nanocarriers and nanoparticles for skin care and dermatological treatments. Indian Dermatol Online J 4:267–272
Guttmann P, Bittencourt C (2015) Overview of nanoscale NEXAFS performed with soft X-ray microscopes. Beilstein J Nanotechnol 6:595–604
Hegenbarth R, Steinmann A, Mastel S, Amarie S, Huber AJ, Hillenbrand R, Sarkisov SY, Giessen H (2014) High-power femtosecond mid-IR sources for s-SNOM applications. J Opt 16:094003
Henke BL, Gullikson EM, Davis JC (1993) X-ray interactions - photoabsorption, scattering, transmission, and reflection at E=50-30,000 eV, Z=1-92. At Data Nucl Data Tables 54:181–342
Hirvonen LM, Suhling K (2020) Fast timing techniques in FLIM applications. Front Physiol 8:161
Hirvonen LM, Nedbal J, Almutairi N, Phillips TA, Becker W, Conneely T, Milnes J, Cox S, Sturzenbaum S, Suhling K (2020) Lightsheet fluorescence lifetime imaging microscopy with wide-field time-correlated single photon counting. J Biophotonics 13:e201960099
Jeong WY, Kwon M, Choi HE, Kim KS (2021) Recent advances in transdermal drug delivery systems: a review. Biomater Res 25:24
Jo JA, Fang QY, Marcu L (2005) Ultrafast method for the analysis of fluorescence lifetime imaging microscopy data based on the Laguerre expansion technique. IEEE J Quantum Electron 11:835–845
Kaeokhamloed N, Legeay S, Roger E (2022) FRET as the tool for in vivo nanomedicine tracking. J Control Release 349:156–173
Kanevche K, Burr D, Elsaesser A, Hass PK, Nuernberg D, Heberle J (2021) Infrared nanoscopy and tomography of intracellular structures. Commun Biol 4:1341
Kästner B, Johnson CM, Hermann P, Kruskopf M, Pierz K, Hoehl A, Hornemann A, Ulrich G, Fehmel J, Patoka P, Rühl E, Ulm G (2018) Infrared nanospectroscopy of phospholipid and surfactin monolayer domains. ACS Omega 3:4141–4147
Keilmann F, Huber AJ, Hillenbrand R (2009) Nanoscale conductivity contrast by scattering-type near-field optical microscopy in the visible, infrared and THz domains. J Infrared Millim Terahertz Waves 30:1255–1268
Kirchberg K, Kim TY, Möller M, Skegro D, Raju GD, Granzin J, Büldt G, Schlesinger R, Alexiev U (2011) Conformational dynamics of helix 8 in the GPCR rhodopsin controls arrestin activation in the desensitization process. Proc Natl Acad Sci U S A 108:18690–18695
Kirejev V, Guldbrand S, Borglin J, Simonsson C, Ericson MB, Multiphoton microscopy. (2012) A powerful tool in skin research and topical drug delivery science. J Drug Deliv Sci Technol 22: 250–259
Klossek A, Thierbach S, Rancan F, Vogt A, Blume-Peytavi U, Rühl E (2017) Studies for improved understanding of lipid distributions in human skin by combining stimulated and spontaneous Raman microscopy. Eur J Pharm Biopharm 116:76–84
Koehler MJ, Zimmermann S, Springer S, Elsner P, Koenig K, Kaatz M (2011) Keratinocyte morphology of human skin evaluated by in vivo multiphoton laser tomography. Skin Res Technol 17:479–486
König K (2020) Review: clinical in vivo multiphoton FLIM tomography. Methods Appl Fluoresc 8: 034002
Koprinarov IN, Hitchcock AP, McCrory CT, Childs RF (2002) Quantitative mapping of structured polymeric systems using singular value decomposition analysis of soft X-ray images. J Phys Chem B 106:5358–5364

Krüger HR, Schütz I, Justies A, Licha K, Welker P, Haucke V, Calderon M (2014) Imaging of doxorubicin release from theranostic macromolecular prodrugs via fluorescence resonance energy transfer. J Control Release 194:189–196
Kurniasih IN, Keilitz J, Haag R (2015) Dendritic nanocarriers based on hyperbranched polymers. Chem Soc Rev 44:4145–4164
Kuschewski F, von Ribbeck HG, Döring J, Winnerl S, Eng LM, Kehr SC (2016) Narrow-band near-field nanoscopy in the spectral range from 1.3 to 8.5 THz. Appl Phys Lett 108: 113102
Lademann J, Caspers PJ, van der Pol A, Richter H, Patzelt A, Zastrow L, Darvin M, Sterry W, Fluhr JW (2009) In vivo Raman spectroscopy detects increased epidermal antioxidative potential with topically applied carotenoids. Laser Phys Lett 6:76–79
Lawrence JR, Swerhone GDW, Dynes JJ, Korber DR, Hitchcock AP (2016) Soft X-ray spectromicroscopy for speciation, quantitation and nano-eco-toxicology of nanomaterials. J Microsc 261:130–147
Le Marois A, Labouesse S, Suhling K, Heintzmann R (2017) Noise-corrected principal component analysis of fluorescence lifetime imaging data. J Biophotonics 10:1124–1133
Lee SC, Kim K, Kim J, Lee S, Yi JH, Kim SW, Ha KS, Cheong C (2001) One micrometer resolution NMR microscopy. J Magn Reson 150:207–213
Legall H et al (2012) Compact x-ray microscope for the water window based on a high brightness laser plasma source. Opt Express 20:18362–18369
Lemaster JE, Jokerst JV (2017) What is new in nanoparticle-based photoacoustic imaging? Wiley Interdiscip Rev Nanomed Nanobiotechnol 9:e1404
Lerotic M, Mak R, Wirick S, Meirer F, Jacobsen C (2014) MANTiS: a program for the analysis of X-ray spectromicroscopy data. J Synchrotron Radiat 21:1206–1212
Leung BO, Chou KC (2011) Review of super-resolution fluorescence microscopy for biology. Appl Spectrosc 65:967–980
Liu LX, Yang QQ, Zhang ML, Wu ZQ, Xue P (2019) Fluorescence lifetime imaging microscopy and its applications in skin cancer diagnosis. J Innov Opt Health Sci 12:1930004
Lu FK, Basu S, Igras V, Hoang MP, Ji MB, Fu D, Holtom GR, Neel VA, Freudiger CW, Fisher DE, Xie XS (2015) Label-free DNA imaging in vivo with stimulated Raman scattering microscopy. Proc Natl Acad Sci U S A 112:11624–11629
Ma X, Fernandez FM (2022) Advances in mass spectrometry imaging for spatial cancer metabolomics. Mass Spectrom Rev:e21804
Mannam V, Zhang YD, Yuan XT, Ravasio C, Howard SS (2020) Machine learning for faster and smarter fluorescence lifetime imaging microscopy. J Phys 2:042005
Mao G, Flach CR, Mendelsohn R, Walters RM (2012) Imaging the distribution of sodium dodecyl sulfate in skin by confocal Raman and infrared microspectroscopy. Pharm Res 29:2189–2201
Mathurin J, Deniset-Besseau A, Bazin D, Dartois E, Wagner M, Dazzi A (2022) Photothermal AFM-IR spectroscopy and imaging: status, challenges, and trends. J Appl Phys 131:010901
Mirakovski D, Damevska K, Simeonovski V, Nikolovska S, Boev B, Petrov A, Sijakova Ivanova T, Zendelska A, Hadzi-Nikolova M, Boev I, Dimov G, Darlenski R, Kazandjieva J, Damevska S, Situm M (2022) Use of SEM/EDX methods for the analysis of ambient particulate matter adhering to the skin surface. J Eur Acad Dermatol Venereol 36:1376–1381
Mitchell MJ, Billingsley MM, Haley RM, Wechsler ME, Peppas NA, Langer R (2021) Engineering precision nanoparticles for drug delivery. Nat Rev Drug Discov 20:101–124
Mitragotri S, Burke PA, Langer R (2014) Overcoming the challenges in administering biopharmaceuticals: formulation and delivery strategies. Nat Rev Drug Discov 13:655–672
Nagano S, Sadeghi M, Balke J, Fleck M, Heckmann N, Psakis G, Alexiev U (2022) Improved fluorescent phytochromes for in situ imaging. Sci Rep 12:5587
Nastiti C, Ponto T, Abd E, Grice JE, Benson HAE, Roberts MS (2017) Topical nano and microemulsions for skin delivery. Pharmaceutics 9:37
Niehaus M, Soltwisch J, Belov ME, Dreisewerd K (2019) Transmission-mode MALDI-2 mass spectrometry imaging of cells and tissues at subcellular resolution. Nat Methods 16:925–931

Noun M, Akoumeh R, Abbas I (2022) Cell and tissue imaging by TOF-SIMS and MALDI-TOF: an overview for biological and pharmaceutical analysis. Microsc Microanal 28:1–26

Ober K, Volz-Rakebrand P, Stellmacher J, Brodwolf R, Licha K, Haag R, Alexiev U (2019) Expanding the scope of reporting nanoparticles: sensing of lipid phase transitions and nanoviscosities in lipid membranes. Langmuir 35:11422–11434

Okay S (2020) Single-molecule characterization of drug delivery systems. Assay Drug Dev Technol 18:56–63

Patra JK, Das G, Fraceto LF, Campos EVR, Rodriguez-Torres MDP, Acosta-Torres LS, Diaz-Torres LA, Grillo R, Swamy MK, Sharma S, Habtemariam S, Shin HS (2018) Nano based drug delivery systems: recent developments and future prospects. J Nanobiotechnol 16:71

Paturi J, Kim HD, Chakraborty B, Friden PM, Banga AK (2010) Transdermal and intradermal iontophoretic delivery of dexamethasone sodium phosphate: quantification of the drug localized in skin. J Drug Target 18:134–140

Pelkmans L, Helenius A (2002) Endocytosis via caveolae. Traffic 3:311–320

Pena A-M, Chen X, Pence IJ, Bornschlögl T, Jeong S, Grégoire S, Luengo GS, Hallegot P, Obeidy P, Feizpour A, Chan KF, Evans CL (2020) Imaging and quantifying drug delivery in skin – part 2: fluorescence and vibrational spectroscopic imaging methods. Adv Drug Deliv Rev 153:147–168

Pischon H, Radbruch M, Ostrowski A, Volz P, Gerecke C, Unbehauen M, Hönzke S, Hedtrich S, Fluhr JW, Haag R, Kleuser B, Alexiev U, Gruber AD, Mundhenk L (2017) Stratum corneum targeting by dendritic core-multishell-nanocarriers in a mouse model of psoriasis. Nanomedicine 13:317–327

Poudel C, Mela I, Kaminski CF (2020) High-throughput, multi-parametric, and correlative fluorescence lifetime imaging. Methods and Applications in Fluorescence 8:024005

Rajes K, Walker KA, Hadam S, Zabihi F, Ibrahim-Bacha J, Germer G, Patoka P, Wassermann B, Rancan F, Rühl E, Vogt A, Haag R (2021) Oxidation-sensitive core-multishell nanocarriers for the controlled delivery of hydrophobic drugs. ACS Biomater Sci Eng 7:2485–2495

Richter C, Schneider C, Quick MT, Volz P, Mahrwald R, Hughes J, Dick B, Alexiev U, Ernsting NP (2015) Dual-fluorescence pH probe for bio-labelling. Phys Chem Chem Phys 17:30590–30597

Ruman U, Fakurazi S, Masarudin MJ, Hussein MZ (2020) Nanocarrier-based therapeutics and theranostics drug delivery systems for next generation of liver cancer nanodrug modalities. Int J Nanomedicine 15:1437–1456

Sahu KS, Raj R, Raj MP, Alpana R (2020) Topical lipid based drug delivery systems for skin diseases: a review. Curr Drug Ther 15:283–298

Schäfer-Korting M, Zoschke C (2021) How qualification of 3D disease models cuts the Gordian knot in preclinical drug development. Handb Exp Pharmacol 265:29–56

Schmitt MV, Lienau P, Fricker G, Reichel A (2019) Quantitation of lysosomal trapping of basic lipophilic compounds using in vitro assays and in silico predictions based on the determination of the full pH profile of the endo-/lysosomal system in rat hepatocytes. Drug Metab Dispos 47: 49–57

Schnell M, Goikoetxea M, Amenabar I, Carney PS, Hillenbrand R (2020) Rapid infrared spectroscopic nanoimaging with nano-FTIR holography. ACS Photonics 7:2878–2885

Schulz R, Yamamoto K, Klossek A, Flesch R, Hönzke S, Rancan F, Vogt A, Blume-Peytavi U, Hedtrich S, Schäfer-Korting M, Rühl E, Netz RR (2017) Data-based modeling of drug penetration relates human skin barrier function to the interplay of diffusivity and free-energy profiles. Proc Natl Acad Sci U S A 114:3631–3636

Scimeca M, Bischetti S, Lamsira HK, Bonfiglio R, Bonanno E (2018) Energy dispersive X-ray (EDX) microanalysis: a powerful tool in biomedical research and diagnosis. Eur J Histochem 62:88–97

Sersa I (2021) Magnetic resonance microscopy of samples with translational symmetry with FOVs smaller than sample size. Sci Rep 11:541

Shapiro DA et al (2020) An ultrahigh-resolution soft x-ray microscope for quantitative analysis of chemically heterogeneous nanomaterials. Sci Adv 6:eabc4904

Sheppard CJR (2020) Multiphoton microscopy: a personal historical review, with some future predictions. J Biomed Opt 25:1–11

Shin CS, Dunnam CR, Borbat PP, Dzikovski B, Barth ED, Halpern HJ, Freed JH (2011) ESR microscopy for biological and biomedical applications. Nanosci Nanotechnol Lett 3:561–567

Smith JT, Yao RY, Sinsuebphon N, Rudkouskaya A, Un N, Mazurkiewicz J, Barroso M, Yan PK, Intes X (2019) Fast fit-free analysis of fluorescence lifetime imaging via deep learning. Proc Natl Acad Sci U S A 116:24019–24030

Stöhr J (1992) NEXAFS sepctroscopy. Springer, Berlin

Stojanov K, Zuhorn IS, Dierckx RAJO, de Vries EFJ (2012) Imaging of cells and nanoparticles: implications for drug delivery to the brain. Pharm Res 29:3213–3234

Tanaka R, Ichimura Y, Kubota N, Konishi R, Nakamura Y, Mizuno S, Takahashi S, Fujimoto M, Nomura T, Okiyama N (2022) The role of PD-L1 on langerhans cells in the regulation of psoriasis. J Investig Dermatol 142:3167–3174.e9

Tenchov R, Bird R, Curtze AE, Zhou QQ (2021) Lipid nanoparticles-from liposomes to mRNA vaccine delivery, a landscape of research diversity and advancement. ACS Nano 15:16982–17015

Ustione A, Piston DW (2011) A simple introduction to multiphoton microscopy. J Microsc 243: 221–226

Valli J, Sanderson J (2021) Super-resolution fluorescence microscopy methods for assessing mouse biology. Curr Protoc 1:e224

van Smeden J, Bouwstra JA (2016) Stratum Corneum lipids: their role for the skin barrier function in healthy subjects and atopic dermatitis patients. Curr Probl Dermatol 49:8–26

Vogt A, Wischke C, Neffe AT, Ma N, Alexiev U, Lendlein A (2016) Nanocarriers for drug delivery into and through the skin - do existing technologies match clinical challenges? J Control Release 242:3–15

Volz P, Boreham A, Wolf A, Kim T-Y, Balke J, Frombach J, Hadam S, Afraz Z, Rancan F, Blume-Peytavi U, Vogt A, Alexiev U (2015) Application of single molecule fluorescence microscopy to characterize the penetration of a large amphiphilic molecule in the Stratum Corneum of human skin. Int J Mol Sci 16:6960–6977

Volz P, Schilrreff P, Brodwolf R, Wolff C, Stellmacher J, Balke J, Morilla MJ, Zoschke C, Schäfer-Korting M, Alexiev U (2017) Pitfalls in using fluorescence tagging of nanomaterials: tecto-dendrimers in skin tissue as investigated by cluster-FLIM. Ann N Y Acad Sci 1405:202–214

Volz P, Brodwolf R, Zoschke C, Haag R, Schäfer-Korting M, Alexiev U (2018) White-light supercontinuum laser-based multiple wavelength excitation for TCSPC-FLIM of cutaneous nanocarrier uptake. Z Phys Chem 232:671–688

Wang LV, Hu S (2012) Photoacoustic tomography: in vivo imaging from organelles to organs. Science 335:1458–1462

Wanjiku B, Yamamoto K, Klossek A, Schumacher F, Pischon H, Mundhenk L, Rancan F, Judd MM, Ahmed M, Zoschke C, Kleuser B, Rühl E, Schäfer-Korting M (2019) Qualifying X-ray and stimulated Raman spectromicroscopy for mapping cutaneous drug penetration. Anal Chem 91:7208–7214

Weissleder R, Ntziachristos V (2003) Shedding light onto live molecular targets. Nat Med 9:123–128

Wirth KG, Linnenbank H, Steinle T, Banszerus L, Icking E, Stampfer C, Giessen H, Taubner T (2021) Tunable s-SNOM for nanoscale infrared optical measurement of electronic properties of bilayer graphene. ACS Photonics 8:418–423

Wolf A, Volz-Rakebrand P, Balke J, Alexiev U (2023) Diffusion analysis of NAnoscopic ensembles: a tracking-free diffusivity analysis for nanoscopic ensembles in biological samples and nanotechnology. Small 19:e2206722

Wong CH, Siah KW, Lo AW (2019) Estimation of clinical trial success rates and related parameters. Biostatistics 20:273–286

Working PK, Dayan AD (1996) Pharmacological-toxicological expert report - Caelyx(TM) - (Stealth(R) liposomal doxorubicin HCl) - foreword. Hum Exp Toxicol 15:751–785

Xia J, Yao JJ, Wang LV (2014) Photoacoustic tomography: principles and advances. Prog Electromagn Res 147:1–22

Yamamoto K, Flesch R, Ohigashi T, Hedtrich S, Klossek A, Patoka P, Ulrich G, Ahlberg S, Rancan F, Vogt A, Blume-Peytavi U, Schrade P, Bachmann S, Schäfer-Korting M, Kosugi N, Rühl E (2015) Selective probing of the penetration of dexamethasone into human skin by soft X-ray spectromicroscopy. Anal Chem 87:6173–6179

Yamamoto K, Klossek A, Flesch R, Ohigashi T, Fleige E, Rancan F, Frombach J, Vogt A, Blume-Peytavi U, Schrade P, Bachmann S, Haag R, Hedtrich S, Schäfer-Korting M, Kosugi N, Rühl E (2016) Core-multishell nanocarriers: transport and release of dexamethasone probed by soft X-ray spectromicroscopy. J Control Release 242:64–70

Yamamoto K, Klossek A, Flesch A, Rancan F, Weigand M, Bykova I, Bechtel M, Ahlberg S, Vogt A, Blume-Peytavi U, Schrade P, Bachmann S, Hedtrich S, Schäfer-Korting M, Rühl E (2017) Influence of the skin barrier on the penetration of topically-applied dexamethasone probed by soft X-ray spectromicroscopy. Eur J Pharm Biopharm 118:30–37

Yamamoto K, Klossek A, Fuchs K, Watts B, Raabe J, Flesch R, Rancan F, Pischon H, Radbruch M, Gruber AD, Mundhenk L, Vogt A, Blume-Peytavi U, Schrade P, Bachmann S, Gurny R, Rühl E (2019) Soft X-ray microscopy for probing of topical tacrolimus delivery via micelles. Eur J Pharm Biopharm 139:68–75

Zavalin A, Todd EM, Rawhouser PD, Yang JH, Norris JL, Caprioli RM (2012) Direct imaging of single cells and tissue at sub-cellular spatial resolution using transmission geometry MALDI MS. J Mass Spectrom 47:1473–1481

Zavalin A, Yang JH, Haase A, Holle A, Caprioli R (2014) Implementation of a Gaussian beam laser and aspheric optics for high spatial resolution MALDI imaging MS. J Am Soc Mass Spectrom 25:1079–1082

Zhang GJ, Moore DJ, Flach CR, Mendelsohn R (2007) Vibrational microscopy and imaging of skin: from single cells to intact tissue. Anal Bioanal Chem 387:1591–1599

Zhang QH, Flach CR, Mendelsohn R, Page L, Whitson S, Bettex MB (2020) Visualization of epidermal reservoir formation from topical diclofenac gels by Raman spectroscopy. J Pain Res 13:1621–1627

Zhang X, Li X, Wang Y, Chen Y, Hu Y, Guo C, Yu Z, Xu P, Ding Y, Mi Q-S, Wu J, Gu J, Shi Y (2022) Abnormal lipid metabolism in epidermal Langerhans cells mediates psoriasis-like dermatitis. JCI Insight 7:e15022

Zheng FF, Xiong WW, Sun SS, Zhang PH, Zhu JJ (2019) Recent advances in drug release monitoring. Nanophotonics 8:391–413

Characterization of Drug Delivery Systems by Transmission Electron Microscopy

Stephanie Hoeppener

Contents

Abstract

The contribution of electron microscopy, and here, in particular transmission electron microscopy (TEM), to the formulation and understanding of the biological action of drug delivery systems has led to a better insight into the design principles of drug delivery systems. TEM can be applied for particle characterization, for the visualization of the uptake and intracellular pathways of drug vehicles in cells and tissues and more recently can be also applied for the high-resolution investigation of drug–receptor interactions with near-atomic resolution. This chapter introduces basic techniques to optimize imaging quality of soft matter samples, highlights possibilities to study certain aspects of drug delivery applications, and finally provides a short introduction to high-resolution characterization possibilities which recently emerged.

S. Hoeppener (✉)
Jena Center for Soft Matter (JCSM), Friedrich Schiller University Jena, Jena, Germany

Laboratory of Organic and Macromolecular Chemistry (IOMC), Friedrich Schiller University Jena, Jena, Germany
e-mail: s.hoeppener@uni-jena.de

M. Schäfer-Korting, U. S. Schubert (eds.), *Drug Delivery and Targeting*,
Handbook of Experimental Pharmacology 284, https://doi.org/10.1007/164_2023_699

Keywords

Cellular uptake · Drug delivery · Particle characterization · Structural analysis · Transmission electron microscopy

Abbreviations

CCD	Charge-coupled device
CPP	Cell penetrating peptides
Cryo-ET	Cryo-electron tomography
cryo-TEM	Cryogenic transmission electron microscopy
DED	Direct electron detector
DNA	Deoxyribonucleic acid
EM	Electron microscopy
mRNA	Messenger ribonucleic acid
PEG	Polyethylene glycol
SEM	Scanning electron microscopy
TEM	Transmission electron microscopy

1 Introduction

Detailed insight into the structure, architecture, and function of drug delivery systems as well as into their interaction with cells and tissues is of tremendous interest for the design and optimization of drug carrier systems. Due to their frequently small size, detailed information on the nanoparticle architecture can be provided only by high-resolution microscopy techniques. While fluorescence, and, more recently, super-resolution fluorescence microscopy, allow the investigation of the intracellular fate of nanoparticle systems in live cell experiments, electron microscopy has ever since been a standard characterization technique for evaluating the architecture of nanomaterials and has contributed enormously to elucidate the structure of cells and drug carrier-cell interactions (Malatesta 2021). As such, electron microscopy, and here in particular transmission electron microscopy, has determined the structure of essential building blocks of cells, their specific architecture, and could help to gain insight into tissues and cells (Jastrow 2014) as well as particle uptake (Reifarth et al. 2018a, b). Moreover, TEM has contributed to the structural characterization of nanostructures, drug delivery vehicles (Kuntsche et al. 2011), etc. These possibilities are strongly linked to steady and continuous developments of better instruments, major improvements in the sample preparation, new concepts for image analysis, dedicated possibilities to improve the image contrast, and new approaches to identify the three-dimensional structure in complex environments. Even, drug–receptor interactions down to the atomic level can be visualized. In the field of soft drug nanocarrier engineering, in particular cryo-TEM is a frequently used methodology for the visualization of drug-free and drug-loaded liposomes and its use is expected to become even more important than today in pharmaceutical applications in future for drug design (Renaud et al. 2018).

Following an introduction to TEM analysis and preparation techniques, the chapter addresses furthermore special considerations for the characterization of drug delivery systems as well as cell and tissue samples. The final section summarizes recent developments of cryo-TEM for high-resolution protein structure determination and studies on drug–protein/drug–receptor interactions.

2 Basics of Transmission Electron Microscopy

Electron microscopy essentially comprises two different techniques: scanning electron microscopy (SEM) and transmission electron microscopy (TEM). Scanning electron microscopy (SEM) can be employed to determine the structure of nanoparticles and their interactions with the surfaces of cells, also in relation to internalization processes and cell shape modifications. Yet SEM is less suitable for studying the intracellular distribution of nanoparticles. This is a domain of TEM investigations.

The technical setup of transmission electron microscopes is closely related to the construction of classical light microscopes. The major difference is the utilization of electrons as alternative light sources and the utilization of electromagnetic lens systems. In general, the resolving power of light microscopes is restricted to approximately half the wavelength of light, i.e., ~300 nm. This value is close to the diameter of small bacteria, but not sufficient to resolve smaller objects like viruses, small compartments in cells, vesicles or nanoparticles, and micelles. In electron microscopy, this problem is circumvented by dramatically decreasing the wavelength of the illumination source by utilizing electrons which are accelerated in an electric field to energies of 80–300 keV. Thus, already at an acceleration voltage of 100 kV the resolution power is theoretically as good as 0.24 nm. The electron beam is then shaped by means of electromagnetic lenses and apertures and finally transmits through the sample while being magnified. The typical setup of a TEM is schematically depicted in Fig. 1, where also the functions of the individual components are summarized. Essential for the image formation in TEM is the interaction of the electrons with the sample material. Some of the electrons of the beam might be scattered when being transmitted through the sample, hence, upon interaction with the sample material they deviate from the beam propagation direction and are missing in the final image which is visualized nowadays by a CCD camera or a direct electron detector (DED). As a consequence, in TEM always a two-dimensional analogue of a magnified shadow image of the sample is obtained.

In general, there are several requirements to be met by the samples which practically limit the applicability of TEM and demand for dedicated preparation procedures to enable visualization of the samples. These restrictions concern, in particular, the sample thickness. Since electrons have to be—at least partially—transmitted through the sample, their thickness is roughly limited to less than approximately 500 nm. Another issue is the mechanism of contrast formation. To

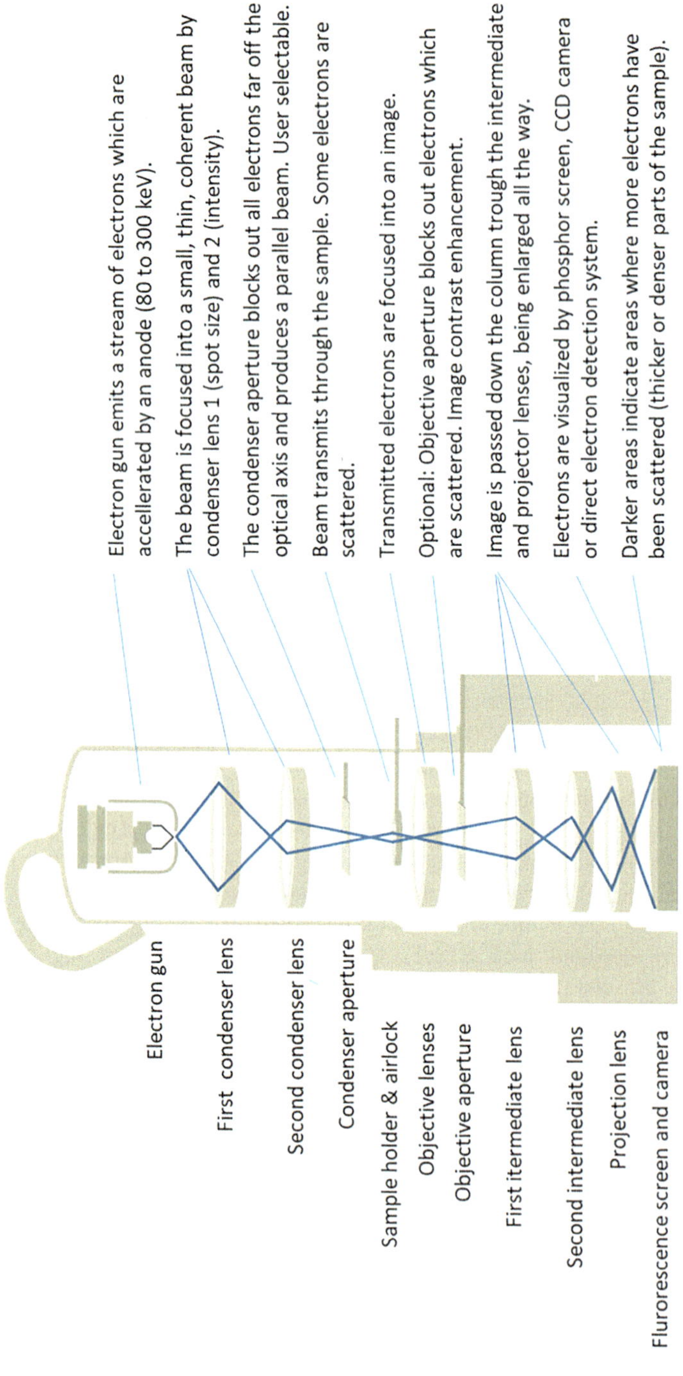

Fig. 1 Setup of a transmission electron microscope and function of the individual components

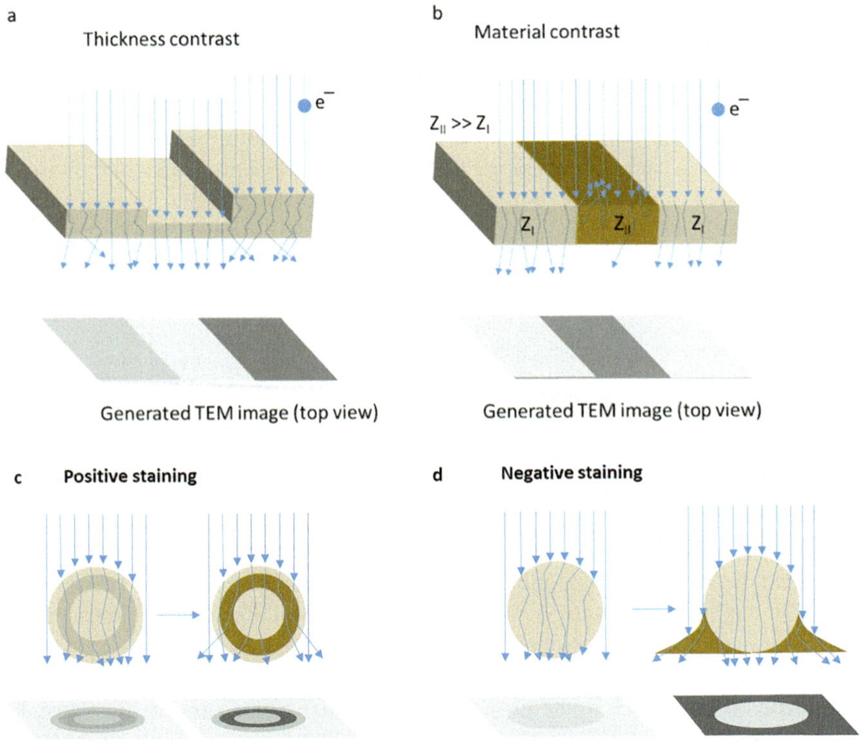

Fig. 2 Contrast generation and image generation in TEM. (**a**) Thickness contrast: Scattering event probability increases with increased thickness. (**b**) Material contrast: Heavier elements cause increased scattering. These electrons do not transmit through the sample. (**c**) Positive staining of functional groups inside the sample structure (core-shell-corona particles) by heavy elements, i.e., uranyl acetate or lead citrate. (**d**) Negative staining introduced by interaction of heavy elements onto the TEM support film

generate sufficient contrast to visualize details of the sample, either thickness variations in the sample (Fig. 2a) or the presence of different local elemental compositions are required, e.g., the presence of heavy metals which show a high scattering probability for electrons (Fig. 2b). This contrast formation has severe consequences for the investigation in particular of biological samples and polymer materials since these samples consist almost exclusively of light elements and, as a consequence, produce only weak contrasts due to a lack of strong differences in the scattering probability of the elements. Hence, biological and polymer specimens require frequently a dedicated processing step which artificially improves the image contrast. This is frequently established by introducing heavy atoms into the chemical structure (positive staining, see Fig. 2c) utilizing functional groups being present in different areas of the sample or are introduced in the background of the structures creating a negative staining effect (Fig. 2d), which helps to identify the structures of interest as bright features in the resulting images. Negative staining can be used, e.g., for the visualization of small isolated objects, like, e.g., viruses.

Another serious issue which imposes limitations to the sample is the requirement of operating electron microscopes under ultrahigh vacuum conditions. As a consequence of this requirement, an essential part of performing electron microscopy investigations is a sample preparation adapted to the special properties of the sample systems. This is crucial for biological specimens and materials formed by soft materials, such as polymers and biomolecules. Such materials frequently suffer from artifacts which are induced if the sample preparation is not carried out with great care.

2.1 Suspensions, Solutions, Bacteria, Viruses, and Proteins

Back in the early days of TEM hardly any strategy was available to cope with the harsh environmental constraints soft matter samples encounter in the ultrahigh vacuum conditions in the electron microscope. For example, virus particle suspensions without proper fixation and staining were utilized and were simply deposited onto a carbon-supported TEM grid and were allowed to dry. This strategy has three main disadvantages: First, the water is removed from the specimens which sometimes can cause severe alterations in the sample structure. Second, the sample interacts with the carbon support, and third, during the drying process, strong forces are involved when the water evaporates. The latter point can be illustrated by estimating the forces which are exerted on small structures during such drying processes which are mainly caused by the surface tension of water (Reimer 1959). A particle with a radius of 1 μm would be exposed to a drying force in the range of 1.4 kg cm^{-2} while a particle with a radius of 10 nm is even exposed to a force of 140 kg cm^{-2}. This certainly can result in the deformation of the particles or can result in extreme flattening of the nanoparticles into almost pancake-like disks. This is particularly critical if the nanoparticles consist of soft materials, i.e., (bio-) polymers or lipids.

This class of specimens is moreover susceptible to other artifacts that impede proper analysis of the sample. These include size sorting effects due to capillary forces experienced during the drying process, preferred orientation of objects (like proteins) due to interaction with the carbon support film, etc. All of these issues should be taken care of when analyzing samples that have been prepared by the conventional blotting technique.

Therefore, the preservation of the sample structure, issues of stability of the specimens under ultrahigh vacuum conditions and the electron beam, enhancement of the contrast of the specimen details as well as the specific visualization of small molecules, i.e., enzymes and proteins, are subject of dedicated sample preparation strategies.

2.1.1 Cryo-TEM

Cryo-TEM investigations have become extremely popular as this method is regarded as an excellent tool that allows investigating aqueous specimen suspensions close to their native, liquid state. It has developed into the standard method of structural biology to determine the structure of proteins and serves as a method to visualize the structure of multicompartment nanoparticles and drug delivery systems, such as polymer micelles, polymersomes, liposomes, hexosomes, and cubosomes. Cryo-TEM preparations were introduced by Dubochet in 1981 and utilize the fact that the vapor pressure of water becomes negligible if it is kept in a frozen state, even at ultrahigh vacuum conditions (Dubochet et al. 1988; Dubochet and McDowall 1981). A serious obstacle is that the formed ice films need to be thin enough to allow for electron transmission (typically thinner than 100 nm) and even more important, the formation of crystalline ice has to be avoided. Not only that crystalline ice would cause problems in TEM imaging, since they produce a strong contrast and even can diffract the electron beam, but more importantly also biological specimens tend to denature and are damaged by the ice crystals. Crystalline ice is formed if the sample cooling is performed slowly. Consequently, Dubochet and coworkers developed a technique to obtain thin amorphous vitrified ice layers. This is achieved by cooling down the sample so rapidly that the water molecules in the liquid film do not have time to organize themselves into a crystalline ice lattice. For this purpose, the liquid samples are deposited on special TEM grids that feature hole structures. Onto these, the sample suspension is applied and excess of the solution is removed by filter paper. The aim here is to span a liquid film in the hole areas which has the desired thickness of 100 nm or even less. Subsequently, the samples are plunge-frozen in a suitable cryogen. These cryogens have to ensure a rapid cooling of the specimens. A cooling rate of $>20{,}000\ \mathrm{K\ s^{-1}}$ can be realized, e.g., with liquid ethane which is kept at its melting point (−182.2°C) by passive nitrogen cooling. As long as temperatures of less than −137°C are maintained, the vitrified ice remains in its amorphous state. Above this temperature, irreversibly crystalline ice is formed. Despite of the fact that vitrified biological samples greatly preserve their structural features the ice embedding moreover reduces radiation damage caused by the electron beam during measurement and protects the sample. Moreover, it locks the water molecules in place around the native samples and, thus, the quaternary structure of molecules is preserved. Today, cryo-TEM investigations are regarded as the standard preparation technique to obtain electron micrographs from biomolecules and drug carrier vehicles and can be even utilized to obtain high-resolution three-dimensional electron density maps of proteins, virus capsids, and macromolecules with nearly atomic resolution.

TEM investigations on particle suspensions of drug delivery vehicles can be a useful tool to determine the size, shape, homogeneity, and size distribution of nanoparticles, albeit it has to be critically mentioned that the statistics obtained from TEM investigations is frequently poor due to the limited number of structures (tens to hundreds) that are usually measured. However, it is the only available microscopic technique that provides insight into the architecture of particles and drug delivery systems at the nanometer scale and can be supplemented with studies

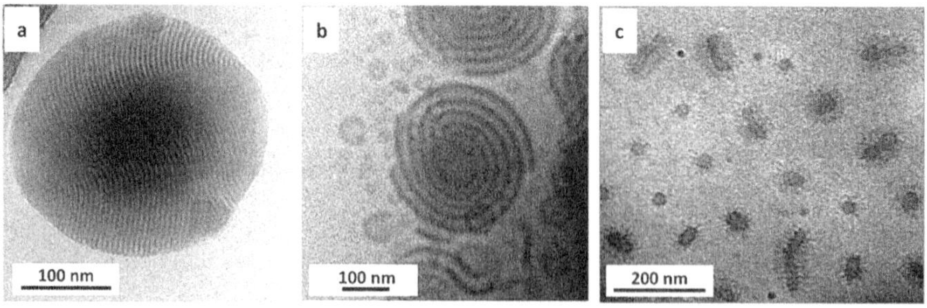

Fig. 3 Cryo-TEM images of particle systems. (**a**) "Rugby ball"-shaped nanoparticles formed by doxorubicin chemically conjugated to D-α-tocopherol succinate through an amide bond to form N-doxorubicin–α-D-tocopherol succinate (N-DOX–TOS) which is stabilized by d-α-tocopherol poly(ethylene glycol) 2,000 succinate. The prodrug self-assembles in water into 250 nm nanostructures. The periodic stripe structure originates from an internal lamellar microphase-separated structure and features a periodicity of 5.5 nm ± 0.5 nm (Duhem et al. 2014). Copyright 2014 American Chemical Society. (**b**) Self-assembled spiral organization of a linear terpoly(2-oxazoline) block copolymer containing fluorinated 2-(2,6-difluorophenyl)-2-oxazoline (ODFOx), lipophilic 2-(1-ethylheptyl)-2-oxazoline (EPOx), and hydrophilic 2-ethyl-2-oxazoline (EtOx) blocks. The worm-like micellar structure forms a superstructure in the form of a spiral-like, planar disk (Kempe et al. 2010). Unpublished result. (**c**) Bottle-brush polymers with resolved grafted side chains. Unpublished result

such as dynamic light scattering, analytical ultracentrifugation, or field-flow-field investigations. Figure 3 summarizes a few illustrative examples of nanoparticles characterized by cryo-TEM investigations.

Figure 3a represents the shape of a chemically modified doxorubicin derivative which forms hollow, rugby ball-shaped nanocapsules (Duhem et al. 2014). Evident is the regular pattern on the surface of the nanoparticles consisting of dark and bright stripes, which suggest that these lamellae contain on the one hand the aromatic part of the doxorubicin and on the other hand the aliphatic areas of the tocopherol succinate. Besides the classical self-organized nanostructures of micelles and vesicles, also more complex features can be found by cryo-TEM investigations. Figure 3b depicts disk-shaped spirals which are formed by a terpolymer consisting of three immiscible polymer blocks (Kempe et al. 2010). It is also well observed that beside the disks, small vesicles are present which appear to be open in close vicinity of the disk structure suggesting that the system remains in a metastable state. While in the previous two examples the water-soluble polyethylene glycol (PEG), added as a stealth layer to nanoparticles to escape the body's immune system, and the 2-ethyl-2-oxazoline moieties utilized for the stabilization and solubilization of the structures is not visible due to a lack of contrast, Fig. 3c depicts an example of a terpolymer system which self-assembled in the form of a bottle-brush system. The water-soluble blocks are clearly visible as a corona of the entire structure while the core and a slightly darker shell are formed by the water-insoluble parts of the polymer system.

Other fields of active research where cryo-TEM contributes valuable information are liposomes or polymersomes (Fig. 4a). Given their ease of preparation, their biocompatibility resulting from their specific membrane structure, and their versatile

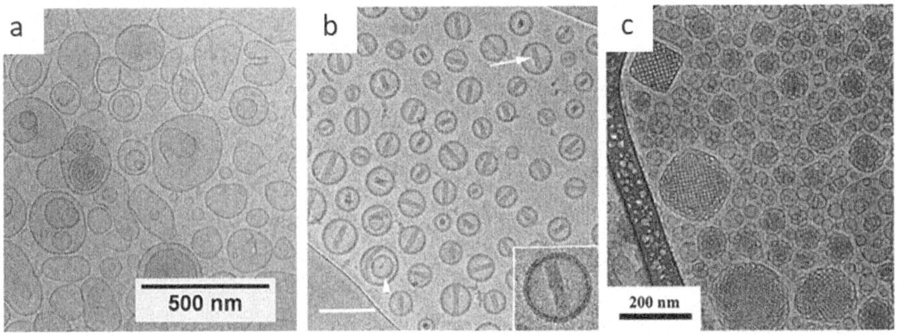

Fig. 4 (**a**) Cryo-TEM investigation of polymersomes. Unpublished result. (**b**) Detailed structural analysis of Doxil®. Clearly visible are the doxorubicin crystals which are located in a unilamellar liposomal carrier (Koifman and Talmon 2021). Published under CCBY 4.0 license. (**c**) Cubosomes (Spicer et al. 2001). Reprinted with permission of the American Chemical Society

potential to encapsulate a variety of molecules these systems can be used as drug delivery systems. In general, liposomes are rather fragile structures and their structure is highly influenced by their preparation and different structures can be found which range from unilamellar to bi- and even multilamellar concentric structures. Cryo-TEM investigations are able to visualize the core as well as the membrane of these structures without the necessity to stabilize the liposomes by fixation. Cryo-TEM images can provide a detailed insight into the structure as well as into the rigidity of the lipid bilayers by evaluating their characteristic appearance and the overall shape of the liposomes: rigid lipid bilayers in the gel state appear to be slightly angular, in particular, if the liposomes are small, while deformation and bilayer invaginations are an indication that the lipid bilayers are highly flexible.

An illustrative example of a liposome-based drug is Doxil®, which consists of PEGylated liposomes encapsulating the anticancer drug doxorubicin (Koifman and Talmon 2021). In this system, the doxorubicin is encapsulated into unilamellar liposomes in the form of crystals, and the crystalline structure can be resolved (Fig. 4b). It is observed that a part of these crystals appears to be featureless, which is an indication for a twisted form of the crystals. In other systems indications of successful drug loading are, e.g., the occurrence of precipitates as discrete structures in the liposome core or an increase of contrast observed inside the liposome core.

Quality control as well as the influence of drug formulation play an essential role in drug delivery investigations. As an example, the anticancer drug paclitaxel (Taxol) is to be mentioned here. Direct imaging by cryo-TEM reveals the formation of complement-activating needles in aqueous solutions as a result of dilution of the drug administration and further dilution in the bloodstream, which was interpreted as a possible cause for adverse reactions observed for this drug (Szebeni et al. 2001).

Cubosomes (Fig. 4c) as an example of promising drug delivery vehicles are another typical sample system to be investigated by cryo-TEM (Spicer et al. 2001). These systems are regarded as self-assembled liquid crystalline particles consisting of a surfactant that self-assembles into a bicontinuous phase and refers to the presence of non-intersecting aqueous regions which are separated by a lipid bilayer that arranges in a space-filling structure. These cubic phases comprise a unique microstructure that is biologically compatible and allows the establishing of controlled release of solubilized drugs and proteins.

Despite the success of cryo-TEM investigations for the determination of the native structure of nanoparticle systems in their liquid-like environment, it has to be mentioned here that cryo-TEM has also its limitations. Issues of careful sample preparation include a complex workflow, which has to be carried out at sufficiently low temperatures, minimizing the exposure of the sample to ambient air after blotting, as well as the blotting process itself, as liquid flow and shear stress might lead to a re-orientation of the dispersed objects or may induce a rearrangement of the self-assembled structures. Moreover, the size sorting phenomenon, which is manifested by the observation that smaller nanoparticles are preferentially located in the thin middle area of the ice layer while larger particles are found in the thicker areas close to the rim of the hole areas of the TEM grid support, has to be avoided. Additionally, water-miscible polymer chains, e.g., PEG, are usually not visible in cryo-TEM due to a lack of imaging contrast (Spicer et al. 2001). A severe limitation for drug internalization studies is that only a snapshot of the internalization mechanism can be obtained. This practically prevents TEM from being a method that can provide, e.g., the uptake rates or quantitative information of other dynamic processes.

2.2 Cells and Tissues

The question of how to prepare a suitable sample for TEM investigations becomes even more complex if the ultrastructural imaging of cell or tissue samples is addressed. Here, several problems are faced: first, cells contain >70% water compared to the entire mass of the cell, and, second, cells feature size of several microns, and, finally, they only provide a poor electron contrast. Thus, they cannot be directly visualized by TEM and dedicated sample preparation techniques have to be used. They have to be fixated, hardened, and sliced into thin sections with a thickness of less than 500 nm. This process is by far not trivial and all preparation steps should be critically reviewed regarding alterations that they might be induced in the specimen, in particular, if proteins, enzymes, or cellular response to nanoparticle uptake is in focus of investigations. In particular, altered osmotic pressures or increased temperatures due to exothermic reactions are here to be critically mentioned.

The most important step in the preparation of cells and tissue samples is fixation. Its main aims are the cross-linking of cellular structures to preserve their structure as close to the native state as possible with a minimum of alterations of the morphology, volume, spatial distribution, and a minimum loss of cellular constituents. Fixation procedures involve chemical reactions that consume time and rely on the diffusion of the fixative components into the sample. Fixation is performed in most cases by glutaraldehyde which mainly crosslinks proteins followed by a postfixation step with osmium tetroxide. The primary aim of postfixation is further stabilization by reacting with unsaturated lipids of the membranes and amino acids. For ultrastructural studies of the cellular compartments and their intracellular structure, the fixation of membranes is regarded as a key requirement to preserve the cell and tissue structure integrity. At the same time, both media can precipitate proteins and DNA and cause undesired aggregation. Without proper prior fixation strong alterations of the cell structure would have to be considered.

Fixation can be alternatively achieved by high-pressure freezing (McDonald and Auer 2006). While plunge freezing similar to the preparation of cryo-TEM samples is only applicable for samples of less than 10 μm, high-pressure freezing permits the vitrification of thicker samples up to 200 μm. Dedicated high-pressure freezing devices provide synchronized pressurization and cooling of the samples in a time span of 20 ms. Cryo-fixation omits the diffusion of chemical reagents into the cell and tissue samples and is thus much faster which helps to maintain the sample integrity. Moreover, by choosing dedicated time points for the vitrification process studying and capturing highly dynamic processes with millisecond precision is possible, e.g., to visualize changes in the fine structure or the dynamics of cellular processes. Compared to chemical fixation, cryo-fixation simultaneously stabilizes all of the cellular components. Cryo-fixated samples can be directly investigated by cryo-TEM only if their sample thickness is well below 1 μm. This is rarely the case. In some instances, focused ion beam slicing is possible at cryogenic temperatures to prepare TEM lamella which are thin enough for TEM investigations. More commonly, chemically fixed as well as samples that have been prepared by high-pressure freezing are embedded into resins. For this purpose, the water has to be removed from the specimens, either by a graded series of increasing ethanol or acetone concentrations for chemically fixed samples or by freeze substitution in case of high-pressure frozen samples. In the following steps, these samples are infiltrated with suitable resins and hardened. Finally, they have to be sliced into thin sections by an ultramicrotome utilizing diamond knives to achieve a slice thickness of 80–100 nm and are subsequently positively stained by uranyl acetate and lead citrate to enhance the contrast of membranes, the nucleus, ribosomes, etc. A mandatory step in the analysis of the obtained imaging data is the critical evaluation of the cellular ultrastructure for indications to verify if artifacts stemming from the preparation process are observable. Typical indications are abnormal structures of cell compartments, i.e., mitochondria swelling, the presence of a large number of vacuoles, etc.

3 Cellular Uptake of Drug Delivery Vehicles

TEM investigations for drug and gene delivery after incubation of particles in cells and tissue can provide valuable information on, e.g., the cell toxicity of nanoparticles. Unlike commonly used methods to determine the cell death rate and viability of the cell culture, sub-lethal cell stress levels or organelle damage are easily detectable at a rather early stage by TEM investigations. These are critical for the application of nanoparticle systems as nanomedical products, as induced cell injury can alter, e.g., tissue homeostasis and trigger inflammatory responses. Here, TEM can significantly contribute due to its superior resolution power and several indicators for different stress levels can be checked (Dussouchaud et al. 2022). These include alterations of the plasma membrane, such as blebbing or loss of surface protrusions, the reorganization of the membranous endoplasmic system, DNA condensation or the rearrangement of the nuclear domains in the cell nucleus, the shrinkage or swelling of mitochondria, changes or loss of their typical cristae structure, the accumulation of residual bodies, or fine changes in the membrane structure such as thickening or rupture. In tissues, the alteration of capillary walls or the restructuring of the extracellular matrix may be indicative of damage and stress levels induced by nanoparticle uptake. Also, viruses can be visualized in the cellular environment, and damage induced by the infection can be visualized in different tissues (Deinhardt-Emmer et al. 2021; Roingeard et al. 2019).

Besides these severe alterations, which become visible as a consequence of adverse effects of nanoparticle internalization, the full strength of TEM investigations is localization and tracking of nanoparticles—starting from their cellular uptake, their intracellular localization up to the intracellular degradation, which are valuable information for the design and optimization of drug and gene delivery systems (Malatesta 2021). The internalization of drug delivery systems can guide already the intracellular pathways and imply possibilities for release and degradation. For example, the possible pathways for nanoparticle uptake are governed by a multitude of physicochemical properties of the drug- and gene-delivery vehicles, i.e., size, shape (Gratton et al. 2008), and charge.

TEM investigations can be easily used to study the internalization mechanism of nanoparticles. This is achieved by investigating the extracellular membrane at places where nanoparticle membrane interactions occur. It is possible to determine if nanoparticles are taken up individually or in the form of larger clusters, which is an important aspect that also influences the mode of uptake. Moreover, characteristic modifications in the membrane are indicative of different uptake mechanisms (Fig. 5a).

Direct penetration pathways are only accessible for individual, small particles with a size in the range of only a few nanometers and include different entry processes, such as diffusion, penetration, membrane fusion of lipids from the nanoparticle with lipids of the membrane, and pore formation. While diffusion and penetration are not associated with characteristic changes in the structure of the extracellular membrane, fusion processes, and the formation of pores are visible by high-resolution ultrastructural investigations of membrane areas, where nanoparticle contact is observed. In all cases, the nanoparticles directly enter into the cytosol of the cell and are not surrounded by any distinct compartments or membranes, which allows further confirmation of the uptake by direct penetration. Nanoparticles, which are coated by cell penetrating peptides (CPP), are also prone to be taken up by direct membrane penetration, though it is not their exclusive route to cell internalization and endocytic pathways are also likely to occur. The later particles are surrounded by an endosomal membrane inside the cell. Lipid or membrane fusion-mediated uptake

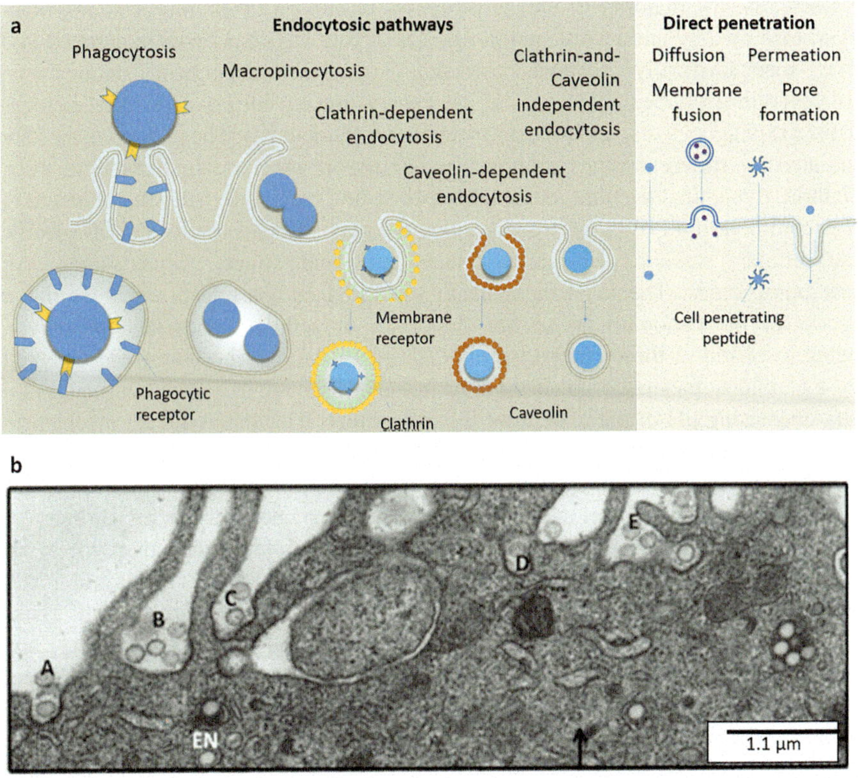

Fig. 5 (**a**) Schematic representation of different uptake mechanisms. All uptake pathways are associated with different membrane interactions and hence characteristic membrane morphologies. Depending on the uptake mechanism also different intracellular distributions of the nanoparticles are found. (**b**) Study on the uptake of 100 nm polystyrene nanoparticles. Multiple endocytic pathways are simultaneously observed in bone marrow-derived macrophages (Firdessa et al. 2014). A: clathrin-mediated endocytosis; B: phagocytosis; C: clathrin and caveolae-in-dependent endocytosis; D: caveolae-mediated endocytosis; and E: micropinocytosis. Moreover, the PS beads that show up with a bright contrast are intercellularly located in endosomal vesicles (EN). Scale bar: 1.1 µm. Reprinted with permission of Elsevier

may take place if particles are coated with some types of bilayers that can fuse with the cell's extracellular membrane. After membrane fusion, the encapsulated cargo of the nanoparticles, e.g., proteins, nucleotides, and small molecules, are directly released into the cytosol. These are, however, frequently not visible by TEM imaging anymore due to a severe lack of contrast as well as a relatively low density. Finally, direct penetration is possible by the formation of small pores in the extracellular membrane which allows the particles to enter the cell. Nanoparticles that are directly transported into the cytosol are freely dispersed and can interact and target subcellular organelles and intracellular structures. This can be beneficial to stimulate biological responses and medical functions.

Actually, the majority of uptake processes of nanoparticles into cells are, however, mediated by endocytotic pathways. These pathways can be differentiated into five mechanistically distinct classes: (a) clathrin-dependent endocytosis; (b) caveolin-dependent endocytosis; (c) clathrin- and caveolin-independent endocytosis; (d) phagocytosis; and (e) macro- and micropinocytosis. These mechanisms are initiated by different types of lipids and transport proteins, such as lipid rafts, clathrin, dynamin, caveolin, and pattern recognition receptors. After internalization, it is common to all of these processes that the nanoparticles are located in specific intracellular vesicle structures, such as endosomes, phagosomes, or macropinosomes. The localization in these closed compartments excludes direct access of the nanoparticles to the cytoplasm or cellular organelles. Moreover, being localized in these compartments determines their further fate inside the cell as, e.g., endosomes undergo ripening processes which are associated with a gradually decreasing pH of the content of the endosomes. The actual uptake mechanism can be investigated by TEM imaging. Here, typical structures of the extracellular membrane, when interacting with the nanoparticles as well as the structure of the intracellular localization in endocytic vesicles can provide valuable insight into the uptake process. After binding to the lipids or transport proteins, the nanoparticles are located in an invagination of the cell membrane which gradually deepens and finally results in the formation of a vesicle that transports the material into the cell. These membrane deformations are typical for endocytosis via clathrin-, caveolin-, and independent uptake. In TEM investigations, phagocytosis is seen as the intake of very large particles by the formation of large protrusions of the extracellular membrane, which engulf the entire nanoparticle. By fusion of the protrusions, the nanoparticle is completely encapsulated and finally dragged into the cell in a large endocytotic vesicle representing a phagosome. Phagosomes can be identified by TEM image by their large size (up to several micrometers). With time, lysosomes attach to the phagosome and the lysosomal enzymes start to digest the content of the phagosome. The formed new structures are so-called phagolysosomes. They can be identified by TEM due to their size which is in sliced samples in the range of 0.3–2 μm, which is considerably larger than a simple lysosome (25–200 nm) and they are surrounded by a characteristic double-layer membrane. The phagolysosomes are more or less spherical and feature variable electron density since it depends much on the material that is being digested. Some heterolysosomes show remains of the attached cells or contain lipid droplets (identified by their round shape and moderate electron density). Due to the continuous digestion of the phagolysosomal content and constant transport of water and usable substances (e.g., amino acids), the size of the phagolysosome gradually decreases and they appear more condensed. Finally, only non-digestible components remain within the phagolysosome which are forming residual bodies at this stage. These are either transported quickly out of the cell by fusion with the extracellular membrane or in rare cases, such as in aged nerve cells or macrophages, reside inside the cell until they die. In TEM images residual bodies can be identified by double-layer membrane and a size of 0.2–0.6 μm in sliced cell specimens, which is significantly smaller than the diameter of the initial phagolysosome. They contain some hardly electron-dense areas, representing lipidic components of the digested material, and are otherwise very electron dense with a granular structure.

Phagolysosomes are also capable of digesting their own cellular compartments if they are damaged. This special form of material recycling is summarized under the term autophagy and the formed respective phagolysosomes are called autophagosomes—they may contain, e.g., damaged mitochondria.

Micropinocytosis is the analog which facilitates the nonspecific internalization of extracellular nutrients, antigens, and soluble molecules present in the extracellular fluid. It is facilitated by cell surface ruffles which finally fuse with the basal membrane. Thereby large, uncoated vesicular structures, so-called micropinosomes, are formed which greatly deviate in size, ranging from 0.2 to 5 μm (Lim and Gleeson 2011). Since most of the content is fluid, they appear frequently as electron transparent vesicles.

In contrast to mechanisms that reach out to the extracellular space by forming pseudopodia and surface ruffles, micropinocytotic uptake is possible in many different kinds of mammalian cells. Micropinocytosis facilitates the uptake of molecular and colloidal substances for which the cell membrane does not provide transporter proteins. Typically, small endocytotic vesicles are produced with a diameter of 50–400 nm, whereby a size of 100 nm is most abundant. One can distinguish between three major forms of micropinocytosis: a) clathrin-mediated, b) caveolin-mediated, and c) clathrin-and-caveolin-independent uptake. Besides visualizing the typical membrane invaginations and the formed vesicles inspection of the vesicles directly after their formation, e.g., close to the extracellular membrane, permits also to identify clathrin-coated vesicles, which can be seen in the form of a thin electron-dense rim. During the phase of direct membrane interaction and membrane invagination, a gap between the membrane and the nanoparticles is visible with a thickness of 20 nm. The clathrin is recycled relatively quickly and the final vesicles do not feature the electron-dense rim anymore.

Thus, TEM imaging can greatly help to determine the cellular uptake of drug delivery vehicles and the intracellular internalization becomes possible, too. This can be used to investigate endosomal release processes in great detail. Here, in particular, the influence of the individual microenvironment in the respective compartments (e.g., pH value) might also have an influence on the particle structure, e.g., for polycationic polymer carriers suitable for endosomal release by the proton sponge effect. Here, the size of the particles can be analyzed in the compartments, and swelling effects can be observed by comparing the particle size inside the endosomes with particles that are present outside the cell. Finally, information on the degradation of nanoparticles in the compartments becomes accessible as well.

Adverse effects of nanoparticles are mostly not directly visible but manifest themselves by abnormal appearances of typical cell compartments. They have to be carefully analyzed in the context of reference cell samples and require a careful characterization of a large number of individual cell and tissue samples.

3.1 Single Particle Reconstruction and Electron Tomography

During the last decade, exciting developments opened up a new application field to TEM investigations in the field of structural biology and drug design. The so-called resolution revolution, fueled by extensive improvement of the TEM equipment, automated image acquisition and analysis, and sophisticated reconstruction algorithms to obtain the three-dimensional structure of proteins, viruses, receptors, etc., allows nowadays the routine characterization of these systems with near atomic resolution in rather short time frames of days. Before, such investigations mainly utilized X-ray diffraction techniques which inevitably required the preparation of ultrapure materials and the formation of crystals. Single particle reconstruction (Fig. 6a) permits the investigation of the volume structure of the objects by acquiring a large number of projections of the object from different viewing angles and reconstructing the obtained information in the form of a 3D model of the structure. Therefore, the structure of 100.000s of particles can be analyzed by automated imaging and analysis routines. Due to their random orientation, different projection axis's are imaged and combined into a three-dimensional model of the protein. This method permits the investigation not only of proteins but also the interaction of drug molecules to specific receptor sites. This approach was successfully applied to determine the structure of a large number of proteins, but also permits studying drug-integral membrane protein interactions, supports structure-based drug design, and can be used for vaccine development. An illustrative example is the development of mRNA vaccines against COVID-19. Two antigens had been identified as promising candidates for developing a novel mRNA-based vaccine that can deliver viral spike protein-coding sequences to cells. While BNT162b1 encoded an

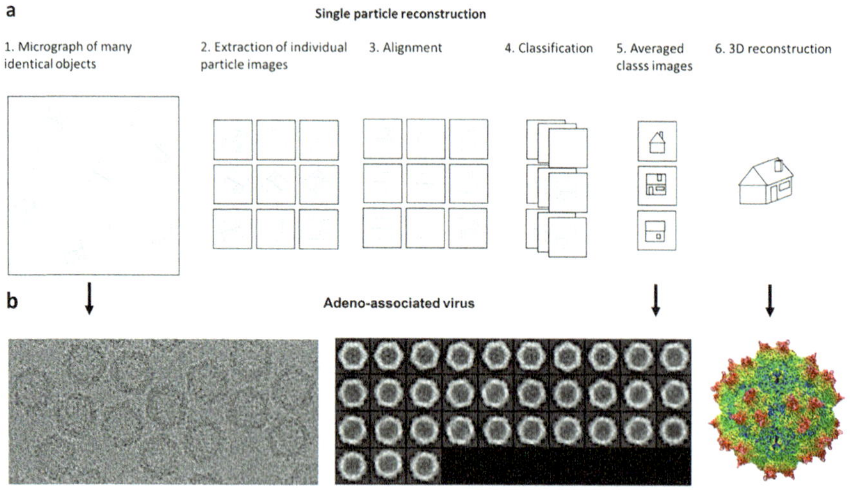

Fig. 6 (**a**) Schematic representation of the fundamentals of single particle reconstruction. (**b**) Example of a single particle reconstruction of an adeno-associated virus with a resolution of 1.56 Å. Adapted from Xie et al. (2020) with permission from MDPI

artificially trimerized spike protein receptor binding domain, BNT162b2 resembled a pre-fusion-stabilized variant of the full-length transmembrane S glycoprotein spike structure. In order to warranty that the correct epitopes are exposed to the patients' immune system single particle analysis was performed. For this purpose, BNT162b1 was attached to the ACE2 receptor for the spike protein to improve its size and rigidity. The formed complex revealed that the trimer adopts an active fold and binds to the receptor through the native interface and activates neutralizing antibody production. Similar investigations on BNT162b2, which is the form that was finally used in the vaccines, demonstrated not only its native conformation but could also highlight the conformational dynamics of the receptor binding domain (Vogel et al. 2021).

In the instance of objects like viruses and nanoparticles interacting eventually with structures, i.e., membranes, single particle analysis is not possible but the sample has to be tilted at rather small increment steps acquiring a so-called tilt series in cryo-electron tomography (cryo-ET). Here, cryo-TEM preparation as well as the introduction of direct electron detectors, which permit acquisition of images at low illumination levels, boosted the development and permitted to investigate, e.g., viruses in their native environment of the cell. Recently, following the COVID-19 outbreak, intensive cryo-EM work allowed structure determination of the virus and contributed significantly to the understanding of the structure of its spike proteins, their orientations and potential functions (Papageorgiou and Mohsin 2020; Rapp et al. 2022; Wrapp et al. 2020). Cryo-electron tomography was utilized to image SARS-CoV-2 viruses and determine the activated and inactivated stages of the protein conformation. New developments combine even cryo-ET and single-particle reconstruction. These developments are regarded as a new era of TEM in structural biology and drug design.

4 Conclusions

TEM investigations can provide valuable information on drug delivery systems and their interaction and mode of action in the context of cells and tissue with an unprecedented high resolution. Detailed insight into the architecture of drug carriers as well as their interaction with cells and tissue, their uptake and intracellular fate provide detailed information on potential optimization routes and allow for a dedicated modification of drug delivery systems. New developments in TEM automation, sensitivity, and analysis are opening up a much faster approach to obtain near atomic structures of proteins and receptors. Besides these developments, the role of TEM cannot be underestimated in future for the development of drug delivery systems.

References

Deinhardt-Emmer S, Wittschieber D, Sanft J, Kleemann S, Elschner S, Haupt KF, Vau V, Häring C, Rödel J, Henke A, Ehrhardt C, Bauer M, Philipp M, Gaßler N, Nietzsche S, Löffler B, Mall G (2021) Early postmortem mapping of SARS-CoV-2 RNA in patients with COVID-19 and the correlation with tissue damage. Elife 10:e60361. https://doi.org/10.7554/eLife.60361

Dubochet J, McDowall AW (1981) Vitrification of pure water for electron microscopy. J Microsc 124:RP3-RP4. https://doi.org/10.1111/j.1365-2818.1981.tb02483.x

Dubochet J, Adrian M, Chang JJ, Homo JC, Lepault J, McDowall AW, Schultz P (1988) Cryo-electron microscopy of vitrified specimens. Q Rev Biophys 21:129–228. https://doi.org/10.1017/s0033583500004297

Duhem N, Danhier F, Pourcelle V, Schumers JM, Bertrand O, Leduff CS, Hoeppener S, Schubert US, Gohy JF, Marchand-Brynaert J, Préat V (2014) Self-assembling doxorubicin-tocopherol succinate prodrug as a new drug delivery system: synthesis, characterization, and in vitro and in vivo anticancer activity. Bioconjug Chem 25:72–81. https://doi.org/10.1021/bc400326y

Dussouchaud A, Jacob J, Secq C, Verbavatz J-M, Moras M, Larghero J, Fader CM, Ostuni MA, Lefevre SD (2022) Transmission electron microscopy to follow ultrastructural modifications of erythroblasts upon ex vivo human erythropoiesis. Front Physiol 12. https://doi.org/10.3389/fphys.2021.791691

Firdessa R, Oelschlaeger TA, Moll H (2014) Identification of multiple cellular uptake pathways of polystyrene nanoparticles and factors affecting the uptake: relevance for drug delivery systems. Eur J Cell Biol 93:323–337. https://doi.org/10.1016/j.ejcb.2014.08.001

Gratton SE, Ropp PA, Pohlhaus PD, Luft JC, Madden VJ, Napier ME, DeSimone JM (2008) The effect of particle design on cellular internalization pathways. Proc Natl Acad Sci U S A 105: 11613–11618. https://doi.org/10.1073/pnas.0801763105

Jastrow H (2014) Electron microscopic Atlas of cells, tissues and organs in the Internet. http://www.drjastrow.de/WAI/EM/EMAtlas.html. Accessed 12 July 2023

Kempe K, Hoogenboom R, Hoeppener S, Fustin C-A, Gohy J-F, Schubert US (2010) Discovering new block terpolymer micellar morphologies. Chem Commun 46:6455–6457. https://doi.org/10.1039/C001629B

Koifman N, Talmon Y (2021) Cryogenic electron microscopy methodologies as analytical tools for the study of self-assembled pharmaceutics. Pharmaceutics 13:1015. https://doi.org/10.3390/pharmaceutics13071015

Kuntsche J, Horst JC, Bunjes H (2011) Cryogenic transmission electron microscopy (cryo-TEM) for studying the morphology of colloidal drug delivery systems. Int J Pharm 417:120–137. https://doi.org/10.1016/j.ijpharm.2011.02.001

Lim JP, Gleeson PA (2011) Macropinocytosis: an endocytic pathway for internalising large gulps. Immunol Cell Biol 89:836–843. https://doi.org/10.1038/icb.2011.20

Malatesta M (2021) Transmission electron microscopy as a powerful tool to investigate the interaction of nanoparticles with subcellular structures. Int J Mol Sci 22. https://doi.org/10.3390/ijms222312789

McDonald KL, Auer M (2006) High-pressure freezing, cellular tomography, and structural cell biology. Biotechniques 41:137–143. https://doi.org/10.2144/000112226

Papageorgiou AC, Mohsin I (2020) The SARS-CoV-2 spike glycoprotein as a drug and vaccine target: structural insights into its complexes with ACE2 and antibodies. Cell 9. https://doi.org/10.3390/cells9112343

Rapp M, Shapiro L, Frank J (2022) Contributions of single-particle cryoelectron microscopy toward fighting COVID-19. Trends Biochem Sci 47:117–123. https://doi.org/10.1016/j.tibs.2021.10.005

Reifarth M, Hoeppener S, Schubert US (2018a) Uptake and intracellular fate of engineered nanoparticles in mammalian cells: capabilities and limitations of transmission electron microscopy – polymer-based nanoparticles. Adv Mater 30:1703704. https://doi.org/10.1002/adma.201703704

Reifarth M, Schubert US, Hoeppener S (2018b) Considerations for the uptake characteristic of inorganic nanoparticles into mammalian cells – insights gained by TEM investigations. Adv Biosyst 2:1700254. https://doi.org/10.1002/adbi.201700254

Reimer L (1959) Elektronenmikroskopische Untersuchungs- und Präparationsmethoden. Springer, Berlin

Renaud J-P, Chari A, Ciferri C, Liu W-t, Rémigy H-W, Stark H, Wiesmann C (2018) Cryo-EM in drug discovery: achievements, limitations and prospects. Nat Rev Drug Discov 17:471–492. https://doi.org/10.1038/nrd.2018.77

Roingeard P, Raynal PI, Eymieux S, Blanchard E (2019) Virus detection by transmission electron microscopy: still useful for diagnosis and a plus for biosafety. Rev Med Virol 29:e2019. https://doi.org/10.1002/rmv.2019

Spicer PT, Hayden KL, Lynch ML, Ofori-Boateng A, Burns JL (2001) Novel process for producing cubic liquid crystalline nanoparticles (Cubosomes). Langmuir 17:5748–5756. https://doi.org/10.1021/la010161w

Szebeni J, Alving CR, Savay S, Barenholz Y, Priev A, Danino D, Talmon Y (2001) Formation of complement-activating particles in aqueous solutions of Taxol: possible role in hypersensitivity reactions. Int Immunopharmacol 1:721–735. https://doi.org/10.1016/S1567-5769(01)00006-6

Vogel AB, Kanevsky I, Che Y, Swanson KA, Muik A, Vormehr M, Kranz LM, Walzer KC, Hein S, Güler A, Loschko J, Maddur MS, Ota-Setlik A, Tompkins K, Cole J, Lui BG, Ziegenhals T, Plaschke A, Eisel D, Dany SC, Fesser S, Erbar S, Bates F, Schneider D, Jesionek B, Sänger B, Wallisch AK, Feuchter Y, Junginger H, Krumm SA, Heinen AP, Adams-Quack P, Schlereth J, Schille S, Kröner C, de la Caridad Güimil Garcia R, Hiller T, Fischer L, Sellers RS, Choudhary S, Gonzalez O, Vascotto F, Gutman MR, Fontenot JA, Hall-Ursone S, Brasky K, Griffor MC, Han S, AAH S, Lees JA, Nedoma NL, Mashalidis EH, Sahasrabudhe PV, Tan CY, Pavliakova D, Singh G, Fontes-Garfias C, Pride M, Scully IL, Ciolino T, Obregon J, Gazi M, Carrion R Jr, Alfson KJ, Kalina WV, Kaushal D, Shi PY, Klamp T, Rosenbaum C, Kuhn AN, Türeci Ö, Dormitzer PR, Jansen KU, Sahin U (2021) BNT162b vaccines protect rhesus macaques from SARS-CoV-2. Nature 592:283–289. https://doi.org/10.1038/s41586-021-03275-y

Wrapp D, Wang N, Corbett KS, Goldsmith JA, Hsieh CL, Abiona O, Graham BS, McLellan JS (2020) Cryo-EM structure of the 2019-nCoV spike in the prefusion conformation. Science 367: 1260–1263. https://doi.org/10.1126/science.abb2507

Xie Q, Yoshioka CK, Chapman MS (2020) Adeno-associated virus (AAV-DJ) – Cryo-EM structure at 1.56 Å resolution. Viruses 12:1194. https://doi.org/10.3390/v12101194

Part III

Target Specific Delivery

Blood-Brain Barrier (BBB)-Crossing Strategies for Improved Treatment of CNS Disorders

Wandong Zhang

Contents

Abstract

Blood-brain barrier (BBB) is a special biological property of the brain neurovascular unit (including brain microvessels and capillaries), which facilitates the transport of nutrients into the central nervous system (CNS) and exchanges metabolites but restricts passage of blood-borne neurotoxic substances and drugs/xenobiotics into CNS. BBB plays a crucial role in maintaining the homeostasis and normal physiological functions of CNS but severely impedes the delivery of drugs and biotherapeutics into CNS for treatment of neurological disorders. A variety of technologies have been developed in the past decade for

W. Zhang (✉)
Human Health Therapeutics Research Centre, National Research Council of Canada, Ottawa, ON, Canada

Department of Cellular and Molecular Medicine, Faculty of Medicine, University of Ottawa, Ottawa, ON, Canada
e-mail: Wandong.Zhang@nrc-cnrc.gc.ca; wzhan2@uOttawa.ca

M. Schäfer-Korting, U. S. Schubert (eds.), *Drug Delivery and Targeting*, Handbook of Experimental Pharmacology 284, https://doi.org/10.1007/164_2023_689

brain drug delivery. Most of these technologies are still in preclinical stage and some are undergoing clinical studies. Only a few have been approved by regulatory agencies for clinical applications. This chapter will overview the strategies and technologies/approaches for brain drug delivery and discuss some of the recent advances in the field.

Keywords

ABC transporters · Adsorptive-mediated transcytosis · AI-assisted drug development · Blood-brain barrier (BBB) · Brain drug delivery · Carrier-mediated transcytosis (CMT) · Cell-/BBB-penetrating peptides · Cell-mediated drug delivery · Focused ultrasound · Intranasal drug delivery · Nanoparticles · Neurovascular unit · Receptor-mediated transcytosis (RMT) · Viral vector and gene delivery

Abbreviations

AAV	Adeno-associated virus
ABC transporter	ATP-binding cassette transporter
ALS	Amyotrophic lateral sclerosis
AMT	Adsorptive-mediated transcytosis
ASO	Antisense oligonucleotide
ATV	Antibody transport vehicle
BBB	Blood-brain barrier
CD98hc	CD98 heavy chain
CMT	Carrier-mediated transcytosis
CNS	Central nervous system
CSF	Cerebral spinal fluid
ETV	Enzyme transport vehicle
FDA	Food and Drug Administration (USA)
GAGs	Glycosaminoglycans
IDS	Iduronate 2-sulfatase
LRP-1	Low-density lipoprotein receptor-related protein-1
MPS II	Mucopolysaccharidosis type II
NSC	Neural stem cells
RMT	Receptor-mediated transcytosis
RVG	Rabies viral glycoprotein
siRNA	small interfering RNA
SLC transporter	Solute carrier transporter
SOD1	Superoxide dismutase type 1
TAT	Trans-activating transcription factor
TfR	Transferrin receptor
TREM2	Triggering receptor expressed on myeloid cells 2

1 Introduction

The blood-brain barrier (BBB) is a special biological property of brain microvessels and capillaries that helps to protect the brain from blood-borne neurotoxic substances, drugs, and xenobiotics while allowing necessary nutrients and oxygen to reach the brain. The functionality of the BBB lies in the neurovascular unit made up of tightly sealed cerebral microvascular and capillary endothelial cells with surrounding pericytes, astrocyte foot processes, microglia, and neuronal innervation (Fig. 1), which forms a barrier restricting the movement of substances between the blood and brain/spinal cord. Polarized expression of ATP-binding cassette (ABC) transporters, solute carrier (SLC) transporters, and various receptors on the luminal and abluminal side of the BBB endothelial cells mediates the efflux of small molecular drugs, the passage of nutrients and metabolism-needed molecules into the central nervous system (CNS) and excretion of metabolic wastes. The BBB is thus critical to maintain the homeostasis environment for normal CNS functions. However, this barrier can also impede the passage or delivery of therapeutics

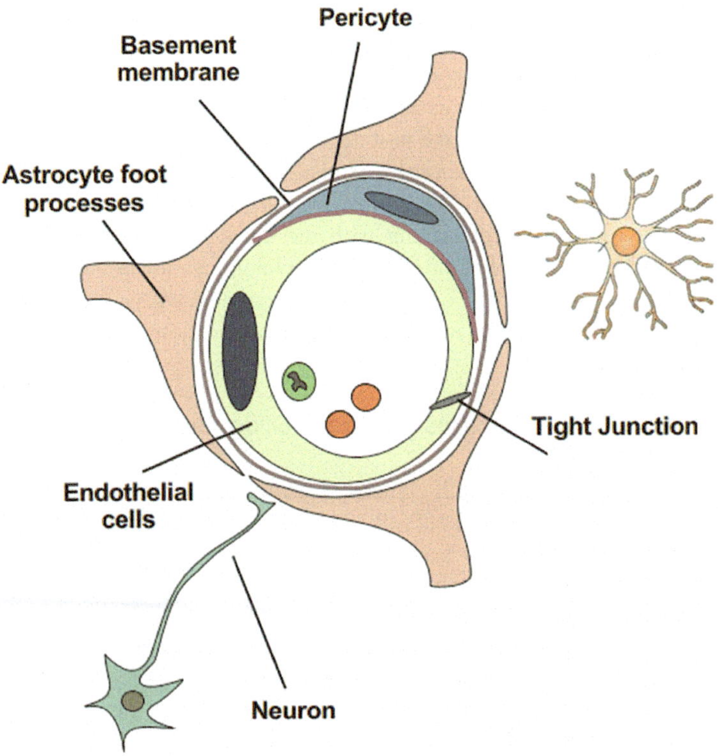

Fig. 1 Schematic diagram for cellular anatomy of the neurovascular unit (modified from Zhang W and Stanimirovic DB 2005. The transport systems of the blood-brain barrier. In. The Blood-Brain Barrier and its Microenvironment: Basic Physiology to Neurological Disease)

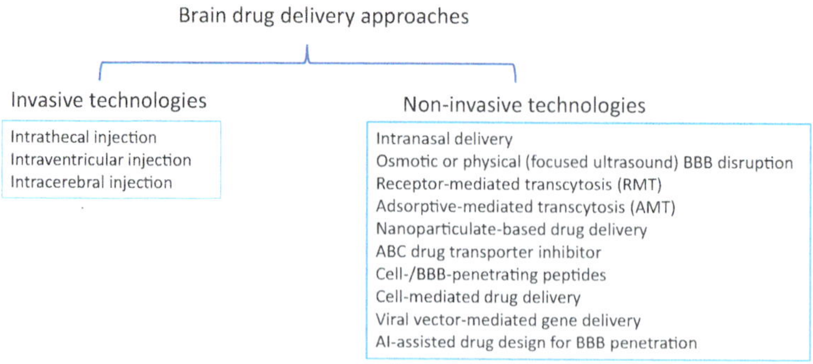

Scheme 1 Brain drug delivery approaches

(including both small molecular drugs and macromolecular biopharmaceutics) to reach the targets in the CNS, which is a challenge for the development of CNS drugs and therapeutics and also for the treatment of neurological disorders. Various factors can influence the permeability of the BBB, including inflammation, injury, and disease. It is important to explore the ways to manipulate the BBB permeability or to take advantage of natural pathways (such as receptor-mediated transcytosis) to develop drug delivery technologies and improve drug delivery to the CNS. This chapter will overview the strategies and approaches for brain drug delivery that have been extensively investigated in the past decade along with the deep understanding of the BBB biology and discuss some recent advances in the field.

Strategies and approaches for brain drug delivery have been extensively investigated in the past decade along with the deep understanding of the BBB biology. There are invasive and non-invasive technologies for brain drug delivery. Many new non-invasive technologies are developed in recent years, but traditional brain drug delivery approaches are still in clinical applications (Scheme 1).

2 Invasive Approaches for Brain Drug Delivery

Some invasive approaches are still clinically used for brain drug delivery, including intracerebral and intracerebroventricular injection and intrathecal injection into cerebral spinal fluid (CSF) (synthetic drugs, siRNA, or gene therapeutics). Intracerebral injection can deliver the therapeutics to a specific region of the brain. For intracerebroventricular and CSF injection, the therapeutics have to penetrate the ependymal layer of epithelial cells to reach the interstitial fluid and neurons which bypasses the blood-brain barrier (Fig. 2). Intracerebral and intracerebroventricular injections are not commonly used while intrathecal delivery of therapeutics is a common clinical practice in many cases (Fig. 2). One example is Qalsody which is an antisense oligonucleotide (ASO) drug recently approved by US Food & Drug Administration (FDA) for intrathecal injection for treatment of amyotrophic lateral

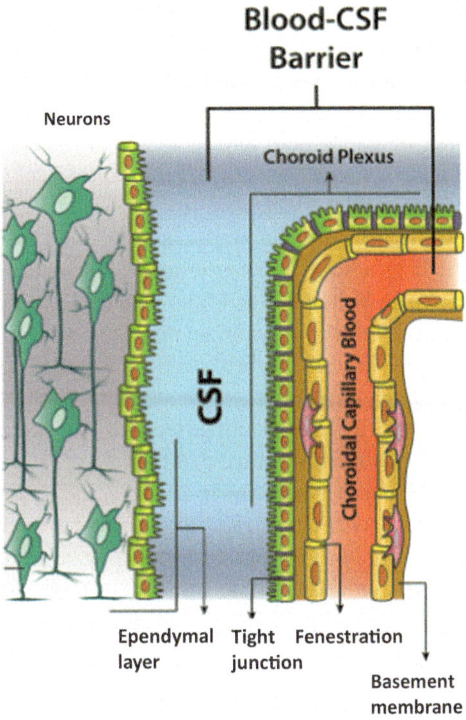

Fig. 2 Structure of the blood–CSF (cerebral spinal fluid) barrier. Partially adopted from D'Agata F et al. Molecules 23: 9, 2018

sclerosis (ALS) associated with a mutation in the SOD1 (superoxide dismutase type 1) gene (FDA 2023).

3 BBB Disruption for Brain Drug Delivery

BBB cells are tightly sealed by tight junctions and adherens junctions, which can be opened or disrupted temporarily with intra-arterial cerebral infusion of mannitol (high dose) or by using focused ultrasound for an access of high molecular weight drugs or chemotherapeutic drugs into the brain. The use of mannitol is a common clinical practice, in particular for brain tumor chemotherapeutics (D'Amico et al. 2020; Chakraborty et al. 2016). Focused ultrasound with microbubbles regionally disrupting the BBB for ~24 h, however, is still in clinical trial stage. In addition to opening the paracellular space of brain endothelial cells, focused ultrasound can also increase transcellular or transcytosis activities for drug delivery (Barzegar-Fallah et al. 2022; Chen et al. 2021). Microvascular bleeding and sterile inflammation in the brain as a result of some focused ultrasound treatment are still concerns and require further investigations and optimization of the technology.

4 Intranasal Drug Delivery

Administering drugs through the nose allows drugs to reach olfactory nerve ends at the olfactory mucosa of nasal cavity (Fig. 3). The drugs will bypass the BBB and enter olfactory bulb and then spread to some deep brain neuronal structure (Erdő et al. 2018; Antunes et al. 2023). Intranasal drug delivery to the brain may reduce systemic side effects and toxicity compared to i.v. or oral administrations of the drugs. Insulin is an important regulator of brain cell function and metabolism affecting neuronal synaptic function and plasticity as well as glucose/lipid/cholesterol metabolism in the brain. Studies have shown clinical correlations between the failure of insulin signaling pathway and AD (Najem et al. 2014). Intranasal insulin is used in several clinical trials for mild cognitive impairment and early-stage Alzheimer's patients; some of the studies showed improved cognitive function. However, the therapeutic effect is still controversial (Craft et al. 2020; Hallschmid 2021). It should be noted that the area of olfactory mucosa in human is small relative to the whole nasal cavity surface, and the amount of the drug delivery via this approach is limited. However, the relative area of olfactory mucosa in rodent is larger and thus the dose delivered may be sufficient to show therapeutic effects in the animal models. Caution should be taken for translation of rodent experimental results into human. Some intranasally delivered drugs have been approved by

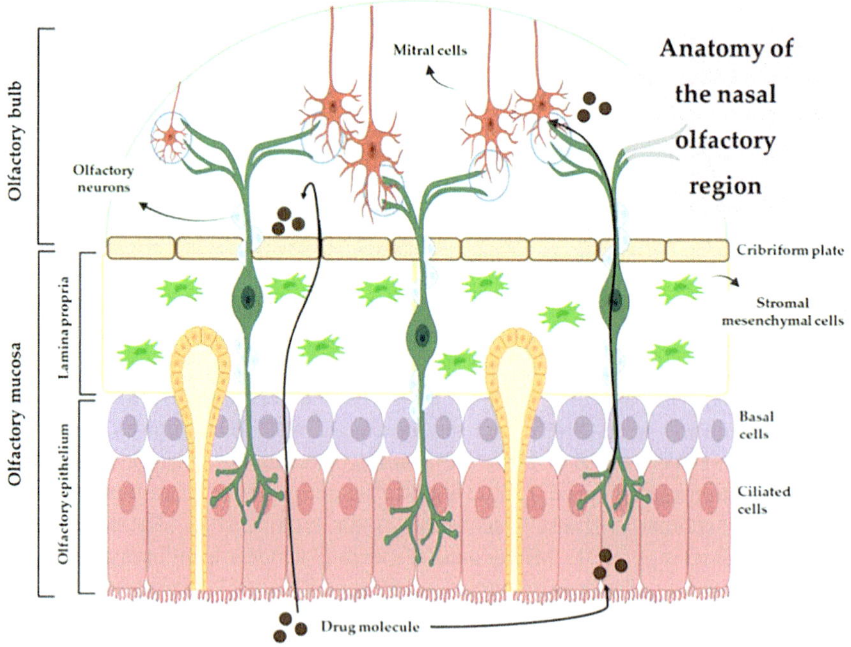

Fig. 3 Structure of the nasal olfactory mucosa. Adopted from Antunes JL, et al. Pharmaceutics 15: 998, 2023

regulatory agencies for treatment of CNS diseases. One example is Spravato (esketamine) nasal spray approved by US FDA in 2019 for add-on therapy with oral antidepressant in treatment-resistant depression in adults (FDA 2019). Another example is ZAVZPRET™ (zavegepant, a CGRP receptor antagonist) recently FDA approved for acute treatment of migraine (Pfizer 2023).

5 Receptor-Mediated Transcytosis (RMT)

This is one of the natural pathways for some proteins to cross the BBB, which is exemplified by transferrin surmounting the BBB via binding to transferrin receptor (TfR) triggering receptor-mediated transcytosis. A molecule binding to or targeting a receptor on the luminal surface of the BBB cells triggers the process of transcytosis to transport the molecule in vesicular ligand-receptor bound structure to the abluminal surface. Once the vesicles carrying ligand (molecule)/receptor complex reach the abluminal side of the BBB, the ligand (such as transferrin) is released from the ligand-receptor complexes and the receptor may recycle back to the luminal surface. RMT has been extensively explored for development of brain drug delivery. If the target protein is a solute carrier protein, the process is known as carrier-mediated transcytosis (CMT). Receptor-mediated transcytosis is a highly regulated process that requires a complex interplay of different molecules and cellular pathways.

Transferrin receptor (TfR) is widely explored for brain drug delivery. TfR is expressed at moderate levels on the BBB cells or in cerebral vessels relative to other receptors (such as LRP-1, CD98hc/SLC3A2) (Uchida et al. 2011; Ito et al. 2011; Zhang et al. 2020). Antibodies and peptides have been developed to target TfR for brain drug delivery (Terstappen et al. 2021). A TfR antibody is fused to its C-terminus with the enzyme iduronate 2-sulfatase (IDS) [Pabinafusp alfa (JR-141)] was i.v. injected for delivery of IDS into the brain to treat the lysosomal storage disease, Hunter syndrome, also known as mucopolysaccharidosis type II (MPS II) (Giugliani et al. 2021; Okuyama et al. 2021). Clinical studies showed reduced levels of glycosaminoglycans (GAGs) in CSF, serum, and urine and improved neurocognitive developments in the patients (Giugliani et al. 2021; Okuyama et al. 2021). Approved by Japan regulatory agency for treatment of Hunter syndrome (Mullard 2021), the fusion protein is the first biologic approved for brain drug delivery via RMT mechanism.

Another recent advance on targeting TfR for brain drug delivery is the development of a transport vehicle (TV) in which an Fc domain was engineered to bind the TfR and enable brain delivery of biotherapeutics via receptor-mediated transcytosis (Kariolis et al. 2020). The transport vehicle was fused to anti-BACE1 (beta-secretase 1) Fabs or a TREM2 (triggering receptor expressed on myeloid cells 2)-activating antibody as an antibody-transport vehicle (ATV) (Kariolis et al. 2020; van Lengerich et al. 2023). By targeting TfR, substantial amount of the fusion protein ATV was delivered to the brains of mouse or/and monkey post i.v. administration (Kariolis et al. 2020; van Lengerich et al. 2023). The ATV: TREM2 fusion enhanced microglial activity and glucose metabolism in an AD mouse model (van Lengerich et al. 2023). Moreover, a bispecific antibody (fusion protein of TREM2 agonist and TfR antibody) boosted microglial clearance of amyloid plaques in the 5XFAD mouse model (Zhao et al. 2022). In addition, the transport vehicle was fused with the enzyme IDS to be the enzyme transport vehicle (ETV) enabling the delivery of the enzyme to the murine brain in a Hunter syndrome model, a lysosomal storage disease. Behavioral and skeletal phenotypes improved (Ullman et al. 2020; Arguello et al. 2021). A phase 2/3 clinical trial is being conducted to evaluate the therapeutic effect of ETV (DNL310) for Hunter syndrome (Denali n.d.)). A couple of other ETVs, including DNL126 for MPS IIIA (Sanfilippo syndrome type A) (ETV: SGSH) and DNL622 (ETV: IDUA) for MPS I, and PTV (PTV: PGRN) for frontotemporal dementia (granulin) (Logan et al. 2021), are being developed using the same approach for delivery of the biotherapeutics into the brain (Denali n.d.). An important note is that several studies have demonstrated that low-to-moderate affinity TfR antibodies or a monovalent TfR antibody is more efficient in crossing the BBB into the brain (Terstappen et al. 2021). A recent study further confirmed superior brain uptake by a monovalent moderate-affinity TfR-binding transport compared to high-affinity bivalent TfR antibody (Arguello et al. 2022).

Recent studies have explored aptamers for drug delivery and also as therapeutics. Aptamers are short single-stranded DNA or RNA molecules that can bind to specific target molecules. Aptamers targeting TfR have been recently developed for brain drug delivery (Li et al. 2020; Kusmierz et al. 2022). One study reported that DNA aptamers targeting TfR and tau protein were developed, respectively, and then both were ligated together by T4 ligase as bifunctional aptamers (Li et al. 2020). Aptamers are emerging as a promising tool for drug delivery, including to the brain.

A number of other receptors and carrier proteins on the BBB cells have been explored or targeted for brain drug delivery, including CD98 heavy chain (CD98hc)/SLC3A2, LRP-1, insulin receptor, IGF-1R, SLC2A1/GLUT1, LDLR, and LRP8 (Zhang et al. 2020; Terstappen et al. 2021). The selection of a target for the development of brain drug delivery technology should consider the following:

- The target protein is expressed at high levels or enriched on the luminal surface of the BBB cells but at low levels on the peripheral endothelial cells, which will enhance brain drug delivery and minimize peripheral toxicity. The relative expression levels of the target protein to other proteins on BBB cells should be quantified (e.g., TfR vs. LRP-1; Zhang et al. 2020).
- Whether the extracellular domain or loop of the receptor/protein is large enough to be targeted by an antibody, peptide, or nanoparticle. One example is SLC7A5 which is highly expressed on BBB cells but its extracellular loops are very small and short and are difficult to be targeted.
- Whether the functionality or signaling of the protein is affected if targeted (such as insulin receptor, IGF-1R, and CD98hc/SLC3A2) which may lead to adverse effects.
- Whether the stability and half-life of the receptor or protein is affected if targeted, leading to insufficient functionality of the receptor/protein.

- Whether targeting the receptor or protein would cause the leakage of the BBB. It is reported that amyloid-β immunotherapy causes BBB leakage or brain edema in animal models and even in some cases of clinical trial patients (Blockx et al. 2016; Roytman et al. 2023). If an antibody is developed to target a BBB receptor/protein for brain drug delivery, the Fc-mediated antibody-dependent cell-mediated cytotoxicity (ADCC) or complement dependent cytotoxicity (CDC) must be taken into consideration.
- The immunogenicity of the BBB carrier with the cargo complex should be considered.

We have compared the relative expression levels of commonly targeted receptors and proteins on human and mouse isolated brain vessels vs. peripheral vessels and tissues by RNA-seq analysis (Zhang et al. 2020). It was found that the expression levels of those targeted receptors and proteins are following in human brain vessels: SLC2A1 > LRP-1 > SLC3A2 > CDC50A > Insulin receptor> TfR > IGF1R > LEPR > LRP-8 > IGF2R; while the expression levels of these receptors and proteins in mouse brain vessels are slightly different from human as following: SLC2A1 > LRP-1 > IGF-1R > SLC3A2 > CDC50A > LRP8 > TfR > Insulin receptor > LDLR > IGF-2R > LEPR (Zhang et al. 2020). All the above factors should be considered when selecting a target for the development of RMT-mediated brain drug delivery.

6 Nanoparticle-Based Drug Delivery to the Brain

This involves using nanoparticles (including liposomes, micelles, exosomes, dendrimers, solid lipid nanoparticles, polymeric nanoparticles or nano-DNA carriers) to transport low molecular weight drugs and biotherapeutics across the BBB into the brain as well as agents for brain imaging (Luo et al. 2020; Xu et al. 2020; Terstappen et al. 2021; Liu et al. 2022; Chen et al. 2022). Nanoparticles can be designed with different formulations, chemical and physical properties to carry a variety of drugs, including small molecule drugs, antibodies, peptides, and nucleic acids. Nanoparticles may be engineered to target-specific regions of the brain or to release drugs slowly over time (Luo et al. 2022). Most of the nanoparticles have to be functionalized with antibodies or peptides targeting the receptors/proteins on the BBB to efficiently enter the CNS (Luo et al. 2022; Terstappen et al. 2021). If nanoparticles are functionalized with BBB-targeting ligands (such as antibodies or peptides), they actually trigger receptor-mediated transcytosis or AMT to cross the BBB (Luo et al. 2022; Xu et al. 2020; Terstappen et al. 2021; Guo et al. 2023). Despite clinical trials for nanoparticle-mediated brain drug delivery, none of the nanoparticle technologies has been approved by regulatory agency for brain drug delivery yet.

DNA Nanocages

In addition to various formulations of nanoparticles for drug delivery, recently, DNA nanocarriers with different structures have been developed for targeting tumors, in vivo imaging as well as for brain drug delivery (Jiang et al. 2016; Tam et al. 2020; Chen et al. 2022). The advantages of DNA nanocarriers are less toxicity and low immunogenicity as compared to other BBB carriers (such as proteins and antibodies). Self-assembled 3D DNA nanocages with or without a BBB-target peptide TGN (12-amino acid peptide) modification penetrated the BBB similarly, and the spherical DNA nanocages were more permeable across the BBB than tubular DNA nanostructures (Tam et al. 2020). The DNA nanocages were capable of delivering doxorubicin across the BBB to inhibit the tumor in a mouse xenograft tumor (U87MG) model (Tam et al. 2020). Larger and softer DNA nanostructures were more BBB permeable than smaller and rigid DNA nanostructures (Chen et al. 2022). Yet, DNA nanocarriers for brain drug delivery is still in the early stage of development, and there is no reported clinical study yet. It is also unknown how efficient DNA nanocarriers-mediated brain drug delivery is in comparison with alternative approaches as well as the specificity, adverse effects, etc. One potential concern is that DNA nanocarriers are negatively charged DNA structures and the BBB cells are also covered with a layer of negatively charged glycocalyx (Dorovini-Zis 2015). The interactions or the attachment of DNA nanocarriers to BBB cell surface may not be efficient due to the negative charges on both.

7 Viral Vector-Mediated Gene Delivery into CNS

Neurotropic viruses have been explored for brain drug delivery, such as adeno-associated virus (AAV) (Bedbrook et al. 2018; Challis et al. 2022; Terstappen et al. 2021). The adeno-associated virus (AAV) is a small, non-pathogenic virus that has been widely used as a vector for gene therapy because of its ability to transduce a wide range of cell types and tissues, its low immunogenicity, and its ability to establish long-term gene expression in target cells (Bedbrook et al. 2018; Fajardo-Serrano et al. 2021; Challis et al. 2022). The AAV9 vector shows the highest tropism for neural tissue and can cross the BBB more efficiently than other AAV vectors (Enomoto et al. 2016; Merkel et al. 2017; Hardcastle et al. 2018). Studies show that AAV serotype AAVrh10 vector can also cross the BBB more efficiently (Fajardo-Serrano et al. 2021). However, one limiting factor for AAV vector-mediated gene delivery is its maximal capacity of carrying a gene around 5 kb, and larger gene fragment cannot be delivered by this approach. In addition to viral vectors for gene delivery, protein fragments were also identified from neurotropic viral proteins as cell-/BBB-penetrating peptides for brain drug delivery, such as TAT peptide derived from HIV viral protein and RVG peptide derived from rabies viral glycoprotein (Green and Loewenstein. 1988; Frankel and Pabo. 1988; Fu et al. 2018) (see below section). There are at least 13 viral vector-mediated gene therapies so far approved by regulatory agencies, and one of them is AAV9-mediated gene therapy for spinal muscular atrophy via intravenous injection (ZOLGENSMA®, Novartis

Gene Therapies). Pediatric SMA patients less than 2 years old with bi-allelic mutation in the survival motor neuron 1 (SMN1) showed significant improvement in their ability to reach developmental motor milestones (e.g., head control and the ability to sit without support).

Furthermore, virus-like particles assembled from recombinant viral capsid proteins or nanoparticles conjugated with viral protein fragment (such as RVG peptide) were investigated for delivery of gene or therapeutics across the BBB into the brain (Ye et al. 2021; Chang et al. 2011; Gao et al. 2014). In addition to AAV, many other neurotropic viruses are also explored for brain drug delivery. Overall, neurotropic viruses hold great promise as a tool for targeted drug/gene delivery to the CNS, and further research is needed to optimize its use for different therapeutic applications for gene therapy and drug delivery. More information can be found elsewhere (Bedbrook et al. 2018; Challis et al. 2022; Terstappen et al. 2021).

8 ABC Drug Efflux Transporters and Inhibitors

ATP-binding cassette (ABC) transporters are a family of transmembrane proteins that play a critical role in the transport of various substances against substance concentration gradient fueled by ATP hydrolysis, including sugars, amino acids, nucleosides, lipids/cholesterol, peptides, ions, metals, drugs, and xenobiotics across cell membranes or cellular barriers (Zhang and Stanimirovic 2005; Shen and Zhang 2010; Zhang et al. 2015, 2023a, b; Sweeney et al. 2019). ABC transporters are expressed in various tissues and cells, including the BBB cells, astrocytes, and pericytes (Sweeney et al. 2019). Several ABC drug efflux transporters are highly expressed in cerebral vessels and BBB cells and play a critical role in forming the BBB for small molecular drugs, also known as transport barrier, including ABCB1/MDR-1 P-glycoprotein (Pgp), ABCG2/BCRP, ABCC1/MRP-1, ABCC4/MRP-4 and ABCC5/MRP-5 (Shen and Zhang 2010; Zhang et al. 2015, 2023a, b; Sweeney et al. 2019). These transporters restrict the entry of drugs and xenobiotics into the brain by actively transporting the drugs back into the bloodstream, known as efflux (Zhang et al. 2015; Sweeney et al. 2019). This efflux can limit the effectiveness of drugs for the treatment of neurological and neurodegenerative disorders (Zhang et al. 2015; Sweeney et al. 2019). Several strategies have been developed to overcome the efflux mechanism of ABC transporters for brain drug delivery. One approach is to design drugs that are not substrates for these transporters or to modify existing drugs to reduce their affinity for ABC transporters as weaker substrates (de Gooijer et al. 2018) or conjugate the drugs to a BBB carrier peptide/antibody to bypass the drug efflux transporters (Drappatz et al. 2013; Cavaco et al. 2021; Zhou et al. 2021). Another approach is to use transporter inhibitors that can block the efflux activity of ABC transporters (Namanja-Magliano et al. 2017; Bauer et al. 2019), thereby increasing the concentration of drugs in the brain. However, there are limitations by targeting ABC transporters for brain drug delivery. Since ABC transporters are widely expressed in human tissues and cells, some of the inhibitors can have toxic effects and safety concerns (Bauer et al. 2019). In addition, long time administrations of drugs that are substrates of ABC drug efflux transporters have the risk of developing drug resistance as a result of inducing overexpression of these ABC drug transporters. There is currently no ABC transporter inhibitor approved clinically for enhancing brain drug delivery. Overall, ABC transporters represent a promising target for brain drug delivery, particularly for small molecular drugs, but further research is needed to fully understand the mechanisms of efflux transport across the BBB and to optimize the design and delivery of drugs or the inhibitors that target these transporters for the treatment of neurological and neurodegenerative disorders (for more information, please see Chapter "Cardiovascular: Heart Failure, Ischemic Heart Disease, Arrhythmia").

9 Cell-/BBB-Penetrating Peptides

Cell-penetrating peptides (CPPs) comprise a large and heterogeneous group of peptide molecules (Räägel & Pooga. 2011; Milletti 2012; Guidotti et al. 2017; Zhou et al. 2021). They were originally discovered from natural proteins, among which the trans-activating transcription factor TAT from human immunodeficiency virus (HIV) was one of the first examples (Green and Loewenstein. 1988; Frankel and Pabo. 1988). Since then, research has been carried out to study the mechanisms of CPP-mediated endocytosis/transcytosis and determine the required amino acid residues in order to develop effective transport vectors. CPPs have also been investigated for brain delivery of therapeutics or imaging agents (Hill et al. 2012; Lim et al. 2015; Tu et al. 2015; Guidotti et al. 2017). BBB cells are covered with a layer of negatively charged molecules such as glycocalyx and proteoglycans (Dorovini-Zis. 2015), and most of the BBB-penetrating CPPs are positively charged (such as TAT and RVG peptides and angiopep-2) (Milletti 2012; Guidotti et al. 2017; Habib and Singh 2022), which enhances their binding to BBB cells. Such CPPs may either directly penetrate the BBB via adsorptive-mediated transcytosis (AMT) pathway (Terstappen et al. 2021) or interact with receptors or other proteins on BBB cells to initiate endo/transcytosis (RMT) or other transport-relevant events. A significant number of peptide–drug conjugates and/or fusion constructs have been explored for brain drug delivery and imaging applications (Maderna et al. 2018; Zhou et al. 2021). Some of the studies employ CPP-/BBB-penetrating peptides to functionalize the nanoparticles for drug delivery into tumors or into the brain (Gao et al. 2014; Morshed et al. 2016; Zhou et al. 2021; Habib and Singh 2022; Thirumurugan et al. 2022). BBB-penetrating peptides have the potential for delivery of drugs/therapeutics and imaging agents to the CNS and provide new treatment options for a wide range of neurological and psychiatric disorders. The development of effective BBB-penetrating peptides is still in its early stages, and significant challenges remain in optimizing their pharmacokinetic properties, improving their stability, and minimizing off-target effects (Zhou et al. 2021). Clinical trials have been conducted for CPP/BBB-penetrating peptide-mediated brain drug delivery (Hill et al. 2012; Terstappen et al. 2021), but there is no CPP-/BBB-penetrating peptide approved for clinical applications at the moment.

10 Cell-Mediated Drug Delivery

Cells (such as macrophages, monocytes, or myeloid-derived cells) can be engineered to carry cargos, such as proteins or other therapeutics to the brain via transmigration across the BBB or directly implanted into a specific region of the brain or spinal cord (Klyachko et al. 2017; Terstappen et al. 2021, Li et al. 2021; Choi et al. 2023; Fauzi et al. 2023; Zhang et al. 2023a, b). Cell-mediated drug delivery into the brain is a promising approach by using cells to transport therapeutics across the BBB into the brain (Klyachko et al. 2017; Li et al. 2021; Choi et al. 2023). The main mechanism of cell-mediated brain drug delivery is to engineer the cells to express a specific therapeutic protein, molecule, or drug (Metz et al. 2013; Choi et al. 2023). These cells can be designed to cross the BBB and migrate to specific regions of the brain where they can express or release the therapeutic molecule (Terstappen et al. 2021). One example of cell-mediated drug delivery into the brain is the use of neural stem cells (NSCs) (Choi et al. 2023). NSCs are multipotent cells that can differentiate into neurons, astrocytes, and oligodendrocytes. The cells can be engineered to express therapeutic proteins or enzymes or to encapsulate the drug-loaded nanoparticles, and used to treat neurological disorders (Sun et al. 2023). Another example is the use of monocytes, which can cross the BBB and migrate to areas of inflammation site in the brain. These cells are engineered to express therapeutic proteins or drugs, such as anti-inflammatory agents, and used to treat neuroinflammatory disorders (Klyachko et al. 2017; Li et al. 2021). In addition, cell membrane are used to coat nanoparticles for brain drug delivery to avoid immune clearance of nanoparticles (Li et al. 2023). Cell-mediated drug delivery into the brain has several advantages over other drug delivery methods, including increased specificity and reduced toxicity. However, there are challenges associated with this approach, including the need for precise cell targeting and the potential for immune response. Direct implantations of stem cells, NSC, or engineered cells into the brain or spinal cord for treatment of neurological diseases or injuries have also been investigated clinically (Kalladka et al. 2016; Muir et al. 2020; Fauzi et al. 2023), but there is little advance in terms of employing BBB transmigration of engineered cells for treatment of neurological disorders. Overall, cell-mediated drug delivery into the brain is a potential approach for the treatment of neurological and neurodegenerative disorders, but further research is needed to address many challenges.

11 AI-Assisted Drug Design

AI-assisted drug design is a rapidly growing field that combines artificial intelligence (AI) and machine learning (ML) with traditional drug discovery methods to develop new and more effective drugs (Yang et al. 2019; Cerchia and Lavecchia 2023). The key benefit of AI-assisted drug design is the ability to quickly identify promising drug candidates from vast libraries of potential molecules, which can save significant time and resources. It can also help to optimize drug candidates for specific targets, predict toxicity, and reduce the likelihood of adverse side effects (Yang et al. 2019;

Cerchia and Lavecchia 2023). AI may assist the design of small molecular drugs that bypass efflux drug transporters or to be weaker substrates of the transporters at the BBB. AI may also help in optimizing the BBB carrier antibodies for more effective penetration across the BBB into the brain. Furthermore, AI may be used to predict the pharmacokinetics of drugs, which can help optimize drug dosing and reduce the risk of toxicity. On the other hand, AI-assisted drug design can help identify new drug targets for neurological diseases and develop more effective treatments. By analyzing large datasets of genetic and molecular data, AI can identify new pathways and targets that can be exploited to develop drugs that can modulate brain function and treat neurological disorders. For an example, Pharma.AI-assisted development of an ALS drug (FB1006) is in phase I clinical trial (4B Technologies n.d.). Overall, AI-assisted drug design has the great potential to speed up drug development, identify new therapeutic targets, and develop new treatments for neurological diseases.

Summary

For brain drug delivery, a number of factors should be considered as described above. The technologies developed should have the capacity of delivering enough therapeutic dose of the drugs to the CNS and be long lasting. If a receptor or a protein is targeted by the drug delivery technology, the receptor/protein should be highly expressed/enriched on the BBB cells or brain vessels but expressed at low levels on the peripheral endothelial cells to avoid peripheral toxicity. The delivery technologies should be site-specific and the cargoes should have target-specific engagement on brain cells after delivered into CNS. The technologies should not damage brain vasculature resulting inflammatory response, microbleeding, and brain edema. The technologies with delivered cargos should have low CNS toxicity, low peripheral toxicity, and low immunogenicity. The choice of delivery approaches/ technologies should depend on the specific drugs/biotherapeutics being used, the disease being treated, whether the BBB permeability is altered in diseased conditions, and the patient's individual needs and circumstances.

Acknowledgment Dr. W. Zhang's research work was supported by the funding from the National Research Council of Canada as well as from CIHR and Heart & Stroke Foundation of Canada.

References

4B Technologies (n.d.). https://www.4btechnologies.com/index.php?c=category&id=3

Antunes JL, Amado J, Veiga F et al (2023) Nanosystems, drug molecule functionalization and intranasal delivery: an update on the most promising strategies for increasing the therapeutic efficacy of antidepressant and anxiolytic drugs. Pharmaceutics 15(3):998

Arguello A, Meisner R, Thomsen ER et al (2021) Iduronate-2-sulfatase transport vehicle rescues behavioral and skeletal phenotypes in a mouse model of hunter syndrome. JCI Insight 6(19): e145445

Arguello A, Mahon CS, Calvert MEK et al (2022) Molecular architecture determines brain delivery of a transferrin receptor-targeted lysosomal enzyme. J Exp Med 219(3):e20211057

Barzegar-Fallah A, Gandhi K, Rizwan SB et al (2022) Harnessing ultrasound for targeting drug delivery to the brain and breaching the blood-brain tumour barrier. Pharmaceutics 14(10):2231
Bauer M, Karch R, Wulkersdorfer B et al (2019) A proof-of-concept study to inhibit ABCG2- and ABCB1-mediated efflux transport at the human blood-brain barrier. J Nucl Med 60(4):486–491
Bedbrook CN, Deverman BE, Gradinaru V (2018) Viral strategies for targeting the central and peripheral nervous systems. Annu Rev Neurosci 41:323–348
Blockx I, Einstein S, Guns PJ et al (2016) Monitoring blood-brain barrier integrity following amyloid-β immunotherapy using gadolinium-enhanced MRI in a PDAPP mouse model. J Alzheimers Dis 54(2):723–735
Cavaco M, Frutos S, Oliete P et al (2021) Conjugation of a blood brain barrier peptide shuttle to an fc domain for brain delivery of therapeutic biomolecules. ACS Med Chem Lett 12(11): 1663–1668
Cerchia C, Lavecchia A (2023) New avenues in artificial-intelligence-assisted drug discovery. Drug Discov Today 28(4):103516
Chakraborty S, Filippi CG, Wong T et al (2016) Superselective intraarterial cerebral infusion of cetuximab after osmotic blood/brain barrier disruption for recurrent malignant glioma: phase I study. J Neurooncol 128(3):405–415
Challis RC, Ravindra Kumar S, Chen X et al (2022) Adeno-associated virus toolkit to target diverse brain cells. Annu Rev Neurosci 45:447–469
Chang CF, Wang M, Ou WC et al (2011) Human JC virus-like particles as a gene delivery vector. Expert Opin Biol Ther 11(9):1169–1175
Chen KT, Wei KC, Liu HL (2021) Focused ultrasound combined with microbubbles in central nervous system applications. Pharmaceutics 13(7):1084
Chen X, Liu D, Wu Y et al (2022) Investigation of the transporting behavior of framework DNA Nano-devices across the artificial blood-brain barrier (BBB). Chembiochem 23(21): e202200459
Choi Y, Lee HK, Choi KC (2023) Engineered adult stem cells: a promising tool for anti-cancer therapy. BMB Rep 56(2):71–77
Craft S, Raman R, Chow TW et al (2020) Safety, efficacy, and feasibility of intranasal insulin for the treatment of mild cognitive impairment and Alzheimer disease dementia: a randomized clinical trial. JAMA Neurol 77(9):1099–1109
D'Agata F, Ruffinatti FA, Boschi S et al (2018) Magnetic nanoparticles in the central nervous system: targeting principles, applications and safety issues. Molecules 23:9
D'Amico RS, Khatri D, Reichman N et al (2020) Super selective intra-arterial cerebral infusion of modern chemotherapeutics after blood-brain barrier disruption: where are we now, and where we are going. J Neurooncol 147(2):261–278
de Gooijer MC, Zhang P, Weijer R et al (2018) The impact of P-glycoprotein and breast cancer resistance protein on the brain pharmacokinetics and pharmacodynamics of a panel of MEK inhibitors. Int J Cancer 142(2):381–391
Denali (n.d.). https://www.denalitherapeutics.com
Dorovini-Zis (2015) The morphology and functional properties of the blood-brain barrier. In: Dorovini-Zis K (ed) The blood-brain barrier in health and disease, vol 1. CRC Press/Taylor & Francis Group, New York, pp 9–10
Drappatz J, Brenner A, Wong ET et al (2013) Phase I study of GRN1005 in recurrent malignant glioma. Clin Cancer Res 19(6):1567–1576
Enomoto M, Hirai T, Kaburagi H, Yokota T (2016) Efficient gene suppression in dorsal root ganglia and spinal cord using adeno-associated virus vectors encoding short-hairpin RNA. Methods Mol Biol 1364:277–290
Erdő F, Bors LA, Farkas D et al (2018) Evaluation of intranasal delivery route of drug administration for brain targeting. Brain Res Bull 143:155–170
Fajardo-Serrano A, Rico AJ, Roda E et al (2021) Adeno-associated viral vectors as versatile tools for Parkinson's research, both for disease modeling purposes and for therapeutic uses. Int J Mol Sci 22(12):6389

Fauzi AA, Thamrin AMH, Permana AT et al (2023) Comparison of the administration route of stem cell therapy for ischemic stroke: a systematic review and meta-analysis of the clinical outcomes and safety. J Clin Med 12(7):2735

FDA (2019). https://www.fda.gov/news-events/press-announcements/fda-approves-new-nasal-spray-medication-treatment-resistant-depression-available-only-certified

FDA (2023). https://www.fda.gov/drugs/news-events-human-drugs/fda-approves-treatment-amyotrophic-lateral-sclerosis-associated-mutation-sod1-gene

Frankel AD, Pabo CO (1988) Cellular uptake of the tat protein from human immunodeficiency virus. Cell 55:1189–1193

Fu C, Xiang Y, Li X, Fu A (2018) Targeted transport of nanocarriers into brain for theranosis with rabies virus glycoprotein-derived peptide. Mater Sci Eng C Mater Biol Appl 87:155–166

Gao Y, Wang ZY, Zhang J et al (2014) RVG-peptide-linked trimethylated chitosan for delivery of siRNA to the brain. Biomacromolecules 15(3):1010–1018

Giugliani R, Martins AM, So S et al (2021) Iduronate-2-sulfatase fused with anti-hTfR antibody, pabinafusp alfa, for MPS-II: a phase 2 trial in Brazil. Mol Ther 29(7):2378–2386

Green M, Loewenstein PM (1988) Autonomous functional domains of chemically synthesized human immunodeficiency virus tat trans-activator protein. Cell 55:1179–1188

Guidotti G, Brambilla L, Rossi D (2017) Cell-penetrating peptides: from basic research to clinics. Trends Pharmacol Sci 38(4):406–424

Guo ZH, Khattak S, Rauf MA et al (2023) Role of nanomedicine-based therapeutics in the treatment of CNS disorders. Molecules 28(3):1283

Habib S, Singh M (2022) Angiopep-2-modified nanoparticles for brain-directed delivery of therapeutics: a review. Polymers (Basel) 14(4):712

Hallschmid M (2021) Intranasal insulin for Alzheimer's disease. CNS Drugs 35(1):21–37

Hardcastle N, Boulis NM, Federici T (2018) AAV gene delivery to the spinal cord: serotypes, methods, candidate diseases, and clinical trials. Expert Opin Biol Ther 18(3):293–307

Hill MD, Martin RH, Mikulis D et al (2012) Safety and efficacy of NA-1 in patients with iatrogenic stroke after endovascular aneurysm repair (ENACT): a phase 2, randomised, double-blind, placebo-controlled trial. Lancet Neurol 11(11):942–950

Ito K, Uchida Y, Ohtsuki S et al (2011) Quantitative membrane protein expression at the blood-brain barrier of adult and younger cynomolgus monkeys. J Pharm Sci 100:3939–3950

Jiang D, Sun Y, Li J et al (2016) Multiple-armed tetrahedral DNA nanostructures for tumor-targeting, dual-modality in vivo imaging. ACS Appl Mater Interfaces 8(7):4378–4384

Kalladka D, Sinden J, Pollock K et al (2016) Human neural stem cells in patients with chronic ischaemic stroke (PISCES): a phase 1, first-in-man study. Lancet 388(10046):787–796

Kariolis MS, Wells RC, Getz JA et al (2020) Brain delivery of therapeutic proteins using an fc fragment blood-brain barrier transport vehicle in mice and monkeys. Sci Transl Med 12(545): eaay1359

Klyachko NL, Polak R, Haney MJ et al (2017) Macrophages with cellular backpacks for targeted drug delivery to the brain. Biomaterials 140:79–87

Kusmierz CD, Callmann CE, Kudruk S et al (2022) Transferrin aptamers increase the *in vivo* blood-brain barrier targeting of protein spherical nucleic acids. Bioconjug Chem 33(10):1803–1810

Li X, Yang Y, Zhao H et al (2020) Enhanced in vivo blood-brain barrier penetration by circular tau-transferrin receptor bifunctional aptamer for tauopathy therapy. J Am Chem Soc 142(8): 3862–3872

Li YJ, Wu JY, Liu J et al (2021) From blood to brain: blood cell-based biomimetic drug delivery systems. Drug Deliv 28(1):1214–1225

Li J, Wei Y, Zhang C et al (2023) Cell-membrane-coated nanoparticles for targeted drug delivery to the brain for the treatment of neurological diseases. Pharmaceutics 15(2):621

Lim S, Kim WJ, Kim YH et al (2015) dNP2 is a blood-brain barrier-permeable peptide enabling ctCTLA-4 protein delivery to ameliorate experimental autoimmune encephalomyelitis. Nat Commun 6:8244

Liu T, Xie Q, Dong Z, Peng Q (2022) Nanoparticles-based delivery system and its potentials in treating central nervous system disorders. Nanotechnology 33:452001

Logan T, Simon MJ, Rana A et al (2021) Rescue of a lysosomal storage disorder caused by Grn loss of function with a brain penetrant progranulin biologic. Cell 184(18):4651–4668.e25

Luo Y, Yang H, Zhou YF, Hu B (2020) Dual and multi-targeted nanoparticles for site-specific brain drug delivery. J Control Release 317:195–215. https://doi.org/10.1016/j.jconrel.2019.11.037. Epub 2019 Nov 30

Luo Y, Yang H, Zhou YF, Hu B (2022) Dual and multi-targeted nanoparticles for site-specific brain drug delivery. J Control Release 317:195–215

Maderna E, Colombo L, Cagnotto A et al (2018) In situ tissue labeling of cerebral amyloid using HIV-related tat peptide. Mol Neurobiol 55(8):6834–6840

Merkel SF, Andrews AM, Lutton EM et al (2017) Trafficking of adeno-associated virus vectors across a model of the blood-brain barrier; a comparative study of transcytosis and transduction using primary human brain endothelial cells. J Neurochem 140(2):216–230

Metz MZ, Gutova M, Lacey SF et al (2013) Neural stem cell-mediated delivery of irinotecan-activating carboxylesterases to glioma: implications for clinical use. Stem Cells Transl Med 2(12):983–992

Milletti F (2012) Cell-penetrating peptides: classes, origin, and current landscape. Drug Discov Today 17(15–16):850–860. https://doi.org/10.1016/j.drudis.2012.03.002. Epub 2012 Mar 23

Morshed RA, Muroski ME, Dai Q et al (2016) Cell-penetrating peptide-modified gold nanoparticles for the delivery of doxorubicin to brain metastatic breast cancer. Mol Pharm 13(6):1843–1854

Muir KW, Bulters D, Willmot M et al (2020) Intracerebral implantation of human neural stem cells and motor recovery after stroke: multicentre prospective single-arm study (PISCES-2). J Neurol Neurosurg Psychiatry 91(4):396–401

Mullard A (2021) Blood-brain barrier-traversing biologic secures regulatory approval, in Japan. Nat Rev Drug Discov 20(5):332

Najem D, Bamji-Mirza M, Chang N, Liu QY, Zhang W (2014) Insulin resistance, neuroinflammation, and Alzheimer's disease. Rev Neurosci 25(4):509–525

Namanja-Magliano HA, Bohn K, Agrawal N et al (2017) Dual inhibitors of the human blood-brain barrier drug efflux transporters P-glycoprotein and ABCG2 based on the antiviral azidothymidine. Bioorg Med Chem 25(19):5128–5132

Okuyama T, Eto Y, Sakai N et al (2021) A phase 2/3 trial of Pabinafusp alfa, IDS fused with anti-human transferrin receptor antibody, targeting neurodegeneration in MPS-II. Mol Ther 29(2): 671–679

Pfizer (2023). https://www.pfizer.com/news/press-release/press-release-detail/pfizers-zavzprettm-zavegepant-migraine-nasal-spray

Räägel H, Pooga M (2011) Peptide and protein delivery with cell-penetrating peptides. In: Van Der Walle C (ed) Peptide and protein delivery. Elsevier, pp 221–246

Roytman M, Mashriqi F, Al-Tawil K et al (2023) Amyloid-related imaging abnormalities: an update. AJR Am J Roentgenol 220(4):562–574

Shen S, Zhang W (2010) ABC transporters and drug efflux at the blood-brain barrier. Rev Neurosci 21(1):29–53

Sun Y, Kong J, Ge X et al (2023) An antisense oligonucleotide-loaded blood-brain barrier penetrable nanoparticle mediating recruitment of endogenous neural stem cells for the treatment of Parkinson's disease. ACS Nano 17(5):4414–4432

Sweeney MD, Zhao Z, Montagne A et al (2019) Blood-brain barrier: from physiology to disease and Back. Physiol Rev 99(1):21–78

Tam DY, Ho JW, Chan MS et al (2020) Penetrating the blood-brain barrier by self-assembled 3D DNA Nanocages as drug delivery vehicles for brain cancer therapy. ACS Appl Mater Interfaces 12(26):28928–28940

Terstappen G, Meyer A, Bell R, Zhang W (2021) Strategies for delivering central nervous system therapeutics across the blood-brain barrier. Nat Rev Drug Discov 20(5):362–383

Thirumurugan S, Dash P, Liu X et al (2022) Angiopep-2-decorated titanium-alloy core-shell magnetic nanoparticles for nanotheranostics and medical imaging. Nanoscale 14(39): 14789–14800

Tu J, Zhang X, Zhu Y et al (2015) Cell-permeable peptide targeting the Nrf2-Keap1 interaction: a potential novel therapy for global cerebral ischemia. J Neurosci 35(44):14727–14739

Uchida Y, Ohtsuki S, Katsukura Y et al (2011) Quantitative targeted absolute proteomics of human blood-brain barrier transporters and receptors. J Neurochem 117:333–345

Ullman JC, Arguello A, Getz JA et al (2020) Brain delivery and activity of a lysosomal enzyme using a blood-brain barrier transport vehicle in mice. Sci Transl Med 12(545):eaay1163

van Lengerich B, Zhan L, Xia D et al (2023) A TREM2-activating antibody with a blood-brain barrier transport vehicle enhances microglial metabolism in Alzheimer's disease models. Nat Neurosci 26(3):416–429

Xu Y, Wei L, Wang H (2020) Progress and perspectives on nanoplatforms for drug delivery to the brain. J Drug Deliv Sci Technol 57:101636

Yang X, Wang Y, Byrne R et al (2019) Concepts of artificial intelligence for computer-assisted drug discovery. Chem Rev 119(18):10520–10594

Ye D, Zimmermann T, Demina V et al (2021) Trafficking of JC virus-like particles across the blood-brain barrier. Nanoscale Adv 3(9):2488–2500

Zhang W, Stanimirovic DB (2005) The transport systems of the blood-brain barrier. In: De Vries E, Prat A (eds) The blood-brain barrier and its microenvironment: basic physiology to neurological disease. Taylor & Francis Group, New York, pp 103–142

Zhang W, Bamji-Mirza M, Chang N et al (2015) Erters at the blood-brain barrier. In: Dorovini-Zis K (ed) The blood-brain barrier in health and disease, vol 1. CRC Press/Taylor & Francis Group, New York, pp 172–214

Zhang W, Liu QY, Haqqani AS et al (2020) Differential expression of receptors mediating receptor-mediated transcytosis (RMT) in brain microvessels, brain parenchyma and peripheral tissues of mouse and human. Fluids Barriers CNS 17:47

Zhang F, Xu Z, Jolly KJ (2023a) Myeloid cell-mediated drug delivery: from nanomedicine to cell therapy. Adv Drug Deliv Rev 197:114827

Zhang W, Liu QY, Haqqani AS, Liu Z, Sodja C, Leclerc S, Baumann E, Delaney CE, Brunette E, Stanimirovic DB (2023b) Differential expression of *ABC* transporter genes in brain vessels vs. peripheral tissues and vessels from human, mouse and rat. Pharmaceutics 15(5):1563

Zhao P, Xu Y, Fan X et al (2022) Discovery and engineering of an anti-TREM2 antibody to promote amyloid plaque clearance by microglia in 5XFAD mice. MAbs 14(1):2107971

Zhou X, Smith QR, Liu X (2021) Brain penetrating peptides and peptide-drug conjugates to overcome the blood-brain barrier and target CNS diseases. Wiley Interdiscip Rev Nanomed Nanobiotechnol 13(4):e1695

Nanomedicine – Immune System Interactions: Limitations and Opportunities for the Treatment of Cancer

Sara Elsafy, Josbert Metselaar, and Twan Lammers

Contents

Abstract

Nanoparticles interact with immune cells in many different ways. These interactions are crucially important for determining nanoparticles' ability to be

S. Elsafy · J. Metselaar · T. Lammers (✉)
Department of Nanomedicine and Theranostics, Institute for Experimental Molecular Imaging (ExMI), Center for Biohybrid Medical Systems (CBMS), University Hospital RWTH Aachen, Aachen, Germany
e-mail: selsafy@ukaachen.de; jmetselaar@ukaachen.de; tlammers@ukaachen.de

M. Schäfer-Korting, U. S. Schubert (eds.), *Drug Delivery and Targeting*, Handbook of Experimental Pharmacology 284, https://doi.org/10.1007/164_2023_685

used for cancer therapy. Traditionally, strategies such as PEGylation have been employed to reduce (the kinetics of) nanoparticle uptake by immune cells, to endow them with long circulation properties, and to enable them to exploit the Enhanced Permeability and Retention (EPR) effect to accumulate in tumors. More recently, with immunotherapy becoming an increasingly important cornerstone in the clinical management of cancer, ever more research efforts in academia and industry are focusing on specifically targeting immune cells with nanoparticles. In this chapter, we describe the barriers and opportunities of immune cell targeting with nanoparticles, and we discuss how nanoparticle-based drug delivery to specific immune cell populations in tumors as well as in secondary myeloid and lymphoid organs (such as bone marrow, lymph nodes, and spleen) can be leveraged to boost the efficacy of cancer immunotherapy.

Keywords

Cancer · Immune cells · Immunotherapy · Macrophage · Nanoparticle

Abbreviations

APC	Antigen-presenting cell
BM	Bone marrow
CAF	Cancer-associated fibroblast
CAR	Chimeric antigen receptor
CSF1	Colony-stimulating factor-1
CTLA-4	Cytotoxic T lymphocyte-associated antigen
DAMP	Damage-associated molecular pattern
DC	Dendritic cell
Dox	Doxorubicin
ECM	Extracellular matrix
EPR	Enhanced permeability and retention
HBV	Hepatitis B
HPV	Human papillomavirus
HSC	Hematopoietic stem cell
ICD	Immunogenic cell death
ICI	Immune checkpoint inhibitor
IDC	Invasive ductal carcinoma
ILC	Invasive lobular carcinoma
LN	Lymph node
LNP	Lipid nanoparticle
MDSC	Myeloid-derived suppressor cell
MPS	Mononuclear phagocyte system
NK	Natural killer
NP	Nanoparticle
PC	Protein corona

PD-1	Programmed cell death protein
PDAC	Pancreatic ductal adenocarcinoma mouse model
PD-L1	Programmed cell death ligand 1
PEG	Poly(ethylene glycol)
RNAi	RNA interference
ROS	Reactive oxygen species
TAA	Tumor-associated antigen
TAMs	Tumor-associated macrophage
TME	Tumor microenvironment
TNF-α	Tumor necrosis factor alpha
Treg	Regulatory T cell
VEGF	Vascular endothelial growth factor

1 Introduction

Better treatment of cancer has arguably been the most important overarching goal for nanomedicine. In the decades that followed the introduction of the first nanomedicinal anticancer drug Doxil®/Caelyx® in 1995, consistent progress has indeed been made in improving cancer therapy via nanocarrier-based drug delivery (He et al. 2019; Barenholz 2012). Using nanomedicine formulations, drug accumulation in tumors can be improved while accumulation in healthy tissues is attenuated (Barenholz 2012). In certain cases, also the rate of drug release can be controlled. Anticancer nanomedicines typically show better safety profiles in the clinic as compared to traditional chemotherapy treatments (Murry and Blaney 2000). However, it is increasingly accepted that real breakthroughs in terms of therapeutic efficacy have not yet come, at least not to the extent that was initially hoped for.

In roughly the same period of time, big strides have been made in the treatment of cancer by harnessing the power of the immune system (Esfahani et al. 2020). Ironically, the immune system was initially always referred to as being a major barrier hampering effective drug delivery via nanomedicines (Tsoi et al. 2016). Nowadays, we are more and more appreciating the enormous potential that nanomedicine formulations have to engage with the immune system to better treat cancer.

In this chapter, we look back at some key historical milestones of nanomedicine in cancer and we summarize what has been learned about the way nanomedicine drug products interact with the immune system. Based on the lessons learnt, we provide the reader with thought-provoking examples on how the immune system can be capitalized on by nanomedicine. We start off examining the mechanisms by which nanoparticles (NPs) target cancer cells and analyze what the major obstacles are that keep NP from reaching their intended sites (typically tumors and metastases). In this part, we mainly focus on the immune system as a barrier toward efficient drug delivery. In the second half, we describe how the natural propensity of NPs to interact with the immune system can be harnessed to overcome delivery barriers to enhance anticancer nanomedicine and we discuss how to use the interplay between NPs and the immune system to boost the efficacy of immunotherapy.

1.1 Passive Tumor Targeting

Tumor-targeted drug delivery has long been one of the most promising applications of nanotechnology in the field of medicine (He et al. 2019). It is still extensively studied in the hope that it can improve existing cancer treatments (Sindhwani et al. 2020). NPs are often used with the aim to deliver drugs directly to tumors, improving drug efficacy and reducing toxicity (Barenholz 2012). The main mechanism by which NPs can deliver drugs to tumors is typically referred to as the Enhanced Permeation and Retention (EPR) effect, which takes advantage of the structural and biological differences between diseased and normal tissue (Maeda and Matsumura 1989). Due to the rapid proliferation of tumor cells, the structure of newly formed tumor blood vessels is immature, with gaps between the endothelial cell walls that can reach up to 1 μm. This allows for the extravasation of circulating NPs into the tumor extravascular space. In addition, lymphatic drainage is impaired in tumors, contributing to the local retention of NPs (Maeda and Matsumura 1989).

The extent to which the EPR phenomenon – also referred to as "passive targeting" – occurs depends on the physicochemical properties of the NP (size, shape, charge, and flexibility). These properties need to be tuned to minimize premature uptake by cells of the mononuclear phagocyte system (MPS), thereby conferring prolonged plasma circulation times (Alexis et al. 2008). However, it is worth noting that EPR-mediated passive targeting of tumors only promotes tumor accumulation and does not actually guarantee efficient delivery to cancer cells. As a matter of fact, it has been revealed that in most cases, tumor-associated macrophages form the ultimate fate for drug-loaded nanoparticles, which can still contribute to efficient therapy by processing the NPs and releasing the drugs for killing neighboring cancer cells (Rosenblum et al. 2018). Passive tumor targeting is the concept employed for the majority of clinically used nanomedicine formulations (Fig. 1).

1.2 Active Targeting to Cancer Cells

Active targeting involves the decoration of the NP surface with targeting moieties such as monoclonal antibodies, engineered antibody fragments, proteins, peptides, carbohydrates, and aptamers to achieve specific binding to target cells (Alexis et al. 2008; Peer et al. 2007). Active targeting is based on the specific interaction between (overexpressed) receptors present on the surface of cancer (or immune) cells and the high affinity ligand on the NP surface. Active targeting mainly helps to facilitate the cellular uptake of NPs (Rosenblum et al. 2018). For active targeting to be successful, several factors need to be considered. These include the conjugation approach used, the ligand density, and the choice of the targeting ligand (Rosenblum et al. 2018; Tammam et al. 2015). It is also important to note that successful targeting doesn't

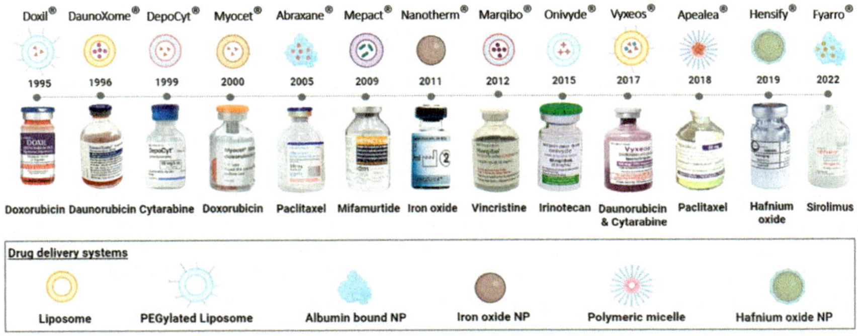

Fig. 1 Overview of clinically used cancer nanomedicine formulations. These FDA/EMA-approved nanomedicine products are developed for various therapeutic purposes. They exploit EPR to passively deliver NP to the tumor site (Doxil, DaunoXome, Myocet, Mepact, Marqibo, Onivyde, and Apealea), alter drug pharmacokinetics for sustained release purposes (DepoCyt), reduce solvent toxicity (e.g., Cremophor in Taxol; vs. Abraxane, Fyarro), co-deliver two drugs in a synergistic ration for combination therapy (Vyxeos), generate heat (Nanotherm), or enhance radiotherapy efficacy (Hensify)

solely depend on the particles' surface properties but will also be affected by barriers in the tumor microenvironment.

While developing nanomedicines that can target specific cells within the body might sound promising, creating a targeted delivery platform with a one-size-fits-all approach is a challenge. In reality, there is high heterogeneity in receptor expression and vascularity among tumors, between individuals, and over the course of the disease. The efficiency of active targeted drug delivery systems can also be affected by receptor recycling kinetics, the ability of the ligand to induce an immune response, and the binding site barrier (which results from strong binding of NPs to cells in close proximity to blood vessels and which thereby limits NP penetration). Importantly, the addition of a targeting moiety on the surface of NPs can facilitate rapid recognition by the MPS in liver and spleen, thereby promoting clearance from the blood stream, suppressing tumor targeting capacity, and reducing therapeutic efficacy (Rosenblum et al. 2018; Salvati et al. 2013; Poon et al. 2020). By doing so, the primary advantage of targeting is lost – it is no longer possible to deliver nanoparticles to primary and disseminated tumors.

In recent years, the utilization of LNPs in RNA delivery has emerged as a promising strategy for treating different types of diseases and malignancies. Hematological malignancies, however, are extremely challenging to treat due to limited nanoparticle uptake by lymphocytes, difficulty to precisely target cells without off-target side effects, and the inherent resistance of lymphocytes to in vivo transfection (Tarab-Ravski et al. 2023). Therefore, in this case, active targeting becomes crucial to effectively deliver nanoparticles to primary and secondary lymphoid organs and to facilitate their internalization by immune cells.

1.3 Immune System Barriers to Tumor-Targeted Drug Delivery

Intravenously administered NPs face a number of physical and biological barriers that limit the fraction of administered dose that reaches the target site. These include shear forces, protein corona formation, rapid clearance by MPS, blood vessel walls, extracellular matrix (ECM), tumor stroma cells, tumor-associated immune cells, and finally cellular and subcellular plasma membranes. Obviously, the NP physicochemical characteristics determine to a large extent how each of these barriers in the circulation and the tumor microenvironment (TME) affect the delivery process. Tissue physiology, which differs in different diseases and disease states, can further alter these barriers, affecting NP accumulation at the target location (Poon et al. 2020).

The journey of NPs along the delivery pathway and their sequential loss in numbers as they move through biological barriers is depicted in a schematic diagram by Chan and colleagues (Poon et al. 2020) (Fig. 2). The authors postulate that only approximately one out of a million administered NPs actually make it to the tumor cell nucleus, illustrating how challenging the delivery process is.

Following systemic administration, serum proteins called opsonins instantly absorb on the NP's surface forming the so-called protein corona (PC). This imparts a new identity to NPs (Poon et al. 2020; Tarab-Ravski et al. 2023). The PC can compromise the efficacy of actively targeted NPs by masking the targeting ligands and preventing them from interacting with the corresponding receptors on cancer cells (Salvati et al. 2013; Tenzer et al. 2013). Opsonins promote the recognition and clearance of the NPs by the MPS in liver and spleen, which present a significant (and early) barrier that is responsible for the clearing of the majority of intravenously administered NPs (Tsoi et al. 2016). MPS clearance typically depends on the NP physical and chemical properties, with stiffer, spherical, and highly charged particles (especially positively charged) getting cleared more rapidly from the circulation than softer, non-spherical, and neutral or slightly negatively charged particles, respectively (Varnamkhasti et al. 2015; Blanco et al. 2015). In the event NPs survive MPS clearance, the formed PC can result in decreased cell adhesion and uptake (Kou et al. 2018). NPs that manage to overcome the above-mentioned hurdles and reach the tumor vasculature are faced by yet another barrier, which is the tumor microenvironment (Poon et al. 2020). Stromal cells within the TME often generate a dense ECM, creating a physical barrier that hinders the diffusion and penetration of NPs and prevents NPs from reaching cancer cells (Lesniak et al. 2012; Miao et al. 2015). Tumor-associated macrophages (TAMs) are myeloid immune cells in the tumor stroma that phagocytose and process PC-covered NPs (Zhu et al. 2019). TAM-uptake may be preferable or prevented depending on the type of drug delivered. In case of small molecule chemotherapeutics like doxorubicin, TAM processing is beneficial for anti-tumor efficacy. In case of genetic drug treatment, e.g. anti-oncogene siRNA, uptake by TAM (and other stromal/immune cells in the microenvironment) is to be prevented, to maximize the amount that is eventually delivered to the target cell type, i.e. cancer cells.

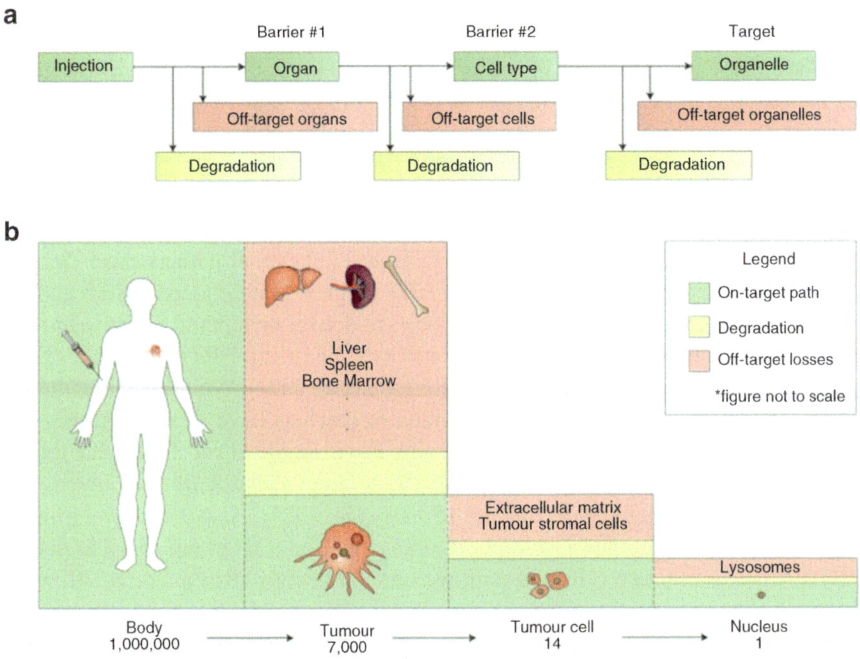

Fig. 2 Graphical illustration of NP transportation in the body. The journey from the site of administration to the pathological destination is depicted, as well as the biological barriers that are encountered along the way. Upon intravenous (IV) injection, NP fall prey to phagocytic cells of the MPS (in liver, spleen, and bone marrow). NP surviving MPS clearance remain in circulation and can reach the tumor site. At the tumor site, the majority of extravasated NPs either get engulfed by tumor stromal cells (most prominently tumor-associated macrophages) or entrapped in the extracellular matrix. Only a very small fraction of IV administered NPs eventually makes it to the primary target site for chemotherapeutic drug action, i.e. the tumor cell nucleus. This highlights how challenging the delivery process actually is. Figure adopted from Poon et al. (2020) with permission from Springer-Nature

1.4 Addressing and Exploiting Immune System Barriers

As indicated above, the impact of the biological barriers on the delivery process is to a large extent dictated by the physicochemical properties of the NPs. NPs should ideally remain in circulation long enough to reach their target site before getting sequestered by phagocytic cells (Barenholz 2012). The literature generally agrees that NPs with a neutral surface charge, surface-coated with poly(ethylene glycol) (PEG), and size of 10–100 nm have the longest residence time in systemic circulation (Barenholz 2012; Korangath et al. 2020; Mitchell et al. 2021).

To avoid PC-mediated MPS clearance, certain NP designs integrate surface modifications. Besides PEGylation these include NP coating with zwitterions (Li et al. 2016; Debayle et al. 2019) and camouflaging NPs with "don't-eat-me" markers, such as the CD47 protein (Estephan et al. 2011). These established strategies rely mostly on reducing particle recognition and interaction with phagocytic immune cells (Barenholz 2012; Li et al. 2016; Debayle et al. 2019).

The emergence of the field of cancer immunotherapy and the better understanding of the role of the PC and immune cells in NP delivery and clearance has led some researchers to rethink the "avoidance approach" and embark on a different strategy, which is to capitalize on the potential of NP to interact with the immune system and to bolster it to enhance immunotherapy. For instance, instead of avoiding PC formation, researchers designed NPs capable of attracting the necessary plasma proteins to guide cellular uptake (Gheibi Hayat et al. 2019). Others have cleverly exploited the natural tendency of immune cells to migrate to inflamed lesions and use their increased interactivity with nanoparticles to deliver therapeutic cargo to tumors. In such setups, immune cells act as Trojan horses, taking up NPs in the bloodstream and delivering them to and into tumors (Johnson et al. 2022). While such hitchhiking approaches help overcome immune barriers, researchers have shown that they can also be exploited to improve immunotherapy. For example, it was found that the PC can be used not only for targeting, but also to polarize macrophage phenotypes as a means to potentiate anticancer efficacy (Sofias et al. 2021). Also the natural propensity of NPs to accumulate in lymphoid organs can be a targeting route to deliver therapeutics to immune cells and improve immunotherapy (Rostam et al. 2020).

2 The Immune System in Cancer

The relationship between the immune system and cancer is a complex one. Navigating the interplay between the innate and adaptive immune system and cancer cells has been the focus of many researchers over many years. In order to understand the relationship between cancer and the immune system, Chen and Mellman proposed the cancer-immunity cycle (Fig. 3), which describes the mechanisms by which anticancer immune responses are generated (Chen and Mellman 2013). The cycle is initiated with the death of cancer cell and the release of tumor-associated antigens (TAA). The released TAA are taken up by antigen-presenting cells (APC) such as macrophages, dendritic cells, and B cells. These cells present antigens to naïve T cells present in secondary lymphoid organs. Upon exposure to antigens, naïve T cells will mature into effector T cells. Educated T cells will then leave the lymph nodes and enter the bloodstream. In the case of liquid tumors, T cells will attack and kill cancer cells carrying the same antigen. For solid tumors, on the other hand, T cells will infiltrate the tumor bed, target and destruct the cancerous cells there. Attacked cancer cells release antigens and co-stimulatory molecules that serve to further amplify the anticancer immune response (Chen and Mellman 2013). However, upon further studying the cancer-immunity cycle, it was discovered that cancer cells can obstruct the cycle leading to immune evasion and dampening of anti-tumor immune responses (Chen and Mellman 2013).

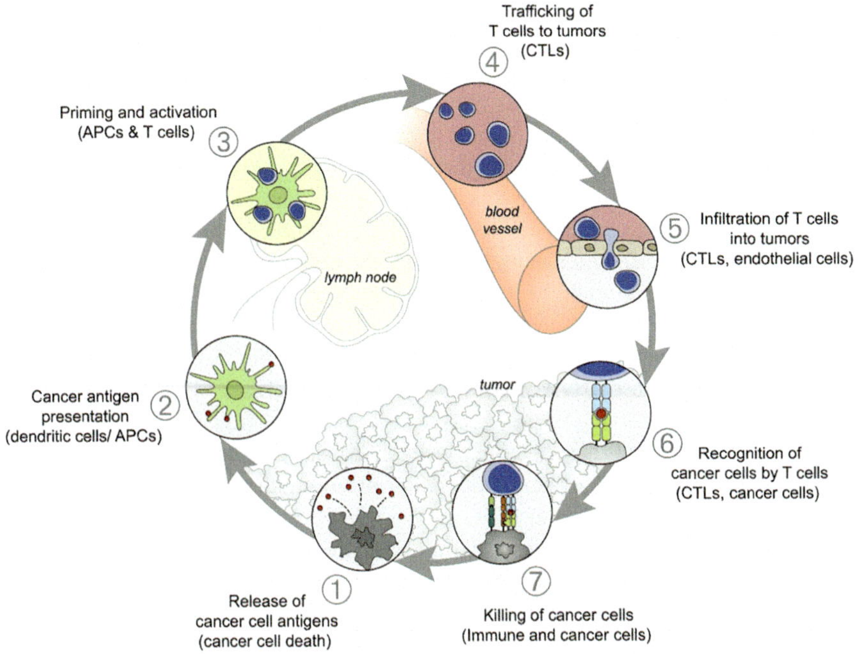

Fig. 3 The cancer-immunity cycle. This cycle describes how the immune system interacts with cancer cells. It begins with the death of the cancer cell and the release of tumor-associated antigens, followed by the priming and education of T cells in the lymph node, then T cells home to the tumor site and to kill cancer cells, which releases antigens amplifying the cycle. Figure adopted from Chen and Mellman (2013), with permission from Elsevier

2.1 Evasion of Immune Detection

In terms of tumor–immune system interaction, cancer cells have developed several strategies to evade the immune response and impair the tumor immunity cycle, allowing tumors to grow and spread (Tang et al. 2020). Many of these strategies exploit normal mechanisms of immune regulation, including the loss of immunogenicity (Tang et al. 2020), the release of immunosuppressive cytokines (Saleh and Elkord 2019), and the activation of regulatory T cells (Tregs) (Saleh and Elkord 2019). The loss of immunogenicity, due to the downregulation of tumor antigens, makes it harder for immune cells to identify the tumor (Mittal et al. 2014). Furthermore, tumor cells release immunosuppressive cytokines and chemo-attractants, such as TGF-β and IL-10, which further hinder the body's defense against them, as these factors cause macrophages to polarize from M1 to M2 (TAMS) and recruit myeloid-derived suppressor cells (MDSC) to the tumor site (Salemme et al. 2021). These MDSCs secrete cytokines that activate immunosuppressive Tregs, which then play a role in suppressing the maturation of dendritic cells (DCs) and interfere with the initiation of anti-tumor immunity (Liu et al. 2018).

Moreover, tumors can exploit immune checkpoint control to induce T-cell exhaustion. Programmed death ligand 1 (PD-L1) is an immune checkpoint protein that is often overexpressed on tumor cells and binds to programmed cell death protein (PD-1) on T cells. The PD-L1/PD-1 signaling axis suppresses T-cell activity, resulting in potent immunesuppression and promoting tumor growth (Sharpe and Pauken 2018). Lastly, the TME is another factor that facilitates tumor progression. It is often characterized by a dense extracellular matrix, immunosuppressive cytokines, and hostile metabolites, which all work together to inhibit immune cell activity and allow cancer cells to survive and proliferate (Valkenburg et al. 2018). The role of the TME in tumor immunity will be described in the next subsection.

2.2 Tumor Microenvironment (TME) Formation

Tumors can be regarded as pathologic tissue that consists of cancer and stromal cells. Stromal cells are a heterogeneous population of non-malignant cells consisting of fibroblasts, vascular endothelial cells, and infiltrated immune cells. This complex network of cells alongside extracellular matrix and soluble mediators form what is collectively known as the TME (Valkenburg et al. 2018).

The crosstalk taking place between cancer cells and the diverse immune cells dictates tumor progression and affects treatment efficacy (Laplagne et al. 2019). Immune cells in TME can be divided into two immunologically active groups: effector (anti-tumor) and protector (pro-tumor) cells. The former include T cells, natural killer (NK) cells, and DCs and are responsible for eradication of tumor cells. The latter protect tumor cells by shielding them from the host's immune surveillance. These include MDSCs, TAMs, and Tregs and cancer-associated fibroblasts (CAFs) (Tesi 2019). Established tumors exploit the host's immune system to recruit protector cells. Protector cells present in TME secrete cytokines and chemokines to either suppress the functions of effector cells or hinder their ability to reach tumor cells altogether. This results in an immunosuppressive environment that supports tumor immune evasion as well as growth, progression, and metastasis. Crucially, the gradual unraveling of this intricate physiology has led to the development of effective anticancer immunotherapy.

3 A Brief History of Cancer Immunotherapy

Immunotherapy is nowadays considered the fourth pillar of cancer therapy. This relatively novel treatment approach doesn't directly target cancer cells but rather modulates and re-educates immune cells to recognize and eradicate tumors. Though immunotherapy is perceived as a recent medical achievement that emerged with the development of immune checkpoint inhibitors (ICI), cancer vaccines, and chimeric antigen receptor (CAR) T-cell therapy, the concept of harnessing the immune system in the fight against cancer goes back more than a century in time.

The first immune-based treatment was a cancer vaccine developed by William Bradley Coley in 1899, who is known today as the Father of Immunotherapy (McCarthy 2006). Despite his success, Coley's inability to explain the anti-tumor response produced by the administration of a mixture of attenuated bacterial strains ("Coley's toxin"), together with the high mortality rate and variability in treatment response led oncologists to abandon this approach (Esfahani et al. 2020; McCarthy 2006).

In the meantime, the field of immunology itself continued to evolve with the discovery of immune cells including granulocytes, macrophages, B cells, T cells, DC, and NK, and their role in immunity was identified (Dobosz and Dzieciątkowski 2019). Yet, the role of these immune cells in cancer was not clear until 1957, when Thomas and Burnet first proposed the theory of "cancer immunosurveillance" which describes the potential role of the immune system in suppressing growth and eliminating genetically transformed somatic cells (Dunn et al. 2002). Unfortunately, further progress in the field was halted due to the lack of relevant technologies to prove the hypothesis.

It wasn't until 1974 that the discovery of cytokine family and their role in enhancing T-cell function re-ignited interest in immunotherapy. This eventually led to the FDA approval of IL-2 as an immunotherapeutic agent for metastatic kidney cancer in 1991, and in metastatic melanoma in 1998 (Morgan et al. 1976). During the same period, advancements in antibody production technology in the lab (Milstein 1999) paved the way for the production of rituximab, the first monoclonal antibody approved by the FDA in 1997 for treating non-Hodgkin lymphoma (Rudnicka et al. 2013).

However, it can be safely stated that the real breakthrough in cancer immunotherapy came about as a result of a better understanding of immunosurveillance. Concretely, the key trigger was the identification of negative immune regulatory pathways (also referred to as immune check points), such as CTLA-4 (cytotoxic T lymphocyte-associated antigen) and programmed death/ligand 1 (PD-1/PD-L1), which allow cancer cells to escape anti-tumor immune responses. This finding laid the basis for understanding the function of T cells and ultimately prompted the development of monoclonal antibodies to inhibit these regulatory pathways. This discovery resulted in the FDA approval of several immune checkpoint inhibitors for various malignancies, and in Allison and Honjo receiving the Nobel Prize in physiology and medicine in 2018 (Ribas and Wolchok 2018).

The use of vaccines to increase immune responses against cancer has also been explored. This work has resulted in the EMA/FDA approval of several cancer-preventing vaccines, such as the human papillomavirus (HPV) vaccine for cervical cancer and the hepatitis B (HBV) vaccine for liver cancer. In spite of these great achievements in a few specific cancer types, the success of this approach in a broader sense was modest, perhaps due to a poor selection of a target antigen, low immunogenicity, or an inadequate selection of patients (Dobosz and Dzieciątkowski 2019).

Cancer vaccines re-emerged in 2010 when the FDA approved sipuleucel-T (Provenge), an anticancer therapeutic vaccine that was used to treat refractory prostate cancer (Kantoff et al. 2010). Therapeutic vaccine works by modifying DC ex vivo before reinfusing them into a patient's blood, as is done with chimeric antigen receptor (CAR) T-cell therapies (Rosenberg and Restifo 2015). However, the implementability of such cell therapies is somewhat hampered by their very high cost (Smith et al. 2017). Therefore, with the success of the COVID mRNA vaccine, researchers are inspired to use NPs as an easier-to-implement alternative for in vivo immune cell modification. This approach will be discussed later on in this chapter.

4 History of Nanomedicine and the Immune System

Drug delivery using NPs was first envisioned in the mid-twentieth century with the development of polymer-drug conjugates (Jatzkewitz 1954). In the following years, liposomes (Bangham and Horne 1964; Bangham et al. 1965) and albumin-based particles (Scheffel et al. 1972) were introduced. After a few decades of intense research into these delivery vehicles, the efforts paved the way for the FDA approval of PEGylated liposomal formulation of doxorubicin (Doxil®) in 1995 (Barenholz 2012) and paclitaxel-associated albumin nanoparticles (Abraxane®) in 2005 (Gradishar et al. 2005), two of the most prominent examples of NPs used in the clinic for cancer therapy.

NP-based drug formulations, however, can be seen as foreign material, much alike bacteria and viruses, which explains their rapid recognition by plasma proteins (opsonin) and their oftentimes swift elimination by the immune system (Fadeel 2019). For this reason, Doxil was featured with the so-called stealth properties, which are based on NP surface coating with polyethylene glycol (PEG) to convey the capacity to escape the immune system detection and reside in the bloodstream for prolonged periods of time, enabling better drug delivery to tumors.

As the 2000s progressed, different NPs for various biomedical applications (hyperthermia, diagnostics, and imaging) began to be clinically investigated (Fig. 1). Also in these cases, polymers for surface coating seemed desirable to avoid immune interactions, like with PEG (Barenholz 2012; Bangham et al. 1965). To further avoid immune detection and clearance, researchers investigated additional approaches such as those mentioned above in Sect. 1.4.

Recent advancements in the fields of immunotherapy made scientists question whether the NP interactions with the immune cells and the immune system could also be beneficial from a therapeutic perspective (Andorko and Jewell 2017; Yousefpour et al. 2023). The discovery of the ability of (nano)biomaterials to exhibit innate immunomodulatory effects and to activate immune pathways, regardless of whether an immune-stimulating molecule is present or not, has caused a shift from considering nanomaterials as pure carrier vehicles that should avoid any interaction with the immune system to a platform technology that can have inherent bioactivity in its own right (regardless of the pharmacologically active content to be delivered) (Sharp et al. 2009; Demento et al. 2009). In the following section, we will provide an overview of this current renewed interest in the engineering of nanomaterials to modify the immune response and enhance therapeutic outcome of current immunotherapies.

5 The Interaction of Nanoparticles with Immune Cells

Understanding the interaction between nanoparticles and immune cells is essential for the optimization of their in vivo performance, the assessment of potential toxicities and eventually for the development of effective nanomedicine therapeutics. As already stated above, the immune system can "recognize" NPs and mount a response to eliminate them (Fadeel 2019). NPs, on the other hand, can also trigger the immune system to produce antibodies and inflammatory cytokines, as well as activate the complement pathway. These interactions can result in inflammation, immune cell activation, and other adverse effects.

The type and severity of the immune response is often determined by the physicochemical properties of the nanomaterials, which include material composition, molecular weight, size, shape, surface charge, and chemical functionality (Andorko and Jewell 2017). It is clear that a better understanding of the interaction between NPs and the immune system could open up new research avenues with the aim to capitalize on the intrinsic immunogenic features of nanomaterials to have them assist in achieving the desired immunological outcome. As macrophages are a major cell population in most tissues, and as they play key roles in cancer progression and treatment response, we will specifically address the NP interaction with macrophages in the following two subsections.

5.1 Macrophage Clearance of NP as a Bio-barrier

Macrophages are key components of the MPS (Biozzi and Stiffel 1965; Ngo et al. 2022). They can be considered the sentinels of the innate immune system in which they contribute to cytokine production and are responsible for the initiation of inflammation (Hirayama et al. 2017). Through phagocytosis, macrophages actively identify, engulf, and break down pathogens to present their features to T cells to mount an immune response against them. Macrophage clearance consequently is a natural process that plays an important role in protecting the body from invading microbes and pathogens (Hirayama et al. 2017).

Not surprisingly, it appeared that macrophages can also very effectively detect and take up NPs. This results in the rapid clearance of NPs and – if no further modification is employed – their massive off-target accumulation in MPS organs (Ngo et al. 2022). Macrophage clearance is organ dependent with liver macrophages (Kupffer cells) contributing the most to off-target NPs sequestration (Ouyang et al. 2022; Zhang et al. 2016; Tavares et al. 2017). This is because the liver is home to most of the body's phagocytic cells (Ngo et al. 2022) and because the highly vascularized liver architecture provides Kupffer cells with direct access to circulating NPs (Tsoi et al. 2016; Ngo et al. 2022). So unless the aim is to treat liver diseases or liver macrophage dysfunction, the accumulation of NPs in liver macrophages is therapeutically undesirable.

For these reasons, earlier delivery strategies adopted by researchers to reduce macrophage uptake involved increasing NP circulation time and reducing liver NP uptake by altering the NP physicochemical properties and surface characteristics (Barenholz 2012; Li et al. 2016; Debayle et al. 2019; Estephan et al. 2011; Mitchell et al. 2021), while other strategies involved depleting liver macrophages (Tavares et al. 2017). Interestingly, while NP residence in the circulation increased after liver macrophage elimination, the percentage of the injected NP dose that accumulated in tumors remained fairly low (2%). This suggests that NPs could potentially be intercepted and sequestered by macrophages in other organs, such as blood, spleen, and bone marrow.

In this context, also the macrophages in and around tumors (TAMs) have long been seen as an undesired target for NP aimed at delivering anticancer drugs to tumor cells (Zhu et al. 2019; Tavares et al. 2017). However, as researchers gained a better insight into the role of TAMs in drug delivery (Ngai et al. 2023) and with the rise of the field of immunotherapy, they started to explore whether it would be therapeutically beneficial to exploit rather than to eliminate or downregulate macrophage activity.

5.2 Macrophage Targeting

Macrophage targeting for cancer immunotherapy applications is an area of growing research interest. Macrophages are nowadays more and more considered target cells to either boost their effectiveness against cancer cells or to take advantage of them to deliver NPs to tumor tissues (Ngai et al. 2023). The former can be achieved by delivering chemical agents to reprogram macrophages (Cheng et al. 2021; Li et al. 2021) and help them recognize cancer cells. The goal of this approach is to mobilize the body's own immune response against cancer and to further improve the efficacy of other treatments.

As an interesting example in this regard, it was demonstrated that single-walled carbon nanotubes (SWCNT) can target specific subsets of circulating monocytes and hitchhike with them to the tumor site via a Trojan horse mechanism (Smith et al. 2014). In line with this, Sofias and colleagues visualized and quantified the homing of RGD-targeted lipid nanoparticles to inflamed lesions using intravital microscopy and identified "NP hitchhiking" with circulating phagocytes as a key contributing mechanism (Sofias et al. 2021). In a similar study setup, Chen and colleagues found that TAMs actively took up extravasated NPs, delivering them deep into tumors with 2-5x greater efficiency than if delivery was solely dependent on NP diffusion (Lin et al. 2022). In these studies, the natural propensity of macrophages to phagocytose NPs and migrate to and into inflamed lesions has been capitalized on to improve NP drug delivery. However, it is important to note that most of these studies focused on macrophages as delivery vehicles for NPs and we should also keep in mind that other phagocytic cells, including neutrophils, are also prominently capable of internalizing and delivering NPs (Sofias et al. 2020; Chu et al. 2015, 2016).

6 How Do Nanoparticles Enable Modulation of the Immune System in Cancer?

Current immunotherapies use biological products, such as proteins and cells, to stimulate the immune system in its fight against tumors. These products, particularly the more advanced ones, such as adoptive cell transfer therapeutics (Rosenberg and Restifo 2015), require complex biotechnological procedures and technical expertise, resulting in high cost of therapy and limited clinical availability (Rosenberg and Restifo 2015; Smith et al. 2017).

The use of NP in principle may enable immune system modulation in a more straightforward way that could be more readily implemented in current clinical care. In addition, being a versatile and adaptable platform, NPs allow for the encapsulation of a variety of molecules or a combination of molecules. Moreover, one of the major benefits of NP is their flexibility in terms of size and surface characteristics, making it possible to tune NPs to efficiently reach lymph nodes, penetrate lymphoid tissues, and deliver therapeutics (Liu et al. 2014; Porter and Trevaskis 2020) to specific immune cells including DC which are a main target for cancer vaccines.

Because of the importance of striking the right balance between generating a desired immune response against tumors while avoiding systemic activation of the immune system, selective targeting of specific immune cells is necessary. In this case, the NP surface can be modified with small molecules, peptides, or antibodies, to achieve increased circulation behavior or enhanced immune cell targeting ability (Yong et al. 2022; Ramishetti et al. 2015; Veiga et al. 2023). Alternatively, NPs can be conjugated to the surface of specific immune cells (such as T cells) prior to reinfusion into patients, via a strategy known as "backpacking," which ensures that NPs get a "free ride" to the desired tissue while continuously expanding T cells in vivo (Tang et al. 2018).

One of the major limitations of current immunotherapeutics is the severe side effects resulting from the need to administer high doses (Ishihara et al. 2019). In some patients, these effects can be life-threatening and may lead to termination of therapy. Indeed, NP can present a relatively straightforward platform to enhance specific interactions between immune-modulatory molecules and the immune cells, while avoiding the potentially toxic effects endured due to systemic exposure to these agents in free form (Ishihara et al. 2019; Xie et al. 2018). In the following subsections, we will explore in detail how nanomaterials can be used to enhance immunotherapy with examples from the literature. The subsections will respectively address the approaches that target immune cells in TME, lymphoid organs, and bone marrow.

6.1 TME Targeting and Modulation

The first step of the cancer-immunity cycle is driven by the release of tumor-associated antigens (TAA). If the released antigens are below a certain threshold, antigen presentation will be insufficient to effectively trigger an immune response, and the cycle stops (Chen and Mellman 2013). Immunogenic cell death (ICD) is a form of regulated cell death that induces the release of damage-associated molecular patterns (DAMPs), which activate the immune system against antigens expressed by the dying cancer cell. Some therapies, such as chemotherapy, radiation, and oncolytic viruses, can trigger ICD (Gao et al. 2020). Chemotherapeutic drugs have been successfully combined with immune checkpoint inhibitors (ICI) in various nanoparticle-based drug delivery systems (Gao et al. 2020; Catanzaro et al. 2022) to induce ICD and turn "cold tumors" into "hot tumors." Cold tumors are those with low immunogenicity and poor infiltration of immune cells. In contrast, hot tumors are highly immunogenic with improved immune cell infiltration. Preclinical studies on nano-delivery systems found that only a fraction of the administered dose (0.7%) reaches the tumor vicinity (Wilhelm et al. 2016). This coupled with the sometimes premature release of chemotherapeutic drugs loaded in NPs means that a considerable fraction of the dose of cytotoxic drug gets delivered to immune cells residing in healthy tissues and in lymphoid organs, resulting in toxicity and systemic immunosuppression (Mathios et al. 2016). Researchers have therefore opted to synthesize prodrugs with enzyme-cleavable linkers for selective delivery to and activation by enzymes overexpressed in tumors (Yang et al. 2021; Moon et al. 2022). Moon et al., for instance, developed PD-L1 targeted doxorubicin (Dox) prodrug nanoparticles. The prodrug NPs consisted of enzyme-specific cleavable peptide conjugated to Dox at one end and to an anti-PD-L1 peptide at the other end. By developing these self-assembling NPs, the team were able to relieve TME immunosuppression by simultaneously blocking PD-L1 and inducing ICD through anti-PD-L1 peptides and Dox, respectively (Moon et al. 2022).

The fact that most solid tumors have an immunosuppressive tumor microenvironment (TME) subdues the ICD-mediated anti-tumor immune response and oftentimes renders ICIs ineffective. This immuno-cold TME typically results from the presence of immunosuppressive molecules or cells. Ectonucleotides are an example of immunosuppressive enzymes that rapidly degrade ATP into adenosine (Ado). Ado is then responsible for inhibiting DC maturation and reducing T-cell function. To overcome this, Moa et al. designed a reactive oxygen species (ROS)-producing NP loaded with the ectonucleotidase inhibitor (ARL6756). Using near-infrared light, the team showed that ROS was produced, which in turn initiated ICD and the release of DAMPs. ROS production further mediated the release of ARL6756 from NPs, which then augmented anti-tumor immunity, enhanced T-cell response, and reprogrammed the TME resulting in an enhanced response to immunotherapy, particularly also in the PD1–resistant 4T1 breast cancer mouse model (Mao et al. 2022).

Immune cells such as Tregs, or stromal cells such as CAF, are among the cells that potently suppress effector immune cell functioning in the TME. The latter is the primary source of TGF-ß, a multifunctional cytokine which knocks down the immune system through inhibiting activation of NK and maturation of DC, decreasing cytokine production, and increasing Tregs production, in addition to its contribution to extracellular matrix formation and remodeling (Ping et al. 2021). Approaches to neutralize or inhibit the production of TGF-ß have involved the use

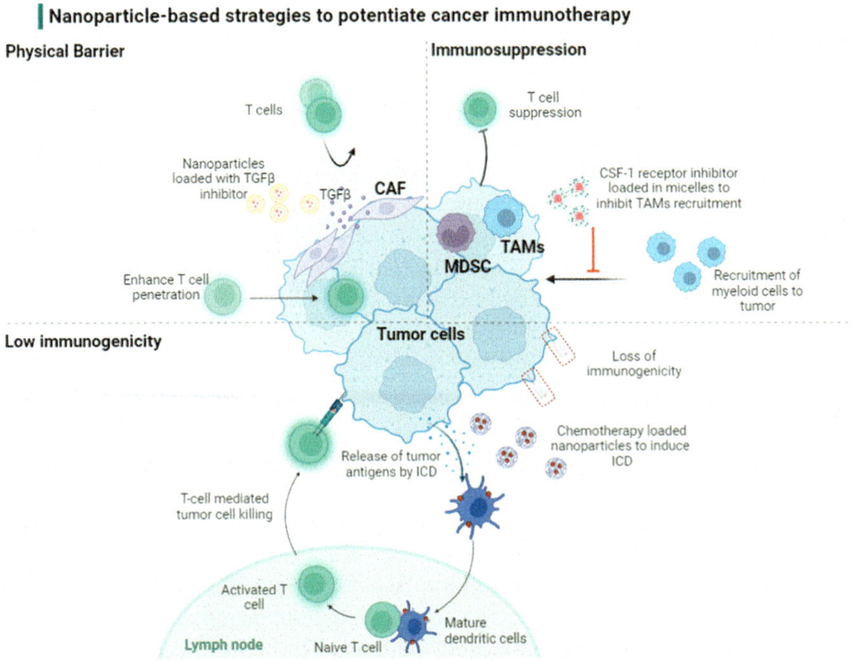

Fig. 4 Strategies adopted by cancer cells to evade immune surveillance and NP-based approaches to combat them. Cancer-specific strategies to avoid immune responses include the creation of a physical barrier to prevent effector T cell from penetrating tumors and attacking the cancer cells, decreasing antigen expression on cancer cells to prevent their recognition by immune cells, and the recruitment of myeloid cells that secrete immunosuppressive cytokines to suppress effector cell function. NPs can be used to deliver TGF-β inhibitor to CAFs to decrease the formation of a fibrotic shield and enhance T-cell penetration. Another potential approach involves the use of NPs to deliver chemotherapeutic agents to induce ICD and thereby release TAAs that can be picked up by DCs which migrate to lymph nodes and activate T cells against cancer cells. Finally, drug-loaded NPs can be delivered to prevent the recruitment of immunosuppressive cells such as TAMs and MDSCs, thereby relieving the immunosuppressive microenvironment and enhancing T-cell function. TGF-β: transforming growth factor beta, CAFs: cancer-associated fibroblasts, DCs: dendritic cells, MDSCs: myeloid-derived suppressor cells, TAMs: tumor-associated macrophages, CSF-1: colony-stimulating growth factor-1, ICD: immunogenic cell death

of chemical inhibitors (Schmid et al. 2017; Zheng et al. 2017) and RNA interference (RNAi) (Wu et al. 2022). In one study, anti-CD90 liposomes were developed to deliver SB525334, a TGF-ß inhibitor, to T cells. The authors showed that, compared to untargeted liposomes, anti-CD90 targeted liposomes enhanced T-cell function and led to a significant reduction in tumor growth and metastasis in the B16F10 melanoma mouse model (Zheng et al. 2017). In another example, Smidt et al. designed a PLGA–PEG NPs decorated with anti-PD-1 antibodies and loaded them with the TGF-β receptor inhibitor SD-208. The NPs successfully targeted and reversed the exhausted state of T cells, delayed tumor growth, and extended survival in the MC38 colon cancer mouse model (Schmid et al. 2017) (Fig. 4).

Among all immunosuppressive cells in the TME, TAMs are the most abundant immune cells, constituting up to 50% of tumor mass and creating an immunosuppressive TME through the release of immunosuppressive cytokines and chemokines (Larionova et al. 2020; Solinas et al. 2009). TAMs can display an array of different phenotypes, but are typically classified into M1 (anti-tumor) or M2 (pro-tumor) phenotypes (Guillot and Tacke 2019). Particularly the pro-tumorigenic M2-like contribute to tumor growth and immunesuppression (Larionova et al. 2020; Solinas et al. 2009). Three prominent strategies to target TAMs to relieve immunosuppression and inhibit tumor growth include depleting TAMs, inhibiting the recruitment of TAMs, and reprogramming TAMs (Cheng et al. 2021). Examples of this are discussed below. A more extensive overview on TAM-targeted nanomedicine strategies to improve immunotherapy outcomes is provided elsewhere (Cheng et al. 2021; Li et al. 2021).

TAMs are recruited to the tumor site as a result of the cancer cells secreting cytokines such as stromal cell–derived factor-1 (SDF1), vascular endothelial growth factor (VEGF), and colony-stimulating growth factor-1 (CSF1). Inhibiting the activity of these molecules seems therapeutically appealing as this will help reduce TAM recruitment to TMEs and inhibit tumor growth. For this reason, Wang et al. incorporated the CSF-1 receptor inhibitor BLZ-945 in a pH-responsive polymeric micelle coated with an erythrocyte-tumor cell hybrid membrane. The resulting micelles depleted TAMs and significantly inhibited 4T1 breast cancer tumor growth in mice (Wang et al. 2020). Another strategy to reverse immunosuppression is via direct elimination of TAMs in the TME. In a recent study by Tian et al. lipid-coated calcium bisphosphonates NPs were developed to deplete TAMs, which indeed resulted in a tumor-suppressing effect (Tian et al. 2018).

The presence of myeloid cells such as TAMs and MDSCs contributes to overall immune system suppression in tumors and it is consequently associated with poor prognosis (Santegoets et al. 2014). While it seems compelling to deplete these cells for therapeutic purposes, caution should be exercised, as unselective depletion of immune cells can potentially worsen clinical outcomes (Kowal et al. 2019; Bercovici et al. 2019). Moreover, data from human and mouse lung cancer found that tumor-infiltrating macrophage populations differ in their prognostic effects depending on their TAM markers, histologic location, and stage of disease (Yi et al. 2023; Casanova-Acebes et al. 2021). The immune landscape of estrogen receptor (ER) positive breast cancer was investigated by analyzing the transcriptional and functional aspects of tumors with invasive ductal carcinomas (IDC) and invasive lobular carcinomas (ILC). Macrophages, not T cells turned out to be the predominant immune cells infiltrating the tumor bed and differences in macrophage functions between IDCs and ILCs became obvious (Onkar et al. 2023). Therefore, a better understanding of the activation modes of infiltrating macrophages in the tumor microenvironment and more accurate delineation of the roles they play in different tumor types will enable the development of NPs that specifically target a subset/phenotype of immune cells within a specific tumor type and location. Fortunately, given the plasticity of these myeloid cells, it is possible to reprogram them and such approaches are increasingly explored. As an example, multiple studies have employed inorganic iron oxide NPs, as well as organic $CaCO_3$ (Chen et al. 2019) and cyclodextrin NPs (Zanganeh et al. 2016; Rodell et al. 2018), to reprogram TAMs and polarize them toward a more benign M1 phenotype.

6.2 Targeting Lymph Nodes (LNs) and Antigen-Presenting Cells (APCs)

While modulating the TME is crucial to facilitate immune cell entry and preserve immune cell effector function, it is also important to boost immune cell functioning in lymphoid organs to promote anticancer immunotherapy efficacy. Consequently, there is growing interest in NPs targeting secondary lymphoid organs, like lymph nodes and the spleen, as they play an important role in antigen presentation and T-cell activation. Indeed, in cancer, the functioning of the immune system in these organs is often impaired (Hiam-Galvez et al. 2021). Nanomedicines can help restore immune system functioning, either indirectly by engaging APCs (Shi and Lammers 2019) or directly by enhancing T-cell function to attack cancer cells (Gong et al. 2021).

Research into the cancer-immunity cycle highlights that cancer cells downregulate antigen expression as a strategy to evade immune surveillance, making effective immunotherapy challenging (Chen and Mellman 2013). Cancer vaccines have emerged as a way to re-sensitize immune cells against cancer cells (Hollingsworth and Jansen 2019). In fact, several studies have used NPs to deliver antigens and adjuvants to APCs in lymph nodes following local (Kuai et al. 2017) or systemic administration (Liu et al. 2014). As a recent example, Moon and colleagues developed PEI-based nanovaccines incorporating neoantigens and CpG adjuvants (Nam et al. 2021). Upon local injection, the nanovaccines efficiently drained to LNs and promoted potent anticancer immunity against locally established and metastatic tumors (Nam et al. 2021).

Given the heterogeneity of tumors, it is generally acknowledged that the delivery of several antigens at the same time is preferable. This can be achieved with the help of lipid nanoparticle (LNP) platform technology. LNPs are composed of a mixture of lipids loaded nucleic acids, and they are typically condensed into 60–100 nm nanospheres. What is unique about LNPs is the incorporation of a special type of lipid, called "ionizable lipids." Ionizable lipids are positively charged at low pH and uncharged at physiological pH. This allows LNPs to efficiently encapsulate highly negatively charged mRNA/siRNA in small lipid pockets when fabricated at low pH. A shift toward neutral pH is applied to the LNPs prior to their injection in vivo which makes them much more biocompatible and enables them to travel safely in the blood.

The versatility of LNPs has enabled the delivery of different forms of RNAs, as well as the co-delivery of nucleic acids plus adjuvants, as a strategy to further increase the potency of vaccines and enhance anti-tumor immune responses. In this context, Oberli et al. used LNPs to encapsulate mRNA encoding gp100 and TRP2 antigens (Oberli et al. 2017). A strong cytotoxic T-cell response was observed

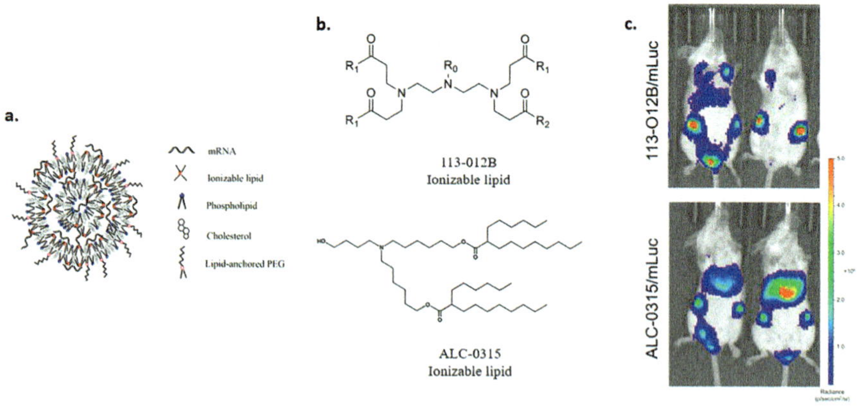

Fig. 5 mRNA LNP for selective lymph node targeting. (**a**) Schematic representation of LNP composition. (**b**) Structure of the ionizable lipids which display high levels of lymph node targeting (113-012B) vs. the structure of the ionizable lipid used in the Pfizer-BioNTech covid vaccine (ALC-0315). (**c**) Representative images of bioluminescence generation at 6 h after the injection of mice with the luciferase mRNA-loaded LNP, exemplifying more specific lymph node expression for 1130012B-containing LNPs. Figure adopted from Chen et al. (2022) with permission from NAS

following the transfection of various APCs (macrophages, DC, and B cells) with LNPs. The team also showcased the possibility of further prolonging survival in the B16F10 melanoma model by delivering an adjuvant alongside multiple antigens in LNPs (Oberli et al. 2017).

To reduce off-target effects and potentiate anti-tumor immunity, specific lymph node (LN) targeting may help. In this context, Chen et al. constructed mRNA-loaded LNPs using ionizable lipids that showed superior LN targeting as compared the more conventional ionizable lipids used in the Pfizer-BioNTech covid vaccine (Fig. 5). The LN-targeted mRNA vaccine elicited robust CD8+ T-cell responses and exhibited protective effects against lung metastasis in the B16F10 melanoma mouse model. The authors also tested the LNPs' capacity to deliver a variety of antigens, ranging from nucleic acids to whole proteins, highlighting the platform's versatility (Chen et al. 2022).

The number of antigens that can be delivered at once remains to be limited, and most NPs have so far served as delivery vehicles for TAA, leaving the opportunity open to explore them also for delivery of neoantigens, which are more immunogenic than TAA. Whole-cell tumor antigens have emerged as a way forward to allow for the delivery of an even broader antigen array and to elicit stronger anti-tumor immune responses (Chen et al. 2021). This strategy eliminates the need for the daunting and costly process of identifying and manufacturing neoantigens. In this context, Zhang and colleagues developed LNPs loaded with melittin, a cationic peptide that exerts its action through the induction of ICD and release of DAMPs. The NPs accumulated in draining LNs upon intratumoral injection and the nanovaccines efficiently promoted the release of whole-tumor antigens, which upon processing by locally present APCs led to a strong systemic anti-tumor immune response (Yu et al. 2020).

Although targeting APCs is a promising approach to activate T cells, some researchers have chosen to circumvent this process and directly target T cells instead. T cells are employed in immunotherapy due to their antigen-specific selectivity and their ability to induce cell death. The specificity of T cells can be further increased by genetically engineering them with chimeric antigen receptors (CARs). CARs allow T cells to specifically bind to antigens expressed on cancer cells, stimulating T-cell activity, proliferation, and cytokine release. The success of CAR T-cell therapy in preclinical and clinical trials has already led to multiple FDA/EMA-approved CAR T-cell therapies for hematopoietic tumors. However, complex procedures and technical expertise needed for ex vivo manipulation of T cells restrict their availability to a few clinical centers worldwide. Furthermore, the substantial cost of such treatment of nearly half a million USD limits its widespread accessibility (Smith et al. 2017).

Nanotechnology may offer possibilities to overcome this limitation by providing a less expensive platform for in vivo T-cell manipulation. For instance, Smith et al. used PLGA NPs encapsulating DNA to specifically target and transduce T cells in vivo. Currently, clinical trials are underway to assess the potential of this nanomaterial-based method of creating CAR T cells in vivo (Gong et al. 2021). An important drawback of this approach is that there is always the risk of DNA incorporation into the host genetic material, resulting in permanent changes. Fortunately, with RNA-LNP technology gradually advancing, researchers are exploring the transfection of T cells with mRNA because it provides nucleotide sequences that are ready for translation into proteins without changing the genetic code of the host cell (Smith et al. 2017). To further boost T-cell expansion in vivo and immunotherapy, mRNA LNP vaccines have also already been co-infused with CAR T cells (Reinhard et al. 2020).

Other approaches for enhancing T-cell functioning using NPs include the delivery of cytokines, such as IL-2 and tumor necrosis factor alpha (TNF-a) (Zheng et al. 2013; Stephan et al. 2010), or pharmacological targeting of the T-cell exhaustion pathways such as STAT3/STAT5 pathway using small molecule inhibitors (Schmid et al. 2017; Zheng et al. 2017). Several studies have utilized NPs to co-deliver immune stimulatory molecules and immunesuppression inhibitors concurrently, because of the separate success of using cytokines to stimulate immune responses and inhibitors to prevent immunesuppression (Kosmides et al. 2017; Park et al. 2012; Zhang et al. 2018). For more selective in vivo T-cell expansion, nanomaterials loaded with cytokines or/and small therapeutic agents can be anchored on the cell wall of T cells, resulting in T-cell expansion in a pseudo-autocrine manner while simultaneously inhibiting tumor growth (Tang et al. 2018).

In solid tumors, the presence of a dense extracellular matrix (ECM) barrier and the immunosuppressive environment hinder T-cell functioning. Therefore, effective strategies to enhance T-cell activity against solid tumors should involve the modulation of tumor microenvironment in terms of reducing the ECM (Huang et al. 2020) as well as blocking immunosuppressive cells (Zhang et al. 2018). The former can be established by using nanomaterials to target and degrade the dense ECM, thus improving the infiltration of T cells within the tumor (Huang et al. 2020). In this context, Goa, Chen, and colleagues developed a core-shell calcium phosphate liposome which they termed "Nano-sapper" and co-loaded it with the antifibrotic agent α-mangostin and plasmid DNA encoding for TNF-α (Fig. 6). The resulting NPs decreased collagen production by activated fibroblasts, made the TME more permeable for T-cell infiltration, and potentiated the anti-tumor effect of checkpoint inhibitors in a pancreatic ductal adenocarcinoma mouse model (PDAC) (Huang et al. 2020).

As an alternative approach, to compensate for the loss of cancer antigens, nanomaterials can be used to decrease the proximity between immune cells and cancer cells, thereby facilitating cancer cell killing by T cells (Yuan et al. 2017). This was shown with the development of nanomaterial-based bispecific T-cell engagers (nBITNEs). These are NP functionalized with antibodies that target both the cytotoxic T cells in the body and the cancer cells, facilitating their interaction leading to the induction of tumor cell death.

6.3 Bone Marrow Targeting

The bone marrow (BM) is responsible for the production and development of blood cells. Apart from its importance in hematopoiesis, the BM also plays a critical role in host immunity. It harbors various immune cells which are essential for protecting the body against infections and cancer. Many malignancies, particularly hematopoietic tumors such as leukemia and lymphoma, affect the bone marrow and result in the overproduction of abnormal blood cells (Sou et al. 2011; Mu et al. 2018). Solid tumors can hijack the hematopoietic system to ensure a continuous supply of TAMs and MDSCs, which promote tumor growth (Wu et al. 2020). Thus, both in hematological and solid cancer types, the BM plays a crucial role, justifying the search for therapeutic strategies that aim at modulating the BM.

Chemotherapeutic agents can efficiently suppress the BM, but their use is limited by their high toxicity and their inability to target specific subsets of cells (Cruz et al. 2022). Although ex vivo gene correction of hematopoietic stem cell (HSC) transfer would be a promising approach, this method is limited by its complexity, the high costs, the need for large numbers of HSC, and the high morbidity associated with the procedure (Cruz et al. 2022). In spite of its potential, the BM thus remains to be a challenging target for targeted drug delivery, due to its relatively low blood volume and its complex environment, which act as biological barriers that restrict NPs from entering the tissue.

The literature shows that nanoformulations can target specific cell types within the BM, either passively by making use of the natural propensity of NPs for uptake by BM cells or actively by using ligands or antibodies on the NPs that recognize receptors expressed on the surface of BM cells (Sou et al. 2011; Cruz et al. 2022). In fact, different NP platforms including lipid-based, polymer-based, and metal-based NPs have shown promising results in this regard in preclinical studies (Cruz et al. 2022). For instance, Mann et al. demonstrated that biodegradable polymeric NPs

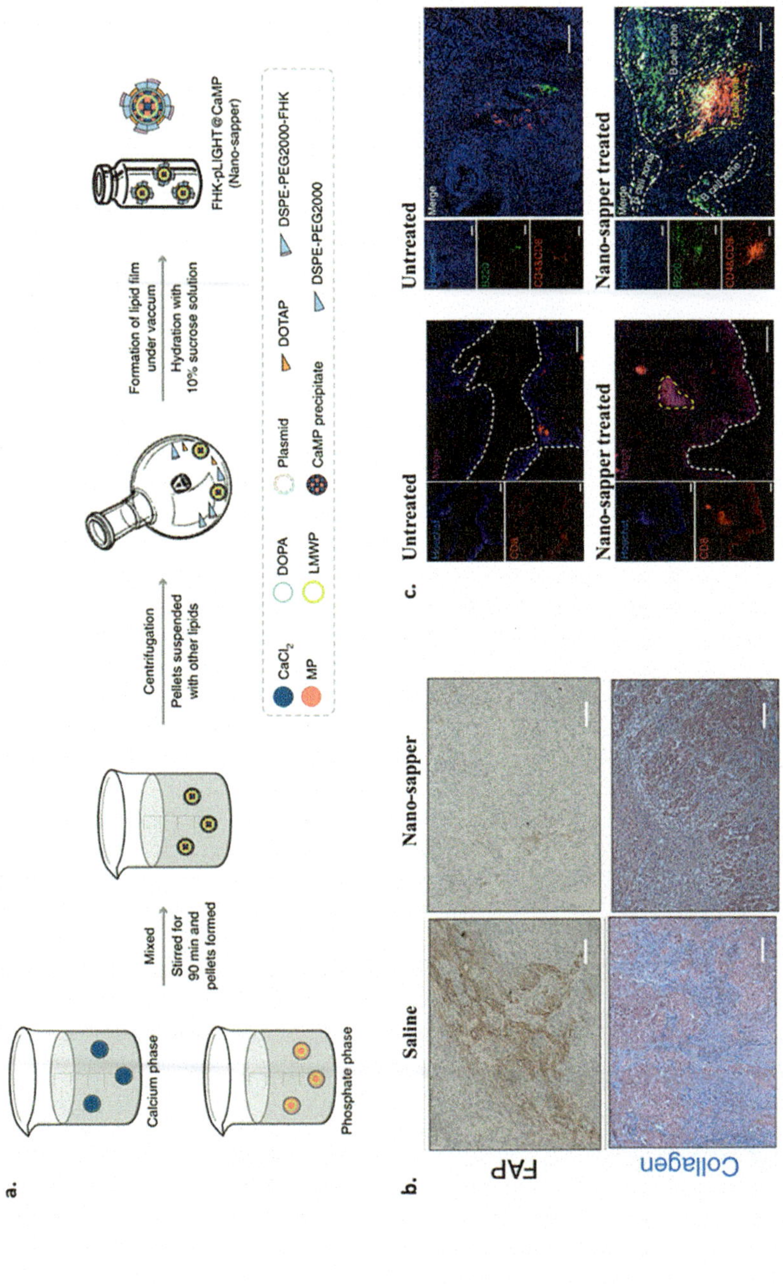

Fig. 6 Use of NPs to prime the TME and promote immune cell infiltration. (**a**) Schematic depiction of the method of preparation of the “Nano-sapper” platform, via reversed-phase microemulsion followed by thin-film hydration. (**b**) Tumor slices stained for fibroblast activation protein (FAP) and collagen demonstrating

Fig. 6 (continued) the ability of the Nano-sapper to reverse CAF activation and reduce collagen deposition in a PDAC mouse model. (**c**) The Nano-sapper formulation enhanced the infiltration of cytotoxic T lymphocytes (CTLs) and initiated the formation of tertiary lymphoid structure (TLSs) in the TME. Figure adopted from Huang et al. (2020)

functionalized with E-selectin ligands preferentially target BM endothelial cells (Mann et al. 2011). Other groups of scientists used LNPs containing siRNA to efficiently silence target genes in the BM microenvironment with the potential of improving the outcome of stem cell transplantation (Sago et al. 2018; Krohn-Grimberghe et al. 2020). Mitchell and colleagues used bisphosphonate lipid-like NPs to deliver mRNA to cells in the BM microenvironment, to make them produce proteins, which could lead to applications such as protein replacement and gene editing Xue et al. (2022). It is expected that these and follow-up developments in the nanomedicine field will open up new treatment paradigms for BM-related diseases and will offer alternatives to conventional ex vivo HSC gene correction therapies.

7 Identifying Optimal Nano-immunotherapy Regimens

Advances in the field of nanomedicine have created many opportunities and approaches for (more) effective immunomodulatory treatment of a range of different cancer types. We now need to be increasingly capable of making rational decisions about when and how to best target a specific subset of immune cells and/or when and how to best target a specific pathway.

Biomarkers offer solutions here, as they help to stratify patients to see who is amenable for which specific targeting approach or immuno-intervention. It is for this reason that the cancer immunogram and the immunoscore were developed, which are scoring systems based on clinical data and histology. These scoring systems allow for patient stratification and prognosis prediction based on a patient's individual tumor immune profile. The immunogram uses seven parameters to describe the interaction between an individual's immune system and cancer (Blank et al. 2016). The immunoscore determines the density of immune cell infiltration within and around tumors, classifying tumors into distinct four phenotypes: absent, altered-excluded, altered-immunosuppressed, and optimal Galon et al. (2006). Based on these phenotypes, a decision can be made as to which (nano)immunotherapy best fits the patient. For instance, patients who present with an altered-excluded tumor phenotype, i.e., who show low levels of cytotoxic T-cell infiltration, may likely benefit from nanomedicines that reshape the TME. Available options could include NPs loaded with agents that reduce the formation of fibrotic shields or NPs that degrade the extracellular matrix, thereby promoting T-cell penetration into the tumor bed.

While biomarkers are undeniably enormously valuable, it is important to acknowledge that cancer is a dynamic disease and that cancer–immune system interactions change during the course of disease progression. As a result, also the physical, metabolic, and cellular microenvironment changes, thereby dynamically impacting immune cell function and the efficacy of (nano)immunotherapy. We consequently have to acknowledge that there is a dire need for new and better biomarkers that will enable pragmatic and specific longitudinal monitoring of besides tumorous features also elements of the local and systemic immune system, to be able to adapt treatment options accordingly.

8 Conclusion

The ability of NPs to interact with the immune system has triggered a great body of research. This is not only aimed at ways to avoid interactions with the immune system, to thereby improving NPs' pharmacokinetic behavior and tumor-targeted drug delivery, but also at ways to actively engage with and modulate immune cells, to boost anti-tumor immune responses. Better understanding how NPs can be optimized for cancer immunotherapy applications should be based on the ever-increasing body of knowledge on NP interactions with different immune cell subsets, including (but certainly not limited to) TAMs, MDSCs, and APCs, as well as B cells and T cells. While T-cell infiltration is currently clinically used as the main parameter to categorize tumors as hot or cold based on their immunogenicity, it is becoming more and more clear that a more extensive assessment and a more detailed characterization of immune cell dynamics (especially in tumors but likely also systemically) is necessary to help further boost (nano)immunotherapy outcomes. The treatment of cancer necessitates a multifaceted approach, with particular emphasis on immunotherapy due to its involvement of diverse immunesuppressive pathways and compensatory mechanisms. A number of clinical trials, including the one combining doxil and ICI yielded rather disappointing results due to the lack of understanding of the immune landscape prior to treatment and the lack of use of predictive biomarkers that could ensure successful treatment allocation for individual patients at the appropriate time. Additionally, it is important to note that the immune phenotype of the TME can undergo dynamic changes during treatment and over time as well as across tumor locations, including metastatic ones. Together, these data illustrate the crucial role biomarkers play in not only stratifying patients for the appropriate treatment (predictive biomarkers), but also in guiding the treatment regime depending on the patient's response to therapy (biomarkers of response). Starting materials used for formulating NPs can be intrinsically immunogenic. For instance, LNPs in vaccines have adjuvant activity, resulting in the production of inflammatory cytokines in lymph node. Comprehensive studies are needed to uncover the mechanisms by which this happens, as well as to understand how the properties of NPs can be tailored to skew immune responses in the right direction, so that eventually nanomaterials with predictable immune responses can be designed.

The success of lipid-based mRNA delivery platforms for vaccination purposes may well make therapeutic gene editing a mainstream treatment option for genetic diseases, thereby sparking hope for cancer patients. However, current LNP formulations still largely accumulate in the liver upon i.v. administration and extrahepatic delivery remains to be challenging. Nonetheless, it is foreseeable that by systematic and effective modifications to the lipid composition of the NPs, as well as by controllably changing critical quality aspects such as particle size, it should be possible to deliver nucleic acids more selectively to other target organs. Beyond this, selective NP delivery to and uptake by non-phagocytic immune cells may require modifications with targeted ligands. To this end, more research is needed to better understand how efficient different NPs are taken up by different immune cells in vivo, and which specific immune cell surface receptors can be addressed to promote NP targeting to and transfection of immune cells.

We consider NP targeting to the bone marrow an important future area of research, as it allows for modulation of immune cells at their origin. Via current advancements regarding the design of NPs that are increasingly able to reach BM (and other lymphoid tissues), it becomes now necessary to get more clarity on how to precisely target specific immune cells there, and how to precisely control the activities of the NPs inside myeloid and lymphoid cells. In this context, it is important to be aware of the fact that there are substantial differences in NP biodistribution and BM targeting between different animal species and humans, cautioning against extrapolating from one species to another and highlighting the importance of carefully choosing the right animal model when targeting the BM and lymphoid tissues with NPs, to obtain results that can be reliably translated into the clinic.

Altogether, despite the obvious need for much more research in multiple different directions, it seems safe to state that nanoformulations hold enormous potential for immunomodulation. This has recently been prominently showcased via the development of highly effective NP vaccines against COVID-19, and it is anticipated that in the very near future, NP formulations will also be widely used to improve immunotherapy responses in patients suffering from cancer.

References

Alexis F, Pridgen E, Molnar LK, Farokhzad OC (2008) Factors affecting the clearance and biodistribution of polymeric nanoparticles. Mol Pharm 5(4):505–515. https://doi.org/10.1021/mp800051m

Andorko JI, Jewell CM (2017) Designing biomaterials with immunomodulatory properties for tissue engineering and regenerative medicine. Bioeng Transl Med 2(2):139–155. https://doi.org/10.1002/btm2.10063

Bangham AD, Horne RW (1964) Negative staining of phospholipids and their structural modification by surface-active agents as observed in the electron microscope. J Mol Biol 8(5):660–668. Available from: https://linkinghub.elsevier.com/retrieve/pii/S0022283664801157

Bangham AD, Standish MM, Watkins JC (1965) Diffusion of univalent ions across the lamellae of swollen phospholipids. J Mol Biol 13(1):238–252. Available from: https://linkinghub.elsevier.com/retrieve/pii/S0022283665800936

Barenholz Y (2012) Doxil® – the first FDA-approved nano-drug: lessons learned. J Control Release 160(2):117–134. Available from: https://linkinghub.elsevier.com/retrieve/pii/S0168365912002301

Bercovici N, Guérin MV, Trautmann A, Donnadieu E (2019) The remarkable plasticity of macrophages: a chance to fight cancer. Front Immunol 10. https://doi.org/10.3389/fimmu.2019.01563/full

Biozzi G, Stiffel C (1965) The physiopathology of the reticuloendothelial cells of the liver and spleen. In: Progress in liver diseases. Elsevier, pp 166–191. Available from: https://linkinghub.elsevier.com/retrieve/pii/B9781483167565500189

Blanco E, Shen H, Ferrari M (2015) Principles of nanoparticle design for overcoming biological barriers to drug delivery. Nat Biotechnol 33(9):941–951. Available from: http://www.nature.com/articles/nbt.3330

Blank CU, Haanen JB, Ribas A, Schumacher TN (2016) The "cancer immunogram". Science 352(6286):658–660. https://doi.org/10.1126/science.aaf2834

Casanova-Acebes M, Dalla E, Leader AM, LeBerichel J, Nikolic J, Morales BM et al (2021) Tissue-resident macrophages provide a pro-tumorigenic niche to early NSCLC cells. Nature 595(7868):578–584. Available from: https://www.nature.com/articles/s41586-021-03651-8

Catanzaro E, Feron O, Skirtach AG, Krysko DV (2022) Immunogenic cell death and role of nanomaterials serving as therapeutic vaccine for personalized cancer immunotherapy. Front Immunol 13. https://doi.org/10.3389/fimmu.2022.925290/full

Chen DS, Mellman I (2013) Oncology meets immunology: the cancer-immunity cycle. Immunity 39(1):1–10. Available from: https://linkinghub.elsevier.com/retrieve/pii/S1074761313002963

Chen Q, Wang C, Zhang X, Chen G, Hu Q, Li H et al (2019) In situ sprayed bioresponsive immunotherapeutic gel for post-surgical cancer treatment. Nat Nanotechnol 14(1):89–97. Available from: http://www.nature.com/articles/s41565-018-0319-4

Chen J, Qiu M, Ye Z, Nyalile T, Li Y, Glass Z et al (2021) In situ cancer vaccination using lipidoid nanoparticles. Sci Adv 7(19). https://doi.org/10.1126/sciadv.abf1244

Chen J, Ye Z, Huang C, Qiu M, Song D, Li Y et al (2022) Lipid nanoparticle-mediated lymph node–targeting delivery of mRNA cancer vaccine elicits robust CD8 + T cell response. Proc Natl Acad Sci 119(34):e2207841119. https://doi.org/10.1073/pnas.2207841119

Cheng Y, Song S, Wu P, Lyu B, Qin M, Sun Y et al (2021) Tumor associated macrophages and TAMs-based anti-tumor nanomedicines. Adv Healthc Mater 10(18):2100590. https://doi.org/10.1002/adhm.202100590

Chu D, Gao J, Wang Z (2015) Neutrophil-mediated delivery of therapeutic nanoparticles across blood vessel barrier for treatment of inflammation and infection. ACS Nano 9(12): 11800–11811. https://doi.org/10.1021/acsnano.5b05583

Chu D, Zhao Q, Yu J, Zhang F, Zhang H, Wang Z (2016) Nanoparticle targeting of neutrophils for improved cancer immunotherapy. Adv Healthc Mater 5(9):1088–1093. https://doi.org/10.1002/adhm.201500998

Cruz LJ, Rezaei S, Grosveld F, Philipsen S, Eich C (2022) Nanoparticles targeting hematopoietic stem and progenitor cells: multimodal carriers for the treatment of hematological diseases. Front Genome Ed 4(2):87–94. Available from: http://www.ncbi.nlm.nih.gov/pubmed/9666682

Debayle M, Balloul E, Dembele F, Xu X, Hanafi M, Ribot F et al (2019) Zwitterionic polymer ligands: an ideal surface coating to totally suppress protein-nanoparticle corona formation? Biomaterials 219:119357. Available from: https://linkinghub.elsevier.com/retrieve/pii/S0142961219304569

Demento SL, Eisenbarth SC, Foellmer HG, Platt C, Caplan MJ, Mark Saltzman W et al (2009) Inflammasome-activating nanoparticles as modular systems for optimizing vaccine efficacy. Vaccine 27(23):3013–3021. Available from: https://linkinghub.elsevier.com/retrieve/pii/S0264410X09004393

Dobosz P, Dzieciątkowski T (2019) The intriguing history of cancer immunotherapy. Front Immunol 10. https://doi.org/10.3389/fimmu.2019.02965/full

Dunn GP, Bruce AT, Ikeda H, Old LJ, Schreiber RD (2002) Cancer immunoediting: from immunosurveillance to tumor escape. Nat Immunol 3(11):991–998. Available from: https://www.nature.com/articles/ni1102-991

Esfahani K, Roudaia L, Buhlaiga N, Del Rincon SV, Papneja N, Miller WH (2020) A review of cancer immunotherapy: from the past, to the present, to the future. Curr Oncol 27(12):87–97. Available from: https://www.mdpi.com/1718-7729/27/12/5223

Estephan ZG, Schlenoff PS, Schlenoff JB (2011) Zwitteration as an alternative to PEGylation. Langmuir 27(11):6794–6800. https://doi.org/10.1021/la200227b

Fadeel B (2019) Hide and Seek: nanomaterial interactions with the immune system. Front Immunol 10. https://doi.org/10.3389/fimmu.2019.00133/full

Galon J, Costes A, Sanchez-Cabo F, Kirilovsky A, Mlecnik B, Lagorce-Pagès C et al (2006) Type, density, and location of immune cells within human colorectal tumors predict clinical outcome. Science 313(5795):1960–1964. https://doi.org/10.1126/science.1129139

Gao J, Wang W, Pei Q, Lord MS, Yu H (2020) Engineering nanomedicines through boosting immunogenic cell death for improved cancer immunotherapy. Acta Pharmacol Sin 41(7): 986–994. Available from: http://www.nature.com/articles/s41401-020-0400-z

Gheibi Hayat SM, Bianconi V, Pirro M, Sahebkar A (2019) Stealth functionalization of biomaterials and nanoparticles by CD47 mimicry. Int J Pharm 569:118628. Available from: https://linkinghub.elsevier.com/retrieve/pii/S0378517319306738

Gong N, Sheppard NC, Billingsley MM, June CH, Mitchell MJ (2021) Nanomaterials for T-cell cancer immunotherapy. Nat Nanotechnol 16(1):25–36. Available from: http://www.nature.com/articles/s41565-020-00822-y

Gradishar WJ, Tjulandin S, Davidson N, Shaw H, Desai N, Bhar P et al (2005) Phase III trial of nanoparticle albumin-bound paclitaxel compared with polyethylated castor oil–based paclitaxel in women with breast cancer. J Clin Oncol 23(31):7794–7803. https://doi.org/10.1200/JCO.2005.04.937

Guillot A, Tacke F (2019) Liver macrophages: old dogmas and new insights. Hepatol Commun 3(6):730–743. Available from: https://journals.lww.com/02009842-201906000-00003

He H, Liu L, Morin EE, Liu M, Schwendeman A (2019) Survey of clinical translation of cancer nanomedicines – lessons learned from successes and failures. Acc Chem Res 52(9):2445–2461. https://doi.org/10.1021/acs.accounts.9b00228

Hiam-Galvez KJ, Allen BM, Spitzer MH (2021) Systemic immunity in cancer. Nat Rev Cancer 21(6):345–359. Available from: https://www.nature.com/articles/s41568-021-00347-z

Hirayama D, Iida T, Nakase H (2017) The phagocytic function of macrophage-enforcing innate immunity and tissue homeostasis. Int J Mol Sci 19(1):92. Available from: https://www.mdpi.com/1422-0067/19/1/92

Hollingsworth RE, Jansen K (2019) Turning the corner on therapeutic cancer vaccines. npj Vaccines 4(1):7. Available from: https://www.nature.com/articles/s41541-019-0103-y

Huang Y, Chen Y, Zhou S, Chen L, Wang J, Pei Y et al (2020) Dual-mechanism based CTLs infiltration enhancement initiated by nano-sapper potentiates immunotherapy against immune-excluded tumors. Nat Commun 11(1):622. Available from: https://www.nature.com/articles/s41467-020-14425-7

Ishihara J, Ishihara A, Sasaki K, Lee SS-Y, Williford J-M, Yasui M et al (2019) Targeted antibody and cytokine cancer immunotherapies through collagen affinity. Sci Transl Med 11(487). https://doi.org/10.1126/scitranslmed.aau3259

Jatzkewitz H (1954) Incorporation of physiologically-active substances into a colloidal blood plasma substitute. I. Incorporation of mescaline peptide into polyvinylpyrrolidone. Hoppe Seylers Z Physiol Chem 297(3–6):149–156. Available from: http://www.ncbi.nlm.nih.gov/pubmed/13221275

Johnson LT, Zhang D, Zhou K, Lee SM, Liu S, Dilliard SA et al (2022) Lipid nanoparticle (LNP) chemistry can endow unique in vivo RNA delivery fates within the liver that alter therapeutic outcomes in a cancer model. Mol Pharm 19(11):3973–3986. https://doi.org/10.1021/acs.molpharmaceut.2c00442

Kantoff PW, Higano CS, Shore ND, Berger ER, Small EJ, Penson DF et al (2010) Sipuleucel-T immunotherapy for castration-resistant prostate cancer. N Engl J Med 363(5):411–422. https://doi.org/10.1056/NEJMoa1001294

Korangath P, Barnett JD, Sharma A, Henderson ET, Stewart J, Yu S-H et al (2020) Nanoparticle interactions with immune cells dominate tumor retention and induce T cell–mediated tumor suppression in models of breast cancer. Sci Adv 6(13). https://doi.org/10.1126/sciadv.aay1601

Kosmides AK, Sidhom J-W, Fraser A, Bessell CA, Schneck JP (2017) Dual targeting nanoparticle stimulates the immune system to inhibit tumor growth. ACS Nano 11(6):5417–5429. https://doi.org/10.1021/acsnano.6b08152

Kou L, Bhutia YD, Yao Q, He Z, Sun J, Ganapathy V (2018) Transporter-guided delivery of nanoparticles to improve drug permeation across cellular barriers and drug exposure to selective cell types. Front Pharmacol 9. https://doi.org/10.3389/fphar.2018.00027/full

Kowal J, Kornete M, Joyce JA (2019) Re-education of macrophages as a therapeutic strategy in cancer. Immunotherapy 11(8):677–689. https://doi.org/10.2217/imt-2018-0156

Krohn-Grimberghe M, Mitchell MJ, Schloss MJ, Khan OF, Courties G, Guimaraes PPG et al (2020) Nanoparticle-encapsulated siRNAs for gene silencing in the haematopoietic stem-cell niche. Nat Biomed Eng 4(11):1076–1089. Available from: https://www.nature.com/articles/s41551-020-00623-7

Kuai R, Ochyl LJ, Bahjat KS, Schwendeman A, Moon JJ (2017) Designer vaccine nanodiscs for personalized cancer immunotherapy. Nat Mater 16(4):489–496. Available from: https://www.nature.com/articles/nmat4822

Laplagne C, Domagala M, Le Naour A, Quemerais C, Hamel D, Fournié J-J et al (2019) Latest advances in targeting the tumor microenvironment for tumor suppression. Int J Mol Sci 20(19):4719. Available from: https://www.mdpi.com/1422-0067/20/19/4719

Larionova I, Tuguzbaeva G, Ponomaryova A, Stakheyeva M, Cherdyntseva N, Pavlov V et al (2020) Tumor-associated macrophages in human breast, colorectal, lung, ovarian and prostate cancers. Front Oncol 10. https://doi.org/10.3389/fonc.2020.566511/full

Lesniak A, Fenaroli F, Monopoli MP, Åberg C, Dawson KA, Salvati A (2012) Effects of the presence or absence of a protein corona on silica nanoparticle uptake and impact on cells. ACS Nano 6(7):5845–5857

Li H-J, Du J-Z, Du X-J, Xu C-F, Sun C-Y, Wang H-X et al (2016) Stimuli-responsive clustered nanoparticles for improved tumor penetration and therapeutic efficacy. Proc Natl Acad Sci 113(15):4164–4169. https://doi.org/10.1073/pnas.1522080113

Li X, Guo X, Ling J, Tang Z, Huang G, He L et al (2021) Nanomedicine-based cancer immunotherapies developed by reprogramming tumor-associated macrophages. Nanoscale 13(9):4705–4727. Available from: http://xlink.rsc.org/?DOI=D0NR08050K

Lin ZP, Nguyen LNM, Ouyang B, MacMillan P, Ngai J, Kingston BR et al (2022) Macrophages actively transport nanoparticles in tumors after extravasation. ACS Nano 16(4):6080–6092. https://doi.org/10.1021/acsnano.1c11578

Liu H, Moynihan KD, Zheng Y, Szeto GL, Li AV, Huang B et al (2014) Structure-based programming of lymph-node targeting in molecular vaccines. Nature 507(7493):519–522. Available from: http://www.nature.com/articles/nature12978

Liu Y, Wei G, Cheng WA, Dong Z, Sun H, Lee VY et al (2018) Targeting myeloid-derived suppressor cells for cancer immunotherapy. Cancer Immunol Immunother 67(8):1181–1195. https://doi.org/10.1007/s00262-018-2175-3

Maeda H, Matsumura Y (1989) Tumoritropic and lymphotropic principles of macromolecular drugs. Crit Rev Ther Drug Carrier Syst 6(3):193–210. Available from: http://www.ncbi.nlm.nih.gov/pubmed/2692843

Mann AP, Tanaka T, Somasunderam A, Liu X, Gorenstein DG, Ferrari M (2011) E-selectin-targeted porous silicon particle for nanoparticle delivery to the bone marrow. Adv Mater 23(36):H278–H282. https://doi.org/10.1002/adma.201101541

Mao C, Yeh S, Fu J, Porosnicu M, Thomas A, Kucera GL et al (2022) Delivery of an ectonucleotidase inhibitor with ROS-responsive nanoparticles overcomes adenosine-mediated cancer immunosuppression. Sci Transl Med 14(648):abh1261. https://doi.org/10.1126/scitranslmed.abh1261

Mathios D, Kim JE, Mangraviti A, Phallen J, Park C-K, Jackson CM et al (2016) Anti–PD-1 antitumor immunity is enhanced by local and abrogated by systemic chemotherapy in GBM. Sci Transl Med 8(370):370ra180. https://doi.org/10.1126/scitranslmed.aag2942

McCarthy EF (2006) The toxins of William B. Coley and the treatment of bone and soft-tissue sarcomas. Iowa Orthop J 26:154–158. Available from: http://www.ncbi.nlm.nih.gov/pubmed/16789469

Miao L, Lin CM, Huang L (2015) Stromal barriers and strategies for the delivery of nanomedicine to desmoplastic tumors. J Control Release 219:192–204. Available from: https://linkinghub.elsevier.com/retrieve/pii/S0168365915300638

Milstein C (1999) The hybridoma revolution: an offshoot of basic research. Bioessays 21(11): 966–973. Available from: http://www.ncbi.nlm.nih.gov/pubmed/10517870

Mitchell MJ, Billingsley MM, Haley RM, Wechsler ME, Peppas NA, Langer R (2021) Engineering precision nanoparticles for drug delivery. Nat Rev Drug Discov 20(2):101–124. Available from: http://www.nature.com/articles/s41573-020-0090-8

Mittal D, Gubin MM, Schreiber RD, Smyth MJ (2014) New insights into cancer immunoediting and its three component phases – elimination, equilibrium and escape. Curr Opin Immunol 27: 16–25. Available from: https://linkinghub.elsevier.com/retrieve/pii/S0952791514000053

Moon Y, Shim MK, Choi J, Yang S, Kim J, Yun WS et al (2022) Anti-PD-L1 peptide-conjugated prodrug nanoparticles for targeted cancer immunotherapy combining PD-L1 blockade with immunogenic cell death. Theranostics 12(5):1999–2014. Available from: https://www.thno.org/v12p1999.htm

Morgan DA, Ruscetti FW, Gallo R (1976) Selective in vitro growth of T lymphocytes from normal human bone marrows. Science 193(4257):1007–1008. https://doi.org/10.1126/science.181845

Mu C-F, Shen J, Liang J, Zheng H-S, Xiong Y, Wei Y-H et al (2018) Targeted drug delivery for tumor therapy inside the bone marrow. Biomaterials 155:191–202. Available from: https://linkinghub.elsevier.com/retrieve/pii/S0142961217307640

Murry DJ, Blaney SM (2000) Clinical pharmacology of encapsulated sustained-release cytarabine. Ann Pharmacother 34(10):1173–1178. https://doi.org/10.1345/aph.19347

Nam J, Son S, Park KS, Moon JJ (2021) Modularly programmable nanoparticle vaccine based on polyethyleneimine for personalized cancer immunotherapy. Adv Sci 8(5):2002577. https://doi.org/10.1002/advs.202002577

Ngai J, MacMillan P, Kingston BR, Lin ZP, Ouyang B, Chan WCW (2023) Delineating the tumour microenvironment response to a lipid nanoparticle formulation. J Control Release 353:988–1001. Available from: https://linkinghub.elsevier.com/retrieve/pii/S0168365922008355

Ngo W, Ahmed S, Blackadar C, Bussin B, Ji Q, Mladjenovic SM et al (2022) Why nanoparticles prefer liver macrophage cell uptake in vivo. Adv Drug Deliv Rev 185:114238. Available from: https://linkinghub.elsevier.com/retrieve/pii/S0169409X22001284

Oberli MA, Reichmuth AM, Dorkin JR, Mitchell MJ, Fenton OS, Jaklenec A et al (2017) Lipid nanoparticle assisted mRNA delivery for potent cancer immunotherapy. Nano Lett 17(3): 1326–1335. https://doi.org/10.1021/acs.nanolett.6b03329

Onkar S, Cui J, Zou J, Cardello C, Cillo AR, Uddin MR et al (2023) Immune landscape in invasive ductal and lobular breast cancer reveals a divergent macrophage-driven microenvironment. Nat Cancer. Available from: https://www.nature.com/articles/s43018-023-00527-w

Ouyang B, Kingston BR, Poon W, Zhang Y-N, Lin ZP, Syed AM et al (2022) Impact of tumor barriers on nanoparticle delivery to macrophages. Mol Pharm 19(6):1917–1925. https://doi.org/10.1021/acs.molpharmaceut.1c00905

Park J, Wrzesinski SH, Stern E, Look M, Criscione J, Ragheb R et al (2012) Combination delivery of TGF-β inhibitor and IL-2 by nanoscale liposomal polymeric gels enhances tumour immunotherapy. Nat Mater 11(10):895–905. Available from: https://www.nature.com/articles/nmat3355

Peer D, Karp JM, Hong S, Farokhzad OC, Margalit R, Langer R (2007) Nanocarriers as an emerging platform for cancer therapy. Nat Nanotechnol 2(12):751–760. Available from: http://www.nature.com/articles/nnano.2007.387

Ping Q, Yan R, Cheng X, Wang W, Zhong Y, Hou Z et al (2021) Cancer-associated fibroblasts: overview, progress, challenges, and directions. Cancer Gene Ther 28(9):984–999. Available from: https://www.nature.com/articles/s41417-021-00318-4

Poon W, Kingston BR, Ouyang B, Ngo W, Chan WCW (2020) A framework for designing delivery systems. Nat Nanotechnol 15(10):819–829. Available from: https://www.nature.com/articles/s41565-020-0759-5

Porter CJH, Trevaskis NL (2020) Targeting immune cells within lymph nodes. Nat Nanotechnol 15(6):423–425. Available from: http://www.nature.com/articles/s41565-020-0663-z

Ramishetti S, Kedmi R, Goldsmith M, Leonard F, Sprague AG, Godin B et al (2015) Systemic gene silencing in primary T lymphocytes using targeted lipid nanoparticles. ACS Nano 9(7): 6706–6716. https://doi.org/10.1021/acsnano.5b02796

Reinhard K, Rengstl B, Oehm P, Michel K, Billmeier A, Hayduk N et al (2020) An RNA vaccine drives expansion and efficacy of claudin-CAR-T cells against solid tumors. Science 367(6476): 446–453. https://doi.org/10.1126/science.aay5967

Ribas A, Wolchok JD (2018) Cancer immunotherapy using checkpoint blockade. Science 359(6382):1350–1355. https://doi.org/10.1126/science.aar4060

Rodell CB, Arlauckas SP, Cuccarese MF, Garris CS, Li R, Ahmed MS et al (2018) TLR7/8-agonist-loaded nanoparticles promote the polarization of tumour-associated macrophages to enhance cancer immunotherapy. Nat Biomed Eng 2(8):578–588. Available from: https://www.nature.com/articles/s41551-018-0236-8

Rosenberg SA, Restifo NP (2015) Adoptive cell transfer as personalized immunotherapy for human cancer. Science 348(6230):62–68. https://doi.org/10.1126/science.aaa4967

Rosenblum D, Joshi N, Tao W, Karp JM, Peer D (2018) Progress and challenges towards targeted delivery of cancer therapeutics. Nat Commun 9(1):1410. Available from: https://www.nature.com/articles/s41467-018-03705-y

Rostam HM, Fisher LE, Hook AL, Burroughs L, Luckett JC, Figueredo GP et al (2020) Immune-instructive polymers control macrophage phenotype and modulate the foreign body response in vivo. Matter 2(6):1564–1581. Available from: https://linkinghub.elsevier.com/retrieve/pii/S2590238520301314

Rudnicka D, Oszmiana A, Finch DK, Strickland I, Schofield DJ, Lowe DC et al (2013) Rituximab causes a polarization of B cells that augments its therapeutic function in NK-cell–mediated antibody-dependent cellular cytotoxicity. Blood 121(23):4694–4702. Available from: https://ashpublications.org/blood/article/121/23/4694/31468/Rituximab-causes-a-polarization-of-B-cells-that

Sago CD, Lokugamage MP, Islam FZ, Krupczak BR, Sato M, Dahlman JE (2018) Nanoparticles that deliver RNA to bone marrow identified by in vivo directed evolution. J Am Chem Soc 140(49):17095–17105. https://doi.org/10.1021/jacs.8b08976

Saleh R, Elkord E (2019) Treg-mediated acquired resistance to immune checkpoint inhibitors. Cancer Lett 457:168–179. Available from: https://linkinghub.elsevier.com/retrieve/pii/S0304383519302794

Salemme V, Centonze G, Cavallo F, Defilippi P, Conti L (2021) The crosstalk between tumor cells and the immune microenvironment in breast cancer: implications for immunotherapy. Front Oncol 11. https://doi.org/10.3389/fonc.2021.610303/full

Salvati A, Pitek AS, Monopoli MP, Prapainop K, Bombelli FB, Hristov DR et al (2013) Transferrin-functionalized nanoparticles lose their targeting capabilities when a biomolecule corona adsorbs on the surface. Nat Nanotechnol 8(2):137–143. Available from: http://www.nature.com/articles/nnano.2012.237

Santegoets SJ, Stam AG, Lougheed SM, Gall H, Jooss K, Sacks N et al (2014) Myeloid derived suppressor and dendritic cell subsets are related to clinical outcome in prostate cancer patients treated with prostate GVAX and ipilimumab. J Immunother Cancer 2(1):31. https://doi.org/10.1186/s40425-014-0031-3

Scheffel U, Rhodes BA, Natarajan TK, Wagner HN (1972) Albumin microspheres for study of the reticuloendothelial system. J Nucl Med 13(7):498–503. Available from: http://www.ncbi.nlm.nih.gov/pubmed/5033902

Schmid D, Park CG, Hartl CA, Subedi N, Cartwright AN, Puerto RB et al (2017) T cell-targeting nanoparticles focus delivery of immunotherapy to improve antitumor immunity. Nat Commun 8(1):1747. Available from: https://www.nature.com/articles/s41467-017-01830-8

Sharp FA, Ruane D, Claass B, Creagh E, Harris J, Malyala P et al (2009) Uptake of particulate vaccine adjuvants by dendritic cells activates the NALP3 inflammasome. Proc Natl Acad Sci 106(3):870–875. https://doi.org/10.1073/pnas.0804897106

Sharpe AH, Pauken KE (2018) The diverse functions of the PD1 inhibitory pathway. Nat Rev Immunol 18(3):153–167. Available from: https://www.nature.com/articles/nri.2017.108

Shi Y, Lammers T (2019) Combining nanomedicine and immunotherapy. Acc Chem Res 52(6): 1543–1554. https://doi.org/10.1021/acs.accounts.9b00148

Sindhwani S, Syed AM, Ngai J, Kingston BR, Maiorino L, Rothschild J et al (2020) The entry of nanoparticles into solid tumours. Nat Mater 19(5):566–575. Available from: https://www.nature.com/articles/s41563-019-0566-2

Smith BR, Ghosn EEB, Rallapalli H, Prescher JA, Larson T, Herzenberg LA et al (2014) Selective uptake of single-walled carbon nanotubes by circulating monocytes for enhanced tumour delivery. Nat Nanotechnol 9(6):481–487. Available from: http://www.nature.com/articles/nnano.2014.62

Smith TT, Stephan SB, Moffett HF, McKnight LE, Ji W, Reiman D et al (2017) In situ programming of leukaemia-specific T cells using synthetic DNA nanocarriers. Nat Nanotechnol 12(8): 813–820. Available from: http://www.nature.com/articles/nnano.2017.57

Sofias AM, Toner YC, Meerwaldt AE, van Leent MMT, Soultanidis G, Elschot M et al (2020) Tumor targeting by α v β 3 -integrin-specific lipid nanoparticles occurs via phagocyte hitchhiking. ACS Nano 14(7):7832–7846. https://doi.org/10.1021/acsnano.9b08693

Sofias AM, Bjørkøy G, Ochando J, Sønstevold L, Hegvik M, de Davies CL et al (2021) Cyclic arginine–glycine–aspartate-decorated lipid nanoparticle targeting toward inflammatory lesions involves hitchhiking with phagocytes. Adv Sci 8(13):2100370. https://doi.org/10.1002/advs.202100370

Solinas G, Germano G, Mantovani A, Allavena P (2009) Tumor-associated macrophages (TAM) as major players of the cancer-related inflammation. J Leukoc Biol 86(5):1065–1073. Available from: https://academic.oup.com/jleukbio/article/86/5/1065/6959976

Sou K, Goins B, Oyajobi BO, Travi BL, Phillips WT (2011) Bone marrow-targeted liposomal carriers. Expert Opin Drug Deliv 8(3):317–328. https://doi.org/10.1517/17425247.2011.553218

Stephan MT, Moon JJ, Um SH, Bershteyn A, Irvine DJ (2010) Therapeutic cell engineering with surface-conjugated synthetic nanoparticles. Nat Med 16(9):1035–1041. Available from: http://www.nature.com/articles/nm.2198

Tammam SN, Azzazy HME, Lamprecht A (2015) Biodegradable particulate carrier formulation and tuning for targeted drug delivery. J Biomed Nanotechnol 11(4):555–577. Available from: http://openurl.ingenta.com/content/xref?genre=articleandissn=1550-7033andvolume=11andissue=4andspage=555

Tang L, Zheng Y, Melo MB, Mabardi L, Castaño AP, Xie Y-Q et al (2018) Enhancing T cell therapy through TCR-signaling-responsive nanoparticle drug delivery. Nat Biotechnol 36(8): 707–716. Available from: http://www.nature.com/articles/nbt.4181

Tang S, Ning Q, Yang L, Mo Z, Tang S (2020) Mechanisms of immune escape in the cancer immune cycle. Int Immunopharmacol 86:106700. Available from: https://linkinghub.elsevier.com/retrieve/pii/S1567576920311140

Tarab-Ravski D, Hazan-Halevy I, Goldsmith M, Stotsky-Oterin L, Breier D, Naidu GS et al (2023) Delivery of therapeutic RNA to the bone marrow in multiple myeloma using CD38-targeted lipid nanoparticles. Adv Sci. https://doi.org/10.1002/advs.202301377

Tavares AJ, Poon W, Zhang Y-N, Dai Q, Besla R, Ding D et al (2017) Effect of removing Kupffer cells on nanoparticle tumor delivery. Proc Natl Acad Sci 114(51). https://doi.org/10.1073/pnas.1713390114

Tenzer S, Docter D, Kuharev J, Musyanovych A, Fetz V, Hecht R et al (2013) Rapid formation of plasma protein corona critically affects nanoparticle pathophysiology. Nat Nanotechnol 8(10): 772–781. Available from: http://www.nature.com/articles/nnano.2013.181

Tesi RJ (2019) MDSC; the most important cell you have never heard of. Trends Pharmacol Sci 40(1):4–7

Tian L, Yi X, Dong Z, Xu J, Liang C, Chao Y et al (2018) Calcium bisphosphonate nanoparticles with chelator-free radiolabeling to deplete tumor-associated macrophages for enhanced cancer radioisotope therapy. ACS Nano 12(11):11541–11551. https://doi.org/10.1021/acsnano.8b06699

Tsoi KM, MacParland SA, Ma X-Z, Spetzler VN, Echeverri J, Ouyang B et al (2016) Mechanism of hard-nanomaterial clearance by the liver. Nat Mater 15(11):1212–1221. Available from: https://www.nature.com/articles/nmat4718

Valkenburg KC, de Groot AE, Pienta KJ (2018) Targeting the tumour stroma to improve cancer therapy. Nat Rev Clin Oncol 15(6):366–381. Available from: http://www.nature.com/articles/s41571-018-0007-1

Varnamkhasti BS, Hosseinzadeh H, Azhdarzadeh M, Vafaei SY, Esfandyari-Manesh M, Mirzaie ZH et al (2015) Protein corona hampers targeting potential of MUC1 aptamer functionalized SN-38 core–shell nanoparticles. Int J Pharm 494(1):430–444. Available from: https://linkinghub.elsevier.com/retrieve/pii/S0378517315301575

Veiga N, Diesendruck Y, Peer D (2023) Targeted nanomedicine: lessons learned and future directions. J Control Release 355:446–457. Available from: https://linkinghub.elsevier.com/retrieve/pii/S0168365923001049

Wang Y, Luan Z, Zhao C, Bai C, Yang K (2020) Target delivery selective CSF-1R inhibitor to tumor-associated macrophages via erythrocyte-cancer cell hybrid membrane camouflaged pH-responsive copolymer micelle for cancer immunotherapy. Eur J Pharm Sci 142:105136. Available from: https://linkinghub.elsevier.com/retrieve/pii/S0928098719304099

Wilhelm S, Tavares AJ, Dai Q, Ohta S, Audet J, Dvorak HF et al (2016) Analysis of nanoparticle delivery to tumours. Nat Rev Mater 1(5):16014. Available from: https://www.nature.com/articles/natrevmats201614

Wu C, Hua Q, Zheng L (2020) Generation of myeloid cells in cancer: the spleen matters. Front Immunol 11. https://doi.org/10.3389/fimmu.2020.01126/full

Wu F, Xu X, Li W, Hong Y, Lai H, Zhang J et al (2022) Nanoparticle-delivered transforming growth factor-β1 siRNA induces PD-1 against gastric cancer by transforming the phenotype of the tumor immune microenvironment. Pharmaceuticals 15(12):1487. Available from: https://www.mdpi.com/1424-8247/15/12/1487

Xie Y, Wei L, Tang L (2018) Immunoengineering with biomaterials for enhanced cancer immunotherapy. WIREs Nanomed Nanobiotechnol 10(4):e1506. https://doi.org/10.1002/wnan.1506

Xue L, Gong N, Shepherd SJ, Xiong X, Liao X, Han X et al (2022) Rational design of bisphosphonate lipid-like materials for mRNA delivery to the bone microenvironment. J Am Chem Soc 144(22):9926–9937. https://doi.org/10.1021/jacs.2c02706

Yang S, Shim MK, Kim WJ, Choi J, Nam G-H, Kim J et al (2021) Cancer-activated doxorubicin prodrug nanoparticles induce preferential immune response with minimal doxorubicin-related toxicity. Biomaterials 272:120791. Available from: https://linkinghub.elsevier.com/retrieve/pii/S0142961221001472

Yi B, Cheng Y, Chang R, Zhou W, Tang H, Gao Y et al (2023) Prognostic significance of tumor-associated macrophages polarization markers in lung cancer: a pooled analysis of 5105 patients. Biosci Rep 43(2) Available from: https://portlandpress.com/bioscirep/article/43/2/BSR20221659/232437/Prognostic-significance-of-tumor-associated

Yong S, Ramishetti S, Goldsmith M, Diesendruck Y, Hazan-Halevy I, Chatterjee S et al (2022) Dual-targeted lipid nanotherapeutic boost for chemo-immunotherapy of cancer. Adv Mater 34(13):2106350. https://doi.org/10.1002/adma.202106350

Yousefpour P, Ni K, Irvine DJ (2023) Targeted modulation of immune cells and tissues using engineered biomaterials. Nat Rev Bioeng 1(2):107–124. Available from: https://www.nature.com/articles/s44222-022-00016-2

Yu X, Dai Y, Zhao Y, Qi S, Liu L, Lu L et al (2020) Melittin-lipid nanoparticles target to lymph nodes and elicit a systemic anti-tumor immune response. Nat Commun 11(1):1110. Available from: https://www.nature.com/articles/s41467-020-14906-9

Yuan H, Jiang W, von Roemeling CA, Qie Y, Liu X, Chen Y et al (2017) Multivalent bi-specific nanobioconjugate engager for targeted cancer immunotherapy. Nat Nanotechnol 12(8):763–769. Available from: http://www.nature.com/articles/nnano.2017.69

Zanganeh S, Hutter G, Spitler R, Lenkov O, Mahmoudi M, Shaw A, et al (2016) Iron oxide nanoparticles inhibit tumour growth by inducing pro-inflammatory macrophage polarization in tumour tissues. Nat Nanotechnol [Internet]. 11(11):986–994. Available from: http://www.nature.com/articles/nnano.2016.168

Zhang Y-N, Poon W, Tavares AJ, McGilvray ID, Chan WCW (2016) Nanoparticle–liver interactions: cellular uptake and hepatobiliary elimination. J Control Release 240:332–348. Available from: https://linkinghub.elsevier.com/retrieve/pii/S0168365916300190

Zhang F, Stephan SB, Ene CI, Smith TT, Holland EC, Stephan MT (2018) Nanoparticles that reshape the tumor milieu create a therapeutic window for effective T-cell therapy in solid malignancies. Cancer Res 78(13):3718–3730. Available from: https://aacrjournals.org/cancerres/article/78/13/3718/625172/Nanoparticles-That-Reshape-the-Tumor-Milieu-Create

Zheng Y, Stephan MT, Gai SA, Abraham W, Shearer A, Irvine DJ (2013) In vivo targeting of adoptively transferred T-cells with antibody- and cytokine-conjugated liposomes. J Control Release 172(2):426–435. Available from: https://linkinghub.elsevier.com/retrieve/pii/S0168365913003295

Zheng Y, Tang L, Mabardi L, Kumari S, Irvine DJ (2017) Enhancing adoptive cell therapy of cancer through targeted delivery of small-molecule Immunomodulators to internalizing or noninternalizing receptors. ACS Nano 11(3):3089–3100. https://doi.org/10.1021/acsnano.7b00078

Zhu Y, Yu F, Tan Y, Yuan H, Hu F (2019) Strategies of targeting pathological stroma for enhanced antitumor therapies. Pharmacol Res 148:104401. Available from: https://linkinghub.elsevier.com/retrieve/pii/S1043661819306814

Progress in Ocular Drug Delivery: Challenges and Constraints

Ilva D. Rupenthal and Priyanka Agarwal

Contents

Abstract

The eye has several dynamic and static barriers in place to limit the entry of foreign substances including therapeutics. As such, efficient drug delivery, especially to posterior segment tissues, has been challenging. This chapter describes the anatomical and physiological challenges associated with ocular drug delivery before discussing constraints with regard to formulation parameters. Finally, it gives an overview of advanced drug delivery technologies with a specific focus on recently marketed and late-stage clinical trial products.

I. D. Rupenthal (✉) · P. Agarwal
Buchanan Ocular Therapeutics Unit, Department of Ophthalmology, New Zealand National Eye Centre, Faculty of Medical and Health Sciences, The University of Auckland, Auckland, New Zealand
e-mail: i.rupenthal@auckland.ac.nz

M. Schäfer-Korting, U. S. Schubert (eds.), *Drug Delivery and Targeting*,
Handbook of Experimental Pharmacology 284, https://doi.org/10.1007/164_2023_693

Keywords

Dynamic barriers · Eye · Eyedrops · Intracameral implants · Intravitreal implants · Mucus-penetrating particles · Ocular drug delivery · Port delivery system · Punctum plug · Static barriers · Suprachoroidal injection

Abbreviations

BAB	Blood–aqueous barrier
BRB	Blood–retinal barrier
CNTF	Ciliary neurotrophic factor
EVA	Ethylene vinyl acetate
FA	Fluocinolone acetonide
FDA	Food and Drug Administration
MIGS	Micro-invasive glaucoma surgery
MPP	Mucus-penetrating particles
NDA	New drug application
PCL	Polycaprolactone
PDUFA	Prescription Drug User Fee Act
PLGA	Poly(lactic-co-glycolic)acid
PVA	Polyvinyl alcohol
RPE	Retinal pigment epithelium

1 Introduction

Eyedrops are the most commonly used therapeutics to treat ocular conditions, particularly those affecting the front of the eye, due to the eye's easy accessibility and constraints associated with systemic drug delivery to this rather isolated organ. Nevertheless, the unique dynamic and static barriers of the eye render it difficult to achieve effective drug concentrations from eyedrops at target sites other than the ocular surface, especially in the posterior segment of the eye. This is mainly due to fast nasolacrimal drainage limiting the formulation's precorneal residence time to less than 2 min (Gaudana et al. 2010) as well as the poor penetration across the outer ocular tissues further reducing the amount of drug penetrated. As such, drug bioavailability from conventional eyedrops is generally less than 10% (Le Bourlais et al. 1995) leading not only to low efficacy, but also posing potential risks due to systemic absorption of most of the given dose due to nasolacrimal drainage and subsequent absorption in the nasal cavity.

To overcome some of the limitations associated with conventional ocular drug delivery systems, efforts have mainly focussed on two strategies:

(i) to circumvent the dynamic barriers, particularly the fast precorneal clearance, by using particulate (Kim et al. 2015), mucoadhesive (Ruponen and Urtti 2015), viscosity enhancing (Pahuja et al. 2012) or in situ gelling systems (Rupenthal et al. 2011a, b; Thrimawithana et al. 2012) as well as utilizing drug-device combinations (Rupenthal 2017); and

(ii) to increase penetration across the static ocular barriers, particularly the cornea, using prodrugs (Taskar et al. 2017), penetration enhancers and colloidal systems, such as nanoparticles (Joseph and Venkatraman 2017), liposomes (Agarwal et al. 2016), or micelles (Mandal et al. 2017).

However, even when combining these two strategies, topically applied systems are generally unable to deliver sufficient drug to the back of the eye, which is why other delivery routes, such as intravitreal (Thakur et al. 2014), periocular (Agban et al. 2019), and suprachoroidal (Jung et al. 2019) have emerged to treat posterior segment conditions.

This book chapter will give an overview of the anatomical and physiological challenges associated with ocular drug delivery, highlighting dynamic and static ocular barriers, and discussing general approaches to overcome these. Constraints regarding formulation parameters are then further discussed before highlighting advanced delivery approaches and technologies with a focus on recently marketed and late-stage clinical trial products.

2 Anatomical and Physiological Challenges

Although a few drugs used to treat ocular conditions may be taken up via active transport, the majority of molecules penetrate into the ocular tissues via passive diffusion. As such, maintaining a high concentration gradient at the application site by circumventing some of the dynamic barriers is pertinent to facilitate passive diffusion into the ocular tissues. Yet, drug and formulation characteristics described below still need to be taken into account to efficiently overcome the static ocular barriers (Agarwal et al. 2021).

2.1 Dynamic Barriers

Dynamic barriers refer to clearance mechanisms that reduce the drug concentration at the site of administration as well as in ocular tissues. After application of an eyedrop to the ocular surface, the first dynamic barriers encountered include blinking, nasolacrimal drainage as well as basal and reflex tearing. The conjunctival sac, which serves as a reservoir for the applied eyedrop, usually holds about 7–8 μl of tear fluid but can extend to a maximum capacity of 30 μl (Järvinen et al. 1995). Yet, the drop volume dispensed from conventional droppers is generally more than 40 μl (Lederer and Harold 1986), although dependent on the surface tension of the eyedrop vehicle, resulting in immediate overflow which leads to drug loss as well as systemic drug absorption due to nasolacrimal drainage and subsequent absorption in the nasal cavity (Järvinen et al. 1995; Lee and Robinson 1986). It is thought that less than 10 μl of the applied volume remains on the ocular surface following a single blink, leaving a short window of approximately 5–7 min for drug absorption, especially when rapid tear fluid turnover (19.7 ± 6.5%/min) is taken into account (Pearce et al. 2011). Dynamic ocular processes aim to achieve ocular surface homeostasis immediately after eyedrop instillation by reflex blinking and tearing, especially if formulation parameters, as discussed in the next section, are not optimal.

Since many chronic ocular conditions require administration of more than one eyedrop several times a day, washout phenomena also need to be considered (Saarinen-Savolainen et al. 1998), with a negative correlation between time interval and corneal drug concentrations of concurrently administered drugs (Leibowitz and Kupferman 1977; Yamada et al. 2003). Corneal drug concentrations after administration of a single eyedrop containing two drugs, on the other hand, are similar to those observed after administration of each eyedrop individually (Leibowitz and Kupferman 1977). This suggests that combination eyedrops capable of simultaneously treating more than one underlying disease pathology may improve overall treatment efficacy compared to the individual eyedrops administered concurrently.

Besides ocular surface-related barriers, other dynamic processes also play a significant role. These include aqueous humor production and drainage (Goel et al. 2010) as well as diffusive and convective flow in the vitreous (Laude et al. 2010). Moreover, several studies have demonstrated that drugs in many ocular tissues are cleared rapidly via blood and lymphatic vessels (Gausas et al. 1999; Singh 2003), especially via choroidal blood flow, which accounts for 85% of total blood flow in the eye (Kim et al. 2008). Finally, efflux pumps and other transporters in the retinal pigment epithelium (RPE) may decrease ocular drug concentrations, particularly in the retina, by expelling solutes toward the choroid from where they get cleared (Dey and Mitra 2005; Jordán and Ruíz-Moreno 2013; Sellner 1986), although the physical barrier properties of the RPE, as discussed in the next section, may play a more significant role.

2.2 Static Barriers

Static barriers are formed by the various ocular tissues (Fig. 1), which due to their complex structure, with often alternating lipophilic and hydrophilic layers, further limit drug penetration into the eye, depending on the ocular drug delivery route utilized.

The first penetration barrier encountered after application of an eyedrop is the tear film, which comprises a superficial lipid "blanket" covering the aqueous layer with higher concentrations of membrane-associated mucins closer to the corneal surface (Georgiev et al. 2019). Often described as a "sticky net," particles may interact with surface mucins which increases their precorneal retention (Han et al. 2021), although they ultimately need to traverse the entire mucus layer for the drug to penetrate into the corneal epithelium (Lai et al. 2009). Once drugs and/or drug delivery systems have overcome the tear film, they encounter the cornea, with the hydrophobic

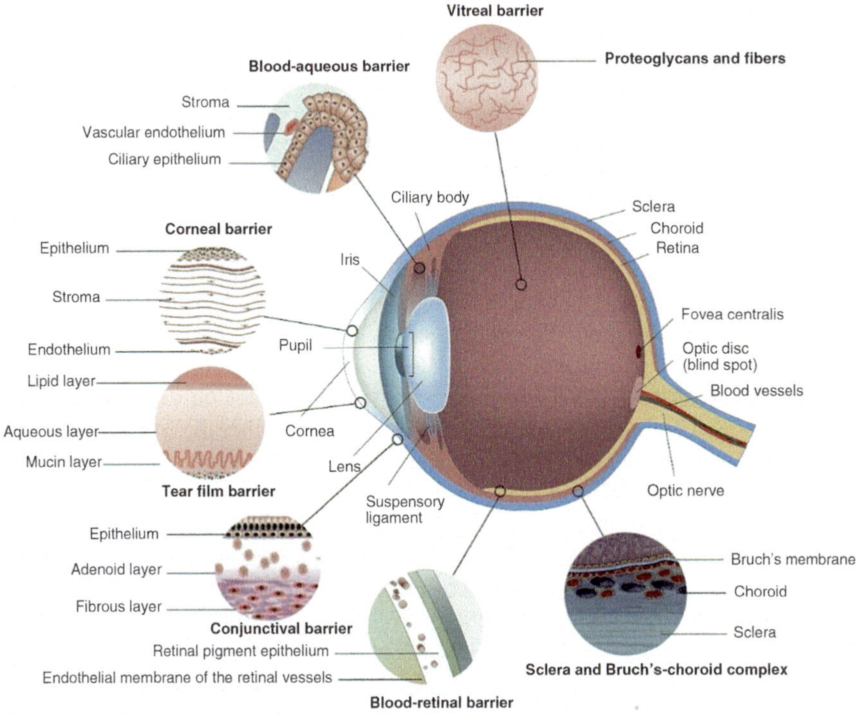

Fig. 1 Schematic of the static ocular barriers. Adapted with permission from (Huang et al. 2018)

corneal epithelium being the major barrier to drug penetration. The corneal epithelium is composed of 5–7 cell layers with intercellular tight junctions allowing only small hydrophilic molecules to traverse paracellularly, while transcellular transport is limited to smaller lipophilic drugs (Ghate and Edelhauser 2008). Overall, it is thought that less than 10% of a topically applied dose eventually traverses the cornea (Koevary 2003).

While traditionally not considered a major drug delivery route, drug penetration may also occur via the conjunctival-scleral pathway which provides a 17-fold larger surface area for drug absorption (Prausnitz and Noonan 1998). Moreover, the conjunctival epithelium is more hydrophilic and leakier, with intercellular spaces being about 230-fold larger than those of the cornea (Geroski and Edelhauser 2001; Hamalainen et al. 1997). In fact, comparing conjunctival and corneal penetration of 25 drugs in porcine tissues ex vivo revealed that the conjunctiva is 8.6 ± 4.4 times leakier than the cornea (Ramsay et al. 2018). However, as discussed above, conjunctival/episcleral clearance via blood and lymphatic vessels is significant, with a large proportion of drug absorbed via this route being lost to the systemic circulation (Urtti 2006). With tight junctions in the blood–aqueous barrier (BAB; Fig. 1), ciliary body epithelium, iris, and Schlemm's canal endothelium, systemic drug administration to treat anterior segment conditions, particularly those of the ocular surface, is thought to be impractical (Coca-Prados 2014). Moreover, the BAB limits drug passage from the anterior to the posterior segment due to continuous drainage of aqueous humor with a turnover rate of 2–3 ml/min (Barar et al. 2008). As such, even if a topically applied drug is able to penetrate the cornea to reach the anterior segment, it is often unable to reach the posterior segment in sufficiently high concentrations.

Static barriers relevant to posterior segment delivery include the sclera and Bruch's-choroid complex, vitreous, and blood–retinal barrier (BRB). The surface area of the sclera is approximately 16.3 cm^2 (Olsen et al. 1998) and thus much larger than that of the cornea. It mainly comprises extracellular matrix consisting of collagen fibrils and glycoproteins (Olsen et al. 1998) and is generally more permeable than the cornea and conjunctiva. This is particularly true for hydrophilic compounds, with transscleral transport primarily dependent on diffusion through an aqueous medium of proteoglycans or porous spaces within the collagen network (25–300 nm in diameter) rather than diffusion across cell membranes (Ambati and Adamis 2002; Cruysberg et al. 2002). The vitreous is a clear gel-like substance that fills the space between the lens and retina and helps maintain the eye's structural integrity. It is composed of collagen fibrils, hyaluronan, and proteoglycans (Bishop 2000) and due to its relatively high viscosity, can act as a diffusion barrier especially to intravitreally injected positively charged molecules that interact with the negatively charged vitreous components (Martens et al. 2013). Finally, the BRB, divided into the inner and outer BRB, mainly hinders substance diffusion from the systemic circulation into ocular tissues (Runkle and Antonetti 2011) again highlighting that systemic treatment of ocular conditions affecting even the highly vascularized posterior segment tissues is limited.

As evident from the above discussion, the eye's dynamic and static barriers form a complex of alternating lipophilic and hydrophilic layers with sophisticated elimination mechanisms that restrict the entry of foreign substances including drugs. Thus, physicochemical properties of not only the drug, but also the delivery vehicle, play a significant role. As such, to enhance ocular drug bioavailability, ocular formulation efforts have mainly focussed on two strategies: i) to circumvent dynamic barriers by increasing ocular retention and ii) to increase penetration across static barriers. The following sections will highlight formulation constraints as well as recent advances in ocular drug delivery.

3 Formulation Constraints

3.1 Physicochemical Drug Properties

While the chemical nature and concentration of a drug can cause ocular irritation, inducing reflex tearing, and therefore reducing the retention time on the ocular surface, physicochemical drug properties also significantly influence tissue penetration (Table 1). Here, important factors include the lipophilicity of the drug as reflected by its n-octanol/water partition coefficient (logP) or its logD, more relevant

Table 1 Effect of physicochemical drug properties on penetration across static ocular barriers. Adapted with permission from Huang et al. (2018)

Ocular tissue	Molecular size	Lipophilicity	Charge
Cornea	Decreases with increasing molecular radius (Edwards and Prausnitz 2001)	Preference for lipophilic molecules (log *D* 2 to 3) (Balla et al. 2021; Huang et al. 1983)	Preference for positively charged molecules (Liaw et al. 1992)
Conjunctiva	Decreases with increasing molecular radius (Hamalainen et al. 1997)	Preference for lipophilic molecules (Balla et al. 2021; Prausnitz and Noonan 1998)	Not studied
Blood–aqueous barrier	Decreases with increasing molecular weight (Freddo 2001; Grabner et al. 1978)	Preference for lipophilic molecules (Urtti 2006)	Not studied
Sclera	Decreases with increasing molecular radius (Ambati et al. 2000)	Preference for hydrophilic molecules (Cruysberg et al. 2002)	Preference for negatively charged molecules (Kim et al. 2007; Maurice and Polgar 1977)
Bruch's-choroid complex	Decreases with increasing molecular weight (Hussain et al. 2002)	Preference for hydrophilic molecules (Cheruvu and Kompella 2006)	Preference for negatively charged molecules (Cheruvu and Kompella 2006)
Blood–retinal barrier	Decreases with increasing molecular radius (Freilich et al. 1966; Pitkanen et al. 2005)	Preference for lipophilic molecules (Kansara and Mitra 2006)	Not studied

to ionizable compounds (Schoenwald and Huang 1983), the molecular size and shape (Grass et al. 1985), and the charge (Liaw et al. 1992), again more relevant to ionizable drugs and determined by the pKa (Sieg and Robinson 1975). Optimal corneal absorption is found for drugs with a logP between 2 and 3 (Schoenwald and Huang 1983; Schoenwald and Ward 1978), while more hydrophilic molecules penetrate preferentially across the sclera (Cruysberg et al. 2002). However, recent studies have found that the spatial drug distribution in ocular surface tissues is much more complex, with lipophilicity affecting drug penetration into the corneal stroma and conjunctiva to a much lesser extent than into the corneal epithelium (Balla et al. 2021). For ionizable compounds (weak acids and bases), drug uptake depends on the chemical equilibrium between the ionized (more hydrophilic) and unionized (more lipophilic) form, both in the delivery system itself and in the tear fluid, with the unionized form penetrating lipid cell membranes more readily. As for the charge, cationic drugs tend to penetrate the cornea more easily than anionic compounds, which are repelled by the negatively charged surface mucins, pores present in the corneal epithelium, and the membrane potential (Järvinen et al. 1995; Le Bourlais et al. 1998; Loftssona and Jarvinen 1999; Rojanasakul and Robinson 1989). However, a positive charge may also decrease penetration, due to possible ionic interactions of the drug with the negatively charged carboxylic acid groups of tight junction proteins (Hornof et al. 2005; Palmgren et al. 2002). Finally, the molecular size of the drug has a significant effect on ocular absorption. While the cornea is generally impermeable to molecules larger than 5,000 Da, the conjunctiva allows compounds of up to 20,000 Da to penetrate (Greaves and Wilson 1993; Huang et al. 1989). Generally, an increase in molecular weight and/or radius is thought to decrease penetration across static ocular barriers. For an in-depth analysis of the effect of drug properties on tissue permeability, please refer to a recent in silico study defining the "Rule of Thumb" for developability assessment of new topical ophthalmic drug candidates (Karami et al. 2021).

3.2 Excipient Limitations

The normal tear fluid pH value is 7.4. As such, ocular formulations should ideally be formulated between pH 7.0 and 7.7 using buffering agents to avoid irritation and thus reflex tearing (Van Ooteghem 1993), although the pH necessary for maximal drug solubility and/or stability is often outside of this range. The osmolarity of the tear fluid normally ranges between 310 and 350 mOsm/kg (Ludwig 2005), although formulations with an osmolarity between 260 and 480 mOsm/kg may still be tolerated without inducing reflex tearing and blinking (Ludwig and Van Ooteghem 1987). As discussed above, reflex tearing and blinking due to poor formulation tolerability should be avoided as these dynamic processes ultimately reduce drug bioavailability.

Polymer addition is one way to partially circumvent the dynamic processes on the ocular surface. These may either be simple viscosity enhancing agents (Pahuja et al. 2012), mucoadhesive polymers that interact with ocular surface mucins (Ruponen and Urtti 2015), or in situ gelling polymers (Rupenthal et al. 2011a, b; Thrimawithana et al. 2012) which undergo sol-to-gel phase transition upon exposure to the physiological conditions (ions, pH, and temperature) in the eye.

The overarching approach to overcome static tissue barriers is to incorporate penetration enhancers such as surfactants or developing colloidal delivery systems such as nanoparticles (Joseph and Venkatraman 2017), liposomes (Agarwal et al. 2016), or micelles (Mandal et al. 2017). However, the tolerability of such systems must be considered, especially with the high surfactant level in micelles, nano-/microemulsions, liposomes, and nanoparticles (Abdelkader et al. 2015; Prow et al. 2008). Surfactants can transiently disrupt the tear film (Cho and Brown 1998) and induce epithelial cell lysis and apoptosis (Kapoor et al. 2009), ultimately causing ocular surface damage upon prolonged use.

Similar observations have been made with preservatives present in most multidose eyedrops. Benzalkonium chloride (BAK), the most commonly used preservative in topical eyedrops, has repeatedly been shown to be toxic to the ocular surface (Baudouin 1998; Ishibashi et al. 2003). BAK disrupts the integrity of corneal tight junctions thus compromising the barrier properties and even elevating the toxicity potential of other excipients. Although less toxic than BAK, significant toxicity is also seen with other preservatives, including Polyquad®, Purite®, OcuPure®, and Sofzia® (Brignole-Baudouin et al. 2011; Kahook and Noecker 2008; Labbé et al. 2006; Lee et al. 2015), especially on prolonged use. As such, preservative-free eyedrops, available in single-use containers or with specialized multidose preservative-free dosing systems (Campolo et al. 2022), are recommended for chronic conditions requiring prolonged eyedrop use, although this may increase treatment costs by 5- to 10-folds (Furrer et al. 2002). Considering the above formulation limitations, it is no surprise that several novel drug delivery systems discovered in the laboratory fail to enter the market due to significant safety concerns, as further highlighted by specific examples in the next section. A list of currently approved excipients and their commonly used concentrations can be found in the Food and Drug Administration (FDA) inactive ingredient database by filtering for the "ophthalmic" route (FDA 2023).

4 Recent Progress in Ocular Drug Delivery

Although many effective drugs exist to treat ocular conditions, their delivery over prolonged periods with minimal side effects remains a challenge. Here, novel drug delivery systems offer great opportunities, especially when using already approved drugs with well-known safety and efficacy (O'Rourke 2014). Although there had been limited progress in terms of marketed advanced ocular drug delivery systems over decades, this has changed significantly over the past 5 years, with many novel products currently in late-stage clinical trials or recently approved. To be marketed successfully, novel products need to offer clear advantages over existing therapies, no matter which delivery route is chosen, especially with regard to therapeutic efficacy, lowered toxicity, and increased patient compliance (Peyman and Hosseini 2011). Figure 2 gives a schematic overview of advanced ocular drug delivery systems currently on the market or in (pre-)clinical studies with some of these further discussed below.

4.1 Novel Drug Delivery Systems for Anterior Segment Diseases

The first advanced drug delivery system for anterior segment delivery dates back to the 1970s when Ocusert® (Alza), a membrane-controlled reservoir system of pilocarpine in an alginate core, sandwiched between two ethylene vinyl acetate (EVA) membranes, was approved for the treatment of glaucoma. While it allowed continuous drug diffusion over 1 week, insertion difficulty, foreign-body sensation, and accidental loss ultimately resulted in its market withdrawal. It took over four decades until another advanced ocular surface device, the bimatoprost containing Helios™ ring developed by ForSight VISION5, which sits under the eyelids and can release drug for up to 6 months, was investigated. Although it showed good retention and efficacy in a Phase 2 randomized, double-masked controlled study (Brandt et al. 2016), clinical development seems to have stalled. This is likely due to Allergan,

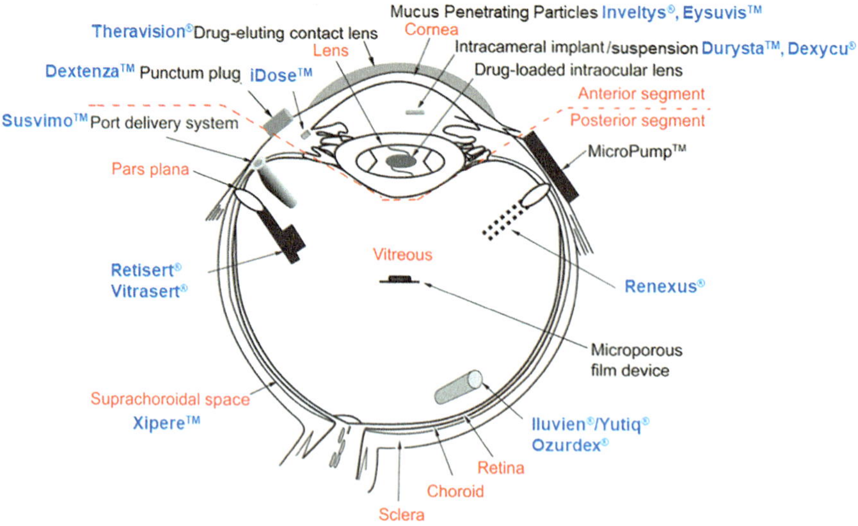

Fig. 2 Advanced ocular drug delivery systems. Schematic overview of general delivery strategies (*black*), marketed product names (*blue*), and anatomical structures (*red*). Adapted with permission from (Rupenthal 2017)

who acquired this periocular ring technology, simultaneously completing Phase 3 clinical studies with another technology, bimatoprost SR (Medeiros et al. 2020). This is a biodegradable, intracameral implant based on the poly(lactic-co-glycolic) acid (PLGA) NOVADUR® matrix system that had demonstrated favorable efficacy and safety for up to 6 months in a Phase 1/2 clinical study (Lewis et al. 2017) and was ultimately approved as Durysta™ in 2020. Interestingly, due to the potential for implant dislocation and the slow degradation profile, this intracameral implant is currently not approved for repeated use (Belamkar et al. 2022). To overcome these shortcomings, PolyActiva and Ripple Therapeutics are currently investigating polymeric prodrug-based intracameral implants with more favorable degradation profiles. PolyActiva's latanoprost implant based on the Prezia™ technology is currently in Phase 2 clinical trials (PolyActiva 2023), while Ripple's intracameral Epidel® prodrug technology is still in preclinical studies, although intravitreal implants based on Epidel have entered Phase 2 clinical trials (Ripple 2023). Another intracameral implant investigated by Envisia Therapeutics utilized a Particle Replication In Non-Wetting Templates (PRINT®)-based PLGA rod for sustained travoprost delivery (ENV515; travoprost XR) (Navratil et al. 2014), with a single rod administration having shown clinically meaningful reduction in intraocular pressure for 11 months. The technology was acquired by Aerie Pharmaceuticals in 2017, which subsequently was acquired by Alcon in 2022, but no further update could be found regarding the clinical development of travoprost XR.

Interesting drug delivery systems for anterior segment delivery based on devices previously approved for surgical applications have also recently emerged. For example, the iStent®, Glaukos' first micro-invasive glaucoma surgery (MIGS) device approved by the FDA in 2012, has been tailored for delivery of travoprost (iDose® TR), with two devices with different drug elution rates having completed Phase 3 clinical trials and a New Drug Application (NDA) submitted in 2023 (Glaukos 2023). Travoprost has also been incorporated into a medicated punctum plug (OTX-TR, Ocular Therapeutix), which failed to achieve a primary endpoint in Phase 3 clinical trials (Vantipalli et al. 2020), but investigations into an intracameral implant based on the same technology continue in Phase 2 clinical studies. The dexamethasone-containing punctum plug (Dextenza™), on the other hand, met the primary endpoints in Phase 3 clinical studies for post-operative inflammation (Gira et al. 2017) and was approved for post-operative inflammation and allergic conjunctivitis in 2021. Punctum plugs were previously used to reduce tear fluid drainage in patients with aqueous-deficient dry eye disease, but were reworked to contain micronized drug particles that slowly release as the polyethylene glycol hydrogel matrix resorbs as well as a visualization aid to monitor plug retention (Yellepeddi et al. 2015). The technology seems to have great promise, with a cyclosporin A-containing punctum plug currently in Phase 2 clinical trials for the management of dry eye disease, while the hydrogel platform is also being investigated for sustained intravitreal drug delivery (Therapeutix 2023).

Collagen shields and contact lenses have also been investigated for prolonged drug delivery to anterior segment tissues. Once applied to the ocular surface, collagen shields gradually dissolve into a gel beneficial for dry eye management or wound healing (Marmer 1988). Moreover, dehydrated shields can be soaked in a drug solution before insertion, thus serving as drug reservoirs. However, the non-transparent nature and marginal improvement in drug delivery duration have rendered them less suitable (Lee et al. 2001). The reservoir principle has also been explored with contact lenses, which have shown better acceptance due to their transparency, although the improvement in precorneal drug residence has remained minimal when simply soaking lenses in the drug solution (Bengani et al. 2013). Thus, other loading techniques such as molecular imprinting, "piggybacking," or incorporation of nanocarriers have been investigated over the years (Carvalho et al. 2015; González-Chomón et al. 2013; Maulvi et al. 2016), with a ketotifen eluting contact lens (ACUVUE® Theravision™) approved in 2022 (Novack 2023). While this is currently the first and only drug-eluting contact lens on the market, there is no doubt that this technology holds great promise for the future. Similar drug loading techniques can also be used for silicon-based intraocular lenses (Liu et al. 2013), while implantation of a refillable capsule device into the lens has also been investigated (Molokhia et al. 2010). Although these technologies have great promise in conjunction with cataract surgery, they currently remain at the preclinical stage.

Much simpler than many of the devices discussed above is the use of nanocarriers to improve precorneal retention and tissue penetration (Agarwal et al. 2018a; Bisht et al. 2018; Joseph and Venkatraman 2017; Kang-Mieler et al. 2017; Mandal et al. 2017). Among the most clinically advanced nanoparticle technologies are the mucus-penetrating particles (MPP), developed by Kala Pharmaceutical, based on micronized drug particles coated with polyethylene glycol which efficiently penetrate the tear film mucin layer, the first defense mechanism encountered after topical eyedrop administration (Schopf et al. 2015). In a recent Phase 3 study delivering loteprednol etabonate (KPI-121) following cataract surgery, twice-daily administration of the MPP-formulation was as effective as four daily doses of the conventional drug suspension (Kim et al. 2019). The 1% loteprednol etabonate formulation (Inveltys®) approved for post-operative inflammation and pain in 2018 and the 0.25% loteprednol etabonate eyedrop (Eysuvis®) approved for the management of dry eye disease in 2020 were sold to Alcon in 2022. Finally, another potential paradigm shift has been seen with the development of non-aqueous eyedrops, especially for the delivery of hydrophobic drugs, since they not only enhance ocular drug penetration (Agarwal et al. 2018b, 2019a), but may have additional benefits in the management of ocular surface conditions due to their emollient effect (Agarwal et al. 2019b; Agarwal and Rupenthal 2023). The most advanced formulation here is a cyclosporin A-containing eyedrop based on semifluorinated alkanes, which has completed Phase 3 clinical trials (Akpek et al. 2023; Sheppard et al. 2021) and was approved as VEVYE™ in June 2023. Nevertheless, while many promising delivery technologies have been approved or are in late-stage clinical trials for the treatment of anterior segment condition in recent year, the majority of these are still unable to deliver sufficiently high drug concentrations to treat back-of-the-eye conditions.

4.2 Novel Drug Delivery Systems for Posterior Segment Diseases

Advanced drug delivery to the back of the eye started with Vitrasert® (Chiron) in 1996, a ganciclovir containing scleral implant for the treatment of *cytomegalovirus retinitis*, and was continued with Retisert® (Bausch+Lomb), containing fluocinolone acetonide (FA) approved for the treatment of non-infectious posterior uveitis in 2005. Both implants are based on the same technology, with a drug pellet coated by two non-biodegradable polymer layers, although Retisert is much smaller as it contains a more potent drug. In Vitrasert, the inner polyvinyl alcohol (PVA) coating allows drug permeation for up to 8 months from one side while the other sides are covered by impermeable EVA (Martin et al. 1994). In Retisert, the drug is released for up to 30 months via a PVA suture tab spared by the impermeable silicon coating (Jaffe et al. 2000). Iluvien® (Alimera Sciences, approved for diabetic macular edema in 2014) and Yutiq® (EyePoint Pharmaceuticals, approved for chronic non-infectious uveitis in 2018), based on the DURASERT™ technology (pSivida), are also non-biodegradable but are injected into the vitreous rather than sutured into the *pars plana* region. They contain FA in a PVA matrix inside a polyimide tube with membrane caps to control drug release (Kane et al. 2008). Although implant injection is generally preferable over surgical implantation, the fate of such implants after drug depletion remains uncertain which highlights the potential advantage of bioerodible implants.

Ozurdex® (Allergan), the first biodegradable intravitreal implant approved in 2009, is based on the NOVADUR technology (which is the same as discussed for Durysta in the previous section) containing dexamethasone in a PLGA matrix for the treatment of diabetic macular edema, retinal vein occlusion, and posterior uveitis. While biodegradability has its advantages, it also leads to variable drug release compared to the almost zero-order release kinetics seen with the non-biodegradable implants discussed in the previous paragraph. As such, Ozurdex exhibits relatively fast drug diffusion over the first 2 months with polymer degradation responsible for slower drug release thereafter (Whitcup and Robinson 2015). The previously mentioned PRINT technology has also been used to prepare intravitreal formulations, with 1 μm PRINT cylinders composed of trehalose/bevacizumab incorporated into biodegradable hydrogels having shown sustained protein release for up to 25 days (Herlihy et al. 2014). By adjusting implant size, shape, porosity, chemical composition, and surface functionality, the PRINT technology allows customizable drug delivery, an advantage over conventional implants (Navratil et al. 2014). Customizable intravitreal implants are also possible with Ocular Therapeutix's hydrogel technology as well as Ripple Therapeutics' Epidel technology, both discussed for anterior segment delivery in the previous section.

Similar to Vitrasert/Retisert but fully biodegradable, a film device consisting of a drug pellet, sandwiched between two thin layers of impermeable polycaprolactone (PCL) membrane with specific membrane pores has also been investigated for drug delivery to the retina (Bernards et al. 2014). Adjusting PCL film porosity and thickness, drug release can be tailored with sustained rapamycin delivery shown for up to 4 months (Lance et al. 2015). Since PCL eventually degrades, device removal is not required. Interestingly, this technology has also recently been investigated for delivery of anti-glaucoma medications into the anterior chamber (Samy et al. 2019) as well as protein delivery to the back of the eye (Schlesinger et al. 2019), highlighting the versatility of this reservoir-based delivery device. Protein delivery over prolonged periods is also possible with the bioerodible oxidized meso-porous silicon-based Tethadur™ technology (pSivida). Unlike most other polymer-based drug delivery systems, the Tethadur system does not require complex chemistry, with the heat and radiation stable biosilicon simplifying the manufacturing and sterilization process (Ashton 2015). Using UV light to photo-crosslink biodegradable polymers to either form an implant in situ (OcuLief®) or create a preformed implant for injection (EyeLief®) is currently being investigated in preclinical studies by Re-Vana Therapeutics, allowing delivery of both small molecular weight drugs and biologics for over 6 months (Thakur Singh and Jones 2018).

Although biodegradable implants have become more favorable over recent years, a number of non-biodegradable systems have also been under investigation. These include the encapsulated cell technology implant, Renexus® (Neurotech), containing recombinant human ciliary neurotrophic factor (CNTF)-secreting human retinal pigment epithelial cells within a non-biodegradable polyethylene terephthalate yarn (Emerich and Thanos 2008). The outer polyether sulfone shell allows nutrients to flow in and CNTF to exit while preventing immune cell attack. Clinically effective amounts of CNTF can be released over 18 months (Birch et al. 2013), with Renexus being granted orphan drug designation by the FDA for retinitis pigmentosa and macular telangiectasia as well as fast-track designation for retinitis pigmentosa and dry age-related macular degeneration over recent years.

Refillable non-biodegradable implants have also gained attention due to their increased life span. The port delivery system developed by ForSight VISION4 and acquired by Roche/Genentech in 2017 comprises a vessel, a semi-permeable non--biodegradable membrane with a refill port and exit ports to release the drug into the vitreous humor (Ranade et al. 2022). The device was well tolerated in a Phase 1 clinical trial (Loewenstein et al. 2020), with the Phase 2 LADDER (Campochiaro et al. 2019) and Phase 3 Archway (Holekamp et al. 2022) trials, delivering ranibizumab for the treatment of wet age-related macular degeneration for up to 6 months showing favorable results, ultimately leading to its FDA approval (Susvimo™) in 2021. However, only 1 year after entering the market it was recalled voluntarily due to manufacturing issues, but is expected to enter the market again after a redesign. One advantage of the port delivery system includes its flushability, allowing abortion of drug delivery if required; however, the overall drug release rate, determined by the semi-permeable membrane, is fixed. Tunable drug delivery devices have thus received some attention as they allow patient-specific drug delivery (Yasin et al. 2014). The MicroPump™ by Replenish, for example, enables precisely programmable drug release for up to 5 years by volume expansion due to conversion of water into gas increasing the pressure on the drug reservoir, thus pushing more drug out (Lo et al. 2009), with first-in-man safety and feasibility studies completed a few years back (Humayun et al. 2014), although no further update regarding its clinical advancement could be found.

Finally, using physical forces to enhance ocular drug delivery has also become of great interest. This includes the use of electrical fields, sonophoresis, and microneedles, which can enhance penetration efficiency by transiently disrupting the static ocular barriers in a minimally or non-invasive manner (Huang et al. 2018). The EyeGate II iontophoresis eye cup, for example, relies on electrorepulsion and electroosmosis of the drug and has been investigated for dexamethasone delivery (EGP-437, EyeGate Pharma) in the treatment of anterior uveitis (Cohen et al. 2012), with this technique also able to achieve back-of-the-eye delivery. A patented electrotransfection system is also currently being tested for non-viral gene therapy of various posterior segment conditions (Evensys 2023). Microneedles, on the other hand, create transport pathways of micro-dimensions and can come in a variety of shapes, sizes, materials, and configurations (Donnelly et al. 2010). They can be used for transcorneal or transscleral drug delivery. A special microinjector developed by Clearside Biomedical delivers drug directly into the suprachoroidal space, spreading around the circumference of the posterior segment. Delivering triamcinolone acetonide using this microinjector, safety and preliminary efficacy in the treatment of non-infectious uveitis was shown a few years back (Goldstein et al. 2016), with the technology (Xipere™) ultimately approved in 2021. Clearside has many commercial collaborations to bring this technology to other markets while also investigating it for gene therapy which has received significant attention since the first ocular viral gene therapy, subretinal voretigene neparvovec-rzyl (Luxturna®), was approved in 2017. With the suprachoroidal space being a potential space between the sclera and choroid that traverses the circumference of the posterior segment, which is easier to access than the vitreous or subretinal space, this technology offers high drug bioavailability in the choroid, RPE, and retina, while maintaining low levels elsewhere in the eye (Chiang et al. 2018; Jung et al. 2019). It could thus offer great advantages to deliver other drugs including gene therapies to the posterior segment, although the suprachoroidal space is not known to have the same immune privilege status as the subretinal space. For an overview of ocular gene therapies currently in clinical trials, the reader is referred to a recent review (Ghoraba et al. 2022).

5 Future Directions in Ocular Drug Delivery

The past decade has shown great success with regard to approved advanced ocular drug delivery systems. Most of these have been able to circumvent some of the dynamic ocular barriers, leading to improved retention and sustained drug release on the ocular surface, ultimately resulting in reduced application frequency and increased efficacy. Similarly, sustained drug release systems for posterior segment delivery have reduced the need for frequent specialist visits, thus lowering the overall treatment burden. However, size restrictions within the eye limit some of these approaches to highly potent drugs such as steroids, while drug–device interactions, biocompatibility, clinical translation, and regulatory approval remain challenging. In general, it seems that simpler systems have a greater chance to make it to the market than highly complicated approaches. Overall, while a number of constraints with regard to anterior segment delivery have been overcome, sustained delivery of large molecular weight drugs to the back of the eye remains a challenge still to be tackled.

References

Abdelkader H, Pierscionek B, Carew M, Wu Z, Alany RG (2015) Critical appraisal of alternative irritation models: three decades of testing ophthalmic pharmaceuticals. Br Med Bull 113:59–71

Agarwal P, Rupenthal ID (2023) Non-aqueous formulations in topical ocular drug delivery – a paradigm shift? Adv Drug Deliv Rev:114867

Agarwal R, Iezhitsa I, Agarwal P, Abdul Nasir NA, Razali N, Alyautdin R, Ismail NM (2016) Liposomes in topical ophthalmic drug delivery: an update. Drug Deliv 23:1075–1091

Agarwal P, Huang D, Thakur SS, Rupenthal ID (2018a) Nanotechnology for ocular drug delivery. In: Design of nanostructures for versatile therapeutic applications, pp 137–188

Agarwal P, Scherer D, Günther B, Rupenthal ID (2018b) Semifluorinated alkane based systems for enhanced corneal penetration of poorly soluble drugs. Int J Pharm 538:119–129

Agarwal P, Craig JP, Krösser S, Eickhoff K, Swift S, Rupenthal ID (2019a) Topical semifluorinated alkane-based azithromycin suspension for the management of ocular infections. Eur J Pharm Biopharm 142:83–91

Agarwal P, Khun D, Krosser S, Eickhoff K, Wells FS, Willmott GR, Craig JP, Rupenthal ID (2019b) Preclinical studies evaluating the effect of semifluorinated alkanes on ocular surface and tear fluid dynamics. Ocul Surf 17:241–249

Agarwal P, Craig JP, Rupenthal ID (2021) Formulation considerations for the management of dry eye disease. Pharmaceutics 13

Agban Y, Thakur SS, Mugisho OO, Rupenthal ID (2019) Depot formulations to sustain periocular drug delivery to the posterior eye segment. Drug Discov Today 24:1458–1469
Akpek EK, Wirta DL, Downing JE, Tauber J, Sheppard JD, Ciolino JB, Meides AS, Krösser S (2023) Efficacy and safety of a water-free topical cyclosporine, 0.1%, solution for the treatment of moderate to severe dry eye disease: the ESSENCE-2 randomized clinical trial. JAMA Ophthalmol
Ambati J, Adamis AP (2002) Transscleral drug delivery to the retina and choroid. Prog Retin Eye Res 21:145–151
Ambati J, Canakis CS, Miller JW, Gragoudas ES, Edwards A, Weissgold DJ, Kim I, Delori FC, Adamis AP (2000) Diffusion of high molecular weight compounds through sclera. Invest Ophthalmol Vis Sci 41:1181–1185
Ashton P (2015) pSivida and ophthalmic drug delivery. ONdrugDelivery 2015:18–19
Balla A, Auriola S, Grey AC, Demarais NJ, Valtari A, Heikkinen EM, Toropainen E, Urtti A, Vellonen KS, Ruponen M (2021) Partitioning and spatial distribution of drugs in ocular surface tissues. Pharmaceutics 13
Barar J, Javadzadeh AR, Omidi Y (2008) Ocular novel drug delivery: impacts of membranes and barriers. Expert Opin Drug Deliv 5:567–581
Baudouin C (1998) Short term comparative study of topical 2% carteolol with and without benzalkonium chloride in healthy volunteers. Br J Ophthalmol 82:39–42
Belamkar A, Harris A, Zukerman R, Siesky B, Oddone F, Verticchio Vercellin A, Ciulla TA (2022) Sustained release glaucoma therapies: novel modalities for overcoming key treatment barriers associated with topical medications. Ann Med 54:343–358
Bengani LC, Hsu KH, Gause S, Chauhan A (2013) Contact lenses as a platform for ocular drug delivery. Expert Opin Drug Deliv 10:1483–1496
Bernards DA, Bhisitkul RB, Desai TA (2014) Zero-order sustained drug delivery to the retina from a nanoporous film device. ONdrugDelivery:20–21
Birch DG, Weleber RG, Duncan JL, Jaffe GJ, Tao W, Ciliary Neurotrophic Factor Retinitis Pigmentosa Study Groups (2013) Randomized trial of ciliary neurotrophic factor delivered by encapsulated cell intraocular implants for retinitis pigmentosa. Am J Ophthalmol 156:283–292.e1
Bishop PN (2000) Structural macromolecules and supramolecular organisation of the vitreous gel. Prog Retin Eye Res 19:323–344
Bisht R, Mandal A, Jaiswal JK, Rupenthal ID (2018) Nanocarrier mediated retinal drug delivery: overcoming ocular barriers to treat posterior eye diseases. WIREs Nanomed Nanobiotechnol 10: e1473
Brandt JD, Sall K, DuBiner H, Benza R, Alster Y, Walker G, Semba CP (2016) Six-month intraocular pressure reduction with a topical bimatoprost ocular insert: results of a phase II randomized controlled study. Ophthalmology 123:1685–1694
Brignole-Baudouin F, Riancho L, Liang H, Nakib Z, Baudouin C (2011) In vitro comparative toxicology of polyquad-preserved and benzalkonium chloride-preserved travoprost/timolol fixed combination and latanoprost/timolol fixed combination. J Ocul Pharmacol Ther 27:273–280
Campochiaro PA, Marcus DM, Awh CC, Regillo C, Adamis AP, Bantseev V, Chiang Y, Ehrlich JS, Erickson S, Hanley WD, Horvath J, Maass KF, Singh N, Tang F, Barteselli G (2019) The port delivery system with ranibizumab for neovascular age-related macular degeneration: results from the randomized phase 2 ladder clinical trial. Ophthalmology 126:1141–1154
Campolo A, Crary M, Shannon P (2022) A review of the containers available for multi-dose preservative-free eye drops. Biomed J Sci Tech Res 45
Carvalho IM, Marques CS, Oliveira RS, Coelho PB, Costa PC, Ferreira DC (2015) Sustained drug release by contact lenses for glaucoma treatment – a review. J Control Release 202:76–82
Cheruvu NP, Kompella UB (2006) Bovine and porcine transscleral solute transport: influence of lipophilicity and the choroid-Bruch's layer. Invest Ophthalmol Vis Sci 47:4513–4522

Chiang B, Jung JH, Prausnitz MR (2018) The suprachoroidal space as a route of administration to the posterior segment of the eye. Adv Drug Deliv Rev 126:58–66

Cho P, Brown B (1998) Disruption of the tear film by the application of small drops of saline and surfactant. Cont Lens Anterior Eye 21:73–80

Coca-Prados M (2014) The blood-aqueous barrier in health and disease. J Glaucoma 23:S36–S38

Cohen AE, Assang C, Patane MA, From S, Korenfeld M, Avion Study Investigators (2012) Evaluation of dexamethasone phosphate delivered by ocular iontophoresis for treating noninfectious anterior uveitis. Ophthalmology 119:66–73

Cruysberg LPJ, Nuijts RMMA, Geroski DH, Koole LH, Hendrikse F, Edelhauser HF (2002) In vitro human scleral permeability of fluorescein, dexamethasone-fluorescein, methotrexate-fluorescein and rhodamine 6G and the use of a coated coil as a new drug delivery system. J Ocul Pharmacol Ther 18:559–569

Dey S, Mitra AK (2005) Transporters and receptors in ocular drug delivery: opportunities and challenges. Taylor & Francis

Donnelly RF, Raj Singh TR, Woolfson AD (2010) Microneedle-based drug delivery systems: microfabrication, drug delivery, and safety. Drug Deliv 17:187–207

Edwards A, Prausnitz MR (2001) Predicted permeability of the cornea to topical drugs. Pharm Res 18:1497–1508

Emerich DF, Thanos CG (2008) NT-501: an ophthalmic implant of polymer-encapsulated ciliary neurotrophic factor-producing cells. Curr Opin Mol Ther 10:506–515

Evensys (2023). https://eyevensys.com/pipeline/. Accessed 6 June 2023

FDA (2023). https://www.fda.gov/drugs/drug-approvals-and-databases/inactive-ingredients-database-download. Accessed 6 June 2023

Freddo TF (2001) Shifting the paradigm of the blood-aqueous barrier. Exp Eye Res 73:581–592

Freilich DB, Lee PF, Freeman HM (1966) Experimental retinal detachment. Arch Ophthalmol 76: 432–436

Furrer P, Mayer JM, Gurny R (2002) Ocular tolerance of preservatives and alternatives. Eur J Pharm Biopharm 53:263–280

Gaudana R, Ananthula H, Parenky A, Mitra A (2010) Ocular drug delivery. AAPS J 12:348–360

Gausas RE, Gonnering RS, Lemke BN, Dortzbach RK, Sherman DD (1999) Identification of human orbital lymphatics. Ophthal Plast Reconstr Surg 15:252–259

Georgiev GA, Eftimov P, Yokoi N (2019) Contribution of mucins towards the physical properties of the tear film: a modern update. Int J Mol Sci 20

Geroski DH, Edelhauser HF (2001) Transscleral drug delivery for posterior segment disease. Adv Drug Deliv Rev 52:37–48

Ghate D, Edelhauser HF (2008) Barriers to glaucoma drug delivery. J Glaucoma 17:147–156

Ghoraba HH, Akhavanrezayat A, Karaca I, Yavari N, Lajevardi S, Hwang J, Regenold J, Matsumiya W, Pham B, Zaidi M, Mobasserian A, DongChau AT, Or C, Yasar C, Mishra K, Do D, Nguyen QD (2022) Ocular gene therapy: a literature review with special focus on immune and inflammatory responses. Clin Ophthalmol 16:1753–1771

Gira JP, Sampson R, Silverstein SM, Walters TR, Metzinger JL, Talamo JH (2017) Evaluating the patient experience after implantation of a 0.4 mg sustained release dexamethasone intracanalicular insert (Dextenza): results of a qualitative survey. Patient Prefer Adherence 11: 487–494

Glaukos (2023). https://investors.glaukos.com/investors/news/news-details/2023/Glaukos-Submits-New-Drug-Application-to-U.S.-FDA-for-iDose-TR/default.aspx. Accessed 4 May 2023

Goel M, Picciani RG, Lee RK, Bhattacharya SK (2010) Aqueous humor dynamics: a review. Open Ophthalmol J 4:52–59

Goldstein DA, Do D, Noronha G, Kissner JM, Srivastava SK, Nguyen QD (2016) Suprachoroidal corticosteroid administration: a novel route for local treatment of noninfectious uveitis. Transl Vis Sci Technol 5:14

González-Chomón C, Concheiro A, Alvarez-Lorenzo C (2013) Soft contact lenses for controlled ocular delivery: 50 years in the making. Ther Deliv 4:1141–1161
Grabner G, Zehetbauer G, Bettelheim H, Honigsmann C, Dorda W (1978) The blood-aqueous barrier and its permeability for proteins of different molecular weight. Graefes Arch Clin Exp Ophthalmol 207:137–148
Grass GM, Wood RW, Robinson JR (1985) Effects of calcium chelating agents on corneal permeability. Invest Ophthalmol Vis Sci 26:110–113
Greaves JL, Wilson CG (1993) Treatment of diseases of the eye with mucoadhesive delivery systems. Adv Drug Deliv Rev 11:349–383
Hamalainen KM, Kananen K, Auriola S, Kontturi K, Urtti A (1997) Characterization of paracellular and aqueous penetration routes in cornea, conjunctiva, and sclera. Invest Ophthalmol Vis Sci 38: 627–634
Han X, Zhao Y, Liu H, Li H, Liu S, Rupenthal ID, Yang F, Lv Z, Chen Y, Zang L, Li W, Ping Q, Tao Q, Hou D (2021) Micro-interaction of mucin tear film interface with particles: the inconsistency of pharmacodynamics and precorneal retention of ion-exchange, functionalized, Mt-embedded nano- and microparticles. Colloids Surf B Biointerfaces 197:111355
Herlihy KP, Williams S, Owens G, Savage J, Gardner L, Robeson R, Maynor B, Navratil T, Gilger BC, Yerxa BR (2014) Extended release of microfabricated protein particles from biodegradable hydrogel implants for the treatment of age related macular degeneration. Invest Ophthalmol Vis Sci 55:1960–1960
Holekamp NM, Campochiaro PA, Chang MA, Miller D, Pieramici D, Adamis AP, Brittain C, Evans E, Kaufman D, Maass KF, Patel S, Ranade S, Singh N, Barteselli G, Regillo C, On Behalf ofall Archway Investigators (2022) Archway randomized phase 3 trial of the port delivery system with ranibizumab for neovascular age-related macular degeneration. Ophthalmology 129:295–307
Hornof M, Toropainen E, Urtti A (2005) Cell culture models of the ocular barriers. Eur J Pharm Biopharm 60:207–225
Huang HS, Schoenwald RD, Lach JL (1983) Corneal penetration behavior of beta-blocking agents II: assessment of barrier contributions. J Pharm Sci 72:1272–1279
Huang AJW, Tseng SCG, Kenyon KR (1989) Paracellular permeability of corneal and conjunctival epithelia. Invest Ophthalmol Vis Sci 30:684–689
Huang D, Chen YS, Rupenthal ID (2018) Overcoming ocular drug delivery barriers through the use of physical forces. Adv Drug Deliv Rev 126:96–112
Humayun M, Santos A, Altamirano JC, Ribeiro R, Gonzalez R, de la Rosa A, Shih J, Pang C, Jiang F, Calvillo P, Huculak J, Zimmerman J, Caffey S (2014) Implantable MicroPump for drug delivery in patients with diabetic macular Edema. Transl Vis Sci Technol 3:5
Hussain AA, Rowe L, Marshall J (2002) Age-related alterations in the diffusional transport of amino acids across the human Bruch's-choroid complex. J Opt Soc Am 19:166–172
Ishibashi T, Yokoi N, Kinoshita S (2003) Comparison of the short-term effects on the human corneal surface of topical timolol maleate with and without benzalkonium chloride. J Glaucoma 12:486–490
Jaffe GJ, Yang CH, Guo H, Denny JP, Lima C, Ashton P (2000) Safety and pharmacokinetics of an intraocular fluocinolone acetonide sustained delivery device. Invest Ophthalmol Vis Sci 41: 3569–3575
Järvinen K, Järvinen T, Urtti A (1995) Ocular absorption following topical delivery. Adv Drug Deliv Rev 16:3–19
Jordán J, Ruíz-Moreno JM (2013) Advances in the understanding of retinal drug disposition and the role of blood–ocular barrier transporters. Expert Opin Drug Metab Toxicol 9:1181–1192
Joseph RR, Venkatraman SS (2017) Drug delivery to the eye: what benefits do nanocarriers offer? Nanomedicine 12:683–702
Jung JH, Chae JJ, Prausnitz MR (2019) Targeting drug delivery within the suprachoroidal space. Drug Discov Today 24:1654–1659

Kahook MY, Noecker RJ (2008) Comparison of corneal and conjunctival changes after dosing of travoprost preserved with sofZia, latanoprost with 0.02% benzalkonium chloride, and preservative-free artificial tears. Cornea 27:339–343

Kane FE, Burdan J, Cutino A, Green KE (2008) Iluvien: a new sustained delivery technology for posterior eye disease. Expert Opin Drug Deliv 5:1039–1046

Kang-Mieler JJ, Dosmar E, Liu W, Mieler WF (2017) Extended ocular drug delivery systems for the anterior and posterior segments: biomaterial options and applications. Expert Opin Drug Deliv 14:611–620

Kansara V, Mitra AK (2006) Evaluation of an *ex vivo* model implication for carrier-mediated retinal drug delivery. Curr Eye Res 31:415–426

Kapoor Y, Howell BA, Chauhan A (2009) Liposome assay for evaluating ocular toxicity of surfactants. Invest Ophthalmol Vis Sci 50:2727–2735

Karami TK, Hailu S, Feng S, Graham R, Gukasyan HJ (2021) Eyes on Lipinski's rule of five: a new "Rule of Thumb" for physicochemical design space of ophthalmic drugs. J Ocul Pharmacol Ther 38:43–55

Kim SH, Lutz RJ, Wang NS, Robinson MR (2007) Transport barriers in transscleral drug delivery for retinal diseases. Ophthalmic Res 39:244–254

Kim SH, Csaky KG, Wang NS, Lutz RJ (2008) Drug elimination kinetics following subconjunctival injection using dynamic contrast-enhanced magnetic resonance imaging. Pharm Res 25:512–520

Kim J, Schlesinger EB, Desai TA (2015) Nanostructured materials for ocular delivery: nanodesign for enhanced bioadhesion, transepithelial permeability and sustained delivery. Ther Deliv 6: 1365–1376

Kim T, Sall K, Holland EJ, Brazzell RK, Coultas S, Gupta PK (2019) Safety and efficacy of twice daily administration of KPI-121 1% for ocular inflammation and pain following cataract surgery. Clin Ophthalmol 13:69–86

Koevary SB (2003) Pharmacokinetics of topical ocular drug delivery: potential uses for the treatment of diseases of the posterior segment and beyond. Curr Drug Metab 4:213–222

Labbé A, Pauly A, Liang H, Brignole-Baudouin F, Martin C, Warnet JM, Baudouin C (2006) Comparison of toxicological profiles of benzalkonium chloride and polyquaternium-1: an experimental study. J Ocul Pharmacol Ther 22:267–278

Lai SK, Wang YY, Hanes J (2009) Mucus-penetrating nanoparticles for drug and gene delivery to mucosal tissues. Adv Drug Deliv Rev 61:158–171

Lance KD, Good SD, Mendes TS, Ishikiriyama M, Chew P, Estes LS, Yamada K, Mudumba S, Bhisitkul RB, Desai TA (2015) In vitro and in vivo sustained zero-order delivery of rapamycin (sirolimus) from a biodegradable intraocular device. Invest Ophthalmol Vis Sci 56:7331–7337

Laude A, Tan LE, Wilson CG, Lascaratos G, Elashry M, Aslam T, Patton N, Dhillon B (2010) Intravitreal therapy for neovascular age-related macular degeneration and inter-individual variations in vitreous pharmacokinetics. Prog Retin Eye Res 29:466–475

Le Bourlais CA, Treupel-Acar L, Rhodes CT, Sado PA, Leverge R (1995) New ophthalmic drug delivery systems. Drug Dev Ind Pharm 21:19–59

Le Bourlais C, Acar L, Zia H, Sado PA, Needham T, Leverge R (1998) Ophthalmic drug delivery systems – recent advances. Prog Retin Eye Res 17:33–58

Lederer CM, Harold RE (1986) Drop size of commercial glaucoma medications. Am J Ophthalmol 101:691–694

Lee VH, Robinson JR (1986) Topical ocular drug delivery: recent developments and future challenges. J Ocul Pharmacol 2:67–108

Lee CH, Singla A, Lee Y (2001) Biomedical applications of collagen. Int J Pharm 221:1–22

Lee HJ, Jun RM, Cho MS, Choi K-R (2015) Comparison of the ocular surface changes following the use of two different prostaglandin F2α analogues containing benzalkonium chloride or polyquad in rabbit eyes. Cutan Ocul Toxicol 34:195–202

Leibowitz HM, Kupferman A (1977) Drug interaction in the eye: concurrent corticosteroid-antibiotic therapy for inflammatory keratitis. Arch Ophthalmol 95:682–685

Lewis RA, Christie WC, Day DG, Craven ER, Walters T, Bejanian M, Lee SS, Goodkin ML, Zhang J, Whitcup SM, Robinson MR, Aung T, Beck AD, Christie WC, Coote M, Crane CJ, Craven ER, Crichton A, Day DG, Durcan FJ, Flynn WJ, Gagné S, Goldberg DF, Jinapriya D, Johnson CS, Kurtz S, Lewis RA, Mansberger SL, Perera SA, Rotberg MH, Saltzmann RM, Schenker HI, Tepedino ME, Yap-Veloso MIR, Uy HS, Walters TR (2017) Bimatoprost sustained-release implants for glaucoma therapy: 6-month results from a phase I/II clinical trial. Am J Ophthalmol 175:137–147

Liaw J, Rojanasakul Y, Robinson JR (1992) The effect of drug charge type and charge density on corneal transport. Int J Pharm 88:111–124

Liu YC, Wong TT, Mehta JS (2013) Intraocular lens as a drug delivery reservoir. Curr Opin Ophthalmol 24:53–59

Lo R, Li PY, Saati S, Agrawal RN, Humayun MS, Meng E (2009) A passive MEMS drug delivery pump for treatment of ocular diseases. Biomed Microdevices 11:959–970

Loewenstein A, Laganovska G, Bressler NM, Vanags J, Alster Y, De Juan E, Stewart JM, Kardatzke D, Singh N, Erickson S (2020) Phase 1 clinical study of the port delivery system with ranibizumab for continuous treatment of neovascular age-related macular degeneration. Invest Ophthalmol Vis Sci 61:4201–4201

Loftssona T, Jarvinen T (1999) Cyclodextrins in ophthalmic drug delivery. Adv Drug Deliv Rev 36: 59–79

Ludwig A (2005) The use of mucoadhesive polymers in ocular drug delivery. Adv Drug Deliv Rev 57:1595–1639

Ludwig A, Van Ooteghem M (1987) The influence of the osmolality on the precorneal retention of ophthalmic solutions. J Pharm Belg 42:259–266

Mandal A, Bisht R, Rupenthal ID, Mitra AK (2017) Polymeric micelles for ocular drug delivery: from structural frameworks to recent preclinical studies. J Controlled Release 248:96–116

Marmer RH (1988) Therapeutic and protective properties of the corneal collagen shield. J Cataract Refract Surg 14:496–499

Martens TF, Vercauteren D, Forier K, Deschout H, Remaut K, Paesen R, Ameloot M, Engbersen JFJ, Demeester J, De Smedt SC, Braeckmans K (2013) Measuring the intravitreal mobility of nanomedicines with single-particle tracking microscopy. Nanomedicine 8:1955–1968

Martin DF, Parks DJ, Mellow SD, Ferris FL, Walton RC, Remaley NA, Chew EY, Ashton P, Davis MD, Nussenblatt RB (1994) Treatment of cytomegalovirus retinitis with an intraocular sustained-release ganciclovir implant. A randomized controlled clinical trial. Arch Ophthalmol 112:1531–1539

Maulvi FA, Lakdawala DH, Shaikh AA, Desai AR, Choksi HH, Vaidya RJ, Ranch KM, Koli AR, Vyas BA, Shah DO (2016) In vitro and in vivo evaluation of novel implantation technology in hydrogel contact lenses for controlled drug delivery. J Control Release 226:47–56

Maurice DM, Polgar J (1977) Diffusion across the sclera. Exp Eye Res 25:577–582

Medeiros FA, Walters TR, Kolko M, Coote M, Bejanian M, Goodkin ML, Guo Q, Zhang J, Robinson MR, Weinreb RN, AS Group (2020) Phase 3, randomized, 20-month study of bimatoprost implant in open-angle glaucoma and ocular hypertension (ARTEMIS 1). Ophthalmology 127:1627–1641

Molokhia SA, Sant H, Simonis J, Bishop CJ, Burr RM, Gale BK, Ambati BK (2010) The capsule drug device: novel approach for drug delivery to the eye. Vision Res 50:680–685

Navratil T, Maynor B, Yerxa B (2014) Improving outcomes in ophthalmology via sustained drug delivery. ONdrugDelivery:10–13

Novack GD (2023) US regulatory approval of a drug-eluting contact lens. Eye Contact Lens 49: 136–138

Olsen TW, Aaberg SY, Geroski DH, Edelhauser HF (1998) Human sclera: thickness and surface area. Am J Ophthalmol 125:237–241

O'Rourke M (2014) Next generation ocular drug delivery platforms, Eye on innovation. The Official Publication of OIS, pp 1–7

Pahuja P, Arora S, Pawar P (2012) Ocular drug delivery system: a reference to natural polymers. Expert Opin Drug Deliv 9:837–861
Palmgren JJ, Toropainen E, Auriola S, Urtti A (2002) Liquid chromatographic-electrospray ionization mass spectrometric analysis of neutral and charged polyethylene glycols. J Chromatogr A 976:165–170
Pearce EI, Dorman M, Wilkinson BC, Oliver KM (2011) Effect of blink frequency on tear turnover rate. Invest Ophthalmol Vis Sci 52:3726–3726
Peyman GA, Hosseini K (2011) Combination therapies in ophthalmology: implications for intravitreal delivery. J Ophthalmic Vis Res 6:36–46
Pitkanen L, Ranta VP, Moilanen H, Urtti A (2005) Permeability of retinal pigment epithelium: effects of permeant molecular weight and lipophilicity. Invest Ophthalmol Vis Sci 46:641–646
PolyActiva (2023). https://polyactiva.com/pipeline/. Accessed 4 May 2023
Prausnitz MR, Noonan JS (1998) Permeability of cornea, sclera, and conjunctiva: a literature analysis for drug delivery to the eye. J Pharm Sci 87:1479–1488
Prow TW, Bhutto I, Kim SY, Grebe R, Merges C, McLeod DS, Uno K, Mennon M, Rodriguez L, Leong K, Lutty GA (2008) Ocular nanoparticle toxicity and transfection of the retina and retinal pigment epithelium. Nanomedicine 4:340–349
Ramsay E, del Amo EM, Toropainen E, Tengvall-Unadike U, Ranta V-P, Urtti A, Ruponen M (2018) Corneal and conjunctival drug permeability: systematic comparison and pharmacokinetic impact in the eye. Eur J Pharm Sci 119:83–89
Ranade SV, Wieland MR, Tam T, Rea JC, Horvath J, Hieb AR, Jia W, Grace L, Barteselli G, Stewart JM (2022) The port delivery system with ranibizumab: a new paradigm for long-acting retinal drug delivery. Drug Deliv 29:1326–1334
Ripple (2023). https://www.rippletherapeutics.com/practice_area#Pipeline. Accessed 4 May 2023
Rojanasakul Y, Robinson JR (1989) Transport mechanisms of the cornea: characterization of barrier permselectivity. Int J Pharm 55:237–246
Runkle EA, Antonetti DA (2011) The blood-retinal barrier: structure and functional significance. The blood-brain and other neural barriers. Springer, pp 133–148
Rupenthal ID (2017) Drug-device combination approaches for delivery to the eye. Curr Opin Pharmacol 36:44–51
Rupenthal ID, Green CR, Alany RG (2011a) Comparison of ion-activated in situ gelling systems for ocular drug delivery. Part 1: physicochemical characterisation and in vitro release. Int J Pharm 411:69–77
Rupenthal ID, Green CR, Alany RG (2011b) Comparison of ion-activated in situ gelling systems for ocular drug delivery. Part 2: precorneal retention and in vivo pharmacodynamic study. Int J Pharm 411:78–85
Ruponen M, Urtti A (2015) Undefined role of mucus as a barrier in ocular drug delivery. Eur J Pharm Biopharm 96:442–446
Saarinen-Savolainen P, Järvinen T, Araki-Sasaki K, Watanabe H, Urtti A (1998) Evaluation of cytotoxicity of various ophthalmic drugs, eye drop excipients and cyclodextrins in an immortalized human corneal epithelial cell line. Pharm Res 15:1275–1280
Samy KE, Cao Y, Kim J, Konichi da Silva NR, Phone A, Bloomer MM, Bhisitkul RB, Desai TA (2019) Co-delivery of timolol and brimonidine with a polymer thin-film intraocular device. J Ocul Pharmacol Ther 35:124–131
Schlesinger EB, Bernards DA, Chen HH, Feindt J, Cao J, Dix D, Romano C, Bhisitkul RB, Desai TA (2019) Device design methodology and formulation of a protein therapeutic for sustained release intraocular delivery. Bioeng Transl Med 4:152–163
Schoenwald RD, Huang HS (1983) Corneal penetration behavior of beta-blocking agents I: physiochemical factors. J Pharm Sci 72:1266–1272
Schoenwald RD, Ward RL (1978) Relationship between steroid permeability across excised rabbit cornea and octanol-water partition coefficients. J Pharm Sci 67:786–788

Schopf LR, Popov AM, Enlow EM, Bourassa JL, Ong WZ, Nowak P, Chen H (2015) Topical ocular drug delivery to the back of the eye by mucus-penetrating particles. Transl Vis Sci Technol 4:11

Sellner PA (1986) The movement of organic solutes between the retina and pigment-epithelium. Exp Eye Res 43:631–639

Sheppard JD, Wirta DL, McLaurin E, Boehmer BE, Ciolino JB, Meides AS, Schlüter T, Ousler GW, Usner D, Krösser S (2021) A water-free 0.1% cyclosporine A solution for treatment of dry eye disease: results of the randomized phase 2B/3 ESSENCE study. Cornea 40:1290–1297

Sieg JW, Robinson JR (1975) Vehicle effects on ocular drug bioavailability i: evaluation of fluorometholone. J Pharm Sci 64:931–936

Singh D (2003) Conjunctival lymphatic system. J Cataract Refract Surg 29:632–633

Taskar P, Tatke A, Majumdar S (2017) Advances in the use of prodrugs for drug delivery to the eye. Expert Opin Drug Deliv 14:49–63

Thakur Singh RR, Jones D (2018) Biodegradable implants for sustained intraocular delivery of small and large molecules. ONdrugDelivery 2018:28–31

Thakur SS, Barnett NL, Donaldson MJ, Parekh HS (2014) Intravitreal drug delivery in retinal disease: are we out of our depth? Expert Opin Drug Deliv 11:1575–1590

Therapeutix O (2023). https://www.ocutx.com/research/pipeline/. Accessed 4 May 2023

Thrimawithana TR, Rupenthal ID, Young SA, Alany RG (2012) Environment-sensitive polymers for ophthalmic drug delivery. J Drug Deliv Sci Technol 22:117–124

Urtti A (2006) Challenges and obstacles of ocular pharmacokinetics and drug delivery. Adv Drug Deliv Rev 58:1131–1135

Van Ooteghem MMM (1993) Formulation of ophthalmic solutions and suspensions. Problems and advantages. In: Edman P (ed) Biopharmaceutics of ocular drug delivery. CRC Press, Boca Raton, pp 27–42

Vantipalli S, Sall KN, Stein E, Schenker H, Mulaney J, Smyth-Medina R, Day D, Benza R, Dixon E-R, Rissman N, Metzinger JL, Goldstein MH (2020) Evaluation of the safety and efficacy of OTX-TP, an intracanalicular travoprost insert, for the treatment of patients with open-angle glaucoma or ocular hypertension: a phase 3 study. Invest Ophthalmol Vis Sci 61:3488–3488

Whitcup SM, Robinson MR (2015) Development of a dexamethasone intravitreal implant for the treatment of noninfectious posterior segment uveitis. Ann N Y Acad Sci 1358:1–12

Yamada M, Mochizuki H, Yamada K, Kawai M, Mashima Y (2003) Aqueous humor levels of topically applied levofloxacin, norfloxacin, and lomefloxacin in the same human eyes. J Cataract Refract Surg 29:1771–1775

Yasin MN, Svirskis D, Seyfoddin A, Rupenthal ID (2014) Implants for drug delivery to the posterior segment of the eye: a focus on stimuli-responsive and tunable release systems. J Control Release 196:208–221

Yellepeddi VK, Sheshala R, McMillan H, Gujral C, Jones D, Raghu Raj Singh T (2015) Punctal plug: a medical device to treat dry eye syndrome and for sustained drug delivery to the eye. Drug Discov Today 20:884–889

New Therapeutic Options in Pulmonal Diseases: Sphingolipids and Modulation of Sphingolipid Metabolism

Burkhard Kleuser, Fabian Schumacher, and Erich Gulbins

Contents

Abstract

Sphingolipids are crucial molecules in the respiratory airways. As in most other tissues and organs, in the lung sphingolipids play an essential role as structural constituents as they regulate barrier function and fluidity of cell membranes. A lung-specific feature is the occurrence of sphingolipids as minor structural components in the surfactant. However, sphingolipids are also key signaling molecules involved in airway cell signaling and their dynamical formation and metabolism are important for normal lung physiology. Dysregulation of sphingolipid metabolism and signaling is involved in altering lung tissue and

B. Kleuser (✉) · F. Schumacher
Institute of Pharmacy, Pharmacology and Toxicology, Freie Universität Berlin, Berlin, Germany
e-mail: Burkhard.Kleuser@fu-berlin.de

E. Gulbins (✉)
Institute of Molecular Biology, University Hospital Essen, University of Duisburg-Essen, Essen, Germany
e-mail: erich.gulbins@uk-essen.de

M. Schäfer-Korting, U. S. Schubert (eds.), *Drug Delivery and Targeting*,
Handbook of Experimental Pharmacology 284, https://doi.org/10.1007/164_2023_700

initiates inflammatory processes promoting the pathogenesis of pulmonal diseases including cystic fibrosis (CF), chronic obstructive pulmonary disease (COPD), and asthma.

In the present review, the important role of specific sphingolipid species in pulmonal diseases will be discussed. Only such an understanding opens up the possibility of developing new therapeutic strategies with the aim of correcting the imbalance in sphingolipid metabolism and signaling. Such delivery strategies have already been studied in animal models of these lung diseases, demonstrating that targeting the sphingolipid profile represents new therapeutic opportunities for lung disorders.

Keywords

Asthma bronchiale · Ceramides · COPD · Cystic fibrosis · Sphingolipids · Sphingosine · Sphingosine 1-phosphate

Abbreviations

CerS	Ceramide synthase
CERT	Ceramide transporter
CF	Cystic fibrosis
CFTR/Cftr	Cystic fibrosis transmembrane conductance regulator
COPD	Chronic obstructive pulmonary disease
IL	Interleukin
NF-κB	Nuclear factor-κB
ORMDL	Orosomucoid-like
S1P	Sphingosine 1-phosphate
S1PR	S1P-Specific G-protein-coupled receptor
SPHK	Sphingosine kinase
TNF-α	Tumor necrosis factor α

1 Sphingolipid Homeostasis

Sphingolipids are one of the main classes of eukaryotic lipids, which were discovered by the German physician Johann Ludwig Thudicum in the cerebrum at the end of the nineteenth century (Thudhicum 1884). However, the elucidation of the molecular structure proved to be difficult and so he introduced the name "sphingosin" in homage to the Greek mythological creature, the sphinx, in view of the many enigmas which it posed to the researcher. Nowadays, sphingolipid structures are well elucidated, the backbone of most sphingolipids is sphingosine ((*E*,2*S*,3*R*)-2-aminooctadec-4-ene-1,3-diol) from which more complex sphingolipids such as sphingomyelins and glycosphingolipids can be formed (Fig. 1) (Fahy et al. 2005). Especially those complex sphingolipids are ubiquitous

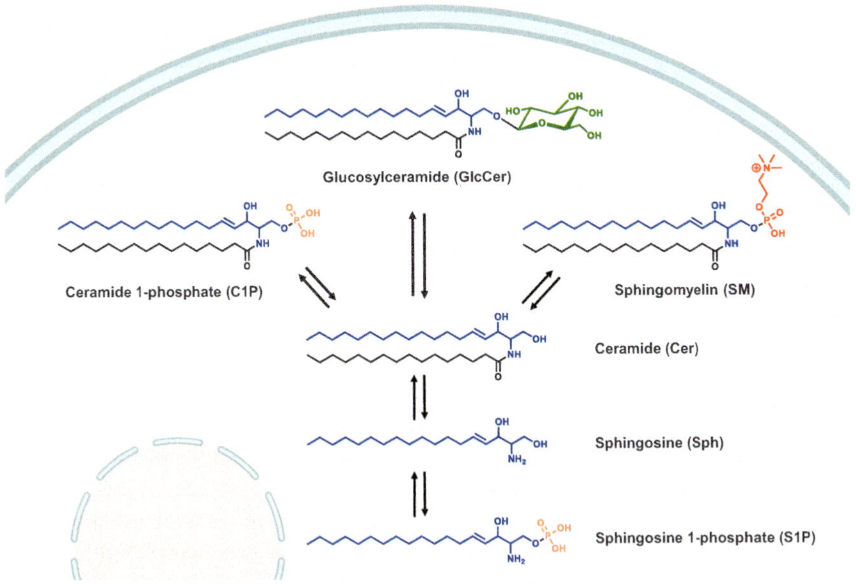

Fig. 1 Chemical structures of bioactive sphingolipid species. Ceramides (Cer), the central representatives of the complex sphingolipid network, consist of a sphingosine (Sph) (d18:1; S) backbone (blue colored) and an N-linked fatty acid (black colored) with chain lengths ranging from C12 to C26 (shown is C16 palmitic acid). To the polar head group, the hydroxyl group at the 1-position, additional functionalities can be attached resulting in more complex sphingolipids. The addition of phosphocholine (in red) leads to sphingomyelins (SM), linkage with glucose (in green) yields glucosylceramides (GlcCer), and after phosphorylation (highlighted orange) ceramide 1-phosphate (C1P) is obtained. Deacylation of ceramides releases sphingosine (Sph), which can be metabolized to sphingosine 1-phosphate (S1P) after phosphorylation (in orange)

components of cell membranes and as such play a crucial role in membrane biophysical characteristics regulating a variety of biological processes through membrane properties (Harayama and Riezman 2018). According to the length of their fatty acid chains and their saturation level, sphingolipids distinctly influence membrane characteristics such as fluidity and rigidity, and thus enable diverse interactions with membrane proteins or cytoskeletal proteins to form signaling platforms in a dynamic and spatiotemporally structured nature (Barrera et al. 2013; Bieberich 2018; Bollinger et al. 2005; Gulbins and Kolesnick 2003). However, sphingolipid species not only structurally support the interaction and crosstalk with their signalosome assemblies, but also function intrinsically as highly potent signaling molecules that regulate a plethora of cellular processes, in particular cell growth and migration as well as inflammation and immune cell modulation (Hannun and Obeid 2008). The most prominent bioactive sphingolipids are ceramides, sphingosine, sphingosine 1-phosphate (S1P), and ceramide 1-phosphate (Fig. 1).

In the sphingolipid metabolic network ceramides act as a center nexus for the formation of complex sphingolipids and bioactive sphingolipid species. A close interaction between ceramide formation and apoptosis has been identified (Siskind et al. 2010). Ceramides are generated via a highly coordinated system, which includes the de novo synthesis of ceramides and their formation from complex sphingolipids by either lysosomal or non-lysosomal degradation (Hannun and Obeid 2011). The sphingolipid de novo synthesis is initiated in the endoplasmic reticulum by serine palmitoyl-transferase, which catalyzes the condensation of the activated C16 fatty acid palmitoyl-CoA with the amino acid *L*-serine. Further enzymatic steps (see Fig. 2) lead to the formation of ceramides with distinct biophysical characteristics and various biological functions (Wegner et al. 2016). Created with BioRender.com.

After transfer to the Golgi compartment via the ceramide transporter CERT, ceramides are metabolized by glycosylation to glucosylceramides or by acquiring a phosphocholine head group via sphingomyelin synthase to sphingomyelins. Glucosylceramides and sphingomyelins are trafficked by vesicular exocytosis to the plasma membrane, where they are localized predominantly to the outer cell membrane leaflet (Doktorova et al. 2020).

Sphingolipid catabolism is initiated by the generation of ceramides as a result of the activity of sphingomyelinases or, in the specific case of glycosphingolipids, by dedicated hydrolases. Sphingomyelinases are classified into neutral, acidic, and alkaline isoforms depending on their pH optimum. Ceramide levels are strictly controlled, as evidenced by its prompt conversion to ceramide 1-phosphate or deacylation by ceramidases to sphingosine, which has been discussed also as a bioactive sphingolipid molecule and is the precursor for the formation of S1P (Pruett et al. 2008). Phosphorylation of sphingosine is catalyzed by either sphingosine kinase 1 (SPHK1) or 2 (SPHK2), thereby producing S1P (Maceyka et al. 2005).

S1P is able to stimulate five S1P-specific G-protein-coupled receptors (S1PR1-5), which are cell-specific expressed thereby leading to a plethora of sometimes contradictory cellular and physiological responses (Fig. 2) (Cartier and Hla 2019; Kano et al. 2022; Sanchez and Hla 2004). A most important function of S1P has been shown in immune cell circulation. Thus, the egress of T cells is directed by an S1P gradient between lymph nodes, lymph, and plasma (Benechet et al. 2016; Hla et al. 2008). The S1PR1 expressed on lymphocytes is able to respond to this gradient, leading to the migration of lymphocytes from lymphoid tissues into the circulation (Cyster and Schwab 2012). This mechanism can be interrupted via S1PR modulators resulting in an immunosuppressive action. Actually, four S1PR modulators (fingolimod, siponimod, ozanimod, and ponesimod) have regulatory approval for multiple sclerosis and in the case of ozanimod also for the treatment of ulcerative colitis (McGinley and Cohen 2021; Paik 2022). S1P can be reversibly cleaved to sphingosine or irreversibly degraded via an S1P lyase leading to the formation of phosphoethanolamine and hexadecenal (Fig. 2) (Bektas et al. 2010; Hagen-Euteneuer et al. 2012; Le Stunff et al. 2007).

This sophisticated metabolic network can undergo significant adjustments in response to metabolic and external challenges. It is therefore not surprising that a disturbance of the dynamic equilibrium in sphingolipid metabolism is associated with a dysfunction of cellular processes. Indeed, a disturbed sphingolipid

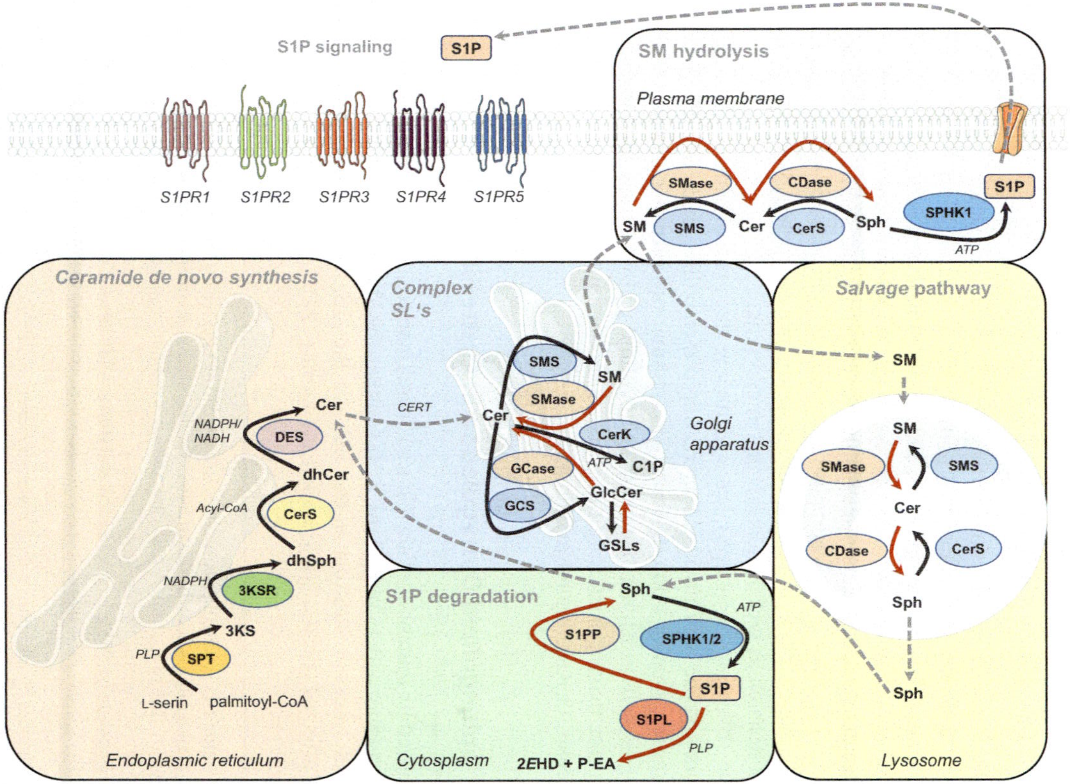

Fig. 2 Cellular compartmentalization of the sphingolipid metabolism. The ceramide de novo synthesis takes place at the outer membrane of the endoplasmic reticulum and starts with the condensation of palmitoyl-CoA and L-serine via the PLP-dependent serine SPT. The formed 3KS is reduced to dhSph by the NADPH-dependent 3KSR. DhSph is further metabolized to dhCer by N-acylation via CerS. Subsequently, a C4-5 double bond is introduced by the NADPH/NADH-dependent DES to form the central molecule Cer. After transport to the Golgi apparatus via CERT, Cer is provided for the synthesis of complex

metabolism is detected in pulmonary disorders and modulation of the sphingolipid metabolism may be an effective target for treatment of those diseases.

2 Sphingolipid Dysregulation in Pulmonal Diseases

The lung is rarely considered an organ of lipid metabolism. Nevertheless, in addition to their essential role as surfactants and structural components, sphingolipids also exert various signaling functions in the physiological and pathophysiological processes of the lung (Ghidoni et al. 2015). Inflammation of the lung may be accompanied by excessive surfactant and mucus production, epithelial cell reactivity, endothelial permeability, immune responses as well as parenchymal and matrix damage. Leukocyte infiltration results in the release of harmful molecules such as radicals and proteases. The pathophysiological consequences are tissue edema and fibrosis, small terminal airway damage with oxygen deficiency, capillary damage, and hypertension as well as necrosis and emphysema.

In the following paragraphs, we will review the involvement of sphingolipid mediators and the adjustments of sphingolipid metabolism in the setting of major lung diseases, namely cystic fibrosis (CF), chronic obstructive pulmonary disease (COPD) as well as asthma. Targeting sphingolipid pathways may hold therapeutic potential for treating such lung disorders by modulating inflammation, promoting tissue repair, or restoring normal lung function.

2.1 Sphingolipid Dysregulation in Cystic Fibrosis

CF is caused by mutations of the CF transmembrane conductance regulator (human: CFTR, murine: Cftr). With 1 of 2,500 births, the disease is the most common autosomal recessive disorder in the EU and the US with approximately 80,000 persons affected (Elborn 2016; Ratjen and Doring 2003).

Fig. 2 (continued) sphingolipids such as SM by SMS, GlcCer by GCS or C1P by CerK. These complex sphingolipids are further shuttled to the plasma membrane or lysosomes. There the breakdown of SM to Cer takes place by SMase. Ceramide can be degraded by CDase to form Sph. S1P can be formed by phosphorylation via SphK1/2. S1P is reversibly degraded by S1PP to Sph or irreversibly by S1PL to yield 2EHD and P-EA. ATP, adenosine triphosphate; C1P, ceramide 1-phosphate; CDase, ceramidase; Cer, ceramide; CerK, ceramide kinase; CerS, ceramide synthases; CERT, ceramide transporter; CoA, coenzyme A; DES, dihydroceramide desaturase; dhCer, dihydroceramide; dhSph, dihydrosphingosine; 2EHD, (2E)-hexadecenal; GCase, glucosylceramidase; GCS, glucosylceramide synthase; GlcCer, glucosylceramide; GSLs, glycosphingolipids; 3KS, 3-ketosphinganine; 3KSR, 3-ketosphinganine reductase; NADH, nicotinamide adenine dinucleotide; NADPH, nicotinamide adenine dinucleotide phosphate; P-EA, phosphoethanolamine; PLP, pyridoxal 5′-phosphate; S1P, sphingosine 1-phosphate; S1PL, S1P lyase; S1PP, S1P phosphatase; S1PR, S1P receptors; SL's, sphingolipids; SM, sphingomyelin; SMase, sphingomyelinase; SMS, sphingomyelin synthase; Sph, sphingosine; SPHK, sphingosine kinases; SPT, serine palmitoyl-transferase. Created with BioRender.com

CFTR encodes a chloride channel and defective CFTR function is linked to alterations of the airway mucus resulting in impaired mucociliary clearance and a lack of functions of defensins and cathelicidins, most likely due to a change of mucus viscosity, but this concept is difficult to demonstrate in vivo (Shah et al. 2016; Vital et al. 2013). Therefore, to understand the pathophysiology of the disease, the balance between pro- and anti-inflammatory cytokines in the airways of CF patients has been intensively investigated. Indeed, concentrations of pro-inflammatory cytokines are increased whereas the release of anti-inflammatory cytokines is reduced in the lungs of Cftr-deficient mice and human CF patients (Oceandy et al. 2002; Schultz et al. 2002; Verhaeghe et al. 2007).

In addition, CF patients show, for unknown reasons, a massive recruitment of neutrophils into the airways. The accumulation of neutrophils might further contribute to the high viscosity of the mucus, since dead neutrophils release DNA, which is a very viscous biomolecule (Whitchurch et al. 2002; Worlitzsch et al. 2002).

Moreover, a dysregulation of sphingolipids has been identified in CF. A progressive elevation of ceramide concentrations in the airways of CF patients and mice has been observed (Liessi et al. 2020; Loberto et al. 2020; Signorelli et al. 2021). Collectively, the studies indicated an increased ceramide concentration in bronchial and tracheal epithelial cells and in alveolar macrophages of CF patients and mice (Teichgraeber et al. 2008; Brodlie et al. 2010; Becker et al. 2010; Pewzner-Jung et al. 2014; Caretti et al. 2014, 2016; Grassme et al. 2017). Acid sphingomyelinase and ceramide affect CFTR function (Cottrill et al. 2021). Increased ceramide concentrations in the bronchial epithelial cells contribute to the high susceptibility of *Cftr*-deficient mice to acute pulmonary infections with *P. aeruginosa* and trigger chronic pulmonary inflammation and deposition of DNA released from dead cells in bronchi (Grassme et al. 2017; Teichgraber et al. 2008).

The basis for ceramide elevation in CF epithelial cells is not fully understood, but several independent studies have shown that the activity and expression of acid ceramidase is downregulated in cells from CF mice and patients, which may result in ceramide accumulation (Gardner et al. 2021; Grassme et al. 2017). Activation of de novo ceramide synthesis has also been shown in association with CF, and it is certainly possible that several pathways lead to the observed changes in ceramide concentrations in CF lungs (Caretti et al. 2017).

In addition to elevated ceramide levels, CF mice and patients exhibit a severe reduction of sphingosine concentrations in airway epithelial cells. Normally, sphingosine is abundantly expressed on the luminal surface of normal human nasal epithelial cells and of tracheal and bronchial epithelial cells of wild-type mice, whereas it is almost undetectable on the surface of nasal epithelial cells from CF patients and on tracheal and bronchial cells from CF mice (Tavakoli Tabazavareh et al. 2016). In vitro studies have indicated that sphingosine is bactericidal for many bacterial species including *P. aeruginosa*, *S. aureus*, and Methicillin-resistant *S. aureus* strains (Martin et al. 2017; Rice et al. 2016; Tavakoli Tabazavareh et al. 2016). Sphingosine induces almost instant permeabilization of the cell membrane in *P. aeruginosa* and *S. aureus*, resulting in leakiness, loss of ATP, loss of bacterial metabolic activity, and death (Fischer et al. 2013; Verhaegh et al. 2020).

Mechanistically, the protonated amino group of sphingosine binds to the highly negatively charged lipid cardiolipin in bacterial cell membranes leading to a rapid permeabilization. It is of interest, that *E. coli* or *P. aeruginosa* strains that lack cardiolipin synthase are resistant to sphingosine (Verhaegh et al. 2020).

Due to diminished sphingosine levels it is not astonishing that individuals with CF suffer mainly from pulmonary problems, which include besides chronic inflammation and fibrosis also recurrent and chronic infections with a variety of bacteria. Especially, *P. aeruginosa* and *S. aureus* are ubiquitous and opportunistic pathogens that cause severe respiratory tract and systemic infections (Sadikot et al. 2005).

There is no cure for cystic fibrosis, but treatment can ease symptoms and reduce complications. Antibiotics, anti-inflammatory drugs, mucus-thinning medications, and bronchodilators are used to treat CF. A major innovation in the therapy of CF is CFTR modulators as they act by improving the production, intracellular processing, and function of the defective CFTR protein. It is of interest that CFTR modulators might influence sphingolipid dysregulation in patients with CF (Westholter et al. 2022). Thus, treatment of patients with elexacaftor/tezacaftor/ivacaftor resulted in a decrease of long-chain ceramides, whereas S1P levels were increased. However, many *P. aeruginosa* and *S. aureus* strains are highly resistant to existing antibiotics, and attempts to eradicate these bacteria usually fail. Even the great success of CFTR modulators does not lead to sufficient elimination of pathogens. Thus, it is necessary to develop novel strategies for treating pulmonary infections with *P. aeruginosa* and *S. aureus*.

2.2 Sphingolipid Dysregulation in COPD

COPD is an inflammatory respiratory disease leading to more than three million deaths worldwide each year. COPD ranked third on the list of leading causes of death in 2020, after ischemic heart disease and cerebrovascular disease (Christenson et al. 2022). The Global Initiative for Chronic Obstructive Lung Disease (GOLD) defines COPD as a common preventable and treatable disease, which is characterized by airflow limitation that is usually progressive and associated with an enhanced chronic inflammatory response in the airways and the lung to noxious particles or gases (Global Initiative for Chronic Obstructive Lung Disease 2002). COPD is closely linked to exposure to cigarette smoking and environmental pollutants, however, genetic and epigenetic environmental risk factors are also clearly involved in the etiology of the disease (Hogg and Timens 2009; Terzikhan et al. 2016). The triggering causes are connected to inflammation and airway obstruction. In the emphysema phenotype of COPD, ongoing damage of the small airways and alveoli is accompanied by chronic respiratory failure as a result of irreversible loss of functional lung units. Chronic inflammation along with oxidative stress, an imbalance of local protease and antiprotease activity, fibrosis, and altered angiogenesis have been identified in the pathophysiological process of COPD. The consequences are a thickened, dysfunctional epithelial layer, an increased thickness of the smooth muscle layer of the airway, disruption of the alveolar walls with varying levels of fibrosis, and hypoxic vasoconstriction leading to emphysematous destruction of the lung tissue (Christenson et al. 2022). Originally, the disbalance between proteases and antiproteases that occurs during inflammation was thought to be the main mechanism for the development of emphysema and COPD (Rabe and Watz 2017). However, recent research has shown that an increased apoptosis and an impaired autophagy of epithelial and endothelial cells in coincidence with chronic inflammatory stress are the main factors responsible for lung destruction (Christenson et al. 2022).

In accordance with these findings, metabolic changes that influence cell fate can be considered as one of the triggering causes for the etiology of COPD. In particular, bioactive sphingolipids appear to play a crucial role in the dynamic processes of injury, repair, and resilience of the lung structure in COPD (Chakinala et al. 2019). The balance between intracellular ceramide levels and its downstream metabolite S1P is critical to lung cell fate (Diab et al. 2010; Petrache et al. 2005). Indeed, even in the early stages of COPD, ceramide levels are elevated while S1P levels are depressed. This disbalance is accompanied by the loss of endothelial cell barrier function (Presson et al. 2011; Schweitzer et al. 2015; Schweitzer et al. 2011). In response to oxidative stress and nicotine, increased ceramide levels induce cytoskeletal changes leading to endothelial barrier dysfunction. Moreover, the enhanced ceramide formation induces apoptosis in lung microvascular endothelial cells (Schweitzer et al. 2011). The critical role of ceramides can be impressively demonstrated in COPD animal models in which pulmonary emphysema is induced by subcutaneous delivery of the VEGF receptor inhibitor SU5416. This inhibitor induces the accumulation of ceramides in alveolar septal cells rather than bronchial cells, which is accompanied by caspase-3 activation leading to an alveolar enlargement and destruction (Petrache et al. 2005). This effect can be diminished in the presence of myriocin suggesting that de novo synthesis at least in part is involved in ceramide formation. Therefore, it is not surprising that ceramide levels in the lungs of smokers with emphysema are higher than those without emphysema (Berdyshev et al. 2021).

In fact, ceramides are also involved in the amplification of lung injury in response to cigarette smoking. The formation of reactive oxygen species due to cigarette smoking is associated with an inhibition of antioxidant enzymes such as superoxide dismutase, leading to accumulation of superoxide radicals, which in turn activate acid sphingomyelinase (Petrache et al. 2008). Additionally, neutral sphingomyelinase 2 is increased in response to cigarette smoking (Filosto et al. 2011). Activation of both enzymes is accompanied by a further increase in ceramide levels indicating that there is a positive feedback loop between oxidative stress and ceramide formation (Fig. 2).

Conversely, S1P possesses opposing effects to ceramides as this sphingolipid species alleviates endothelial barrier dysfunction and induces proliferation, which may be important in the repair phase of injury induced by cigarette smoke (De Cunto et al. 2020). The S1PR1 receptor subtype seems to be involved in this protective and regenerative action (Goel et al. 2022). Consistent with these findings, a decreased SPHK1 activity, the crucial enzyme for the formation of S1P, has been detected in lung tissues of individuals with COPD. Indeed, an inverse correlation between SPHK1 and the severity of emphysema is visible in those tissues (Berdyshev et al. 2021).

The effective clearance of apoptotic epithelial cells by alveolar macrophages, a process known as efferocytosis, is also diminished in smokers. Enhanced ceramide levels decrease efferocytosis by impairing cytoskeletal functions and thus phagocytic capacity, whereas S1P signaling is implicated in an enhanced phagocytic function (Petrusca et al. 2010; Tran et al. 2016).

As typical signs of COPD are airway obstruction and inflammation, current medications include bronchodilators, corticosteroids, and antibiotics (Christenson et al. 2022). However, those drugs are not very effective in reversing the alveolar structure demise. As aberrations in the sphingolipid metabolism and signaling contribute to the initiation and progression of pathogenic processes culminating in emphysema, targeting the sphingolipid rheostat may be an innovative approach for COPD therapy.

2.3 Sphingolipid Dysregulation in Asthma

Asthma is a chronic inflammatory disease that is characterized by episodic shortness of breath with wheezing and cough. Airflow obstruction, airway hyperreactivity, and increased mucus production are typical signs of the disease. It is estimated that more than 330 million people worldwide suffer from the disease, and asthma is in the world's top 20 most important disorders, especially due to the chronicity of the disease (Papi et al. 2018; Porsbjerg et al. 2023). Starting with an inflammatory reaction of the airways, bronchial hyperreactivity, and even bronchial obstruction can occur.

Besides environmental trigger factors, there is also a strong genetic component to asthma. Indeed, asthma seems to be most likely inherited through multiple genes, with some variation in locus heterogeneity and polygenic inheritance. However, several genome-wide association studies have indicated that polymorphisms can occur in genes that exert an influence on sphingolipid metabolism. Those studies have identified the orosomucoid-like (ORMDL) genes as those that are associated with an enhanced asthma risk (Ono et al. 2020; Toncheva et al. 2015). Three mammalian *ORMDL* genes exist (ORMDL1-3) and they encode small transmembrane proteins located in the endoplasmic reticulum (Hjelmqvist et al. 2002). The ORMDL proteins can interact with the serine palmitoyl-transferase thereby inhibiting the entry of the de novo synthesized sphingolipid substrate into the sphingolipid biosynthetic pathway (Davis et al. 2019; Siow et al. 2015). Polymorphisms in all three *ORMDL* genes are associated with asthma and it has been indicated that those polymorphisms lead to increased ORMDL levels in asthmatics (Worgall 2022). The identification of *ORMDL* genes as genes susceptible to asthma has ushered in a new era of research in genetics and sphingolipid regulation in asthma. As ORMDL polymorphisms are associated with its high expression and ORMDL inhibits serine palmitoyl-transferase, it would be expected that sphingolipids are decreased in asthma patients. However, an opposing effect is visible as elevated ceramide and S1P levels have been found in asthma (Masini et al. 2008; Reinke et al. 2017). This controversy can be explained by the fact that a high expression of ORMDL in lung epithelial cells may increase ceramide production through the recycling and salvage pathway (Oyeniran et al. 2015).

Exacerbations are phases of a progressive increase in asthma symptoms and a decrease in lung function, which can be divided into two phases. The early phase is mediated by IgE antibodies which are responsive to environmental factors such as house dust mites, animal allergens, mold, or farm animals. Consequently, inhalation of such a pollutant leads to an activation of mast cells via the bound IgE antibodies and a subsequent degranulation. The released mediators such as histamine, prostaglandins, and leukotrienes induce a contraction of smooth muscle cells and airway tightening (Bush 2019). The late phase, which occurs after a few hours, is characterized by the migration of further immune cells into the lungs such as eosinophils, basophils, neutrophils, and helper and memory T-cells which perpetuates bronchoconstriction and inflammation. It is now well appreciated that mast cells, apart from IgE signaling, play a crucial and multifaceted role in the pathophysiology of asthma. Mast cells not only produce several chemokines and cytokines that recruit neutrophils and eosinophils but also act as antigen-presenting cells for naïve T cells and enhance B cell IgE production by upregulating CD40L (Hong et al. 2013). Consequently, the local TH2 immune response in the lung is further enhanced.

It is of interest that sphingolipids are involved in a variety of mast cell functions. Especially the interplay between S1P and mast cell biology is now appreciated. Mast cells express the high-affinity receptor for IgE, FcεRI. Activation of FcεRI facilitates the recruitment of both, SPHK1 and SPHK2, which is connected with an increase of S1P (Kulinski et al. 2016). Abrogation of SPHK1 indicates that the enzyme is critical for FcεRI-mediated mast cell degranulation and cytokine generation (Pushparaj et al. 2009). S1P generated in mast cells can be released to the extracellular environment, where the bioactive lipid can exert its function after binding to its receptors (Mitra et al. 2006). The activation of S1PR1 can enhance the migration of mast cells toward antigens, while the activation of S1PR2 is able to trigger mast cell degranulation (Jolly et al. 2004). Moreover, the S1PR3 is a crucial receptor subtype in allergic reactions as its activation promotes pulmonary inflammation and fibrosis via the formation of connective tissue growth factor (Murakami et al. 2014). Most recently, also the S1PR4 receptor subtype has been found to be involved in the activation of mast cell degranulation. In contrast, sphingosine and ceramide can be considered to have an opposite role on mast cell activation than S1P (Chiba et al. 2007; Itakura et al. 2002; Izawa et al. 2012; Prieschl et al. 1999).

Long-term asthma control medications such as long-acting beta-agonists, corticosteroids, leukotriene modifiers, and immunomodulators are the cornerstone of asthma treatment. However, the involvement of sphingolipid metabolism and signaling in mast cells may provide valuable insights for the development of new therapeutic options for the treatment of the disease.

3 Therapeutic Options

Since substantial dysregulation of sphingolipid metabolism appears to be central to the pathophysiology of CF, COPD, and asthma, it could be of interest to determine whether drugs approved for parenteral or oral administration for the treatment of other diseases but affecting sphingolipid metabolism can be used to treat patients with such lung diseases by inhalation. The ultimate goal would be to administer drugs targeting sphingolipid metabolism by inhalation to achieve a local effect in the lung without systemic side effects.

3.1 Therapeutic Options in Cystic Fibrosis

Dysregulation of sphingolipids is a critical factor in the pathophysiology of CF. Ceramide levels are markedly increased, while sphingosine levels are drastically decreased. Normalization of sphingolipid levels could be a therapeutic option. Since ceramide generation occurs via different pathways, several possibilities are conceivable to reduce their levels (Fig. 1). In fact, with tricyclic antidepressants, there exist already drugs that interfere with ceramide formation. These are currently used systemically for the treatment of depression, but inhalation would also be a new therapeutic option in the case of CF. In the following, these possibilities as well as the delivery of sphingolipids such as sphingosine will be discussed in more detail.

Inhibition of acid sphingomyelinase is an elegant possibility to reduce ceramide levels. Several antidepressants such as amitriptyline inhibit acid sphingomyelinase as they induce a degradation of acid sphingomyelinase in lysosomes (Gulbins et al. 2013; Kornhuber et al. 2008, 2010). Thus, amitriptyline has been used in several studies to examine its role in CF. In murine CF models systemic treatment with amitriptyline improved lung functions, reduced inflammation, and prevented *P. aeruginosa* infections (Adams et al. 2016; Nahrlich et al. 2013). Similar effects were seen with other approved antidepressant drugs (Becker et al. 2010). Thus, a first clinical approach was conducted in 4 adult CF patients. Oral treatment with 37.5 mg of amitriptyline twice daily for 14 days significantly increased lung function (Riethmuller et al. 2009). A phase IIa safety study indicated no severe and only a few and mild adverse effects related to oral amitriptyline treatment and a subsequent phase IIb study confirmed an increase of the forced expiratory volume in 1 s (FEV_1) compared to placebo (Nahrlich et al. 2013). Efficacy and safety of amitriptyline administration were also demonstrated in CF patients applying 25 mg of amitriptyline twice daily for up to 3 years. Amitriptyline significantly increased lung function, reduced ceramide levels in lung cells and increased weight of CF patients without serious adverse effects (Adams et al. 2016). However, since any treatment of CF should be started as early as possible, i.e., in children, the systemic application of amitriptyline should be replaced by inhalation of the drug to minimize potential systemic adverse effects.

Indeed, inhalation studies in CF mice using functional acid sphingomyelinase inhibitors such as amitriptyline, trimipramine, desipramine, chlorprothixene, fluoxetine, or sertraline have already been performed and indicated that the drugs reduce ceramide concentrations in epithelial cells of the trachea and bronchi, diminish inflammation and prevent *P. aeruginosa* pulmonal infection. Most interestingly, systemic effects were not detected (Becker et al. 2010). However, many inhibitors of acid sphingomyelinase also inhibit ceramidase activity (Elojeimy et al. 2006) and thus prolonged use could counteract the positive effect on ceramide levels. For this reason, it would be interesting to develop specific competitive inhibitors of acid sphingomyelinase, which could then be used by inhalation.

Ceramide levels can also be downregulated via an increased acid ceramidase activity as the enzyme is responsible for breaking down excess ceramides. Thus, transgenic overexpression of acid ceramidase in CF mice normalizes ceramide and sphingosine levels in bronchial and tracheal epithelial cells and rescues CF mice from pulmonary infections with *P. aeruginosa* (Becker et al. 2021). Consequently, inhalation of recombinant acid ceramidase might also be an elegant approach to lower the ceramide level in the lung. Indeed, systemic administration of recombinant acid ceramidase has already been tested in a mouse model of Farber's disease, which is characterized by genetic mutations that disrupt normal acid ceramidase function. The disease is characterized by severe inflammation and neurodegeneration (He et al. 2017). In the case of CF, inhalative delivery of recombinant acid ceramidase would specifically target the airway epithelial cells, which require much smaller amounts of the enzyme than a systemic treatment of Farber's patients. This particular concept has already been tested in airway epithelial cells obtained from donors with CF. Cells were infected with *P. aeruginosa*. Treatment of these cells with recombinant acid ceramidase ameliorated pivotal features of CF, namely inflammation and infection. In addition, nebulization of recombinant acid ceramidase in murine CF models reduced airway inflammation, pointing to a therapeutic approach that merits further investigation (Gardner et al. 2020).

Intervention in the de novo synthesis of sphingolipids represents another possibility for lowering ceramide levels. Myriocin inhibits serine palmitoyl-transferase, and is thus the first step in the de novo synthesis of sphingolipids. Myriocin reduces the accumulation of ceramide in broncho-epithelial cells derived from a CF patient indicating that inhalation of myriocin could be an innovative therapeutic strategy for CF (Signorelli et al. 2021). For this purpose, a solid lipid nanoparticle formulation containing myriocin was developed (Caretti et al. 2017). Inhalation of the myriocin-containing formulation reduced ceramide concentrations in the lungs of CF mice, thereby diminishing inflammation and preventing infection (Caretti et al. 2014, 2017). However, it must be noted that inhibition of serine palmitoyl-transferase not only alters ceramide levels but also modulates sphingolipids that may have a protective effect. In addition, myriocin has a rather high toxicity when administered systemically (Zhang et al. 2018). Thus, there is a demand for the development of an appropriate carrier systems for the inhalative delivery of myriocin.

Inhalation of sphingosine is a novel concept for CF treatment as sphingosine concentrations in airway epithelial cells are significantly reduced, and sphingosine is bactericidal to relevant species. Indeed, sphingosine inhalation in CF mice rescued mice from acute and chronic pulmonary *P. aeruginosa* infections and prevented new

P. aeruginosa or *S. aureus* infections (Grassme et al. 2017; Pewzner-Jung et al. 2014). This demonstrates that sphingosine plays a key role in the innate and immediate antibacterial defense of the respiratory tract and might also serve as novel therapeutics to treat bacterial pneumonia. It is of interest, that histology studies indicated no acute toxicity in mice up to an inhalation of a 1-mM sphingosine solution (Martin et al. 2017).

Preclinical studies have already extended to bacterial pneumonia in mini pigs (Carstens et al. 2019). Inhalation of sphingosine solutions twice daily over 14 days increased the concentration of this sphingolipid in bronchial epithelial cells. The inhalation had no local side effects, such as cell death, inflammation, or fibrosis. In addition, the inhalation induced no systemic adverse effects such as lack of activity, reduced food intake, adverse behavior, or any other change in the general health status. Likewise, unwanted effects were not seen in ex vivo ventilated and perfused pig lungs. Most interestingly, inhalation of sphingosine greatly reduced the number of bacteria in ex vivo ventilated and perfused pig lungs that were infected with *P. aeruginosa* (Carstens et al. 2021, 2022). These results support the notion that sphingosine might serve to treat pulmonary bacterial infections, especially in CF. Moreover, sphingosine could be preferably combined with acid sphingomyelinase inhibitors such as amitriptyline which would decrease ceramide levels and increase sphingosine. The combined inhalative use should alleviate both pneumonia and susceptibility to reinfection in CF.

3.2 Therapeutic Options in COPD

As outlined, there are some common features between CF and COPD with regard to changes in sphingolipid levels. Increased ceramide levels induce the development of epithelial and endothelial cell damage, inflammation, and emphysema. Interestingly, similar to CF, COPD is very commonly associated with chronic infections with *P. aeruginosa*. Accordingly, approaches similar to those used in CF decreasing ceramide levels are conceivable in COPD therapy.

As acid sphingomyelinase activity is increased in COPD, inhalation of antidepressants such as amitriptyline, which inhibits acid sphingomyelinase, could also be an approach in the treatment of COPD. However, differing from CF, COPD is also characterized by an activation of neutral sphingomyelinase. Notably, neutral sphingomyelinase appears also involved in cigarette smoke-related airway injury mediated by ceramide. As the antioxidant *N*-acetyl cysteine downregulates neutral sphingomyelinase this appears to be an option in COPD therapy (Filosto et al. 2011). In fact, a randomized controlled trial suggests the benefit of *N*-acetyl cysteine in the prevention of acute exacerbations of COPD (Zheng et al. 2014).

In addition, inhibition of de novo synthesis of sphingolipids by myriocin is another option to lower ceramide levels. This approach has also been tested in animal studies of COPD. These studies indicated that ceramide levels are increased in lung epithelial cells after exposure to a cigarette smoke mixture, which is accompanied by increased expression of inflammatory cytokines. Pretreatment with myriocin prevented smoke-induced damage (Zulueta et al. 2017). This is consistent with myriocin-loaded nanocarriers administered intratracheally to mice significantly reducing an *A. fumigatus*-induced inflammatory response in the lung as well as the invasion of the fungus into the lung (Caretti et al. 2016).

As S1P possesses a protective effect in COPD, increasing the S1P concentration or stimulating the S1P signaling cascade could be therapeutic options, too. Both strategies have already been investigated in animal studies and show remarkable results. In a COPD animal model using a VEGF receptor inhibitor, intraperitoneal administration of sphingosine increased S1P levels in a dose-dependent manner leading to a markedly diminished lung injury (Diab et al. 2010). Here, it would be interesting to investigate whether inhalation of sphingosine also reduces lung injury. At the same time, inhalation of sphingosine would also be a way of combating the infections that frequently occur in COPD. As the S1PR1 receptor subtype is involved in the protective function, treatment with S1PR1 agonists would be another option to rescue lung injury. Indeed, S1PR1 agonists ameliorated cigarette smoke-induced lung parenchymal apoptosis and airspace enlargement as well as loss of body weight in a mouse model of emphysema (Goel et al. 2022). These data support an important role for the S1P/S1PR1 axis in maintaining the structural integrity of alveoli opening up new therapeutic options in COPD.

3.3 Therapeutic Options in Asthma

Altered sphingolipid metabolism has also been demonstrated in asthma patients, however, there are fundamental differences between CF and COPD. Both, S1P and ceramide, have been shown to be elevated in the airways of asthma patients (Oyeniran et al. 2015; Rosenfeldt et al. 2003). S1P plasma levels in adult asthma patients correlate with severity of the disease (Reinke et al. 2017).

In contrast to CF and COPD, it seems likely that ceramides possess a protective effect on asthma. In fact, intratracheal myriocin, which decreases ceramide levels, exacerbates airway inflammation and allergen-induced airway hyper-responsiveness in a murine model of asthma (Edukulla et al. 2016). Therefore, the administration of ceramides could be a therapeutic intervention in asthma. Nanoscale formulations are shown to dramatically improve the pharmacokinetic and toxicological profiles of ceramide delivery to cells. To this end, initial studies have been conducted in an asthma animal model. To enable intratracheal application, ceramides were incorporated into nanoliposomal formulations. Most interestingly, the degree of airway remodeling was significantly decreased in response to the nanoliposomal ceramide formulation compared to ceramide-free liposomes. Especially, the inhibition of mucosal accumulation and goblet cell hyperplasia in the airways should be emphasized (Sakae et al. 2023). An indirect method to modulate ceramide formation is the administration of fenretinide, which targets dihydroceramide desaturase leading to an increase in dihydroceramide levels. Moreover, this vitamin A derivative is able to increase, especially very long-chain ceramides. LAU-7b is a proprietary oral drug candidate based on fenretinide, which has been tested in a murine asthma model. Indeed, LAU-7b effectively lowered the airway hyper-responsiveness and protected against inflammatory cell infiltration and mucus accumulation induced by house dust mites in mice (Youssef et al. 2020).

Intervention in S1P formation as well S1P signaling cascade represents another strategy in asthma therapy. This is mainly due to the fact that S1P modulates mast cell function. As activation of FcεRI of mast cells is connected with recruitment of SPHK1/2, it was hypothesized that SPHK inhibition could ameliorate lung inflammation in asthma. To test this hypothesis, SPHK inhibitors were used in an asthmatic mouse model. Indeed, inhalation of SPHK inhibitors prevented eosinophil inflammation and goblet hyperplasia suggesting a novel therapeutic strategy to treat bronchial asthma (Nishiuma et al. 2008). Most interestingly, these results were confirmed with more specific SPHK1 inhibitors in an asthmatic animal model (Price et al. 2013).

Besides inhibition of S1P formation, modulation of S1P receptors can also be considered for therapeutic application. Here, an inhibition of the S1PR2 could be at the center of attention as the receptor has been described to enhance FcεRI-induced degranulation and is able to reduce serum histamine levels in a mouse model of anaphylaxis (Olivera et al. 2006, 2013). However, also the S1PR4 could represent a therapeutic target as this receptor subtype is involved in mast cell degranulation and increases an allergen-induced inflammatory response. Therefore, it is not surprising that the S1PR4 antagonist CYM50358, administered via intraperitoneal injection, reduces immune cell accumulation in a murine asthma model (Jeon et al. 2021). An inhalation could also be considered as a possible administration.

In view of the mast cell degranulation sphingosine is assumed as an opponent of S1P, as exogenous sphingosine is able to diminish FcεRI-mediated SPHK1 activation by preventing activation of the mitogen-activated protein kinase pathway (Prieschl et al. 1999). In this respect, inhalation of this sphingolipid would also be conceivable for a therapeutic use. However, it must be proven that sphingosine is not further metabolized to S1P in the lung, which would counteract this action.

Taken together, sphingolipids are significantly involved in the pathophysiology of asthma. Therapeutic options include increasing ceramide levels on the one hand and decreasing S1P levels or inhibiting its signaling pathways on the other. However, for clinical use, the efficacy and tolerability of sphingolipids in asthma must be appropriate to the benefit/risk ratio of current drugs.

4 Conclusion

Recently, many discoveries elucidate the essential role of sphingolipids in lung diseases. Dysregulation of sphingolipid metabolism is considered to be one of the most important factors that are involved in the development and progression of lung disorders such as CF, COPD, and asthma. Preclinical studies have demonstrated the potential of targeting sphingolipid metabolism as a therapeutic strategy for lung diseases. Several drugs that interfere with sphingolipid metabolism are approved for parenteral or oral use in other diseases and, when administered by inhalation, could expand therapeutic options in CF, COPD, or asthma. Initial clinical studies are promising. However, suitable delivery systems still need to be developed.

References

Adams C, Icheva V, Deppisch C, Lauer J, Herrmann G, Graepler-Mainka U, Heyder S, Gulbins E, Riethmueller J (2016) Long-term Pulmonal therapy of cystic fibrosis-patients with amitriptyline. Cell Physiol Biochem 39:565–572. https://doi.org/10.1159/000445648

Barrera NP, Zhou M, Robinson CV (2013) The role of lipids in defining membrane protein interactions: insights from mass spectrometry. Trends Cell Biol 23:1–8. https://doi.org/10.1016/j.tcb.2012.08.007

Becker KA, Riethmuller J, Luth A, Doring G, Kleuser B, Gulbins E (2010) Acid sphingomyelinase inhibitors normalize pulmonary ceramide and inflammation in cystic fibrosis. Am J Respir Cell Mol Biol 42:716–724. https://doi.org/10.1165/rcmb.2009-0174OC

Becker KA, Verhaegh R, Verhasselt HL, Keitsch S, Soddemann M, Wilker B, Wilson GC, Buer J, Ahmad SA, Edwards MJ, Gulbins E (2021) Acid ceramidase rescues cystic fibrosis mice from pulmonary infections. Infect Immun 89. https://doi.org/10.1128/IAI.00677-20

Bektas M, Allende ML, Lee BG, Chen W, Amar MJ, Remaley AT, Saba JD, Proia RL (2010) Sphingosine 1-phosphate lyase deficiency disrupts lipid homeostasis in liver. J Biol Chem 285: 10880–10889. https://doi.org/10.1074/jbc.M109.081489

Benechet AP, Menon M, Xu D, Samji T, Maher L, Murooka TT, Mempel TR, Sheridan BS, Lemoine FM, Khanna KM (2016) T cell-intrinsic S1PR1 regulates endogenous effector T-cell egress dynamics from lymph nodes during infection. Proc Natl Acad Sci U S A 113:2182–2187. https://doi.org/10.1073/pnas.1516485113

Berdyshev EV, Serban KA, Schweitzer KS, Bronova IA, Mikosz A, Petrache I (2021) Ceramide and sphingosine-1 phosphate in COPD lungs. Thorax. https://doi.org/10.1136/thoraxjnl-2020-215892

Bieberich E (2018) Sphingolipids and lipid rafts: novel concepts and methods of analysis. Chem Phys Lipids 216:114–131. https://doi.org/10.1016/j.chemphyslip.2018.08.003

Bollinger CR, Teichgraber V, Gulbins E (2005) Ceramide-enriched membrane domains. Biochim Biophys Acta 1746:284–294. https://doi.org/10.1016/j.bbamcr.2005.09.001

Brodlie M, McKean MC, Johnson GE, Gray J, Fisher AJ, Corris PA, Lordan JL, Ward C (2010) Ceramide is increased in the lower airway epithelium of people with advanced cystic fibrosis lung disease. Am J Respir Crit Care Med 182:369–375. https://doi.org/10.1164/rccm.200905-0799OC

Bush A (2019) Pathophysiological mechanisms of asthma. Front Pediatr 7:68. https://doi.org/10.3389/fped.2019.00068

Caretti A, Bragonzi A, Facchini M, De Fino I, Riva C, Gasco P, Musicanti C, Casas J, Fabrias G, Ghidoni R, Signorelli P (2014) Anti-inflammatory action of lipid nanocarrier-delivered myriocin: therapeutic potential in cystic fibrosis. Biochim Biophys Acta 1840:586–594. https://doi.org/10.1016/j.bbagen.2013.10.018

Caretti A, Torelli R, Perdoni F, Falleni M, Tosi D, Zulueta A, Casas J, Sanguinetti M, Ghidoni R, Borghi E, Signorelli P (2016) Inhibition of ceramide de novo synthesis by myriocin produces the double effect of reducing pathological inflammation and exerting antifungal activity against A. fumigatus airways infection. Biochim Biophys Acta 1860:1089–1097. https://doi.org/10.1016/j.bbagen.2016.02.014

Caretti A, Vasso M, Bonezzi FT, Gallina A, Trinchera M, Rossi A, Adami R, Casas J, Falleni M, Tosi D, Bragonzi A, Ghidoni R, Gelfi C, Signorelli P (2017) Myriocin treatment of CF lung infection and inflammation: complex analyses for enigmatic lipids. Naunyn Schmiedebergs Arch Pharmacol 390:775–790. https://doi.org/10.1007/s00210-017-1373-4

Carstens H, Schumacher F, Keitsch S, Kramer M, Kuhn C, Sehl C, Soddemann M, Wilker B, Herrmann D, Swaidan A, Kleuser B, Verhaegh R, Hilken G, Edwards MJ, Dubicanac M, Carpinteiro A, Wissmann A, Becker KA, Kamler M, Gulbins E (2019) Clinical development of sphingosine as anti-bacterial drug: inhalation of sphingosine in mini pigs has no adverse side effects. Cell Physiol Biochem 53:1015–1028. https://doi.org/10.33594/000000194

Carstens H, Kalka K, Verhaegh R, Schumacher F, Soddemann M, Wilker B, Keitsch S, Sehl C, Kleuser B, Wahlers T, Reiner G, Koch A, Rauen U, Gulbins E, Kamler M (2021) Inhaled sphingosine has no adverse side effects in isolated ventilated and perfused pig lungs. Sci Rep 11: 18607. https://doi.org/10.1038/s41598-021-97708-3

Carstens H, Kalka K, Verhaegh R, Schumacher F, Soddemann M, Wilker B, Keitsch S, Sehl C, Kleuser B, Hubler M, Rauen U, Becker AK, Koch A, Gulbins E, Kamler M (2022) Antimicrobial effects of inhaled sphingosine against Pseudomonas aeruginosa in isolated ventilated and perfused pig lungs. PloS One 17:e0271620. https://doi.org/10.1371/journal.pone.0271620

Cartier A, Hla T (2019) Sphingosine 1-phosphate: lipid signaling in pathology and therapy. Science 366. https://doi.org/10.1126/science.aar5551

Chakinala RC, Khatri A, Gupta K, Koike K, Epelbaum O (2019) Sphingolipids in COPD. Eur Respir Rev 28. https://doi.org/10.1183/16000617.0047-2019

Chiba N, Masuda A, Yoshikai Y, Matsuguchi T (2007) Ceramide inhibits LPS-induced production of IL-5, IL-10, and IL-13 from mast cells. J Cell Physiol 213:126–136. https://doi.org/10.1002/jcp.21101

Christenson SA, Smith BM, Bafadhel M, Putcha N (2022) Chronic obstructive pulmonary disease. Lancet 399:2227–2242. https://doi.org/10.1016/S0140-6736(22)00470-6

Cottrill KA, Peterson RJ, Lewallen CF, Koval M, Bridges RJ, McCarty NA (2021) Sphingomyelinase decreases transepithelial anion secretion in airway epithelial cells in part by inhibiting CFTR-mediated apical conductance. Physiol Rep 9:e14928. https://doi.org/10.14814/phy2.14928

Cyster JG, Schwab SR (2012) Sphingosine-1-phosphate and lymphocyte egress from lymphoid organs. Annu Rev Immunol 30:69–94. https://doi.org/10.1146/annurev-immunol-020711-075011

Davis DL, Gable K, Suemitsu J, Dunn TM, Wattenberg BW (2019) The ORMDL/Orm-serine palmitoyltransferase (SPT) complex is directly regulated by ceramide: reconstitution of SPT regulation in isolated membranes. J Biol Chem 294:5146–5156. https://doi.org/10.1074/jbc.RA118.007291

De Cunto G, Brancaleone V, Riemma MA, Cerqua I, Vellecco V, Spaziano G, Cavarra E, Bartalesi B, D'Agostino B, Lungarella G, Cirino G, Lucattelli M, Roviezzo F (2020) Functional contribution of sphingosine-1-phosphate to airway pathology in cigarette smoke-exposed mice. Br J Pharmacol 177:267–281. https://doi.org/10.1111/bph.14861

Diab KJ, Adamowicz JJ, Kamocki K, Rush NI, Garrison J, Gu Y, Schweitzer KS, Skobeleva A, Rajashekhar G, Hubbard WC, Berdyshev EV, Petrache I (2010) Stimulation of sphingosine 1-phosphate signaling as an alveolar cell survival strategy in emphysema. Am J Respir Crit Care Med 181:344–352. https://doi.org/10.1164/rccm.200906-0826OC

Doktorova M, Symons JL, Levental I (2020) Structural and functional consequences of reversible lipid asymmetry in living membranes. Nat Chem Biol 16:1321–1330. https://doi.org/10.1038/s41589-020-00688-0

Edukulla R, Rehn KL, Liu B, McAlees JW, Hershey GK, Wang YH, Lewkowich I, Lindsley AW (2016) Intratracheal myriocin enhances allergen-induced Th2 inflammation and airway hyper-responsiveness. Immun Inflamm Dis 4:248–262. https://doi.org/10.1002/iid3.110

Elborn JS (2016) Cystic fibrosis. Lancet 388:2519–2531. https://doi.org/10.1016/S0140-6736(16)00576-6

Elojeimy S, Holman DH, Liu X, El-Zawahry A, Villani M, Cheng JC, Mahdy A, Zeidan Y, Bielwaska A, Hannun YA, Norris JS (2006) New insights on the use of desipramine as an inhibitor for acid ceramidase. FEBS Lett 580:4751–4756. https://doi.org/10.1016/j.febslet.2006.07.071

Fahy E, Subramaniam S, Brown HA, Glass CK, Merrill AH Jr, Murphy RC, Raetz CR, Russell DW, Seyama Y, Shaw W, Shimizu T, Spener F, van Meer G, VanNieuwenhze MS, White SH, Witztum JL, Dennis EA (2005) A comprehensive classification system for lipids. J Lipid Res 46:839–861. https://doi.org/10.1194/jlr.E400004-JLR200

Filosto S, Castillo S, Danielson A, Franzi L, Khan E, Kenyon N, Last J, Pinkerton K, Tuder R, Goldkorn T (2011) Neutral sphingomyelinase 2: a novel target in cigarette smoke-induced apoptosis and lung injury. Am J Respir Cell Mol Biol 44:350–360. https://doi.org/10.1165/rcmb.2009-0422OC

Fischer CL, Walters KS, Drake DR, Blanchette DR, Dawson DV, Brogden KA, Wertz PW (2013) Sphingoid bases are taken up by Escherichia coli and Staphylococcus aureus and induce ultrastructural damage. Skin Pharmacol Physiol 26:36–44. https://doi.org/10.1159/000343175

Gardner AI, Haq IJ, Simpson AJ, Becker KA, Gallagher J, Saint-Criq V, Verdon B, Mavin E, Trigg A, Gray MA, Koulman A, McDonnell MJ, Fisher AJ, Kramer EL, Clancy JP, Ward C, Schuchman EH, Gulbins E, Brodlie M (2020) Recombinant acid ceramidase reduces inflammation and infection in cystic fibrosis. Am J Respir Crit Care Med 202:1133–1145. https://doi.org/10.1164/rccm.202001-0180OC

Gardner AI, Wu Y, Verhaegh R, Liu Y, Wilker B, Soddemann M, Keitsch S, Edwards MJ, Haq IJ, Kamler M, Becker KA, Brodlie M, Gulbins E (2021) Interferon regulatory factor 8 regulates expression of acid ceramidase and infection susceptibility in cystic fibrosis. J Biol Chem 296: 100650. https://doi.org/10.1016/j.jbc.2021.100650

Ghidoni R, Caretti A, Signorelli P (2015) Role of sphingolipids in the pathobiology of lung inflammation. Mediators Inflamm 2015:487508. https://doi.org/10.1155/2015/487508

Global Initiative for Chronic Obstructive Lung Disease (2002) Global strategy for the diagnosis, management and prevention of COPD. http://goldcopd.org

Goel K, Schweitzer KS, Serban KA, Bittman R, Petrache I (2022) Pharmacological sphingosine-1 phosphate receptor 1 targeting in cigarette smoke-induced emphysema in mice. Am J Physiol Lung Cell Mol Physiol 322:L794–L803. https://doi.org/10.1152/ajplung.00017.2022

Grassme H, Henry B, Ziobro R, Becker KA, Riethmuller J, Gardner A, Seitz AP, Steinmann J, Lang S, Ward C, Schuchman EH, Caldwell CC, Kamler M, Edwards MJ, Brodlie M, Gulbins E (2017) beta1-integrin accumulates in cystic fibrosis luminal airway epithelial membranes and decreases sphingosine, promoting bacterial infections. Cell Host Microbe 21:707–718 e8. https://doi.org/10.1016/j.chom.2017.05.001

Gulbins E, Kolesnick R (2003) Raft ceramide in molecular medicine. Oncogene 22:7070–7077. https://doi.org/10.1038/sj.onc.1207146

Gulbins E, Palmada M, Reichel M, Luth A, Bohmer C, Amato D, Muller CP, Tischbirek CH, Groemer TW, Tabatabai G, Becker KA, Tripal P, Staedtler S, Ackermann TF, van Brederode J, Alzheimer C, Weller M, Lang UE, Kleuser B, Grassme H, Kornhuber J (2013) Acid sphingomyelinase-ceramide system mediates effects of antidepressant drugs. Nat Med 19: 934–938. https://doi.org/10.1038/nm.3214

Hagen-Euteneuer N, Lutjohann D, Park H, Merrill AH Jr, van Echten-Deckert G (2012) Sphingosine 1-phosphate (S1P) lyase deficiency increases sphingolipid formation via recycling at the expense of de novo biosynthesis in neurons. J Biol Chem 287:9128–9136. https://doi.org/10.1074/jbc.M111.302380

Hannun YA, Obeid LM (2008) Principles of bioactive lipid signalling: lessons from sphingolipids. Nat Rev Mol Cell Biol 9:139–150. https://doi.org/10.1038/nrm2329

Hannun YA, Obeid LM (2011) Many ceramides. J Biol Chem 286:27855–27862. https://doi.org/10.1074/jbc.R111.254359

Harayama T, Riezman H (2018) Understanding the diversity of membrane lipid composition. Nat Rev Mol Cell Biol 19:281–296. https://doi.org/10.1038/nrm.2017.138

He X, Dworski S, Zhu C, DeAngelis V, Solyom A, Medin JA, Simonaro CM, Schuchman EH (2017) Enzyme replacement therapy for Farber disease: proof-of-concept studies in cells and mice. BBA Clin 7:85–96. https://doi.org/10.1016/j.bbacli.2017.02.001

Hjelmqvist L, Tuson M, Marfany G, Herrero E, Balcells S, Gonzalez-Duarte R (2002) ORMDL proteins are a conserved new family of endoplasmic reticulum membrane proteins. Genome Biol 3:RESEARCH0027. https://doi.org/10.1186/gb-2002-3-6-research0027

Hla T, Venkataraman K, Michaud J (2008) The vascular S1P gradient-cellular sources and biological significance. Biochim Biophys Acta 1781:477–482. https://doi.org/10.1016/j.bbalip.2008.07.003

Hogg JC, Timens W (2009) The pathology of chronic obstructive pulmonary disease. Annu Rev Pathol 4:435–459. https://doi.org/10.1146/annurev.pathol.4.110807.092145

Hong GU, Park BS, Park JW, Kim SY, Ro JY (2013) IgE production in CD40/CD40L cross-talk of B and mast cells and mediator release via TGase 2 in mouse allergic asthma. Cell Signal 25: 1514–1525. https://doi.org/10.1016/j.cellsig.2013.03.010

Itakura A, Tanaka A, Aioi A, Tonogaito H, Matsuda H (2002) Ceramide and sphingosine rapidly induce apoptosis of murine mast cells supported by interleukin-3 and stem cell factor. Exp Hematol 30:272–278. https://doi.org/10.1016/s0301-472x(01)00790-1

Izawa K, Yamanishi Y, Maehara A, Takahashi M, Isobe M, Ito S, Kaitani A, Matsukawa T, Matsuoka T, Nakahara F, Oki T, Kiyonari H, Abe T, Okumura K, Kitamura T, Kitaura J (2012) The receptor LMIR3 negatively regulates mast cell activation and allergic responses by binding to extracellular ceramide. Immunity 37:827–839. https://doi.org/10.1016/j.immuni.2012.08.018

Jeon WJ, Chung KW, Lee JH, Im DS (2021) Suppressive effect of CYM50358 S1P(4) antagonist on mast cell degranulation and allergic asthma in mice. Biomol Ther (Seoul) 29:492–497. https://doi.org/10.4062/biomolther.2020.206

Jolly PS, Bektas M, Olivera A, Gonzalez-Espinosa C, Proia RL, Rivera J, Milstien S, Spiegel S (2004) Transactivation of sphingosine-1-phosphate receptors by FcepsilonRI triggering is required for normal mast cell degranulation and chemotaxis. J Exp Med 199:959–970. https://doi.org/10.1084/jem.20030680

Kano K, Aoki J, Hla T (2022) Lysophospholipid mediators in health and disease. Annu Rev Pathol 17:459–483. https://doi.org/10.1146/annurev-pathol-050420-025929

Kornhuber J, Tripal P, Reichel M, Terfloth L, Bleich S, Wiltfang J, Gulbins E (2008) Identification of new functional inhibitors of acid sphingomyelinase using a structure-property-activity relation model. J Med Chem 51:219–237. https://doi.org/10.1021/jm070524a

Kornhuber J, Tripal P, Reichel M, Muhle C, Rhein C, Muehlbacher M, Groemer TW, Gulbins E (2010) Functional inhibitors of acid sphingomyelinase (FIASMAs): a novel pharmacological group of drugs with broad clinical applications. Cell Physiol Biochem 26:9–20. https://doi.org/10.1159/000315101

Kulinski JM, Munoz-Cano R, Olivera A (2016) Sphingosine-1-phosphate and other lipid mediators generated by mast cells as critical players in allergy and mast cell function. Eur J Pharmacol 778: 56–67. https://doi.org/10.1016/j.ejphar.2015.02.058

Le Stunff H, Giussani P, Maceyka M, Lepine S, Milstien S, Spiegel S (2007) Recycling of sphingosine is regulated by the concerted actions of sphingosine-1-phosphate phosphohydrolase 1 and sphingosine kinase 2. J Biol Chem 282:34372–34380. https://doi.org/10.1074/jbc.M703329200

Liessi N, Pesce E, Braccia C, Bertozzi SM, Giraudo A, Bandiera T, Pedemonte N, Armirotti A (2020) Distinctive lipid signatures of bronchial epithelial cells associated with cystic fibrosis drugs, including Trikafta. JCI Insight 5. https://doi.org/10.1172/jci.insight.138722

Loberto N, Mancini G, Bassi R, Carsana EV, Tamanini A, Pedemonte N, Dechecchi MC, Sonnino S, Aureli M (2020) Sphingolipids and plasma membrane hydrolases in human primary bronchial cells during differentiation and their altered patterns in cystic fibrosis. Glycoconj J 37: 623–633. https://doi.org/10.1007/s10719-020-09935-x

Maceyka M, Sankala H, Hait NC, Le Stunff H, Liu H, Toman R, Collier C, Zhang M, Satin LS, Merrill AH Jr, Milstien S, Spiegel S (2005) SphK1 and SphK2, sphingosine kinase isoenzymes with opposing functions in sphingolipid metabolism. J Biol Chem 280:37118–37129. https://doi.org/10.1074/jbc.M502207200

Martin GE, Boudreau RM, Couch C, Becker KA, Edwards MJ, Caldwell CC, Gulbins E, Seitz A (2017) Sphingosine's role in epithelial host defense: a natural antimicrobial and novel therapeutic. Biochimie 141:91–96. https://doi.org/10.1016/j.biochi.2017.03.014

Masini E, Giannini L, Nistri S, Cinci L, Mastroianni R, Xu W, Comhair SA, Li D, Cuzzocrea S, Matuschak GM, Salvemini D (2008) Ceramide: a key signaling molecule in a Guinea pig model of allergic asthmatic response and airway inflammation. J Pharmacol Exp Ther 324:548–557. https://doi.org/10.1124/jpet.107.131565

McGinley MP, Cohen JA (2021) Sphingosine 1-phosphate receptor modulators in multiple sclerosis and other conditions. Lancet 398:1184–1194. https://doi.org/10.1016/S0140-6736(21)00244-0

Mitra P, Oskeritzian CA, Payne SG, Beaven MA, Milstien S, Spiegel S (2006) Role of ABCC1 in export of sphingosine-1-phosphate from mast cells. Proc Natl Acad Sci U S A 103:16394–16399. https://doi.org/10.1073/pnas.0603734103

Murakami K, Kohno M, Kadoya M, Nagahara H, Fujii W, Seno T, Yamamoto A, Oda R, Fujiwara H, Kubo T, Morita S, Nakada H, Hla T, Kawahito Y (2014) Knock out of S1P3 receptor signaling attenuates inflammation and fibrosis in bleomycin-induced lung injury mice model. PloS One 9:e106792. https://doi.org/10.1371/journal.pone.0106792

Nahrlich L, Mainz JG, Adams C, Engel C, Herrmann G, Icheva V, Lauer J, Deppisch C, Wirth A, Unger K, Graepler-Mainka U, Hector A, Heyder S, Stern M, Doring G, Gulbins E, Riethmuller J (2013) Therapy of CF-patients with amitriptyline and placebo – a randomised, double-blind, placebo-controlled phase IIb multicenter, cohort-study. Cell Physiol Biochem 31:505–512. https://doi.org/10.1159/000350071

Nishiuma T, Nishimura Y, Okada T, Kuramoto E, Kotani Y, Jahangeer S, Nakamura S (2008) Inhalation of sphingosine kinase inhibitor attenuates airway inflammation in asthmatic mouse model. Am J Physiol Lung Cell Mol Physiol 294:L1085–L1093. https://doi.org/10.1152/ajplung.00445.2007

Oceandy D, McMorran BJ, Smith SN, Schreiber R, Kunzelmann K, Alton EW, Hume DA, Wainwright BJ (2002) Gene complementation of airway epithelium in the cystic fibrosis mouse is necessary and sufficient to correct the pathogen clearance and inflammatory abnormalities. Hum Mol Genet 11:1059–1067. https://doi.org/10.1093/hmg/11.9.1059

Olivera A, Urtz N, Mizugishi K, Yamashita Y, Gilfillan AM, Furumoto Y, Gu H, Proia RL, Baumruker T, Rivera J (2006) IgE-dependent activation of sphingosine kinases 1 and 2 and secretion of sphingosine 1-phosphate requires Fyn kinase and contributes to mast cell responses. J Biol Chem 281:2515–2525. https://doi.org/10.1074/jbc.M508931200

Olivera A, Dillahunt SE, Rivera J (2013) Interrogation of sphingosine-1-phosphate receptor 2 function in vivo reveals a prominent role in the recovery from IgE and IgG-mediated anaphylaxis with minimal effect on its onset. Immunol Lett 150:89–96. https://doi.org/10.1016/j.imlet.2013.01.005

Ono JG, Kim BI, Zhao Y, Christos PJ, Tesfaigzi Y, Worgall TS, Worgall S (2020) Decreased sphingolipid synthesis in children with 17q21 asthma-risk genotypes. J Clin Invest 130:921–926. https://doi.org/10.1172/JCI130860

Oyeniran C, Sturgill JL, Hait NC, Huang WC, Avni D, Maceyka M, Newton J, Allegood JC, Montpetit A, Conrad DH, Milstien S, Spiegel S (2015) Aberrant ORM (yeast)-like protein isoform 3 (ORMDL3) expression dysregulates ceramide homeostasis in cells and ceramide exacerbates allergic asthma in mice. J Allergy Clin Immunol 136:1035–46 e6. https://doi.org/10.1016/j.jaci.2015.02.031

Paik J (2022) Ozanimod: a review in ulcerative colitis. Drugs 82:1303–1313. https://doi.org/10.1007/s40265-022-01762-8

Papi A, Brightling C, Pedersen SE, Reddel HK (2018) Asthma. Lancet 391:783–800. https://doi.org/10.1016/S0140-6736(17)33311-1

Petrache I, Natarajan V, Zhen L, Medler TR, Richter AT, Cho C, Hubbard WC, Berdyshev EV, Tuder RM (2005) Ceramide upregulation causes pulmonary cell apoptosis and emphysema-like disease in mice. Nat Med 11:491–498. https://doi.org/10.1038/nm1238

Petrache I, Medler TR, Richter AT, Kamocki K, Chukwueke U, Zhen L, Gu Y, Adamowicz J, Schweitzer KS, Hubbard WC, Berdyshev EV, Lungarella G, Tuder RM (2008) Superoxide dismutase protects against apoptosis and alveolar enlargement induced by ceramide. Am J Physiol Lung Cell Mol Physiol 295:L44–L53. https://doi.org/10.1152/ajplung.00448.2007

Petrusca DN, Gu Y, Adamowicz JJ, Rush NI, Hubbard WC, Smith PA, Berdyshev EV, Birukov KG, Lee CH, Tuder RM, Twigg HL 3rd, Vandivier RW, Petrache I (2010) Sphingolipid-mediated inhibition of apoptotic cell clearance by alveolar macrophages. J Biol Chem 285: 40322–40332. https://doi.org/10.1074/jbc.M110.137604

Pewzner-Jung Y, Tavakoli Tabazavareh S, Grassme H, Becker KA, Japtok L, Steinmann J, Joseph T, Lang S, Tuemmler B, Schuchman EH, Lentsch AB, Kleuser B, Edwards MJ, Futerman AH, Gulbins E (2014) Sphingoid long chain bases prevent lung infection by Pseudomonas aeruginosa. EMBO Mol Med 6:1205–1214. https://doi.org/10.15252/emmm.201404075

Porsbjerg C, Melen E, Lehtimaki L, Shaw D (2023) Asthma. Lancet 401:858–873. https://doi.org/10.1016/S0140-6736(22)02125-0

Presson RG Jr, Brown MB, Fisher AJ, Sandoval RM, Dunn KW, Lorenz KS, Delp EJ, Salama P, Molitoris BA, Petrache I (2011) Two-photon imaging within the murine thorax without respiratory and cardiac motion artifact. Am J Pathol 179:75–82. https://doi.org/10.1016/j.ajpath.2011.03.048

Price MM, Oskeritzian CA, Falanga YT, Harikumar KB, Allegood JC, Alvarez SE, Conrad D, Ryan JJ, Milstien S, Spiegel S (2013) A specific sphingosine kinase 1 inhibitor attenuates airway hyperresponsiveness and inflammation in a mast cell-dependent murine model of allergic asthma. J Allergy Clin Immunol 131:501–511 e1. https://doi.org/10.1016/j.jaci.2012.07.014

Prieschl EE, Csonga R, Novotny V, Kikuchi GE, Baumruker T (1999) The balance between sphingosine and sphingosine-1-phosphate is decisive for mast cell activation after Fc epsilon receptor I triggering. J Exp Med 190:1–8. https://doi.org/10.1084/jem.190.1.1

Pruett ST, Bushnev A, Hagedorn K, Adiga M, Haynes CA, Sullards MC, Liotta DC, Merrill AH Jr (2008) Biodiversity of sphingoid bases ("sphingosines") and related amino alcohols. J Lipid Res 49:1621–1639. https://doi.org/10.1194/jlr.R800012-JLR200

Pushparaj PN, Manikandan J, Tay HK, H'Ng SC, Kumar SD, Pfeilschifter J, Huwiler A, Melendez AJ (2009) Sphingosine kinase 1 is pivotal for Fc epsilon RI-mediated mast cell signaling and functional responses in vitro and in vivo. J Immunol 183:221–227. https://doi.org/10.4049/jimmunol.0803430

Rabe KF, Watz H (2017) Chronic obstructive pulmonary disease. Lancet 389:1931–1940. https://doi.org/10.1016/S0140-6736(17)31222-9

Ratjen F, Doring G (2003) Cystic fibrosis. Lancet 361:681–689. https://doi.org/10.1016/S0140-6736(03)12567-6

Reinke SN, Gallart-Ayala H, Gomez C, Checa A, Fauland A, Naz S, Kamleh MA, Djukanovic R, Hinks TS, Wheelock CE (2017) Metabolomics analysis identifies different metabotypes of asthma severity. Eur Respir J 49. https://doi.org/10.1183/13993003.01740-2016

Rice TC, Seitz AP, Edwards MJ, Gulbins E, Caldwell CC (2016) Frontline science: sphingosine rescues burn-injured mice from pulmonary Pseudomonas aeruginosa infection. J Leukoc Biol 100:1233–1237. https://doi.org/10.1189/jlb.3HI0416-197R

Riethmuller J, Anthonysamy J, Serra E, Schwab M, Doring G, Gulbins E (2009) Therapeutic efficacy and safety of amitriptyline in patients with cystic fibrosis. Cell Physiol Biochem 24:65–72. https://doi.org/10.1159/000227814

Rosenfeldt HM, Amrani Y, Watterson KR, Murthy KS, Panettieri RA Jr, Spiegel S (2003) Sphingosine-1-phosphate stimulates contraction of human airway smooth muscle cells. FASEB J 17:1789–1799. https://doi.org/10.1096/fj.02-0836com

Sadikot RT, Blackwell TS, Christman JW, Prince AS (2005) Pathogen-host interactions in Pseudomonas aeruginosa pneumonia. Am J Respir Crit Care Med 171:1209–1223. https://doi.org/10.1164/rccm.200408-1044SO

Sakae H, Ogiso Y, Matsuda M, Shimora H, Deering T, Fox TE, Kester M, Nabe T, Kitatani K (2023) Ceramide nanoliposomes as potential therapeutic reagents for asthma. Cells 12. https://doi.org/10.3390/cells12040591

Sanchez T, Hla T (2004) Structural and functional characteristics of S1P receptors. J Cell Biochem 92:913–922. https://doi.org/10.1002/jcb.20127

Schultz MJ, Rijneveld AW, Florquin S, Edwards CK, Dinarello CA, van der Poll T (2002) Role of interleukin-1 in the pulmonary immune response during Pseudomonas aeruginosa pneumonia. Am J Physiol Lung Cell Mol Physiol 282:L285–L290. https://doi.org/10.1152/ajplung.00461.2000

Schweitzer KS, Hatoum H, Brown MB, Gupta M, Justice MJ, Beteck B, Van Demark M, Gu Y, Presson RG Jr, Hubbard WC, Petrache I (2011) Mechanisms of lung endothelial barrier disruption induced by cigarette smoke: role of oxidative stress and ceramides. Am J Physiol Lung Cell Mol Physiol 301:L836–L846. https://doi.org/10.1152/ajplung.00385.2010

Schweitzer KS, Chen SX, Law S, Van Demark M, Poirier C, Justice MJ, Hubbard WC, Kim ES, Lai X, Wang M, Kranz WD, Carroll CJ, Ray BD, Bittman R, Goodpaster J, Petrache I (2015) Endothelial disruptive proinflammatory effects of nicotine and e-cigarette vapor exposures. Am J Physiol Lung Cell Mol Physiol 309:L175–L187. https://doi.org/10.1152/ajplung.00411.2014

Shah VS, Meyerholz DK, Tang XX, Reznikov L, Abou Alaiwa M, Ernst SE, Karp PH, Wohlford-Lenane CL, Heilmann KP, Leidinger MR, Allen PD, Zabner J, McCray PB Jr, Ostedgaard LS, Stoltz DA, Randak CO, Welsh MJ (2016) Airway acidification initiates host defense abnormalities in cystic fibrosis mice. Science 351:503–507. https://doi.org/10.1126/science.aad5589

Signorelli P, Pivari F, Barcella M, Merelli I, Zulueta A, Dei Cas M, Rosso L, Ghidoni R, Caretti A, Paroni R, Mingione A (2021) Myriocin modulates the altered lipid metabolism and storage in cystic fibrosis. Cell Signal 81:109928. https://doi.org/10.1016/j.cellsig.2021.109928

Siow D, Sunkara M, Morris A, Wattenberg B (2015) Regulation of de novo sphingolipid biosynthesis by the ORMDL proteins and sphingosine kinase-1. Adv Biol Regul 57:42–54. https://doi.org/10.1016/j.jbior.2014.09.002

Siskind LJ, Mullen TD, Romero Rosales K, Clarke CJ, Hernandez-Corbacho MJ, Edinger AL, Obeid LM (2010) The BCL-2 protein BAK is required for long-chain ceramide generation during apoptosis. J Biol Chem 285:11818–11826. https://doi.org/10.1074/jbc.M109.078121

Tavakoli Tabazavareh S, Seitz A, Jernigan P, Sehl C, Keitsch S, Lang S, Kahl BC, Edwards M, Grassme H, Gulbins E, Becker KA (2016) Lack of sphingosine causes susceptibility to pulmonary staphylococcus aureus infections in cystic fibrosis. Cell Physiol Biochem 38:2094–2102. https://doi.org/10.1159/000445567

Teichgraber V, Ulrich M, Endlich N, Riethmuller J, Wilker B, De Oliveira-Munding CC, van Heeckeren AM, Barr ML, von Kurthy G, Schmid KW, Weller M, Tummler B, Lang F, Grassme H, Doring G, Gulbins E (2008) Ceramide accumulation mediates inflammation, cell death and infection susceptibility in cystic fibrosis. Nat Med 14:382–391. https://doi.org/10.1038/nm1748

Terzikhan N, Verhamme KM, Hofman A, Stricker BH, Brusselle GG, Lahousse L (2016) Prevalence and incidence of COPD in smokers and non-smokers: the Rotterdam study. Eur J Epidemiol 31:785–792. https://doi.org/10.1007/s10654-016-0132-z

Thudhicum JL (1884) A treatise on the chemical constitution of the brain. Glasgow Med J 5:363–364

Toncheva AA, Potaczek DP, Schedel M, Gersting SW, Michel S, Krajnov N, Gaertner VD, Klingbeil JM, Illig T, Franke A, Winkler C, Hohlfeld JM, Vogelberg C, von Berg A, Bufe A, Heinzmann A, Laub O, Rietschel E, Simma B, Genuneit J, Muntau AC, Kabesch M (2015) Childhood asthma is associated with mutations and gene expression differences of ORMDL genes that can interact. Allergy 70:1288–1299. https://doi.org/10.1111/all.12652

Tran HB, Barnawi J, Ween M, Hamon R, Roscioli E, Hodge G, Reynolds PN, Pitson SM, Davies LT, Haberberger R, Hodge S (2016) Cigarette smoke inhibits efferocytosis via deregulation of sphingosine kinase signaling: reversal with exogenous S1P and the S1P analogue FTY720. J Leukoc Biol 100:195–202. https://doi.org/10.1189/jlb.3A1015-471R

Verhaegh R, Becker KA, Edwards MJ, Gulbins E (2020) Sphingosine kills bacteria by binding to cardiolipin. J Biol Chem 295:7686–7696. https://doi.org/10.1074/jbc.RA119.012325

Verhaeghe C, Delbecque K, de Leval L, Oury C, Bours V (2007) Early inflammation in the airways of a cystic fibrosis foetus. J Cyst Fibros 6:304–308. https://doi.org/10.1016/j.jcf.2006.12.001

Vital D, Hofer M, Benden C, Holzmann D, Boehler A (2013) Impact of sinus surgery on pseudomonal airway colonization, bronchiolitis obliterans syndrome and survival in cystic fibrosis lung transplant recipients. Respiration 86:25–31. https://doi.org/10.1159/000339627

Wegner MS, Schiffmann S, Parnham MJ, Geisslinger G, Grosch S (2016) The enigma of ceramide synthase regulation in mammalian cells. Prog Lipid Res 63:93–119. https://doi.org/10.1016/j.plipres.2016.03.006

Westholter D, Schumacher F, Wulfinghoff N, Sutharsan S, Strassburg S, Kleuser B, Horn PA, Reuter S, Gulbins E, Taube C, Welsner M (2022) CFTR modulator therapy alters plasma sphingolipid profiles in people with cystic fibrosis. J Cyst Fibros 21:713–720. https://doi.org/10.1016/j.jcf.2022.02.005

Whitchurch CB, Tolker-Nielsen T, Ragas PC, Mattick JS (2002) Extracellular DNA required for bacterial biofilm formation. Science 295:1487. https://doi.org/10.1126/science.295.5559.1487

Worgall TS (2022) Sphingolipids and asthma. Adv Exp Med Biol 1372:145–155. https://doi.org/10.1007/978-981-19-0394-6_10

Worlitzsch D, Tarran R, Ulrich M, Schwab U, Cekici A, Meyer KC, Birrer P, Bellon G, Berger J, Weiss T, Botzenhart K, Yankaskas JR, Randell S, Boucher RC, Doring G (2002) Effects of reduced mucus oxygen concentration in airway Pseudomonas infections of cystic fibrosis patients. J Clin Invest 109:317–325. https://doi.org/10.1172/JCI13870

Youssef M, De Sanctis JB, Shah J, Dumut DC, Hajduch M, Naumova AK, Radzioch D (2020) Treatment of allergic asthma with Fenretinide formulation (LAU-7b) downregulates ORMDL sphingolipid biosynthesis regulator 3 (Ormdl3) expression and normalizes ceramide imbalance. J Pharmacol Exp Ther 373:476–487. https://doi.org/10.1124/jpet.119.263715

Zhang X, Hu Q, Weng Q (2018) Secondary metabolites (SMs) of Isaria cicadae and Isaria tenuipes. RSC Adv 9:172–184. https://doi.org/10.1039/c8ra09039d

Zheng JP, Wen FQ, Bai CX, Wan HY, Kang J, Chen P, Yao WZ, Ma LJ, Li X, Raiteri L, Sardina M, Gao Y, Wang BS, Zhong NS, PANTHEON Study Group (2014) Twice daily N-acetylcysteine 600 mg for exacerbations of chronic obstructive pulmonary disease (PANTHEON): a randomised, double-blind placebo-controlled trial. Lancet Respir Med 2:187–194. https://doi.org/10.1016/S2213-2600(13)70286-8

Zulueta A, Caretti A, Campisi GM, Brizzolari A, Abad JL, Paroni R, Signorelli P, Ghidoni R (2017) Inhibitors of ceramide de novo biosynthesis rescue damages induced by cigarette smoke in airways epithelia. Naunyn Schmiedebergs Arch Pharmacol 390:753–759. https://doi.org/10.1007/s00210-017-1375-2

Targeted Molecular Therapeutics for Pulmonary Diseases: Addressing the Need for Precise Drug Delivery

Simone Carneiro, Joschka T. Müller, and Olivia M. Merkel

Contents

Abstract

Respiratory diseases are a major concern in public health, impacting a large population worldwide. Despite the availability of therapies that alleviate symptoms, selectively addressing the critical points of pathopathways remains a

Simone Carneiro and Joschka T. Müller contributed equally to this work.

S. Carneiro · J. T. Müller
Department of Pharmacy, Pharmaceutical Technology and Biopharmacy, Ludwig-Maximilians-University Munich, Munich, Germany

O. M. Merkel (✉)
Department of Pharmacy, Pharmaceutical Technology and Biopharmacy, Ludwig-Maximilians-University Munich, Munich, Germany

Center for NanoScience (CeNS), Ludwig-Maximilians-University Munich, Munich, Germany

Institute of Lung Health and Immunity (LHI) and Comprehensive Pneumology Center (CPC) with the CPC-M bioArchive, Helmholtz Munich, German Center for Lung Research (DZL), Munich, Germany
e-mail: olivia.merkel@lmu.de

M. Schäfer-Korting, U. S. Schubert (eds.), *Drug Delivery and Targeting*,
Handbook of Experimental Pharmacology 284, https://doi.org/10.1007/164_2023_703

major challenge. Innovative formulations designed for reaching these targets within the airways, enhanced selectivity, and prolonged therapeutic effects offer promising solutions. To provide insights into the specific medical requirements of chronic respiratory diseases, the initial focus of this chapter is directed on lung physiology, emphasizing the significance of lung barriers. Current treatments involving small molecules and the potential of gene therapy are also discussed. Additionally, we will explore targeting approaches, with a particular emphasis on nanoparticles, comparing targeted and non-targeted formulations for pulmonary administration. Finally, the potential of inhaled sphingolipids in the context of respiratory diseases is briefly discussed, highlighting their promising prospects in the field.

Keywords

Gene therapy · Inhalation · Pulmonary administration · Sphingolipids · Targeted nanoparticles

Abbreviations

API	Active pharmaceutical ingredient
CA-IX	Carbonic anhydrase IX
CF	Cystic fibrosis
COPD	Chronic obstructive pulmonary disease
DOTAP	1,2-Dioleoyl-3-trimethylammonium-propane
DPPC	Dipalmitoyl phosphatidylcholine
DSPE	1,2-Distearoyl-sn-glycero-3-phosphorylethanolamine
FA	Folic acid
FR	Folic acid receptor
KRAS	Kirsten rat sarcoma
LNP	Lipid nanoparticle
MCC	Mucociliary clearance
MMAD	Mass median aerodynamic diameter
NHS	N-hydroxysuccinimide
PCLS	Precision-cut lung slices
PEG	Polyethylene glycol
PEI	Polyethyleneimine
PLGA	Poly(lactic-co-glycolic acid)
SP	Surfactant protein
Tf	Human holo-transferrin
TSLP	Thymic stromal lymphopoietin
VIPER	Virus-inspired polymer for endosomal release

1 Introduction: Lung Anatomy, Major Diseases, and Options for Pulmonary Drug Delivery

The leading causes of death worldwide in 2019, according to the WHO, were ischemic heart disease and stroke, followed by chronic obstructive pulmonary disease (COPD) and lower respiratory infections (WHO n.d.-a). Tracheal, bronchial, and lung cancer as well as tuberculosis are also in the top 20 causes of death, highlighting the importance of better treating respiratory diseases. Moreover, the SARS-CoV-2 pandemic that emerged in late 2019 has taken the lives of almost seven million people (WHO n.d.-b). As a result, industry and academia have made numerous attempts to develop effective strategies against lung diseases, which are discussed in the context of this book chapter. However, before embarking on the development of an actual dosage form, the underlying anatomical, physiological, and pathophysiological conditions in the lung are described as different barriers that need to be overcome in drug delivery.

In many first-line therapies for lung diseases, pulmonary administration is the route of choice. The large surface (approximately 100 m^2) of the thin alveolar epithelium and high blood flow rate favor drug absorption resulting in a high concentration of the drug at the target site with less systemic exposure. Moreover, drugs intended for systemic effects are not subject to hepatic first-pass metabolism. Inhalative application also presents fewer practical obstacles for the patient than parenteral therapy and can allow for the use of drugs subject to critical hepatic degradation when delivered orally. In addition, the use of mucoadhesive excipients, for example by encapsulating drugs with chitosan (Zhao et al. 2022), can achieve a prolonged release with a more constant drug level. Disadvantages are mainly characterized by more expensive development work. Moreover, pulmonary application requires special training of the patient by medical or pharmaceutical personnel. For example, inhalation therapy with glucocorticoids can lead to oral thrush or hoarseness if residual drug in the oropharynx is not either rinsed or removed by food after inhalation.

As shown in Fig. 1, airways and their incorporated bifurcations can be compared with an upside-down tree (Baldassi et al. 2021): the upper respiratory tract, represented as a trunk, refers to the conducting or tracheobronchial region consisting of the trachea and the bronchi the former further divides into. The second section represents the lower respiratory tract with the bronchioles and the alveoli (Wang et al. 2022). The thickness of the epithelial layer decreases progressively from 50–60 μm to 0.2 μm from the trachea to the alveoli (Chellappan et al. 2022). The epithelium from the trachea to the bronchi is lined with ciliated cells, club cells, basal cells, and mucus-secreting goblet cells. The directed, coordinated movement of the ciliated cells leads to a process called "mucociliary clearance" (MCC). As a result, particles that impact on mucus are entrapped in the latter, initiating degradation in the oropharynx. MCC represents an initial defense mechanism within the body

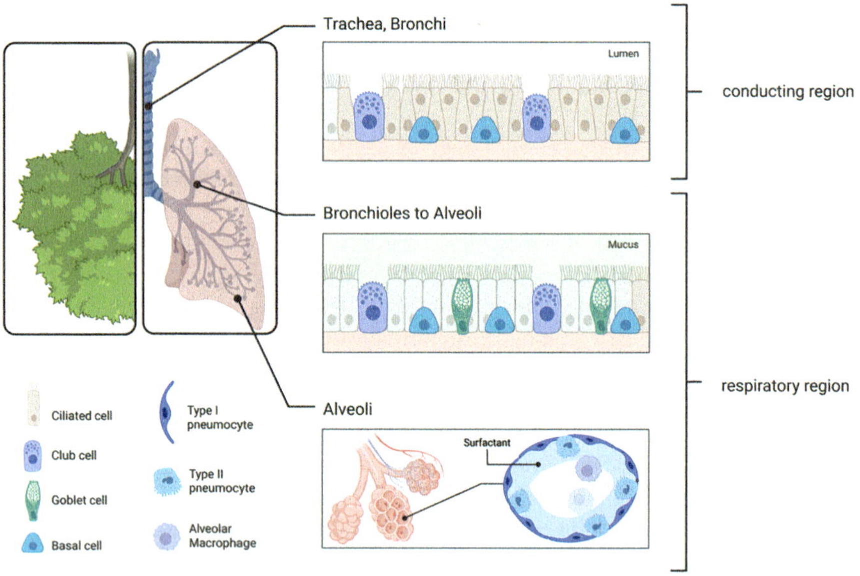

Fig. 1 Lung anatomy (schematic) of the conducting and respiratory regions. Created with BioRender.com

against xenobiotics and pathological microorganisms. In a healthy lung, the complete removal of exogenous particles by MCC occurs within 24 h (Geiser 2010). Type I and type II pneumocytes are found in the alveoli. Type I pneumocytes line up to 95% of the alveolar epithelium; type II pneumocytes perform the important task of producing surfactant.

Inhaled drugs initially impact on the lung lining fluids, and the aerosolized particles need to overcome several physiological hurdles. In order to reach the lower airways, inhaled particles must move along curved and bifurcated paths with the airflow. A mass median aerodynamic diameter (MMAD) of 1–5 μm represents the optimal particle size for deposition by sedimentation in the alveoli. Particles over 10 μm remain in the pharynx and trachea; particles smaller than 0.5 μm are exhaled. However, exceptions are relevant not least with regard to particulate matter (Thompson 2018). For example, β_2-adrenergic receptor agonist-loaded particles 3–6 μm in size and targeting the smooth muscle cells of the trachea and upper airways can be beneficial in asthma bronchiale therapy. Furthermore, ACE2 receptors, relevant in the uptake of SARS-CoV-2, are predominantly expressed in the upper airways; addressing this target may prevent manifestation of the infection (Synowiec et al. 2021).

Mucus (2–5% glycosylated proteins, i.e., mucins plus minor amounts of cell residues such as DNA and cell debris (Guo et al. 2023)) forms a gel-like mesh stabilized by disulfide bridges. Mucus has high viscoelasticity and is a shear-thinning, non-Newtonian fluid. The unstirred layer represents a barrier through which drug particles must necessarily diffuse. As in cystic fibrosis (CF), the dry fraction of mucins is up to 8%, the resulting increase in viscoelasticity of the tenacious fluid inhibits the free movement of immune cells which favors airway infections with *Pseudomonas aeruginosa* or others (Deacon et al. 2015; Ibarra-Sanchez et al. 2022). In addition, cilia motility in MCC is negatively affected. In asthmatic patients, mucus production can be stimulated by the induction of proinflammatory genes. This must be considered when it comes to developing a suitable drug delivery system. For instance, a high concentration of polyethylene glycol (PEG) on nanoparticles can significantly improve mucus penetration (Guo et al. 2023). Due to its polar structures, PEG imitates the surface of proteins and thus passes more easily. Moreover, enhanced mucus penetration of nanoparticles with high PEG density is explained by the fact that in low concentrations, PEG chains adopt a mushroom structure, which does not change the zeta potential of the underlying nanoparticles. Given that the zeta potential reflects the overall charge of the particles and its electrostatic interaction with mucins significantly affects particle retention within the mucus layer, modifying the overall charge could serve as a potential strategy to enhance particle penetration within the mucus. Increasing the concentration of PEG causes this mushroom conformation to unfold into a brush-like structure, which reduces electrostatic interactions with mucus (Guo et al. 2023). In contrast to the observations by Guo et al., we recently described that PEGylation does not have a positive effect on mucus diffusion in sputum from CF patients, however (Conte et al. 2022).

A further lung-specific condition of drug absorption is linked to surfactant production in type II pneumocytes. Surfactant is a surface-active lipid-protein mixture consisting of 92% phospholipids, cholesterol, and other neutral lipids (Parra and Perez-Gil 2015; Xu et al. 2022b), particularly unsaturated phosphatidyl-choline and dipalmitoyl phosphatidylcholine (DPPC). Minor components are the two hydrophilic surfactant proteins (SP) SP-A and SP-D and the strongly hydrophobic proteins SP-B and SP-C. Surfactant prevents the collapse of the alveoli in the continuous cycle of expansion and recoiling during gas exchange. It reduces the surface tension during compression and dilatation at the interface between air and alveolar fluid (Goerke 1998; Wüstneck et al. 1999), for which DPPC in particular is mainly responsible. Surfactant does not merely represent a simple monolayer at the interface between air and liquid, which is normally assumed for surfactants below the critical micelle concentration, but also forms a complex, 3-dimensional network of connected structures (Parra and Perez-Gil 2015).

The main pathophysiological aspects of the target diseases are outlined elsewhere in this handbook. Here, we describe delivery and targeting strategies for pulmonary administration with a special focus on nanoparticles.

2 Pulmonary Diseases: Current and Innovative Drug Delivery

Asthma bronchiale is a heterogeneous chronic lung disorder characterized by a complex pathogenesis, affecting more than 250 million people worldwide (WHO n.d.-c). Based on the advanced understanding of the pathophysiology of asthma, it is presumable that the most promising route to ensure a successful treatment is via pulmonary administration. When using an inhaler, however, breath-inhalation coordination can be challenging, especially among children. Furthermore, not all patients respond favorably to inhaled asthma medications, and side effects of inhaled medication in the oropharynx can affect patient adherence to the treatment (Shukla et al. 2020; WHO n.d.-c). In that regard, the research in the area of asthma therapeutics has advanced toward both designing new drugs and achieving more effective formulations targeting specific asthma biomarkers. For instance, the recombinant monoclonal antibody omalizumab has demonstrated its efficacy in allergic asthmatic patients. The drug specifically binds to free immunoglobulin E, which plays a crucial role in asthma-related inflammation (Busse et al. 2001). Since the bioavailability of inhaled proteins is low, pulmonary administration of these antibodies is so far not available. While the inhalation route offers several benefits for treating respiratory conditions, producing formulations of antibodies for inhalation can be challenging due to stability concerns. Nebulizers require the drug to be dissolved, which may not be ideal as dissolved proteins can undergo changes in conformation and aggregation affecting long-term stability, whereas dry powder antibodies show promise for inhalation purposes. Protein sensitivity to temperature and shearing stress during the spray-drying process can be overcome using suitable excipients and optimized drying parameters resulting in a stable antibody formulation (Mayor et al. 2021; Parray et al. 2021).

Nucleic acid-based therapy is effective in IL-13-mediated asthma. The upregulated transcription factor GATA-3 (Nakamura 1999) is a relevant target due to its role in promoting T_H2 cell activation and as a triggering factor in several asthmatic pathways. It also regulates cell types continuously expressed in asthma, such as eosinophils, basophils, mast cells, and epithelial cells (Keil et al. 2020; Sel et al. 2008). By delivering nucleic acids to downregulate GATA-3, several triggering mechanisms of asthma can be simultaneously blocked. The inhaled formulation SB010 comprises a DNA enzyme (DNAzyme) as active pharmaceutical ingredient (API) known as hgd40, which functions by cleaving and deactivating GATA3 messenger RNA (mRNA). This formulation has undergone clinical trials, including a phase 2a trial in patients with allergic asthma to evaluate the efficacy of inhaled hdg40. The study demonstrated an overall improvement in both early and later stages of the disease (Krug et al. 2015).

Respiratory infectious diseases represent another major public health concern due to the progressively increasing rates of incidence and mortality, especially among vulnerable individuals (WHO n.d.-d). The outbreaks also cause a severe economic burden.

Among viral respiratory infections, influenza viruses are spread worldwide and infect millions of people yearly (WHO n.d.-e); serious diseases and death occur in particular in the elderly and children (Caini et al. 2018; Mattila et al. 2020). The most effective preventive measure for influenza is vaccination. Nonetheless, a few antivirals are available aiming at reducing the exacerbation of symptoms and, therefore, the risk of severe disease. The neuraminidase inhibitors oseltamivir, zanamivir, laninamivir, and peramivir are recommended for specific risk groups.

Neuraminidase inhibitors are available for multiple administration routes. Zanamivir and laninamivir are available as a dry powder for inhalation, while oseltamivir is orally administered. Peramivir must be intravenously injected (Aoki 2015).

Moreover, mRNA loaded in lipid nanoparticles (LNPs) are an innovative approach to fight COVID-19 by vaccination (for details, see Schäfer-Korting, 2023). Redirection of the LNP accumulation away from the liver and toward the lungs was described by using 1,2-dioleoyl-3-trimethylammonium-propane (DOTAP) as an additional cationic lipid. These LNPs also contain DLin-MC3-DMA as an ionizable lipid component, designed to facilitate escape from the endosomes. LNP uptake by the lung was enhanced to around 21%, while 67% was found in the liver and 12% in the spleen (Idris et al. 2021).

A similar approach applying siRNA-based therapy as a possible treatment for COVID-19 was recently published by our group (Baldassi et al. 2022a). First, our collaborators screened sequences to identify the most effective targets within the SARS-CoV-2 genome to be targeted by siRNA and selected the open reading frame 1 (ORF1), which is a highly conserved region and part of the genomic RNA of the virus. An siRNA targeting the sequence (siORF1) was encapsulated in a mix of polyethyleneimine (PEI) and a sophisticated virus-inspired polymer for endosomal release (VIPER) (Ambike et al. 2022). VIPER increases cell permeability in an acidic environment and is therefore suitable as an enhancer of endosomal escape. In addition to various in vitro cell knockdown attempts, virus replication was inhibited by 50% in human precision-cut lung slices (PCLS). In Balb/c mice, preferential uptake in type II pneumocytes and macrophages and a minor increase in proinflammatory molecules in bronchoalveolar lavage fluid indicated low toxicity (Baldassi et al. 2022a).

3 Drug Targeting in Pulmonary Administration

One of the promising approaches to enhance the efficacy and reduce side effects of drugs is to formulate them within encapsulating delivery systems. Various nanocarriers such as liposomes, LNPs, lipo-, and polyplexes are used as drug delivery systems for different active pharmaceutical ingredients (APIs). The utilization of nanoparticles has been the predominant approach for implementing targeting strategies. Consequently, the focus of the following section primarily centers on the use of nanoparticles for this purpose.

For API delivery with nanoparticles in general, and for pulmonary delivery in particular, it is important to consider particle properties. Depending on their size, nanoparticles can be taken up by clathrin-mediated, caveolin-mediated, macropinocytosis, and clathrin- and caveolin-independent pathways (Winkeljann et al. 2022). In addition, targeted nanoparticles can induce receptor-mediated uptake. Alveolar macrophages phagocytose particles particularly sized 1–5 μm (Geiser 2010). Particles sized 500 nm or smaller are more likely to diffuse through the mucus, so that the particles can pass more or less unhindered through the network of mucins (Guo et al. 2023). Yet, negative charged carboxyl and sulfate groups present in mucus glycans tend to repel particles that have a negative zeta potential. Positive zeta potentials, on the other hand, have the tendency to be mucoadhesive, resulting in hampered particles passing through mucus. A strategy to overcome this drawback was recently published by Baldassi et al. (2022b). Since PEI has a positive zeta potential due to its high amine density, the authors aimed to overcome the anticipated lower mucus permeability coating of PEI-siRNA polyplexes with 2.5:1 (*w/w*) Alveofact:PEI. In an alveolar cell model, which was cultured at air–liquid interface, where cells also secrete mucus, the coated poplyplexes had the best mucus-penetrating properties. Moreover, charge distribution, charge density, and particle geometry may also be of relevance.

When administered via aerosol generators such as pressurized metered dose inhalers, dry powder inhalers, or nebulizers, nanoparticulate formulations commonly effectively reach the lungs. However, they are nonspecifically taken up by different cell types present in the respective area. Whereas in the systemic therapy of nanoparticles, the so-called enhanced permeability and retention effect has been described for strongly vascularized tumors, which can result in a passive targeting of nanoparticles in tumor tissue, this effect is not observed in many lung diseases. Therefore, increased effort has been made in recent years to achieve ligand-mediated targeting for nanoparticles. Ligand-mediated targeting exploits intrinsic properties of special cells for nanoparticles to exert their pharmaceutical effect mainly within or at the cell membrane of target cells. For example, receptor overexpression of a certain cell type can lead to an increased uptake of particles through coupling with a receptor ligand. In this section, various methods and nanocarrier systems will be elaborated upon, highlighting the advantages of ligand-mediated targeting. A good overview of different targeting strategies in the lung epithelium can be found here (Abed et al. 2021). For a detailed insight into the coupling of ligands with the corresponding nanoparticles, the reader is referred to (Hermanson 1996; Lu et al. 2021). In the following, various target structures on cells that were selected in recent years for cell-specific targeting will be presented.

3.1 Drug Targeting in Lung Cancer Therapies

Antitumor drugs often exhibit a high number of side effects, primarily due to their inability to discriminate between aberrant and normal cells. Consequently, in cancer therapy, targeted delivery of these drugs to the malignant cells using appropriate strategies has emerged as a crucial objective. Cells with a high division activity require an enormous amount of purine and pyrimidine bases for DNA new synthesis. An important co-factor for the synthesis of purines and other cell components is folic acid (FA). Accordingly, cancer cells overexpress folic acid receptors (FR) up to 100-fold compared to normal cells (Fernandez et al. 2018).

In a recent study, liposomes were prepared according to the film method followed by ultrasound treatment (Zhu et al. 2019). The liposomes were loaded with docetaxel, and 1,2-distearoyl-sn-glycero-3-phosphorylethanolamine (DSPE)-PEG2000-FA was incorporated as a targeting ligand into the lipid bilayer. Particle size was 89 nm for the unloaded liposomes and 100 nm for liposomes loaded with docetaxel, respectively. They were subsequently co-sprayed with mannitol and leucine for improved microparticulate properties, crystallinity and hygroscopicity (Alhajj et al. 2021; Keil et al. 2021). After spray drying, MMAD of the dry powder was 3.1 μm, which is a desirable size for the uptake of particles within the alveoli, as already mentioned in the introduction. However, hydrodynamic diameter of the redispersed liposomes increased significantly. To examine the influence of the targeting ligand, the uptake in SPCA1 cells was analyzed in the presence (FA+) and absence of (FA-) folic acid. Folic acid saturates the FA receptors on the cell, and the advantage of ligand-mediated targeting is lost. Accordingly, the uptake decreased in the FA+ medium. In the FA- medium, however, the liposomes conjugated with folic acid were taken up preferentially compared to the unconjugated counterparts. After spray drying and redispersion, the targeting function was somewhat reduced, which suggests partial destruction of FA coupling.

Another target for anticancer drugs is carbonic anhydrase IX (CA-IX), which is also expressed on the cell surface. Due to the increased oxygen consumption of the tumor tissue, hypoxia-inducible factor is released, enhancing downstream to the CA-IX expression and ultimately contributing to a normalization of the tissue pH (Pastorek and Pastorekova 2015). Lin et al. developed a dual-ligand liposome vector decorated on the surface with an anti-CA-IX antibody and CPP33 (Lin et al. 2018). This tumor cell-penetrating peptide increases the uptake of particles into the tissue. Both ligands were conjugated to DSPE-PEG2000-maleimides via free thiol groups of each peptide as a thiol-ene "click reaction" at different stages of liposome formation. The encapsulated cytostatic drug was triptolide. In a 3D tumor spheroid model developed based on A549 cells (a human lung adenocarcinoma cell line carrying a KRAS mutation), these dual-ligand liposomes significantly reduced cell viability. Lin et al. concluded this to be a synergistic interaction of both the targeting ligand and the cell-penetrating peptide CPP33. Applied to the lungs of tumor-induced rats, the tumor size declined for several weeks following a treatment with the dual-ligand liposomes.

Another approach was taken by Yuan et al., who used N-succinyl-palmitoyl-chitosan as an amphiphilic copolymer, which was coupled with a cRGD motif via N-hydroxysuccinimide (NHS) (Yuan et al. 2015). The conjugated micelles were loaded with paclitaxel. Non-small-cell lung cancer cells overexpress integrin receptor $\alpha_v\beta_3$. Targeting this receptor via cRGD, particles are internalized in luc-A549 cells, and cRGD micelles showed the highest uptake. In a subsequent in vivo experiment, the tumor-bearing mice were i.v. treated with paclitaxel micelles. Despite a loss of the advantages of local application, a significant antitumor effect of the cRGD nanoparticles was observed (Yuan et al. 2015).

3.2 Drug Targeting for Asthma

Airway epithelial cell-specific targeting for asthma was recently attempted by Zhang et al. (2022). In their study, they used LNPs consisting of MC3 lipids, DOPC,

PEG-DMG, and cholesterol. They successfully coupled a cyclic peptide as targeting ligand to cholesterol molecules via an EDC-NHS protocol, which was confirmed via ^{1}H-NMR. The cyclic peptide, derived from rhinovirus, mediates entry into airway epithelial cells after binding to ICAM-1. During inflammatory processes, ICAM-1 receptor is upregulated, especially in asthma, which can therefore be used as a target.

In their study, Zhang et al. used siRNA directed against thymic stromal lymphopoietin, which plays a crucial role in the pathogenesis of asthma. In preliminary experiments, increased uptake of the targeted LNPs was shown in vitro across the three cell lines 16HBE, BEAS-2B, and A549. The highest concentration with a 6.6% content of conjugated cholesterol proved to be the most promising. To test this approach in vivo, an established asthma model was used in mice. On day 35 after the first exposure to ovalbumin, a microspray technique was used to deliver the particles intratracheally to the mice. In LNP-treated mice, the concentration of thymic stromal lymphopoietin almost returned to the baseline value of the control group, while the nanoparticles loaded with non-coding siRNA showed no effect. Downstream, a significant decrease in the cytokine concentration of IL-4 and IL-13 was also observed. Details of the aerosolized LNPs, however, are not provided.

Overexpression of transferrin receptors on activated T cells is another possible target for the treatment of asthma. Utilizing this condition, we were able to develop a promising strategy by linking 5 kDa branched PEI via disulfide linkers to human holo-transferrin (Tf) using SPDP (Kandil et al. 2023). In addition to the targeting protein transferrin, the lytic protein from the European honeybee, melittin, was conjugated to PEI in a similar way. Introducing a disulfide bridge that can be cleaved by an increased glutathione concentration in the cytosol can promote endosomal escape (Mandal et al. 2022). In this approach, PEI with its basic amines encapsulates the siRNA, which targets various GATA-3 sequences. In Jurkat cells, which are considered as difficult to transfect, a GATA-3 knockdown of 65% was achieved. As a sophisticated ex vivo model, human PCLS were chosen from lung explants. CD3/CD28 dynabeads activated the T cells in PCLS and enhanced GATA-3 expression after 5 days. GATA-silencing nanoparticles consisting of Tf-PEI and Tf-melittin-PEI induced a significant knockdown of GATA-3.

3.3 The Management of Respiratory Diseases Beyond Drug Targeting: Sphingolipids

As discussed in Chap. 13, entitled "Looking to the Future: Drug Delivery and Targeting in the Prophylaxis and Therapy of Severe and Chronic Diseases", inhaled sphingolipids offer a promising alternative for treating diseases such as CF and COPD. However, the effective delivery of sphingolipids like sphingosine to the lungs requires overcoming several hurdles. Their inherent lipophilic attributes necessitate the development of strategies not only to ensure the appropriate packaging of these APIs but also to maintain the consistency of dosing and physicochemical stability throughout the manufacturing process and the subsequent repeated administration via aerosolization.

The incorporation of sphingolipids in lipid-containing nanoparticles such as liposomes or LNPs seems, therefore, promising. Carstens et al. recently published the delivery of sphingosine in micelle-like structures along with octylglucopyranoside. Notably, the formation of these nanoparticle systems is expected to achieve polydisperse samples, which would be disadvantageous for a pharmaceutical formulation (Carstens et al. 2019). Moreover, the absence of comprehensive data concerning the impact of nebulization on the structural aspects of the nanoparticle configuration necessitates further investigation. Alternatively, the incorporation of sphingosines into liposomes containing phospholipids such as DPPC or 1,2-distearoyl-*sn*-glycero-3-phosphocholine, utilizing established film hydration or comparable methods, could be a promising approach. Post-homogenization, a monodisperse sample should be achievable for aerosolization via nebulization, even though different formulations might require appropriate nebulizers (Klein et al. 2021; Longest et al. 2019; van Rijn et al. 2023). Recently, liposomal amikacin nebulized by the vibrating mesh nebulizer system LAMIRA®, based on the PARI eFlow® nebulizer, was approved by the EMA, indicating the feasibility of aerosolization of liposomal formulations for commercial products (EMA 2020). In case a prolonged release of the encapsulated lipophilic drug is necessary for pharmacokinetic reasons, an alternative approach may be beneficial. Lipophilic drugs incorporated in the phospholipid bilayer led to a fast release of the API. To overcome this particular hurdle, Zou et al. established a method to encapsulate lipophilic ceramide within biodegradable poly(lactic-co-glycolic acid) (PLGA) nanoparticles (Makadia and Siegel 2011), which could also be used for sphingolipids. PLGA nanoparticles were subsequently encapsulated within a liposomal formulation for prolonged release kinetics (Zou et al. 2014).

Previous research has indicated a connection between an abnormal ceramide level in CF lungs and increased inflammation and infection susceptibility due to the sphingolipids' metabolism (Teichgraber et al. 2008). CF mice treated with nebulized recombinant acid ceramidase exhibited a notable decrease in associated lung inflammatory cells – namely, neutrophils and macrophages (Gardner et al. 2020). The underlying concept was to lower ceramide levels as an anti-inflammatory strategy. However, this approach did not significantly decrease ceramide levels in CF mice compared to normal mice, as demonstrated in the same study. Notably, this effect was evident in airway epithelial cell cultures (Gardner et al. 2020), and further investigations into formulation stability and optimization might be necessary. Utilizing a nanosized delivery system to directly target the lungs holds promise for overcoming these challenges (Munir et al. 2022b). Furthermore, some pharmaceuticals such as Exubera®, Trelstar®, Somatuline®, and Raplixa® serve as instances of protein-based powders produced by spray drying that received approvals from both the EMA and FDA. However, Exubera® was later withdrawn from the market (Pinto et al. 2021).

As an additional approach, employing spray drying to convert particles or drugs into a dry powder for lung administration has been established (Munir et al. 2022a). Fine-tuning aerodynamic properties such as the mass median diameter, fine particle fraction, and residual moisture can enhance the delivery of sphingolipids into the deep lungs. Dry powder formulations also offer improved storage stability, circumventing concerns including coalescence, creaming, or microbiological contamination. Additionally, chemical instabilities are markedly reduced in dry powder formulations due to the absence of liquids that can trigger reactions such as hydrolysis (Chaurasiya and Zhao 2020). For instance, Xu et al. (2022a) spray-dried siRNA-hybrid nanoparticles with suitable physicochemical properties for pulmonary administration. The process preserved the siRNA functionality and achieved a uniform cargo biodistribution in mouse lungs. Such results underscore a promising strategy for optimizing and further developing sphingolipid-based inhalable formulations.

4 Conclusion

As discussed in this chapter, respiratory diseases still pose a risk to millions of lives due to ineffective or lack of medications to treat specific conditions. Despite conventional therapy being highly helpful, the efficacy is limited to low to mild exacerbations of symptoms, and by predefined health criteria of individuals that further determine the eligibility to the therapy, as well as by strong side effects depending on the dose. Despite a long way to reach the market, several promising strategies are currently under investigation to optimize the treatment of respiratory diseases. Therefore, funding and efforts in research to overcome the unmet needs of numerous lung disorders must be scaled up to increase the chances of developing innovative and more efficient formulations. This scenario is presented by several clinical trials that have the potential to generate extremely relevant results to drive the regulatory agencies' decisions on whether or not to implement a new medicine or formulation.

Supported by the medicines that already reached the market in the past few years, nucleic acid-based therapy is a broad research field that offers huge potential to improve challenging diseases. The idea of interfering with the expression of a defective gene in the lungs opens the possibility of optimizing the treatment or even reaching a status of long-term absence of symptoms.

Noteworthy, functionalizing promising carrier systems with targeting molecules that will improve the cargo delivery to the targeted cells not only enhances efficacy but also gives the additional benefit of narrowing down the side effects due to selectivity. Elucidating molecular pathways in lung diseases will certainly contribute to find potent targets in the near future. As demonstrated above, many studies achieved promising results that are worth moving on to the clinics.

Ultimately, inhaled sphingolipids emerge as potent allies for the management of respiratory conditions. Yet, multifaceted parameters to achieve a successful formulation require optimization efforts, with promising outlooks.

References

Abed S, Turner R, Serniuck N, Tat V, Naiel S, Hayat A, Mekhael O, Vierhout M, Ask K, Rullo AF (2021) Cell-specific drug targeting in the lung. Biochem Pharmacol 190:114577. https://doi.org/10.1016/j.bcp.2021.114577

Alhajj N, O'Reilly NJ, Cathcart H (2021) Leucine as an excipient in spray dried powder for inhalation. Drug Discov Today 26:2384–2396. https://doi.org/10.1016/j.drudis.2021.04.009

Ambike S, Cheng CC, Feuerherd M, Velkov S, Baldassi D, Afridi SQ, Porras-Gonzalez D, Wei X, Hagen P, Kneidinger N, Stoleriu MG, Grass V, Burgstaller G, Pichlmair A, Merkel OM, Ko C, Michler T (2022) Targeting genomic SARS-CoV-2 RNA with siRNAs allows efficient inhibition of viral replication and spread. Nucleic Acids Res 50:333–349. https://doi.org/10.1093/nar/gkab1248

Aoki FY (2015) Antiviral drugs for influenza and other respiratory virus infections, pp 531–545.e5. https://doi.org/10.1016/b978-1-4557-4801-3.00044-8

Baldassi D, Gabold B, Merkel O (2021) Air-liquid interface cultures of the healthy and diseased human respiratory tract: promises, challenges and future directions. Adv Nanobiomed Res 1. https://doi.org/10.1002/anbr.202000111

Baldassi D, Ambike S, Feuerherd M, Cheng CC, Peeler DJ, Feldmann DP, Porras-Gonzalez DL, Wei X, Keller LA, Kneidinger N, Stoleriu MG, Popp A, Burgstaller G, Pun SH, Michler T, Merkel OM (2022a) Inhibition of SARS-CoV-2 replication in the lung with siRNA/VIPER polyplexes. J Control Release 345:661–674. https://doi.org/10.1016/j.jconrel.2022.03.051

Baldassi D, Ngo TMH, Merkel OM (2022b) Optimization of lung surfactant coating of siRNA polyplexes for pulmonary delivery. Pharm Res. https://doi.org/10.1007/s11095-022-03443-3

Busse W, Corren J, Lanier BQ, McAlary M, Fowler-Taylor A, Cioppa GD, van As A, Gupta N (2001) Omalizumab, anti-IgE recombinant humanized monoclonal antibody, for the treatment of severe allergic asthma. J Allergy Clin Immunol 108:184–190. https://doi.org/10.1067/mai.2001.117880

Caini S, Kroneman M, Wiegers T, El Guerche-Seblain C, Paget J (2018) Clinical characteristics and severity of influenza infections by virus type, subtype, and lineage: a systematic literature review. Influenza Other Respi Viruses 12:780–792. https://doi.org/10.1111/irv.12575

Carstens H, Schumacher F, Keitsch S, Kramer M, Kuhn C, Sehl C, Soddemann M, Wilker B, Herrmann D, Swaidan A, Kleuser B, Verhaegh R, Hilken G, Edwards MJ, Dubicanac M, Carpinteiro A, Wissmann A, Becker KA, Kamler M, Gulbins E (2019) Clinical development of sphingosine as anti-bacterial drug: inhalation of sphingosine in mini pigs has no adverse side effects. Cell Physiol Biochem 53:1015–1028. https://doi.org/10.33594/000000194

Chaurasiya B, Zhao YY (2020) Dry powder for pulmonary delivery: a comprehensive review. Pharmaceutics 13. https://doi.org/10.3390/pharmaceutics13010031

Chellappan DK, Prasher P, Saravanan V, Vern Yee VS, Wen Chi WC, Wong JW, Wong JK, Wong JT, Wan W, Chellian J, Molugulu N, Prabu SL, Ibrahim R, Darmarajan T, Candasamy M, Singh PK, Mishra V, Shastri MD, Zacconi FC, Chakraborty A, Mehta M, Gupta PK, Dureja H, Gulati M, Singh SK, Gupta G, Jha NK, George Oliver BG, Dua K (2022) Protein and peptide delivery to lungs by using advanced targeted drug delivery. Chem Biol Interact 351:109706. https://doi.org/10.1016/j.cbi.2021.109706

Conte G, Costabile G, Baldassi D, Rondelli V, Bassi R, Colombo D, Linardos G, Fiscarelli EV, Sorrentino R, Miro A, Quaglia F, Brocca P, d'Angelo I, Merkel OM, Ungaro F (2022) Hybrid lipid/polymer nanoparticles to tackle the cystic fibrosis mucus barrier in siRNA delivery to the lungs: does PEGylation make the difference? ACS Appl Mater Interfaces 14:7565–7578. https://doi.org/10.1021/acsami.1c14975

Deacon J, Abdelghany SM, Quinn DJ, Schmid D, Megaw J, Donnelly RF, Jones DS, Kissenpfennig A, Elborn JS, Gilmore BF, Taggart CC, Scott CJ (2015) Antimicrobial efficacy of tobramycin polymeric nanoparticles for Pseudomonas aeruginosa infections in cystic fibrosis: formulation, characterisation and functionalisation with dornase alfa (DNase). J Control Release 198:55–61. https://doi.org/10.1016/j.jconrel.2014.11.022

EMA (2020) Arikayce liposomal epar medicine overview. https://www.ema.europa.eu/en/documents/overview/arikayce-liposomal-epar-medicine-overview_de.pdf. Accessed 14 Aug 2023

Fernandez M, Javaid F, Chudasama V (2018) Advances in targeting the folate receptor in the treatment/imaging of cancers. Chem Sci 9:790–810. https://doi.org/10.1039/c7sc04004k

Gardner AI, Haq IJ, Simpson AJ, Becker KA, Gallagher J, Saint-Criq V, Verdon B, Mavin E, Trigg A, Gray MA, Koulman A, McDonnell MJ, Fisher AJ, Kramer EL, Clancy JP, Ward C, Schuchman EH, Gulbins E, Brodlie M (2020) Recombinant acid ceramidase reduces inflammation and infection in cystic fibrosis. Am J Respir Crit Care Med 202:1133–1145. https://doi.org/10.1164/rccm.202001-0180OC

Geiser M (2010) Update on macrophage clearance of inhaled micro- and nanoparticles. J Aerosol Med Pulm Drug Deliv 23:207–217. https://doi.org/10.1089/jamp.2009.0797

Goerke J (1998) Pulmonary surfactant: functions and molecular composition. Biochim Biophys Acta 1408:79–89. https://doi.org/10.1016/S0925-4439(98)00060-X

Guo Y, Ma Y, Chen X, Li M, Ma X, Cheng G, Xue C, Zuo YY, Sun B (2023) Mucus penetration of surface-engineered nanoparticles in various pH microenvironments. ACS Nano. https://doi.org/10.1021/acsnano.2c11147

Hermanson GT (1996) Bioconjugates techniques. 1 edn. Academic Press

Ibarra-Sanchez LA, Gamez-Mendez A, Martinez-Ruiz M, Najera-Martinez EF, Morales-Flores BA, Melchor-Martinez EM, Sosa-Hernandez JE, Parra-Saldivar R, Iqbal HMN (2022) Nanostructures for drug delivery in respiratory diseases therapeutics: revision of current trends and its comparative analysis. J Drug Deliv Sci Technol 70:103219. https://doi.org/10.1016/j.jddst.2022.103219

Idris A, Davis A, Supramaniam A, Acharya D, Kelly G, Tayyar Y, West N, Zhang P, McMillan CLD, Soemardy C, Ray R, O'Meally D, Scott TA, McMillan NAJ, Morris KV (2021) A SARS-CoV-2 targeted siRNA-nanoparticle therapy for COVID-19. Mol Ther 29:2219–2226. https://doi.org/10.1016/j.ymthe.2021.05.004

Kandil R, Baldassi D, Bohlen S, Muller JT, Keul DC, Bargmann T, Dehmel S, Xie Y, Mehta A, Sewald K, Merkel OM (2023) Targeted GATA3 knockdown in activated T cells via pulmonary siRNA delivery as novel therapy for allergic asthma. J Control Release. https://doi.org/10.1016/j.jconrel.2023.01.014

Keil TWM, Baldassi D, Merkel OM (2020) T-cell targeted pulmonary siRNA delivery for the treatment of asthma. Wiley Interdiscip Rev Nanomed Nanobiotechnol 12:e1634. https://doi.org/10.1002/wnan.1634

Keil TW, Zimmermann C, Baldassi D, Adams F, Friess W, Mehta A, Merkel OM (2021) Impact of crystalline and amorphous matrices on successful spray drying of siRNA polyplexes for inhalation of nano-in-microparticles. Adv Ther (Weinh) 4. https://doi.org/10.1002/adtp.202100073

Klein DM, Poortinga A, Verhoeven FM, Bonn D, Bonnet S, van Rijn CJM (2021) Degradation of lipid based drug delivery formulations during nebulization. Chem Phys:547. https://doi.org/10.1016/j.chemphys.2021.111192

Krug N, Hohlfeld JM, Kirsten AM, Kornmann O, Beeh KM, Kappeler D, Korn S, Ignatenko S, Timmer W, Rogon C, Zeitvogel J, Zhang N, Bille J, Homburg U, Turowska A, Bachert C, Werfel T, Buhl R, Renz J, Garn H, Renz H (2015) Allergen-induced asthmatic responses modified by a GATA3-specific DNAzyme. N Engl J Med 372:1987–1995. https://doi.org/10.1056/NEJMoa1411776

Lin C, Zhang X, Chen H, Bian Z, Zhang G, Riaz MK, Tyagi D, Lin G, Zhang Y, Wang J, Lu A, Yang Z (2018) Dual-ligand modified liposomes provide effective local targeted delivery of lung-cancer drug by antibody and tumor lineage-homing cell-penetrating peptide. Drug Deliv 25:256–266. https://doi.org/10.1080/10717544.2018.1425777

Longest W, Spence B, Hindle M (2019) Devices for improved delivery of nebulized pharmaceutical aerosols to the lungs. J Aerosol Med Pulm Drug Deliv 32:317–339. https://doi.org/10.1089/jamp.2018.1508

Lu L, Duong VT, Shalash AO, Skwarczynski M, Toth I (2021) Chemical conjugation strategies for the development of protein-based subunit nanovaccines. Vaccines (Basel) 9. https://doi.org/10.3390/vaccines9060563

Makadia HK, Siegel SJ (2011) Poly lactic-co-glycolic acid (PLGA) as biodegradable controlled drug delivery carrier. Polymers (Basel) 3:1377–1397. https://doi.org/10.3390/polym3031377

Mandal D, Mohammed EHM, Lohan S, Mandipoor P, Baradaran D, Tiwari RK, Parang K, Aliabadi HM (2022) Redox-responsive disulfide cyclic peptides: a new strategy for siRNA delivery. Mol Pharm 19:1338–1355. https://doi.org/10.1021/acs.molpharmaceut.1c00879

Mattila JM, Vuorinen T, Heikkinen T (2020) Comparative severity of influenza a and B infections in hospitalized children. Pediatr Infect Dis J 39:489–493. https://doi.org/10.1097/INF.0000000000002610

Mayor A, Thibert B, Huille S, Respaud R, Audat H, Heuze-Vourc'h N (2021) Inhaled antibodies: formulations require specific development to overcome instability due to nebulization. Drug Deliv Transl Res 11:1625–1633. https://doi.org/10.1007/s13346-021-00967-w

Munir M, Jena L, Kett VL, Dunne NJ, McCarthy HO (2022a) Spray drying: inhalable powders for pulmonary gene therapy. Biomater Adv 133:112601. https://doi.org/10.1016/j.msec.2021.112601

Munir M, Kett VL, Dunne NJ, McCarthy HO (2022b) Development of a spray-dried formulation of peptide-DNA nanoparticles into a dry powder for pulmonary delivery using factorial design. Pharm Res 39:1215–1232. https://doi.org/10.1007/s11095-022-03256-4

Nakamura YGO, Olivenstein R, Taha RA, Soussi-Gounni A, Zhang D-H, Ray A, Hamid Q (1999) Gene expression of the GATA-3 transcription factor is increased in atopic asthma. J Allergy Clin Immunol 103:215–222. https://doi.org/10.1016/s0091-6749(99)70493-8

Parra E, Perez-Gil J (2015) Composition, structure and mechanical properties define performance of pulmonary surfactant membranes and films. Chem Phys Lipids 185:153–175. https://doi.org/10.1016/j.chemphyslip.2014.09.002

Parray HA, Shukla S, Perween R, Khatri R, Shrivastava T, Singh V, Murugavelu P, Ahmed S, Samal S, Sharma C, Sinha S, Luthra K, Kumar R (2021) Inhalation monoclonal antibody therapy: a new way to treat and manage respiratory infections. Appl Microbiol Biotechnol 105:6315–6332. https://doi.org/10.1007/s00253-021-11488-4

Pastorek J, Pastorekova S (2015) Hypoxia-induced carbonic anhydrase IX as a target for cancer therapy: from biology to clinical use. Semin Cancer Biol 31:52–64. https://doi.org/10.1016/j.semcancer.2014.08.002

Pinto JT, Faulhammer E, Dieplinger J, Dekner M, Makert C, Nieder M, Paudel A (2021) Progress in spray-drying of protein pharmaceuticals: literature analysis of trends in formulation and process attributes. Drying Technol 39:1415–1446. https://doi.org/10.1080/07373937.2021.1903032

Schäfer-Korting M (2023) Looking to the future – drug delivery and targeting in the prophylaxis and therapy of severe and chronic diseases, Handbook of experimental pharmacology, vol x. Springer Nature

Sel S, Wegmann M, Dicke T, Sel S, Henke W, Yildirim AO, Renz H, Garn H (2008) Effective prevention and therapy of experimental allergic asthma using a GATA-3-specific DNAzyme. J Allergy Clin Immunol 121:910–916 e5. https://doi.org/10.1016/j.jaci.2007.12.1175

Shukla SD, Swaroop Vanka K, Chavelier A, Shastri MD, Tambuwala MM, Bakshi HA, Pabreja K, Mahmood MQ, O'Toole RF (2020) Chronic respiratory diseases: an introduction and need for novel drug delivery approaches. Targeting chronic inflammatory lung diseases using advanced drug delivery systems, pp 1–31

Synowiec A, Szczepański A, Barreto-Duran E, Lie LK, Pyrc K (2021) Severe acute respiratory syndrome coronavirus 2 (SARS-CoV-2): a systemic infection. Clin Microbiol Rev 34:e00133–e00120. https://doi.org/10.1128/CMR.00133-20

Teichgraber V, Ulrich M, Endlich N, Riethmuller J, Wilker B, De Oliveira-Munding CC, van Heeckeren AM, Barr ML, von Kurthy G, Schmid KW, Weller M, Tummler B, Lang F, Grassme H, Doring G, Gulbins E (2008) Ceramide accumulation mediates inflammation, cell death and infection susceptibility in cystic fibrosis. Nat Med 14:382–391. https://doi.org/10.1038/nm1748

Thompson JE (2018) Airborne particulate matter: human exposure and health effects. J Occup Environ Med 60:392–423. https://doi.org/10.1097/JOM.0000000000001277

van Rijn CJM, Vlaming KE, Bem RA, Dekker RJ, Poortinga A, Breit T, van Leeuwen S, Ensink WA, van Wijnbergen K, van Hamme JL, Bonn D, Geijtenbeek TBH (2023) Low energy nebulization preserves integrity of SARS-CoV-2 mRNA vaccines for respiratory delivery. Sci Rep 13:8851. https://doi.org/10.1038/s41598-023-35872-4

Wang W, Huang Z, Huang Y, Zhang X, Huang J, Cui Y, Yue X, Ma C, Fu F, Wang W, Wu C, Pan X (2022) Pulmonary delivery nanomedicines towards circumventing physiological barriers: strategies and characterization approaches. Adv Drug Deliv Rev 185:114309. https://doi.org/10.1016/j.addr.2022.114309

WHO (n.d.-a) Global summary estimates. https://www.who.int/data/gho/data/themes/mortality-and-global-health-estimates/ghe-leading-causes-of-death. Accessed 11 Feb 2023

WHO (n.d.-b) WHO Coronavirus (COVID-19) Dashboard. https://covid19.who.int/. Accessed 05 Dec 2023

WHO (n.d.-c) Asthma. https://www.who.int/news-room/fact-sheets/detail/asthma. Accessed 17 Feb 2023

WHO (n.d.-d) Infectious diseases. https://www.who.int/teams/integrated-health-services/clinical-services-and-systems/surgical-care/infectious-diseases. Accessed 17 Feb 2023

WHO (n.d.-e) Influenza seasonal. https://www.who.int/health-topics/influenza-seasonal#tab=tab_1. Accessed 17 Feb 2023

Winkeljann B, Keul DC, Merkel OM (2022) Engineering poly- and micelleplexes for nucleic acid delivery – a reflection on their endosomal escape. J Control Release. https://doi.org/10.1016/j.jconrel.2022.12.008

Wüstneck R, Wüstneck N, Grigoriev DO, Pison U, Miller R (1999) Stress relaxation behaviour of dipalmitoyl phosphatidylcholine monolayers spread on the surface of a pendant drop. Colloids Surf B Biointerfaces 15:275–288. https://doi.org/10.1016/S0927-7765(99)00094-6

Xu Y, Harinck L, Lokras AG, Gerde P, Selg E, Sjoberg CO, Franzyk H, Thakur A, Foged C (2022a) Leucine improves the aerosol performance of dry powder inhaler formulations of siRNA-loaded nanoparticles. Int J Pharm 621:121758. https://doi.org/10.1016/j.ijpharm.2022.121758

Xu Y, Parra-Ortiz E, Wan F, Canadas O, Garcia-Alvarez B, Thakur A, Franzyk H, Perez-Gil J, Malmsten M, Foged C (2022b) Insights into the mechanisms of interaction between inhalable lipid-polymer hybrid nanoparticles and pulmonary surfactant. J Colloid Interface Sci 633:511–525. https://doi.org/10.1016/j.jcis.2022.11.059

Yuan ZQ, Li JZ, Liu Y, Chen WL, Yang SD, Zhang CG, Zhu WJ, Zhou XF, Liu C, Zhang XN (2015) Systemic delivery of micelles loading with paclitaxel using N-succinyl-palmitoyl-chitosan decorated with cRGDyK peptide to inhibit non-small-cell lung cancer. Int J Pharm 492:141–151. https://doi.org/10.1016/j.ijpharm.2015.07.022

Zhang M, Jiang H, Wu L, Lu H, Bera H, Zhao X, Guo X, Liu X, Cun D, Yang M (2022) Airway epithelial cell-specific delivery of lipid nanoparticles loading siRNA for asthma treatment. J Control Release 352:422–437. https://doi.org/10.1016/j.jconrel.2022.10.020

Zhao D, Li D, Cheng X, Zou Z, Chen X, He C (2022) Mucoadhesive, antibacterial, and reductive nanogels as a mucolytic agent for efficient nebulized therapy to combat allergic asthma. ACS Nano. https://doi.org/10.1021/acsnano.2c03993

Zhu X, Kong Y, Liu Q, Lu Y, Xing H, Lu X, Yang Y, Xu J, Li N, Zhao D, Chen X, Lu Y (2019) Inhalable dry powder prepared from folic acid-conjugated docetaxel liposomes alters pharmacodynamic and pharmacokinetic properties relevant to lung cancer chemotherapy. Pulm Pharmacol Ther 55:50–61. https://doi.org/10.1016/j.pupt.2019.02.001

Zou P, Stern ST, Sun D (2014) PLGA/liposome hybrid nanoparticles for short-chain ceramide delivery. Pharm Res 31:684–693. https://doi.org/10.1007/s11095-013-1190-5

RNA Delivery to Mitochondria

Yuma Yamada and Hideyoshi Harashima

Contents

Abstract

The approval of mRNA-containing lipid nanoparticles (LNPs) for use in a vaccine against the severe acute respiratory syndrome coronavirus 2 (SARS-CoV-2) and the clinical utility of RNA-loaded nanocapsules has stimulated a rapid acceleration in research in this area. The development of mRNA-containing LNP vaccines has been rapid, not only because of regulatory adjustments, but also to the advances made in nucleic acid delivery as the result of efforts by many basic researchers. RNA functions, not only in the nucleus and cytoplasm, but also in mitochondria, which have their own genomic apparatus. Mitochondrial diseases caused by mutations or defects in the mitochondrial genome, mitochondrial DNA (mtDNA) are intractable and are mainly treated symptomatically, but gene therapy as a fundamental treatment is expected to soon be a reality. To

Y. Yamada (✉)
Faculty of Pharmaceutical Sciences, Hokkaido University, Sapporo, Japan

Japan Science and Technology Agency (JST) Fusion Oriented Research for Disruptive Science and Technology (FOREST) Program, Kawaguchi, Japan
e-mail: u-ma@pharm.hokudai.ac.jp

H. Harashima
Faculty of Pharmaceutical Sciences, Hokkaido University, Sapporo, Japan

M. Schäfer-Korting, U. S. Schubert (eds.), *Drug Delivery and Targeting*,
Handbook of Experimental Pharmacology 284, https://doi.org/10.1007/164_2023_650

realize this therapy, a drug delivery system (DDS) that delivers nucleic acids including RNA to mitochondria is required, but efforts in this area have been limited compared to research targeting the nucleus and cytoplasm. This contribution provides an overview of mitochondria-targeted gene therapy strategies and discusses studies that have attempted to validate mitochondria-targeted RNA delivery therapies. We also present the results of 'RNA delivery to mitochondria' based on the use of our mitochondria-targeted DDS (MITO-Porter) that was developed in our laboratory.

Keywords

Gene therapy · Mitochondria · Mitochondrial drug delivery · MITO-Porter · RNA delivery · RNA knockdown

Abbreviations

DDS	Drug delivery system
LHON	Leber hereditary optic neuropathy
LNPs	Lipid nanoparticles
MELAS	Mitochondrial myopathy, encephalopathy, lactic acidosis and stroke-like episodes
MERRF	Mitochondria of myoclonus epilepsy associated with ragged-red fibres
mtDNA	Mitochondrial DNA
MTS	Mitochondrial targeting signal
ND	NADH dehydrogenase
RIC	*RNA* import *complex*
SARS-CoV-2	Severe acute respiratory syndrome coronavirus 2

1 Mitochondria-Targeted RNA Delivery Therapeutic Strategies

An increase in the ratio of mutant mtDNA leads to an increase in dysfunctional mitochondria within the cell, making it difficult to maintain cellular function and disease development. There are currently two main therapeutic strategies at the gene level: introducing therapeutic genes to increase the number of normal mtDNAs, or using functional molecules to inhibit replication, repair or degrade mutant mtDNAs, thus reducing the number of mutant mtDNAs (Yamada et al. 2020e). Given the fact that there has been a recent trend towards using RNA as a therapeutic molecule in gene therapy targeting the nucleus and cytoplasm, delivering RNA to mitochondria will also likely play an important role in mitochondria-targeted gene therapy in the future.

Mitochondrial gene therapy strategies that use RNA as a therapeutic nucleic acid are expected to supplement the mitochondria of defect cells with mRNA, tRNA and

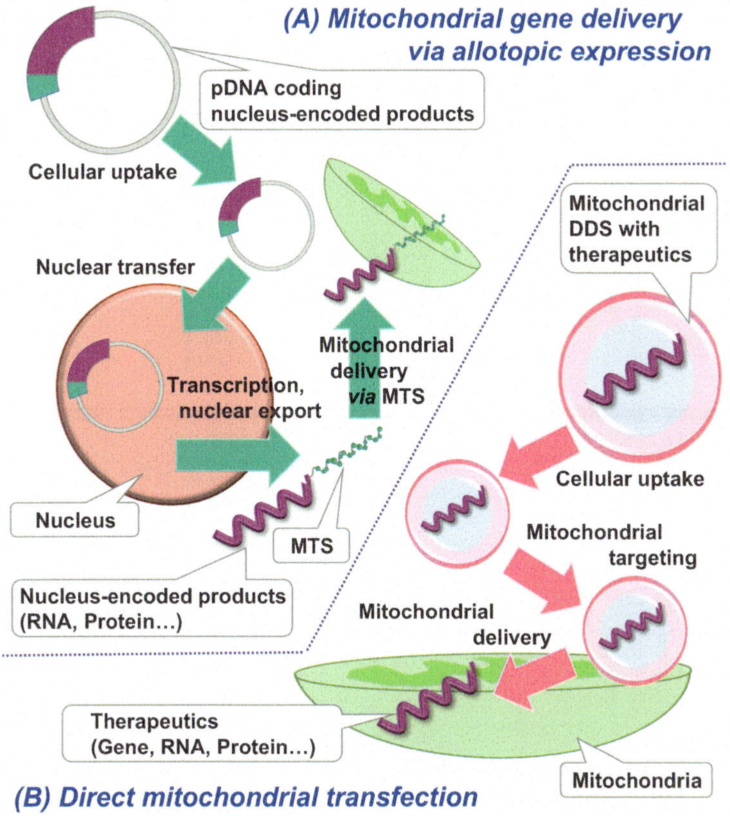

Fig. 1 Two strategies for the delivery of therapeutics to mitochondria. (**a**) Mitochondrial delivery via allotopic expression, (**b**) direct mitochondrial transfection. This figure is used with permission from Taylor & Francis (Yamada et al. 2022c)

rRNA encoded by mtDNA. Supplementation therapy, delivering normal mitochondrial RNA could be an effective strategy for treating mitochondrial diseases that are induced by mtDNA mutations or deletions. Methods for delivering RNA to mitochondria include delivering pDNA to the nucleus and using allotopic expression from the nucleus to deliver RNA to mitochondria (mitochondrial gene delivery via allotopic expression), direct mitochondrial transfection, a strategy that delivers RNA directly to the mitochondria of target cells, has been reported. In the case of allotopic expression, pDNA encoding a therapeutic RNA (or protein) containing a mitochondrial targeting signal (MTS) is delivered to the nucleus and, via transcription (or translation), the MTS-fusion therapeutic molecule is delivered to the mitochondria (Yamada et al. 2022c). Details of each strategy are summarized in Fig. 1. Table 1 summarizes research progress related to the validation of mitochondria-targeted RNA delivery therapies for these strategies.

Table 1 Strategies for delivering RNA to mitochondria for mitochondrial gene therapy

Category	Device	Cargoes to mitochondria	To cytosol	To mitochondria	Target cells (Model diseases)	Outcome	References
Allotopic expression using pDNA vector	pDNA coding nuclear encoded RNA	Wild-type mitochondrial tRNA	Lipofection for pDNA/tRNA with Lipofectamine2000	Mitochondrial tRNA import machinery	MELAS syndrome with a $tRNA^{Leu}$ (A3243G)/ MELAS cybrid cells	Improvement of mitochondrial translation, increased levels of mitochondrial DNA-encoded respiratory complexes subunits and rescue of respiration	(Karicheva et al. 2011)
		mRNA (ND1)/mRNA (ND4)	Lipofection for pDNA with FuGENE 6	Mitochondrial delivery via MTS (cis-acting elements of the COX10 gene)	LHON fibroblasts with mutant ND1 (G3460A)/ ND4 (G11778A)	Restoration of complex I activity	(Bonnet et al. 2008)
Direct mitochondrial transfection	RNA signal tag and RIC1	Therapeutic tRNA	Complexed RNA particle with RIC1 (caveola-medicated pathway)	Mitochondrial tRNA import machinery	MERRF with a $tRNA^{Lys}$ (A8344G)/ MERRF cybrid cells	Restoration of mitochondrial function	(Mahata et al. 2006)
	MITO-Porter (vesicles for mitochondrial delivery)	$tRNA^{Phe}$ mRNA (ND3) 12S rRNA	Macropinocytosis, endosomal escape via membrane fusion	Mitochondrial membrane fusion	G625A fibroblasts with mutant $tRNA^{Phe}$ (G625A)	Rate of mutated RNA reduced and the mitochondrial respiratory activity increased	(Kawamura et al. 2020; Yamada et al. 2020f;

					Leigh syndrome with mutant ND3 (T10158C) A mitochondrial disease's cell with mutant a 12S rRNA (A1555G)		Yamada et al. 2020b)

In recent years, numerous reports have shown that cytoplasmic RNA is transported through mitochondrial membrane carriers into mitochondria (Tarassov et al. 2007; Endo et al. 2010). Therapy using this mechanism has been attempted, with allotopic expression from the nucleus successfully supplementing mitochondria with normal-type tRNA in mutant cells and in maintaining the mitochondrial translation machinery (Kolesnikova et al. 2000; Kolesnikova et al. 2004). Karicheva et al. reported on the design of a $tRNA^{Leu}$ derivative corresponding to the A3243G mutation in mtDNA, a major cause of mitochondrial myopathy, encephalopathy, lactic acidosis and stroke-like episodes (MELAS), and introduced a pDNA encoding a therapeutic RNA into MELAS cells by lipofection (Karicheva et al. 2011). Bonnet et al. reported that skin fibroblasts from two Leber hereditary optic neuropathy (LHON) patients with different point mutations encoding the NADH dehydrogenase (ND)1 and ND4 regions within mtDNA were transfected with a pCMV-Tag 4A vector which is designed to transcribe ND1/ND4 mRNA. They reported that introducing normal mRNA into mitochondria by allotopic expression resulted in the mitochondrial respiratory chain (Complex I activity), which was defective in patient cells, to be restored (Bonnet et al. 2008).

2 Validation of Mitochondrial RNA Therapeutic Strategies by Direct Mitochondrial Transfection

2.1 Mitochondrial Delivery via Direct Mitochondrial Transfection

Methods for mitochondria-targeted drug delivery mainly include the use of MTS, liposomes and transport proteins. Direct mitochondrial transfection for RNA delivery to mitochondria includes the use of RNA transport complexes isolated from Leishmania tropica (RNA import complex (RIC) 1). While problems have arisen regarding the use of tRNAs such as the low efficiency of mitochondrial delivery and toxicity of the transporter, Adhya et al. reported on the efficient delivery of $tRNA^{Lys}$ using RIC 1 (Mahata et al. 2006). Using this technique, tRNA was transported by the transport protein RIC 1 into the mitochondria of myoclonus epilepsy associated with ragged-red fibres (MERRF) patient cells and this increased the respiratory activity of mitochondrial mutations in the disease cells (Mahata et al. 2006).

The MITO-Porter system is another example of therapeutic RNA delivery using liposome-based mitochondrial DDS. Focusing on the fact that mitochondria actively fuse and undergo fission within cells and share biomolecules with each other, we developed a mitochondrial targeting nano device, a MITO-Porter, which is mitochondrial fusogenic liposome (Yamada et al. 2008, 2019, 2020e; Hibino et al. 2019). In this strategy, the physical properties and size of the cargoes are not restricted because the enclosed cargoes are delivered directly to the mitochondria via membrane fusion (Fig. 2a). The lipid composition of the MITO-Porter differs from that of the LNPs used in mRNA vaccines. Therapeutic targets of nanomedicines based on a MITO-Porter include mitochondrial gene therapy (Kawamura et al. 2020; Yamada et al. 2020b, d, f), cancer therapy (Satrialdi et al. 2020; Yamada et al. 2020c, 2022d;

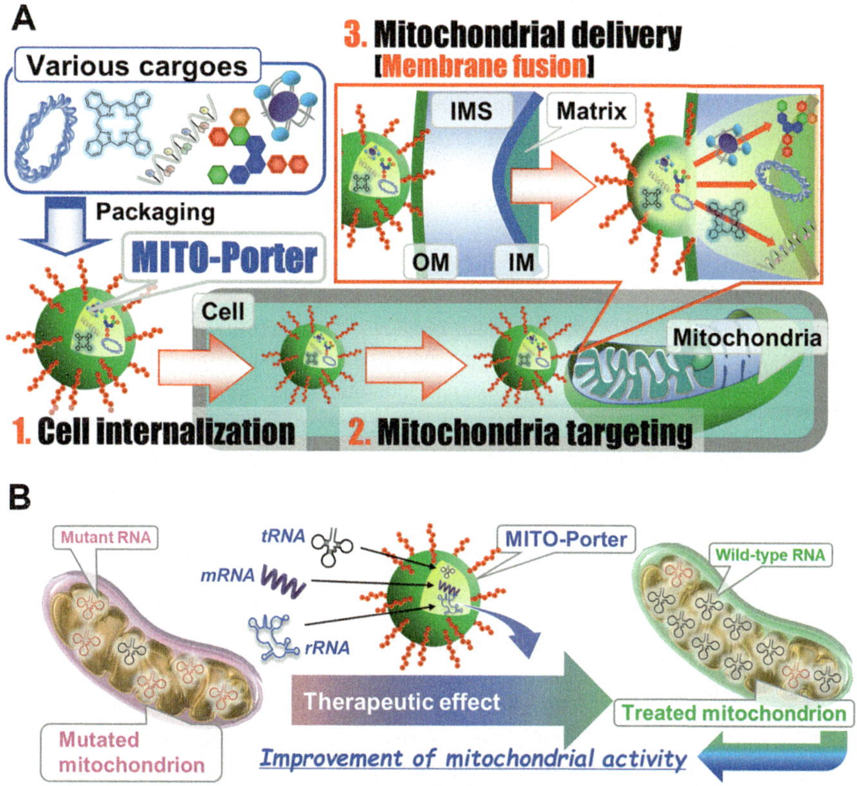

Fig. 2 Summary of direct mitochondrial transfection using the MITO-Porter system. (**a**) Schematic image of mitochondrial delivery using the MITO-Porter system. This figure is used with permission from Elsevier (Yamada et al. 2020d). (**b**) Schematic image of mitochondrial RNA therapy targeting mutated mitochondria is shown. Mitochondrial transfection of RNA in defect cells is achieved via a MITO-Porter system in order to decrease the ratio of mutated RNA in mitochondria, resulting in improved mitochondrial activity. This figure is reproduced with permission from Elsevier (Yamada et al. 2020d)

Satrialdi et al. 2021; Kubota et al. 2022), ischemic diseases therapy (Yamada et al. 2020g, 2022a, b) and cell therapy (Sasaki et al. 2022; Yamada et al. 2020a). Here, we summarize our efforts regarding mitochondrial RNA delivery including mitochondrial RNA knockdown and therapeutic mitochondrial RNA delivery.

2.2 Mitochondrial Therapeutic RNA Delivery Using MITO-Porter System

In this section, we summarize our efforts to develop mitochondria RNA therapy by the direct mitochondrial transfection of therapeutic RNA using the MITO-Porter system (Fig. 2b). In our initial validation, we used cells from a patient with a mitochondrial disease (G625A cells), which have a G625A point mutation in the $tRNA^{Phe}$ region of the mtDNA. In order to reduce the ratio of mutant $tRNA^{Phe}$ in mitochondria, we examined the possibility of delivering wild-type mitochondrial pre-$tRNA^{Phe}$ (pre-WT-$tRNA^{Phe}$) to mitochondria using the MITO-Porter system. The results showed that the mutation rate of $tRNA^{Phe}$ was decreased after the mitochondrial transfection of pre-WT-$tRNA^{Phe}$. In addition, when mitochondrial function was evaluated in relation to the reduction in the mutation rate of $tRNA^{Phe}$, the mitochondrial respiratory activity of the disease cells was increased after the transfection of therapeutic pre-WT-$tRNA^{Phe}$ (Kawamura et al. 2020).

As the next challenge, we used this system to deliver therapeutic mRNA into mitochondria in LS^{ND3} cells, dermal fibroblasts from a patient with Leigh's encephalopathy. This subject carries a large amount of mtDNA with a T10158C point mutation located in the ND3 gene, which constitutes the mitochondrial respiratory chain complex I. After a series of studies, we successfully delivered therapeutic mRNA (ND3) into the mitochondria of LS^{ND3} cells, thus reducing the mutation rate of mRNA (ND3) to 10%. We also observed an increase in the rate of mitochondrial oxygen consumption (mitochondrial function) as the mutation rate of mRNA (ND3) decreased (Yamada et al. 2020f).

A1555G mutant cells derived from a patient with mitochondria-associated hearing loss were used for the validation of a mitochondrial rRNA therapeutic strategy using the MITO-Porter system. A1555G in mtDNA coding rRNA (12S) causes a mutation that results in the loss of hearing (del Castillo et al. 2003; el-Schahawi et al. 1997; Zhu et al. 2014). Through various investigations, we succeeded in preparing an rRNA-MITO-Porter encapsulating wild-type rRNA (12S) for use as a therapeutic RNA. The rRNA-MITO-Porter was added to A1555G mutant cells and the mutation rate of rRNA (12S) was then quantified. The results showed that a significant reduction in the mutation rate was observed. We also observed that the rRNA-MITO-Porter treatment resulted in an increase in mitochondrial respiratory capacity (Yamada et al. 2020b).

In a series of studies, it was shown that the MITO-Porter strategy is useful for the delivery of all three types of RNA encoded by mtDNA: tRNA, mRNA and rRNA. All mtDNA mutations could, in theory, be treated using this approach, suggesting that the MITO-Porter provides a potentially useful innovative therapeutic method for the treatment of mitochondrial diseases.

3 Conclusions

In this contribution, we focused on our research concerning the delivery of RNA to mitochondria with regard to mitochondria-targeted gene therapy research. We also summarize our efforts regarding the validation of mitochondria-targeted RNA therapy based on the MITO-Porter that was developed in our laboratory. Mitochondria-targeted gene therapy has the potential to open up the next generation of therapies. As such, it has the potential to serve as a major weapon against urgent and unknown diseases such as SARS-CoV-2. Our hope is that this contribution will draw attention to this research area, stimulate advances in this research field and provide support for the development of mitochondria-targeted nucleic acid medicines. Our hope is that this will be one of the weapons for use in protecting humankind from future, currently unknown threats.

Acknowledgements This work was supported, in part, by a Grant-in-Aid for Scientific Research (B) (Grant No. 20H04523 to Y.Y.) from the Ministry of Education, Culture, Sports, Science and Technology, the Japanese Government (MEXT), Fusion Oriented Research for disruptive Science and Technology (FOREST) Program (Grant No. JPMJFR203X to Y.Y.) from Japan Science and Technology Agency (JST). We also wish to thank Dr. Milton Feather for his helpful advice in writing the manuscript.

References

Bonnet C, Augustin S, Ellouze S, Benit P, Bouaita A, Rustin P, Sahel JA, Corral-Debrinski M (2008) The optimized allotopic expression of ND1 or ND4 genes restores respiratory chain complex I activity in fibroblasts harboring mutations in these genes. Biochim Biophys Acta 1783(10):1707–1717. https://doi.org/10.1016/j.bbamcr.2008.04.018

del Castillo FJ, Rodriguez-Ballesteros M, Martin Y, Arellano B, Gallo-Teran J, Morales-Angulo C, Ramirez-Camacho R, Cruz Tapia M, Solanellas J, Martinez-Conde A, Villamar M, Moreno-Pelayo MA, Moreno F, del Castillo I (2003) Heteroplasmy for the 1555A>G mutation in the mitochondrial 12S rRNA gene in six Spanish families with non-syndromic hearing loss. J Med Genet 40(8):632–636. https://doi.org/10.1136/jmg.40.8.632

el-Schahawi M, Lopez de Munain A, Sarrazin AM, Shanske AL, Basirico M, Shanske S, DiMauro S (1997) Two large Spanish pedigrees with nonsyndromic sensorineural deafness and the mtDNA mutation at nt 1555 in the 12s rRNA gene: evidence of heteroplasmy. Neurology 48(2):453–456. https://doi.org/10.1212/wnl.48.2.453

Endo T, Yamano K, Yoshihisa T (2010) Mitochondrial matrix reloaded with RNA. Cell 142(3): 362–363. https://doi.org/10.1016/j.cell.2010.07.024

Hibino M, Yamada Y, Fujishita N, Sato Y, Maeki M, Tokeshi M, Harashima H (2019) The use of a microfluidic device to encapsulate a poorly water-soluble drug CoQ10 in lipid nanoparticles and an attempt to regulate intracellular trafficking to reach mitochondria. J Pharm Sci. https://doi.org/10.1016/j.xphs.2019.04.001

Karicheva OZ, Kolesnikova OA, Schirtz T, Vysokikh MY, Mager-Heckel AM, Lombes A, Boucheham A, Krasheninnikov IA, Martin RP, Entelis N, Tarassov I (2011) Correction of the consequences of mitochondrial 3243A>G mutation in the MT-TL1 gene causing the MELAS syndrome by tRNA import into mitochondria. Nucleic Acids Res 39(18):8173–8186. https://doi.org/10.1093/nar/gkr546

Kawamura E, Maruyama M, Abe J, Sudo A, Takeda A, Takada S, Yokota T, Kinugawa S, Harashima H, Yamada Y (2020) Validation of gene therapy for mutant mitochondria by delivering mitochondrial RNA using a MITO-Porter. Mol Ther-Nucl Acids 20:687–698. https://doi.org/10.1016/j.omtn.2020.04.004

Kolesnikova OA, Entelis NS, Mireau H, Fox TD, Martin RP, Tarassov IA (2000) Suppression of mutations in mitochondrial DNA by tRNAs imported from the cytoplasm. Science 289(5486): 1931–1933

Kolesnikova OA, Entelis NS, Jacquin-Becker C, Goltzene F, Chrzanowska-Lightowlers ZM, Lightowlers RN, Martin RP, Tarassov I (2004) Nuclear DNA-encoded tRNAs targeted into mitochondria can rescue a mitochondrial DNA mutation associated with the MERRF syndrome in cultured human cells. Hum Mol Genet 13(20):2519–2534. https://doi.org/10.1093/hmg/ddh267

Kubota F, Satrialdi TY, Maeki M, Tokeshi M, Harashima H, Yamada Y (2022) Fine-tuning the encapsulation of a photosensitizer in nanoparticles reveals the relationship between internal structure and phototherapeutic effects. J Biophotonics:e202200119. https://doi.org/10.1002/jbio.202200119

Mahata B, Mukherjee S, Mishra S, Bandyopadhyay A, Adhya S (2006) Functional delivery of a cytosolic tRNA into mutant mitochondria of human cells. Science 314(5798):471–474. https://doi.org/10.1126/science.1129754

Sasaki D, Abe J, Takeda A, Harashima H, Yamada Y (2022) Transplantation of MITO cells, mitochondria activated cardiac progenitor cells, to the ischemic myocardium of mouse enhances the therapeutic effect. Sci Rep 12(1):4344. https://doi.org/10.1038/s41598-022-08583-5

Satrialdi MR, Biju V, Takano Y, Harashima H, Yamada Y (2020) The optimization of cancer photodynamic therapy by utilization of a pi-extended porphyrin-type photosensitizer in combination with MITO-Porter. Chem Commun (Camb) 56(7):1145–1148. https://doi.org/10.1039/c9cc08563g

Satrialdi TY, Hirata E, Ushijima N, Harashima H, Yamada Y (2021) The effective in vivo mitochondrial-targeting nanocarrier combined with a π-extended porphyrin-type photosensitizer. Nanoscale Adv 3:5919–5927. https://doi.org/10.1039/D1NA00427A

Tarassov I, Kamenski P, Kolesnikova O, Karicheva O, Martin RP, Krasheninnikov IA, Entelis N (2007) Import of nuclear DNA-encoded RNAs into mitochondria and mitochondrial translation. Cell Cycle 6(20):2473–2477. https://doi.org/10.4161/cc.6.20.4783

Yamada Y, Akita H, Kamiya H, Kogure K, Yamamoto T, Shinohara Y, Yamashita K, Kobayashi H, Kikuchi H, Harashima H (2008) MITO-Porter: a liposome-based carrier system for delivery of macromolecules into mitochondria via membrane fusion. Biochim Biophys Acta 1778(2):423–432. https://doi.org/10.1016/j.bbamem.2007.11.002

Yamada Y, Daikuhara S, Tamura A, Nishida K, Yui N, Harashima H (2019) Enhanced autophagy induction via the mitochondrial delivery of methylated beta-cyclodextrin-threaded polyrotaxanes using a MITO-Porter. Chem Commun (Camb) 55(50):7203–7206. https://doi.org/10.1039/c9cc03272j

Yamada Y, Ito M, Arai M, Hibino M, Tsujioka T, Harashima H (2020a) Challenges in promoting mitochondrial transplantation therapy. Int J Mol Sci 21(17). https://doi.org/10.3390/ijms21176365

Yamada Y, Maruyama M, Kita T, Usami SI, Kitajiri SI, Harashima H (2020b) The use of a MITO-Porter to deliver exogenous therapeutic RNA to a mitochondrial disease's cell with a A1555G mutation in the mitochondrial 12S rRNA gene results in an increase in mitochondrial respiratory activity. Mitochondrion 55:134–144. https://doi.org/10.1016/j.mito.2020.09.008

Yamada Y, Munechika R, Satrialdi KF, Sato Y, Sakurai Y, Harashima H (2020c) Mitochondrial delivery of an anticancer drug via systemic administration using a mitochondrial delivery system that inhibits the growth of drug-resistant cancer engrafted on mice. J Pharm Sci. https://doi.org/10.1016/j.xphs.2020.04.020

Yamada Y, Sato Y, Nakamura T, Harashima H (2020d) Evolution of drug delivery system from viewpoint of controlled intracellular trafficking and selective tissue targeting toward future nanomedicine. J Control Release 327:533–545. https://doi.org/10.1016/j.jconrel.2020.09.007

Yamada Y, Satrialdi HM, Sasaki D, Abe J, Harashima H (2020e) Power of mitochondrial drug delivery systems to produce innovative nanomedicines. Adv Drug Deliv Rev 154-155:187–209. https://doi.org/10.1016/j.addr.2020.09.010

Yamada Y, Somiya K, Miyauchi A, Osaka H, Harashima H (2020f) Validation of a mitochondrial RNA therapeutic strategy using fibroblasts from a Leigh syndrome patient with a mutation in the mitochondrial ND3 gene. Sci Rep 10(1):7511. https://doi.org/10.1038/s41598-020-64322-8

Yamada Y, Takano Y, Satrialdi AJ, Hibino M, Harashima H (2020g) Therapeutic strategies for regulating mitochondrial oxidative stress. Biomol Ther 10(1). https://doi.org/10.3390/biom10010083

Yamada Y, Ishimaru T, Harashima H (2022a) Validation of a therapeutic strategy involving the mitochondrial delivery of thiamine pyrophosphate using brain damage induced mouse model. Clin Transl Disc 2:e43

Yamada Y, Ishimaru T, Ikeda K, Harashima H (2022b) Validation of the mitochondrial delivery of vitamin B1 to enhance ATP production using SH-SY5Y cells, a model neuroblast. J Pharm Sci 111(2):432–439. https://doi.org/10.1016/j.xphs.2021.08.033

Yamada Y, Ishizuka S, Arai M, Maruyama M, Harashima H (2022c) Recent advances in delivering RNA-based therapeutics to mitochondria. Expert Opin Biol Ther:1–11. https://doi.org/10.1080/14712598.2022.2070427

Yamada Y, Sato Y, Nakamura T, Harashima H (2022d) Innovative cancer nanomedicine based on immunology, gene editing, intracellular trafficking control. J Control Release. https://doi.org/10.1016/j.jconrel.2022.05.033

Zhu Y, Huang S, Kang D, Han M, Wang G, Yuan Y, Su Y, Yuan H, Zhai S, Dai P (2014) Analysis of the heteroplasmy level and transmitted features in hearing-loss pedigrees with mitochondrial 12S rRNA A1555G mutation. BMC Genet 15:26. https://doi.org/10.1186/1471-2156-15-26

Part IV

Concerted Actions – Thinking the Drug from the Beginning

Advanced Formulation Approaches for Emerging Therapeutic Technologies

Nour Allahham, Ines Colic, Melissa L. D. Rayner, Pratik Gurnani, James B. Phillips, Ahad A. Rahim, and Gareth R. Williams

Contents

Nour Allahham, Ines Colic, Melissa L.D. Rayner, and Pratik Gurnani contributed equally to this work.

N. Allahham · I. Colic · M. L. D. Rayner · P. Gurnani · J. B. Phillips · A. A. Rahim · G. R. Williams (✉)
UCL School of Pharmacy, University College London, London, UK
e-mail: g.williams@ucl.ac.uk

M. Schäfer-Korting, U. S. Schubert (eds.), *Drug Delivery and Targeting*, Handbook of Experimental Pharmacology 284, https://doi.org/10.1007/164_2023_695

Abstract

In addition to proteins, discussed in the Chapter "Advances in Vaccine Adjuvants: Nanomaterials and Small Molecules", there are a wide range of alternatives to small molecule active ingredients. Cells, extracellular vesicles, and nucleic acids in particular have attracted increasing research attention in recent years. There are now a number of products on the market based on these emerging technologies, the most famous of which are the mRNA-based vaccines against SARS-COV-2. These advanced therapeutic moieties are challenging to formulate however, and there remain significant challenges for their more widespread use. In this chapter, we consider the potential and bottlenecks for developing further medical products based on these systems. Cells, extracellular vesicles, and nucleic acids will be discussed in terms of their mechanism of action, the key requirements for translation, and how advanced formulation approaches can aid their future development. These points will be presented with selected examples from the literature, and with a focus on the formulations which have made the transition to clinical trials and clinical products.

Keywords

Cell therapy · Drug delivery · Extracelluar vesicle · Nucleic acid

Abbreviations

AAPC	Autologous antigen-presenting cell
AAVs	Adeno-associated viruses
ATMP	Advanced therapy medicinal product
CAR	Chimeric antigen receptor
Cas	CRISPR associated nuclease enzyme
CRISPR	Clustered regularly interspaced short palindromic repeats
CSD	Sickle cell disease
DC	Dendritic cell
DNA	Deoxyribonucleic acid
EMA	European Medicines Agency
EV	Extracellular vesicle
FDA	US Food and Drug Administration
GMP	Good manufacturing practice
HSC	Haematopoietic stem cell
LNP	Lipid nanoparticle
miRNA	Micro-ribonucleic acid

MSC	Mesenchymal stem cell
NK	Natural killer
OMV	Outer membrane vesicle
OTC	Over the counter
RES	Reticuloendothelial system
RMAT	Regenerative medicine advanced therapy
RNA	Ribonucleic acid
sCTMP	Somatic-cell therapy medicinal product
siRNA	Small interfering ribonucleic acid
TDT	Transfusion-dependent β-thalassemia

1 Introduction

Decades of research into ground-breaking biologics and Advanced Therapeutic Medicinal Products (ATMPs) has led to their establishment as powerful additions to conventional pharmaceuticals. Recent years have seen a number of these therapeutic modalities enter the market as licensed drugs providing life-saving or life-changing benefits to patients. Such modalities include: cell and gene therapies that are revolutionising regenerative medicine and offer curative solutions to inherited diseases; gene editing and mRNA and siRNA approaches to treat or prevent a broad range of conditions; and the widespread introduction of nucleic acid-based vaccines. With some notable exceptions, most of these types of treatments are classified as ATMPs by regulators. The ATMP classification includes gene therapies, cell therapies where cells or tissues have been manipulated, tissue-engineered products, and products containing combinations of these different components (Rayner and Phillips 2022). Exceptions are synthetic nucleic acid therapies, vaccines, and therapeutic cells that have been minimally manipulated or are used for their original function (Iglesias-Lopez et al. 2019). Regardless of regulatory classification, it is clear that these types of therapies that use complex new technologies present a significant challenge in terms of formulation in addition to the regulatory and logistical challenges that surround their production and testing.

Advanced formulation research is critical to the successful development and clinical translation of these new therapeutic technologies, many of which are complex and unstable compared with conventional small molecule drugs. Scalable and safe formulation approaches that are cost effective and ensure the reliable protection and delivery of living cells or nucleic acids are required. This chapter aims to capture some of the current considerations and future directions that are pertinent to this rapidly changing and highly innovative area.

2 Cell Therapies

2.1 Somatic-Cell Therapy Medicinal Products

Somatic-cell therapy medicinal products (sCTMPs) are classified as those containing cells or tissues that have been manipulated to change their biological characteristics to cure, diagnose, or prevent disease (European Medicines Agency 2023). A simple selection or enrichment of a population of cells from tissue or transplantation of cells is not considered an ATMP by the European Medicines Agency (EMA) (Buckland and Bobby Gaspar 2014). Manipulated cells can also be combined with biomaterials (combined ATMPs) or engineered tissues (tissue-engineered medicines) with the goal to repair, regenerate, or replace human tissue (EMA 2023). Cells used for such products can be the patient's own cells (autologous), human donor cells (allogeneic), or animal cells (xenogeneic) (Committee for Advanced Therapies 2010), but their intended use should not be the same as the essential function of these cells within the body (EMA 2023). Stem cells, undifferentiated cells that can differentiate into a wide range of cell types, are also characterised as ATMPs as they have capacity to undergo substantial manipulation.

Cell-based therapies are a promising therapeutic modality with major advantages over conventional drug therapies, given their capacity to perform complex biological functions which cannot be achieved with small molecules (Wang et al. 2021). Cell therapies can respond to biological cues to promote tissue regeneration, attack malignancies, restore lost or impaired functions, and support the body's own ability to fight disease (Fischbach et al. 2013). For instance, the formation of missing enzymes can be induced in recipients with inborn errors of metabolism.

2.2 Current Landscape of sCTMPs

Despite the significant amount of research on-going, there are currently only two sCTMPs approved by the EMA and eight by the US Food and Drug Administration (FDA) (Table 1). Unlike the FDA, the EMA does not consider haematopoietic progenitor cell products as an ATMP since they have not undergone substantial manipulation and are intended to be used for the same function in the recipient as the donor (Shukla et al. 2019).

The complex development and regulation associated with translating an ATMP to the market has led to some sCTMPs being withdrawn a couple of years after their initial market launch (Silva et al. 2022), and there are only a few ATMPs that have received an EU market authorisation. This is very low in comparison with other types of medicinal products.

sCTMP regulation does not fall under the standard regulations tailored for small molecules, which has increased the hurdles associated with getting these products to the clinic (Pellegrini et al. 2016). Regulatory concerns include product safety, characterisation of the cells, and the control of their manufacturing process (Cuende

Table 1 Currently approved sCTMPs listed by the EMA and FDA (accessed May 2023). Tissue-engineered medicines, combined ATMPs and CAR-T cell therapies (for example, Yescarta and Kymriah) are excluded

Regulatory body	sCTMP	Active substance	Clinical indication
EMA	Alofisel	Darvadstrocel	Complex anal fistulas in adults with Crohn's disease
	Spherox	Chondrocyte spheroids	Repair cartilage defects
FDA	Allocord Clevecord Ducord Hemacord	Haematopoietic progenitor cells (cord blood)	Blood cell transplantation Unrelated donor haematopoietic progenitor cell transplantation Allogenic transplantation to induce graft-versus-tumour cell effects through the formation of missing enzymes in recipients with inborn errors of metabolism
	Omisirge	Allogeneic stem cell	Haematologic malignancies Enhance neutrophil recovery to reduce infections following umbilical cord transplantation
	Provenge (Sipuleucel-T)	Autologous antigen-presenting cells (AAPCs)	Autologous cellular immunotherapy to stimulate a patient's own immune system against cancer
	Rethymic	Allogeneic thymus tissue	Treatment of symptoms of congenital athymia in children

and Izeta 2010). The formulation and associated challenges in the development of sCTMPs are discussed below.

2.2.1 Cell Source and Immunogenicity

Most starting cells or tissues within sCTMPs are autologous or allogeneic (Fig. 1). The benefit of autologous cells is low to no immunogenicity; however, they are cost prohibitive (Durand and Zubair 2022). In contrast, allogeneic therapies are produced by a streamlined manufacturing process (Durand and Zubair 2022; Salmikangas et al. 2015), improve efficacy and patient accessibility, shorten clinic waiting times, and reduce costs (Salmikangas et al. 2015). The disadvantage to allogeneic cells is immunogenicity, which can result in an adverse immune response to the therapy by the recipient. Extensive in vitro and in silico testing can ameliorate this risk.

Other factors that need to be considered when sourcing cells include the age and health of the donor. This is particularly important when sourcing cells from cancer patients after treatment, as there could be an introduction of tumourigenic or genetically altered cells (Salmikangas et al. 2015). Cells will respond to external signals which may alter their phenotype and functionality: for example, use of medication by the donor and/or the recipient. Detailed documentation about cell source, cell cloning, and cell banking ensures control of the quality of the cells and enables

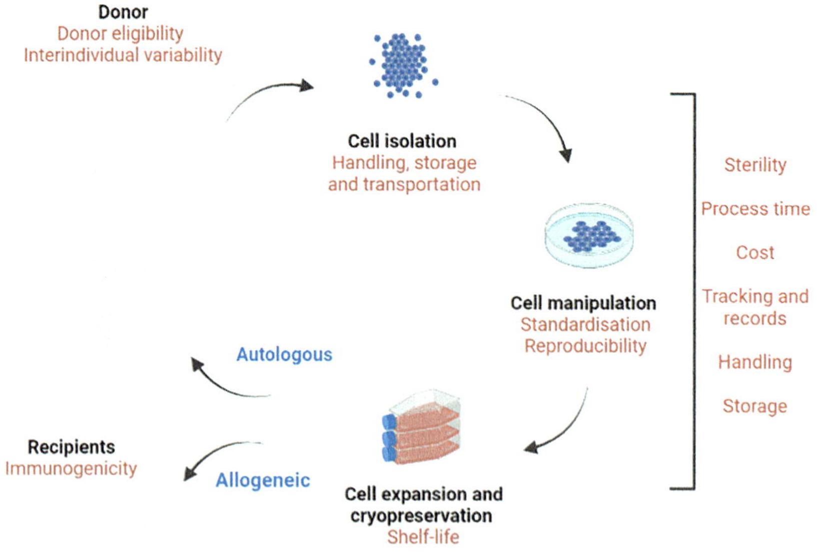

Fig. 1 Schematic of the production of autologous and allogeneic cell products and key factors to consider during the manufacturing process (highlighted in red)

traceability if any issues should arise (Salmikangas et al. 2015). Precise labelling and tracking are vital when using autologous cell therapies (Jere et al. 2021).

2.2.2 Sterility

Microbiological contamination from the starting cells or tissues can instigate major issues and a risk of infection to the recipient. Patients that are receiving an sCTMP are likely to be immunocompromised and at an elevated risk of infection, and therefore safety aspects and microbiological testing are essential (Jere et al. 2021). It can be difficult to remove impurities, as purification methods may affect cell viability or differentiation, and terminal sterilisation is impossible. Stringent efforts should be made to filter or sterilise all excipients before use, and rigorous controls need to be in place to ensure the starting material meets the required standard. This can be achieved through effective standard operating procedures and compliance to appropriate legislation (Salmikangas et al. 2015). Cell-based products needed to be tested for sterility as stated in the United States Pharmacopoeia <1046> and guidelines on Good Manufacturing Practice (GMP) specific to ATMPs (Jere et al. 2021).

2.2.3 Manufacturing

Upscaling sCTMP manufacturing is more difficult than conventional medicinal products owing to more complex manufacturing steps and the need for additional product characterisation and process validation (Rayner and Phillips 2022). Each step of the manufacturing process needs to be defined and validated (Salmikangas et al. 2015). Small changes in one part of the manufacturing process can cause a significant change in the final product (Rayner and Phillips 2022), leading to high validation costs and uncertain value of intellectual property (Morrow et al. 2017). For example, changes to cell density, the frequency of media changes, and freeze/thaw cycles can have a considerable effect on cell proliferation, differentiation, or signalling (Brindley et al. 2011). Where sCTMPs are intended for immediate use after production, more intensive product characterisation is needed as there is no possibility for batch release testing of the finished product (Salmikangas et al. 2015).

2.2.4 Formulation, Storage, and Handling

sCTMPs can be stored as cryopreserved cell suspensions to provide a longer shelf-life (cf. fresh suspensions), enabling multiple dosing. However, the sensitivity of cells to freeze/thaw cycles is a problem (Li et al. 2019) and is difficult to standardise (Aijaz et al. 2018).

When autologous cells are used, they need to be isolated from the patient requiring the treatment, modified, expanded, and quality tested before being administered back to the same patient. For instance, Spherox is an approved autologous product for cartilage regeneration. Its use involves a two-step administration process. First, a cartilage biopsy is obtained from the patient and the cells are expanded to form spheroids over 6–8 weeks. The second step involves the spheroids being delivered back to the same patient via a pre-filled syringe and spread over the affected area (EMA 2023). To ensure success of this process the handling and storage of the cells during the harvest, manufacturing, application, and delivery between sites need to be considered, ensuring there is no loss of cell function. The process is time critical and cost intensive (Jere et al. 2021). There is a need for a systematic approach to the handling and storage of cell-based formulations and any potential impact on cell viability, shelf-life, and patient safety should be studied and well characterised.

2.2.5 Potency

Ultimately the final product needs to be efficacious as well as safe when administered to the patient. Functional assays are used throughout product development not only to characterise the active substance but also to characterise and validate the manufacturing process (Salmikangas et al. 2015). Potency tests are critical for comparability testing and process and product consistency (Bravery et al. 2013). If mixed cell populations are used, potency assays need to ascertain which cells are responsible for the therapeutic effect (Salmikangas et al. 2015).

2.3 Formulating Combined Products

In combined ATMPs, it is rarely the cells alone that are responsible for the therapeutic effect, the additional components such as the biomaterials or scaffolds also being of major relevance. It is required for all the components to be characterised and tested separately and in combination, as it has become evident that bringing the different components together during the manufacturing steps can impact the final product (Salmikangas et al. 2015).

3 Extracellular Vesicles

Extracellular vesicles (EVs) are nano- to micro-sized anuclear vesicles produced by all cell types and released into the extracellular space (Yanez-Mo et al. 2015). They are found in all bodily fluids and they have been isolated from various sources including mammalian and prokaryotic cell cultures and blood plasma (Yanez-Mo et al. 2015). EVs are composed of a lipid membrane encapsulating an aqueous core that contains proteins, lipids, coding and non-coding nucleic acids, and other soluble molecules and metabolites (Yanez-Mo et al. 2015). Their composition generally reflects the state of the parent cell (Yanez-Mo et al. 2015). The most often used classification recognises three main classes of EVs based on their biogenesis – apoptotic bodies, microvesicles, and exosomes, with the latter two being most often studied and described in the literature (Yanez-Mo et al. 2015; Gyorgy et al. 2011). It is important to note EVs represent a fairly heterogeneous population of vesicles where even vesicles released from one cell differ in size, composition, origin, and function (Ferguson and Nguyen 2016; Kalluri and LeBleu 2020). EVs play an important role in cell-to-cell "communication" (information and cargo transfer) between cells, organs, and even between different organisms (Kalluri and LeBleu 2020). Moreover, they act as information mediators in many physiological and pathological processes and as such hold huge potential as diagnostic and therapeutic tools (Kalluri and LeBleu 2020; Cheng and Hill 2022).

3.1 Clinical Applications of EVs

EVs' pharmaceutical potential is reflected in an increasing number of in vivo studies and human clinical trials (Huda et al. 2021; Claridge et al. 2021).

3.1.1 EVs as Diagnostic Tools

The fact that EV composition reflects the state of the cell of origin makes them attractive as minimally invasive diagnostic tools. Taking a small sample of a specific bodily fluid would enable almost real-time monitoring of disease development and the body's response to therapy, and a number of clinical trials are exploring this potential (Huda et al. 2021). One clinically validated product is already available on the market: ExoDx™ Prostate IntelliScore (EPI-CE), a urine-based test assessing a patient's risk of high-grade prostate cancer (McKiernan et al. 2016).

3.1.2 EVs as Therapeutic Tools

In addition, EVs hold huge potential as therapeutic tools since they can interact with or be taken up by a range of target cells, triggering a wide array of effects. The use of EVs as therapeutics has been investigated for tissue regeneration and immunomodulation, as antitumor or prophylactic vaccines and as natural drug delivery vectors (Claridge et al. 2021).

Many pre-clinical studies have demonstrated that native EVs show innate therapeutic activity (Wiklander et al. 2019; Nagelkerke et al. 2021). EVs derived from stem cells (most often mesenchymal stem cells (MSCs)) are known to promote tissue repair and regeneration and their application in various pathologies ranging from cardiovascular, brain, liver, lung, and kidney diseases to wound healing and inflammation treatment is being extensively tested (Cheng and Hill 2022; Nagelkerke et al. 2021; Tsiapalis and O'Driscoll 2020). There is accumulating evidence that EVs derived from stem cells have a comparable therapeutic effect to the parent cells (Nagelkerke et al. 2021; Tsiapalis and O'Driscoll 2020). A major advantage of EV therapeutics compared to live cell therapies is their superior safety profile, since they cannot self-replicate and thus do not pose a risk of uncontrolled proliferation and tumourigenesis (Tsiapalis and O'Driscoll 2020). Moreover, the application of EVs may be less immunogenic than that of parent stem cells, particularly if the cells or EVs used come from non-autologous sources (Zhu et al. 2017; Saleh et al. 2019; Elsharkasy et al. 2020). Unlike cells, EVs can be sterilised by filtration and their transportation and storage are less complicated since biochemical activity can be preserved by storage at −80°C or lyophilisation (Tsiapalis and O'Driscoll 2020).

EVs derived from antigen-presenting cells (most often dendritic cells (DCs)) have immunostimulatory properties and are thus being studied for use as vaccines against tumours and pathogens (Cheng and Hill 2022; Huda et al. 2021; Claridge et al. 2021). EVs released by bacteria, also known as outer membrane vesicles (OMVs), and EVs isolated from pathogen-infected cells are also being tested as vaccines. Indeed, several vaccines against meningococcal serogroup B containing a combination of OMVs and meningococcal recombinant antigens have been licensed for a number of years (Cheng and Hill 2022; van der Pol et al. 2015).

Finally, EVs are being explored as natural drug delivery vectors. EVs have the capacity to encapsulate and protect bioactive cargo and transfer it to target cells even across biological barriers (such as the blood-brain barrier) (Huda et al. 2021; Claridge et al. 2021; Wiklander et al. 2019). They may exhibit inherent targeting characteristics and their surface can be engineered to further enhance target specificity (Wiklander et al. 2019). Additionally, EVs are biocompatible and have been shown to exhibit minimal toxic and immunogenic effects in numerous pre-clinical and clinical studies (Claridge et al. 2021; Zhu et al. 2017; Saleh et al. 2019). The use of EVs as delivery vectors has been explored for cargos ranging from small molecules (e.g. paclitaxel) to complex biopharmaceuticals like proteins, nucleic acids, and viruses (Wiklander et al. 2019; Kooijmans et al. 2021). Therapeutic agents are loaded into or onto EVs either by manipulating a parent cell (endogenous loading) or by manipulating already isolated EVs (exogenous loading) (Joshi et al. 2021). However, clinical translation of EV-based drug delivery vectors is still challenging owing to hurdles with large-scale production and efficient drug loading. An overview of the state of the art can be found in Huda et al. (2021) and Claridge et al. (2021).

The number of pharmaceutical companies looking into clinical application of EV products is growing. Although most of these products are still in development or in pre-clinical phases, several companies have already entered clinical trials (Huda et al. 2021). At the moment of writing there are still no FDA or EMA-approved EV products. However, several EV-based topical products are available on the market as over-the-counter (OTC) products for aesthetic, cosmetic, and dermatological applications: an overview can be found in Nagelkerke et al. (2021) and Davies et al. (2023).

3.2 Regulatory Classification of EV-Based Therapeutics

Regulatory classification of EV-based therapeutics is not straightforward due to their complexity and the intricate nature of the therapeutic effects they induce. EV-based therapeutics are generally classified as biological medicinal products (also referred to as biologicals or biopharmaceuticals), defined as medicines that contain one or more active substances made by or derived from cells (Lener et al. 2015). However, when the functional transgene (RNA or DNA) contained within EVs is responsible for their therapeutic effect, EV-based therapeutics fall under the ATMP regulations (Lener et al. 2015).

3.3 Challenges to Clinical Translation of EV-Based Therapeutics

Clinical translation of EVs remains challenging due to EVs' size and composition heterogeneity, their inherent complexity, and batch-to-batch variability. There is at present a lack of standardised procedures for their production, isolation, quality control, and storage which needs to be carefully considered (Claridge et al. 2021; Herrmann et al. 2021). An overview of the challenges and consideration in manufacturing and clinical translation of EV-based therapeutics is given in Fig. 2.

The first challenge is the selection of EV source and culturing conditions. When selecting parent (donor) cells, the characteristics of the EVs released (innate therapeutic activity and targeting capability, immunogenic, oncogenic, and toxic potential) need to be carefully considered (Claridge et al. 2021; Meng et al. 2020; Paganini et al. 2019). Also, the genetic stability and production yields of the parent cells should be taken into account (Herrmann et al. 2021; Rohde et al. 2019). Culturing conditions must be strictly defined and batch reproducibility ensured, as even small changes in culturing conditions could affect the amount, quality, and potency of the EVs (Claridge et al. 2021; Patel et al. 2017). Moreover, for successful clinical translation EV production has to be scaled up from small-scale manufacturing in flasks to large-scale commercial production (Claridge et al. 2021).

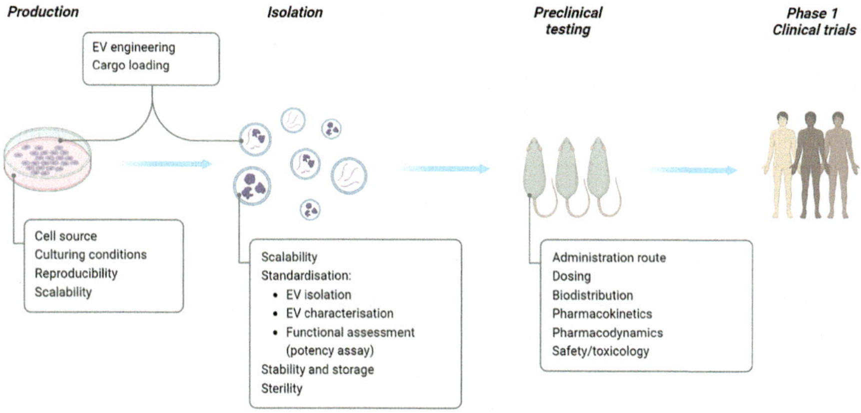

Fig. 2 Schematic of the key challenges and considerations in clinical translation of EV-based products. Created by BioRender.com

There is still no consensus on an appropriate EV isolation technique for large-scale manufacturing, and at present the choice depends on the downstream application of the final product (Paganini et al. 2019; Ramirez et al. 2018; Coumans et al. 2017). Different isolation methods may lead to the enrichment of different subpopulation(s) of EVs, potentially resulting in varied biological activity in the final product (Herrmann et al. 2021). Furthermore, the physicochemical characterisation of EVs relies on bulk analyses since technologies that are able to perform single vesicle analysis have low throughput and are often inaccessible (Herrmann et al. 2021; Ramirez et al. 2018).

The potency of an EV formulation should be determined using assays that measure its therapeutic activity (Nguyen et al. 2020). Today, standardised potency assays do not exist, and again the assays used are chosen based on the downstream application (Nguyen et al. 2020). Although potency assays determine EV functional activity, they do not reveal the underlying mechanism of action (Reiner et al. 2017). A greater understanding of the latter would assist in developing the appropriate assays (Reiner et al. 2017). Additionally, this could lead to further improvements in isolation protocols to enrich vesicles with the greatest functional activity (Claridge et al. 2021).

Finally, storage conditions can affect EVs' stability, resulting in altered physical and functional properties (Ramirez et al. 2018). Due to the heterogeneity of EVs, the impact of different reagents, conditions (time and temperature), and storage containers should be tested, optimised, and validated for every EV-based product.

3.4 Application and Formulation of EVs

EVs are most often applied systemically as prepared, rather than being modified or formulated in any way. Their subsequent biodistribution differs depending on cell source, route of administration, and dose of EVs, and indeed can even differ between different subpopulations (Nagelkerke et al. 2021; Wiklander et al. 2015). Although several reports show native EVs have intrinsic tissue homing capacity, the targeting capabilities of unmodified EVs are relatively low. Following systemic administration, they rapidly and non-specifically accumulate mainly in organs of the reticuloendothelial system (RES; liver, spleen, and lung) regardless of their origin (Claridge et al. 2021; Nagelkerke et al. 2021). To reduce possible side effects and off-target effects of systemic delivery and improve targeting, several approaches are being investigated including modification of the EV surface with and local delivery of EVs to the site of action (possibly loaded into biomaterials).

The presence and complex interplay of different molecules found on EVs' surfaces (integrins, tetraspanins, integrin-associated proteins, glycoproteins, membrane lipids) influence their targeting capabilities, functional cargo delivery, and immune evasion, and therefore play an important role in determining biodistribution (Kooijmans et al. 2021). To improve targeting, EVs can be functionalised with, e.g., antibodies, peptides, sugar moieties, or RNA (Claridge et al. 2021; Richter et al. 2021). This can be achieved either through engineering the EVs to express the species of interest or through chemical modification of the membrane (Kooijmans et al. 2021; Richter et al. 2021). However, although surface modifications are successful in increasing the specificity of targeting, they do not prevent EV accumulation in the RES (Nagelkerke et al. 2021). This leads to loss of dose, but also potentially off-target effects.

Local delivery directly to the site of interest can be employed as an alternative to targeted systemic delivery. Researchers have explored a range of administration routes (e.g., subcutaneous, intraperitoneal, intranasal, intracerebroventricular, intramyocardial) (Nagelkerke et al. 2021). Local delivery should avoid potential off-target effects. Moreover, compared to systemic delivery the dose of EVs applied locally is generally lower. However, locally delivered EVs can leak from the target site into surrounding tissues and vasculature, resulting in their migration to distal organs (Nagelkerke et al. 2021). This problem could be avoided by loading EVs into biomaterial systems. This can result in prolonged residency time at the implant site, and studies also report improved therapeutic effects and lower levels of EVs migration to distal organs compared to local delivery of EVs alone (Nagelkerke et al. 2021). Furthermore, loading EVs into these systems allows the release rate to be tailored. EVs have been successfully incorporated into hydrogels, scaffolds, electrospun fibres, films, and other formulations (Nagelkerke et al. 2021; Leung et al. 2022). To construct these systems a variety of materials were used ranging from natural silk fibroin, hyaluronic acid, gelatine, and collagen to synthetic polymers (e.g., poly(lactic-co-glycolic acid), poly(ethylene glycol), poly(caprolactone)) (Nagelkerke et al. 2021; Leung et al. 2022). The choice of biomaterial system and material depends on the intended application. For instance, hydrogels could be applied in wound healing but not in bone regeneration, as more structural support is required for the latter (Nagelkerke et al. 2021; Leung et al. 2022). Hydrogels are most commonly explored owing to the simplicity of loading – EVs can simply be added immediately prior to gelation (Nagelkerke et al. 2021).

Different formulation strategies are being explored to improve the stability and storage life of EVs (Claridge et al. 2021). The effect of different excipients and storage conditions on integrity and functional activity is being actively investigated (van de Wakker et al. 2022). The recommendation for long-term storage of EVs is storage at −80°C; however, this is challenging in terms of cost, transportation, and other logistics (Claridge et al. 2021; Herrmann et al. 2021; Paganini et al. 2019). Hence, lyophilisation in combination with the use of cryoprotectants is being investigated as an alternative (Frank et al. 2018).

4 Gene Therapies

4.1 Background

Gene therapy refers to the manipulation of the genetic material of a patient's cells via nucleic acids. The term is usually applied to the delivery of genes (DNA). However, it has expanded to include the delivery of mRNA and other regulatory RNAs (such as miRNA and siRNA), as well as gene editing technologies. For nucleic acids to function they need to be taken up into cells. Efficient transfection is required so that nucleic acids can be released into the cytosol (in the case of RNA) or the nucleus (DNA). This is challenging for these molecules because of their large molecular weight and high negative charge, and their susceptibility to degradation by nucleases (Gupta et al. 2021). To overcome these challenges and facilitate cell transfection, genetic materials/nucleic acids are usually encapsulated into a delivery carrier that facilitates their cellular uptake and transfection (Gupta et al. 2021).

4.2 DNA Delivery

There are different approaches to gene delivery, which can be categorised into ex vivo and in vivo approaches. The choice depends on the type of disease and the target tissue (Papanikolaou and Bosio 2021). Viral vectors are mostly used to achieve efficient transfection and delivery to the nucleus. Several ex vivo and in vivo gene therapies have been approved (Table 2) and many more are at various stages of clinical trials.

4.2.1 Ex Vivo Cell Transduction

In this approach, target cells are removed from the patient's body and genetically modified to correct a specific defect or to add a therapeutic gene. The corrected cells are then reintroduced back into the patient's body. This approach is particularly useful for blood cancers and diseases.

CAR-T therapy is one of the first examples of successful ex vivo gene therapy. T-cells are removed from a patient and genetically modified using viral vectors to express chimeric antigen receptors (CARs) on their surface. CARs allow T-cells to recognise and target specific antigens on the surface of cancer cells (Sterner and

Table 2 Examples of approved ex vivo and in vivo gene therapies

Drug	Vector type	Application
Ex vivo – CAR-T		
Yescarta	Lentivirus	Certain types of large B-cell lymphoma
Kymriah	Lentivirus	Acute lymphoblastic leukaemia (ALL)
Breyanzi	Lentivirus	Relapsed or refractory large B-cell lymphoma
Tecartus	Lentivirus	Relapsed or refractory mantle cell lymphoma
Ex vivo – other		
Zynteglo (autologous CD34+ cells transduced to express β-globin)	Lentivirus	Transfusion-dependent beta (β)-thalassemia (TDT)
Libmeldy (autologous CD34+ cells transduced to express ARSA)	Lentivirus	Metachromatic leukodystrophy
Strimvelis (autologous CD34+ cells transduced to express ADA)	Retrovirus (gammaretrovirus)	Severe combined immunodeficiency due to adenosine deaminase deficiency (ADA-SCID)
In vivo transgene delivery		
Luxturna	AAV (via subretinal injection).	Leber's congenital amaurosis
Zolgensma	AAV (through IV infusion).	Spinal muscular atrophy (SMA)

AAV: adeno-associated virus

Sterner 2021). Examples of approved CAR-T therapies are shown in Table 2. Recently there has also been some research into CAR-NK therapy, where NK (natural killer) cells are used to overcome the therapy-induced side effects of T-cells (Albinger et al. 2021).

Other ex vivo gene therapies transduce patients' haematopoietic stem cells (HSCs) to express antigens analogous to a disease. Zynteglo, for example, uses patients' HSCs (specifically autologous CD34+) transduced to produce functional beta-globin for the treatment of β-thalassemia (Thompson et al. 2020). Further examples include Strimvelis and Libmeldy.

Ex vivo gene therapy usually uses lentiviruses (retroviruses) to transduce the target cells. These can transfect non-dividing cells, show prolonged transgene expression and low immunogenicity, and can accommodate a large DNA payload (Bulcha et al. 2021). However, they still pose a risk of insertional mutagenesis. For example, Strimvelis has been shown to cause leukaemia in some patients (Hacein-Bey-Abina et al. 2008). Lentiviruses are generally preferred as they show a better safety profile.

4.2.2 In Vivo Transgene Delivery

Here, the desired gene is encapsulated into a viral vector and injected into the patient's bloodstream, cerebrospinal fluids or into the target tissue. Approved in vivo gene therapies (Table 2) mostly use adeno-associated viruses (AAVs) to deliver the desired genes. AAVs can be used to transfect a wide range of dividing and non-dividing cells (Bulcha et al. 2021). They offer persistent long-term gene expression in non-dividing cells (Nathwani et al. 2014), a good safety profile, and low immunogenicity (Dismuke et al. 2013). However, their efficacy in many patients is hindered by pre-existing neutralising antibodies due to previous exposure to wild-type AAV (Boutin et al. 2010). Various strategies to engineer the AAV capsid to avoid extant immunity are being investigated (Tse et al. 2017). Another widely investigated viral vector is adenovirus (Ad), with a number of early stage clinical trials underway (Bulcha et al. 2021). Non-viral delivery vectors have also been widely investigated for gene delivery (Sung and Kim 2019), but viral vectors remain the gold standard for efficient gene delivery to the nucleus.

4.3 RNA Delivery

mRNA and siRNA have different mechanisms of action. mRNA is used to express desired proteins that are missing, while siRNA is used to downregulate the expression of a target protein. Both function in the cytosol. Non-viral delivery vectors are the most common carriers for RNA delivery, with lipid nanoparticles (LNPs) being the most clinically advanced. Non-viral vectors (LNPs or polymer-based carriers) are usually cationic and depend on electrostatic forces to bind and complex negatively charged RNAs into nanoparticles.

4.3.1 siRNA Delivery

The first approved RNA drug was Patisiran, an LNP-based therapy delivering siRNA for the treatment of hereditary transthyretin-mediated amyloidosis (Yang 2019). LNPs have generally shown potent results for siRNA delivery, but most approved siRNA drugs in the market are in fact based on chemical bioconjugation (Table 3). Bioconjugation involves chemical modification (phosphate- and sugar-based) of siRNA to enhance stability and reduce immunogenicity. Modified siRNA is then covalently conjugated to specific targeting ligands (such as GalNAc) (Zhang et al. 2021a). This approach has been very efficient to achieve targeted delivery and

Table 3 Examples of approved siRNA drugs (Zhang et al. 2021a)

Drug	Delivery platform	Application
Patisiran	LNP	Hereditary transthyretin-mediated amyloidosis
Givosiran	Bioconjugation (GalNAc)	Acute hepatic porphyria
Lumasiran	Bioconjugation (GalNAc)	Primary hyperoxaluria type 1
Inclisiran	Bioconjugation (GalNAc)	Hypercholesterolemia.

GalNAc = N-acetylgalactosamine

Table 4 Examples of siRNA drugs in clinical trials (Saw and Song 2020)

Drug	Delivery platform	Clinical stage	Application	NCT ID
TKM-PLK1	LNP	Phase II	Liver cancer	NCT02191878, NCT01262235, NCT01437007
Atu-27	Cationic lipoplexes	Phase II - III	Carcinoma	NCT01808638
ARB-1467 (TKM HBV)	LNP	Phase II – III	Hepatitis B	NCT02631096
siRNA-EphA2	LNP	Phase I	Advanced cancers	NCT01591356
SIG12D	LODER (biodegradable polymeric matrix)	Phase II	Pancreatic cancer	NCT01676259

prolonged gene silencing, especially to the liver (Nair et al. 2014). Various alternative carriers including lipid- and polymer-based vectors are also being explored (Weng et al. 2019). Selected examples of siRNA therapies in clinical trials are detailed in Table 4.

4.3.2 mRNA Delivery

The field of mRNA delivery has expanded massively with the approval of COVID-19 vaccines (e.g. by BioNTech/Pfizer or Moderna (Corbett et al. 2020; Laczkó et al. 2020)). There are many mRNA therapies in clinical trials at present, largely immunotherapy cancer vaccines (see Sect. 5). While both mRNA and siRNA can both be delivered via non-viral vectors, the structural differences between the two might lead to differences in the behaviour and stability of the formulations (Suzuki and Ishihara 2021). For example, unlike Patisiran, which is stored at 2–8°C, mRNA COVID vaccines require freezing and ultra-freezing storage conditions and thus the addition of cryoprotectants such as sucrose. This is in part due to the instability of mRNA (to prevent hydrolysis) (Schoenmaker et al. 2021). Some studies also suggest that the complexation of mRNA could lead to a reconfiguration of LNP components resulting in inverted-hexagonal internal structures (Yanez Arteta et al. 2018). On the other hand, LNPs containing siRNA seem to have lamellar structures with siRNA being entrapped between the two opposed monolayers (Kulkarni et al. 2018). It is also suggested that the structures of LNPs, affected by their composition, has an impact on the transfection efficiency of the formulations (Eygeris et al. 2020). Therefore, careful design and understanding of the structure and composition of LNPs is needed for the formulation of RNA therapies.

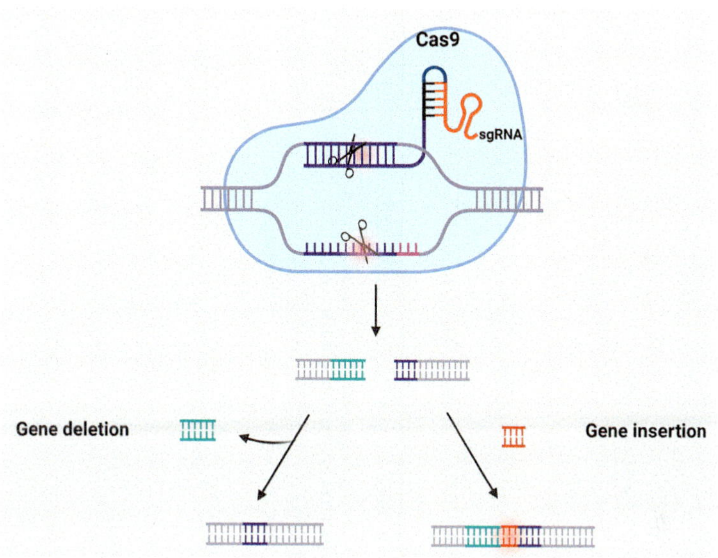

Fig. 3 Schematic diagram showing gene editing mechanism via CRISPR/Cas9. SgRNA = segment RNA. Created with BioRender.com

4.4 Gene Editing

Gene editing is a tool allowing the correction, deletion, or replacement of a gene, or modulation of its expression. It can be applied either in vivo or ex vivo depending on the target tissue. CRISPR is one of the most advanced technologies for this, owing to its simplicity and high precision. Here, an RNA-guided nuclease binds to target DNA in a sequence-specific manner, allowing for the deletion or insertion of a target gene (Fig. 3). CRISPR consists of a specific RNA segment and an associated nuclease enzyme (Cas), with CRISPR-Cas9 being the most investigated (Li et al. 2023).

There are a number of CRISPR-Cas9 therapies in clinical trials (Table 5), using a range of delivery strategies (Li et al. 2023). CTX001 (Exa-cel) is the first CRISPR-Cas9 therapy to be granted Regenerative Medicine Advanced Therapy (RMAT), Fast Track, Orphan Drug, and Rare Paediatric Disease designations from the US Food and Drug Administration for both transfusion-dependent β-thalassemia (TDT) and sickle cell disease (CSD). It functions by genetically modifying patients' HSCs to increase the production of foetal haemoglobin (Frangoul et al. 2020). No viral vector is required: instead, a CRISPR-Cas9 complex is introduced to cells via electroporation. Other examples of gene editing therapies include EDIT-101, an AAV-based gene editing therapy for the retina (Zhang et al. 2021b), and NTLA-2001 which uses LNPs for the delivery of CRISPR-Cas9 therapy to the liver (Gillmore et al. 2021).

Table 5 Examples of CRISPR-Cas9 therapeutics in clinical trials

Drug	Transduction method	Route of administration	Clinical stage	Application	NCT ID
CTX001	Electroporation	Ex vivo (IV infusion).	Phase III	Transfusion-dependent β-thalassemia (TDT) and sickle cell disease (SCD)	NCT03655678 NCT03745287
EDIT-101	AAV	Subretinal injection (in vivo)	Phase 1/II	Leber's congenital amaurosis type 10 (LCA10)	NCT03872479
NTLA-2001	LNP	IV infusion (in vivo)	Phase I	hATTR and transthyretin amyloidosis-related cardiomyopathy (ATTR-CM)	NCT04601051

5 DNA- and RNA-Based Vaccines

In addition to their use as therapeutics, DNA and RNA also have great potential as prophylactics in the form of vaccines against infectious disease (Khoshnood et al. 2022). To overcome some of the challenges with traditional vaccine technologies, nucleic acids can be utilised for vaccination by administering plasmid DNA or messenger RNA constructs that encode for antigens mimicking the surface of the pathogen of interest (Qin et al. 2021). Once the genetic constructs reach their target in the cell nucleus or ribosome, for DNA and mRNA, respectively, they instruct cells at the local injection site to produce these antigens in situ, thus stimulating the immunisation cascade.

Over the last 30 years this technology has matured significantly, with numerous successes at the pre-clinical and clinical trial level, most notably with the commercialisation of three nucleic acid vaccines for protection against severe COVID-19 disease (Pardi et al. 2018). The major advantage of nucleic acid technology is the ability to utilise a single manufacturing platform to produce vaccines against a range of pathogens simply by modifying the nucleic acid sequence, minimising the development time and cost of new vaccines for rapid response scenarios. This was best exemplified through the development of the Moderna SpikeVax mRNA vaccine against COVID-19 which was produced (first clinical batch including fill and finish) within 25 days of the SARS-CoV-2 genome being published (Rosa et al. 2021). Nucleic acid vaccines offer further advantages as both DNA and RNA molecules can stimulate cellular Toll-like receptors (TLRs) to self-adjuvant and maximise the immune response without the risk of pathogenicity from live vaccines. RNA- and DNA-based vaccines are discussed in more detail in Chapter "Advances in Vaccine Adjuvants: Nanomaterials and Small Molecules".

6 Conclusions and Future Outlook

In this chapter, we have considered a range of advanced therapeutic and prophylactic formulation types, ranging from the small (nucleic acid-based systems) through exosomes to cells. These emerging moieties have a wide range of potential benefits in terms of specificity and potency, but all require careful formulation and administration to ensure safe and effective medicines for patients. With a number of recent successes in translating products to the clinic – for instance, not only the cell-based Sperox for cartilage generation, but also the mRNA vaccines against SARS-COV-2 – there has been a dramatic increase in already intense research in this area. It would be fair to say that formulation approaches have lagged behind development of the therapeutic cargo, and more attention will be required in the future to ensure that more products can make it to market. However, a number of powerful formulation and drug delivery approaches have begun to emerge, and research efforts are accelerating. It can be expected that over the coming years rising numbers of increasingly complicated and powerful medicines based on these technologies will become available.

References

Aijaz A et al (2018) Biomanufacturing for clinically advanced cell therapies. Nat Biomed Eng 2(6): 362–376

Albinger N, Hartmann J, Ullrich E (2021) Current status and perspective of CAR-T and CAR-NK cell therapy trials in Germany. Gene Ther 28(9):513–527

Boutin S et al (2010) Prevalence of serum IgG and neutralizing factors against adeno-associated virus (AAV) types 1, 2, 5, 6, 8, and 9 in the healthy population: implications for gene therapy using AAV vectors. Hum Gene Ther 21(6):704–712

Bravery CA et al (2013) Potency assay development for cellular therapy products: an ISCT review of the requirements and experiences in the industry. Cytotherapy 15(1):9–19

Brindley D et al (2011) Bioprocess forces and their impact on cell behavior: implications for bone regeneration therapy. J Tissue Eng 2011:620247

Buckland KF, Bobby Gaspar H (2014) Gene and cell therapy for children – new medicines, new challenges? Adv Drug Deliv Rev 73(100):162–169

Bulcha JT et al (2021) Viral vector platforms within the gene therapy landscape. Signal Transduct Target Ther 6(1):53

Cheng L, Hill AF (2022) Therapeutically harnessing extracellular vesicles. Nat Rev Drug Discov 21(5):379–399

Claridge B et al (2021) Development of extracellular vesicle therapeutics: challenges, considerations, and opportunities. Front Cell Dev Biol 9:734720

Committee for Advanced Therapies (2010) Challenges with advanced therapy medicinal products and how to meet them. Nat Rev Drug Discov 9(3):195–201

Corbett KS et al (2020) SARS-CoV-2 mRNA vaccine design enabled by prototype pathogen preparedness. Nature 586(7830):567–571

Coumans FAW et al (2017) Methodological guidelines to study extracellular vesicles. Circ Res 120(10):1632–1648

Cuende N, Izeta A (2010) Clinical translation of stem cell therapies: a bridgeable gap. Cell Stem Cell 6(6):508–512

Davies OG, Williams S, Goldie K (2023) The therapeutic and commercial landscape of stem cell vesicles in regenerative dermatology. J Control Release 353:1096–1106

Dismuke JD, Tenenbaum L, Samulski JR (2013) Biosafety of recombinant adeno-associated virus vectors. Curr Gene Ther 13(6):434–452

Durand N, Zubair AC (2022) Autologous versus allogeneic mesenchymal stem cell therapy: the pros and cons. Surgery 171(5):1440–1442

Elsharkasy OM et al (2020) Extracellular vesicles as drug delivery systems: why and how? Adv Drug Deliv Rev 159:332–343

European Medicines Agency (2023) Advanced therapy medicinal products: overview. Available from: https://www.ema.europa.eu/en/human-regulatory/overview/advanced-therapy-medicinal-products-overview

European Medicines Agency (2023) Spherox. [cited 2023 June 2023]; Available from: https://www.ema.europa.eu/en/medicines/human/EPAR/spherox

Eygeris Y et al (2020) Deconvoluting lipid nanoparticle structure for messenger RNA delivery. Nano Lett 20(6):4543–4549

Ferguson SW, Nguyen J (2016) Exosomes as therapeutics: the implications of molecular composition and exosomal heterogeneity. J Control Release 228:179–190

Fischbach MA, Bluestone JA, Lim WA (2013) Cell-based therapeutics: the next pillar of medicine. Sci Transl Med 5(179):179ps7

Frangoul H et al (2020) CRISPR-Cas9 gene editing for sickle cell disease and β-thalassemia. N Engl J Med 384(3):252–260

Frank J et al (2018) Extracellular vesicles protect glucuronidase model enzymes during freeze-drying. Sci Rep 8(1):12377

Gillmore JD et al (2021) CRISPR-Cas9 in vivo gene editing for transthyretin amyloidosis. N Engl J Med 385(6):493–502
Gupta A et al (2021) Nucleic acid delivery for therapeutic applications. Adv Drug Deliv Rev 178: 113834
Gyorgy B et al (2011) Membrane vesicles, current state-of-the-art: emerging role of extracellular vesicles. Cell Mol Life Sci 68(16):2667–2688
Hacein-Bey-Abina S et al (2008) Insertional oncogenesis in 4 patients after retrovirus-mediated gene therapy of SCID-X1. J Clin Invest 118(9):3132–3142
Herrmann IK, Wood MJA, Fuhrmann G (2021) Extracellular vesicles as a next-generation drug delivery platform. Nat Nanotechnol 16(7):748–759
Huda MN et al (2021) Potential use of exosomes as diagnostic biomarkers and in targeted drug delivery: progress in clinical and preclinical applications. ACS Biomater Sci Eng 7(6): 2106–2149
Iglesias-Lopez C et al (2019) Regulatory framework for advanced therapy medicinal products in Europe and United States. Front Pharmacol 10:921
Jere D et al (2021) Challenges for cell-based medicinal products from a pharmaceutical product perspective. J Pharm Sci 110(5):1900–1908
Joshi BS, Ortiz D, Zuhorn IS (2021) Converting extracellular vesicles into nanomedicine: loading and unloading of cargo. Mater Today Nano 16:100148
Kalluri R, LeBleu VS (2020) The biology, function, and biomedical applications of exosomes. Science 367(6478)
Khoshnood S et al (2022) Viral vector and nucleic acid vaccines against COVID-19: a narrative review. Front Microbiol 13. https://doi.org/10.3389/fmicb.2022.984536
Kooijmans SAA, de Jong OG, Schiffelers RM (2021) Exploring interactions between extracellular vesicles and cells for innovative drug delivery system design. Adv Drug Deliv Rev 173:252–278
Kulkarni JA et al (2018) On the formation and morphology of lipid nanoparticles containing Ionizable cationic lipids and siRNA. ACS Nano 12(5):4787–4795
Laczkó D et al (2020) A single immunization with nucleoside-modified mRNA vaccines elicits strong cellular and humoral immune responses against SARS-CoV-2 in mice. Immunity 53(4): 724–732.e7
Lener T et al (2015) Applying extracellular vesicles based therapeutics in clinical trials - an ISEV position paper. J Extracell Vesicles 4:30087
Leung KS et al (2022) Biomaterials and extracellular vesicle delivery: current status, applications and challenges. Cell 11(18):2851
Li R et al (2019) Preservation of cell-based immunotherapies for clinical trials. Cytotherapy 21(9): 943–957
Li T et al (2023) CRISPR/Cas9 therapeutics: progress and prospects. Signal Transduct Target Ther 8(1):36
McKiernan J et al (2016) A novel urine exosome gene expression assay to predict high-grade prostate cancer at initial biopsy. JAMA Oncol 2(7):882–889
Meng W et al (2020) Prospects and challenges of extracellular vesicle-based drug delivery system: considering cell source. Drug Deliv 27(1):585–598
Morrow D, Ussi A, Migliaccio G (2017) Addressing pressing needs in the development of advanced therapies. Front Bioeng Biotechnol 5:55
Nagelkerke A et al (2021) Extracellular vesicles for tissue repair and regeneration: evidence, challenges and opportunities. Adv Drug Deliv Rev 175:113775
Nair JK et al (2014) Multivalent N-acetylgalactosamine-conjugated siRNA localizes in hepatocytes and elicits robust RNAi-mediated gene silencing. J Am Chem Soc 136(49):16958–16961
Nathwani AC et al (2014) Long-term safety and efficacy of factor IX gene therapy in hemophilia B. N Engl J Med 371(21):1994–2004
Nguyen VVT et al (2020) Functional assays to assess the therapeutic potential of extracellular vesicles. J Extracell Vesicles 10(1):e12033

Paganini C et al (2019) Scalable production and isolation of extracellular vesicles: available sources and lessons from current industrial bioprocesses. Biotechnol J 14(10):e1800528
Papanikolaou E, Bosio A (2021) The promise and the hope of gene therapy. Front Genome Ed:3
Pardi N et al (2018) mRNA vaccines – a new era in vaccinology. Nat Rev Drug Discov 17(4): 261–279
Patel DB et al (2017) Impact of cell culture parameters on production and vascularization bioactivity of mesenchymal stem cell-derived extracellular vesicles. Bioeng Transl Med 2(2):170–179
Pellegrini G et al (2016) From discovery to approval of an advanced therapy medicinal product-containing stem cells, in the EU. Regen Med 11(4):407–420
Qin F et al (2021) A guide to nucleic acid vaccines in the prevention and treatment of infectious diseases and cancers: from basic principles to current applications. Front Cell Dev Biol 9:9
Ramirez MI et al (2018) Technical challenges of working with extracellular vesicles. Nanoscale 10(3):881–906
Rayner MLD, Phillips JB (2022) Chapter 8 advanced therapy medicinal products (ATMPs). In: Specialised pharmaceutical formulation: the science and technology of dosage forms. The Royal Society of Chemistry, pp 211–229
Reiner AT et al (2017) Concise review: developing best-practice models for the therapeutic use of extracellular vesicles. Stem Cells Transl Med 6(8):1730–1739
Richter M, Vader P, Fuhrmann G (2021) Approaches to surface engineering of extracellular vesicles. Adv Drug Deliv Rev 173:416–426
Rohde E, Pachler K, Gimona M (2019) Manufacturing and characterization of extracellular vesicles from umbilical cord-derived mesenchymal stromal cells for clinical testing. Cytotherapy 21(6): 581–592
Rosa SS et al (2021) mRNA vaccines manufacturing: challenges and bottlenecks. Vaccine 39(16): 2190–2200
Saleh AF et al (2019) Extracellular vesicles induce minimal hepatotoxicity and immunogenicity. Nanoscale 11(14):6990–7001
Salmikangas P et al (2015) Manufacturing, characterization and control of cell-based medicinal products: challenging paradigms toward commercial use. Regen Med 10(1):65–78
Saw PE, Song E-W (2020) siRNA therapeutics: a clinical reality. Sci China Life Sci 63(4):485–500
Schoenmaker L et al (2021) mRNA-lipid nanoparticle COVID-19 vaccines: structure and stability. Int J Pharm 601:120586
Shukla V et al (2019) The landscape of cellular and gene therapy products: authorization, discontinuations, and cost. Hum Gene Ther Clin Dev 30(3):102–113
Silva DN et al (2022) ATMP development and pre-GMP environment in academia: a safety net for early cell and gene therapy development and manufacturing. Immunooncol Technol 16:100099
Sterner RC, Sterner RM (2021) CAR-T cell therapy: current limitations and potential strategies. Blood Cancer J 11(4):69
Sung YK, Kim SW (2019) Recent advances in the development of gene delivery systems. Biomater Res 23(1):8
Suzuki Y, Ishihara H (2021) Difference in the lipid nanoparticle technology employed in three approved siRNA (Patisiran) and mRNA (COVID-19 vaccine) drugs. Drug Metab Pharmacokinet 41:100424
Thompson AA et al (2020) Favorable outcomes in pediatric patients in the phase 3 Hgb-207 (Northstar-2) and Hgb-212 (Northstar-3) studies of betibeglogene autotemcel gene therapy for the treatment of transfusion-dependent β-thalassemia. Blood 136(Supplement 1):52–54
Tse LV et al (2017) Structure-guided evolution of antigenically distinct adeno-associated virus variants for immune evasion. Proc Natl Acad Sci USA 114(24):E4812–e4821
Tsiapalis D, O'Driscoll L (2020) Mesenchymal stem cell derived extracellular vesicles for tissue engineering and regenerative medicine applications. Cell 9(4):991
van de Wakker SI et al (2022) Influence of short term storage conditions, concentration methodsand excipients on extracellular vesicle recovery and function. Eur J Pharm Biopharm 170:59–69

van der Pol L, Stork M, van der Ley P (2015) Outer membrane vesicles as platform vaccine technology. Biotechnol J 10(11):1689–1706

Wang LL et al (2021) Cell therapies in the clinic. Bioeng Transl Med 6(2):e10214

Weng Y et al (2019) RNAi therapeutic and its innovative biotechnological evolution. Biotechnol Adv 37(5):801–825

Wiklander OP et al (2015) Extracellular vesicle in vivo biodistribution is determined by cell source, route of administration and targeting. J Extracell Vesicles 4:26316

Wiklander OPB et al (2019) Advances in therapeutic applications of extracellular vesicles. Sci Transl Med 11:eaav8521

Yanez Arteta M et al (2018) Successful reprogramming of cellular protein production through mRNA delivered by functionalized lipid nanoparticles. Proc Natl Acad Sci USA 115(15): E3351–E3360

Yanez-Mo M et al (2015) Biological properties of extracellular vesicles and their physiological functions. J Extracell Vesicles 4:27066

Yang J (2019) Patisiran for the treatment of hereditary transthyretin-mediated amyloidosis. Expert Rev Clin Pharmacol 12(2):95–99

Zhang MM et al (2021a) The growth of siRNA-based therapeutics: updated clinical studies. Biochem Pharmacol 189:114432

Zhang X et al (2021b) Gene correction of the CLN3 c.175G>A variant in patient-derived induced pluripotent stem cells prevents pathological changes in retinal organoids. Mol Genet Genomic Med 9(3):e1601

Zhu X et al (2017) Comprehensive toxicity and immunogenicity studies reveal minimal effects in mice following sustained dosing of extracellular vesicles derived from HEK293T cells. J Extracell Vesicles 6(1):1324730

Regulatory Aspects for Approval of Advanced Therapy Medicinal Products in the EU

Shayesteh Fürst-Ladani, Anja Bührer, Walter Fürst, and Nathalie Schober-Ladani

Contents

Abstract

In the European Union (EU), advanced therapy medicinal products (ATMPs) undergo evaluation by the European Medicines Agency's (EMA) Committee for Advanced Therapies (CAT) to obtain marketing authorization under the

S. Fürst-Ladani · A. Bührer · W. Fürst · N. Schober-Ladani (✉)
SFL Regulatory Affairs and Scientific Communication GmbH, Basel, Switzerland
e-mail: n.ladani@sfl-services.com

M. Schäfer-Korting, U. S. Schubert (eds.), *Drug Delivery and Targeting*,
Handbook of Experimental Pharmacology 284, https://doi.org/10.1007/164_2023_648

centralized procedure. Because of the diversity and complexity of ATMPs, a tailored approach to the regulatory process is required that needs to ensure the safety and efficacy of each product. Since ATMPs often target serious diseases with unmet medical need, the industry and authorities are interested in providing treatment to patients in a timely manner through optimized and expedited regulatory pathways. EU legislators and regulators have implemented various instruments to support the development and authorization of innovative medicines by offering scientific guidance at early stages, incentives for small developers and products for rare diseases, accelerated evaluation of marketing authorization applications, different types of marketing authorizations, and tailored programs for medicinal products with the orphan drug designation (ODD) and the Priority Medicines (PRIME) scheme. Since the regulatory framework for ATMPs was established, 20 products have been licenced, 15 with orphan drug designation, and 7 supported by PRIME. This chapter discusses the specific regulatory framework for ATMPs in the EU and highlights previous successes and remaining challenges.

Keywords

ATMPs · Centralized procedure · EU · Marketing authorization · PRIME · Risk-based approach

1 Introduction

Advanced therapy medicinal products (ATMPs) are a group of complex and innovative biological medicines that offer novel therapeutic opportunities to treat diseases and injuries. They encompass gene therapy medicinal products (GTMPs), somatic cell therapy medicinal products (sCTMPs), tissue-engineered products (TEPs), and combined ATMPs (cATMPs) including one or more medical devices as an integral part. The potential of these products, commonly referred to as "gene and cell therapies," has been anticipated decades ago when the idea of transferring genetic material or cells to cure genetic diseases was born. Indeed, when the specific regulatory framework for ATMPs was finally established in the European Union (EU) in 2007, cell therapies were already used on a named-patient basis in a number of hospitals (Milazzo et al. 2016). Despite ongoing harmonizing efforts, the regulatory framework lags the fast-paced scientific innovation that drives the development of gene- and cell-based therapy products. This emphasizes the need to further control and standardize the development and regulation of ATMPs to guarantee safe and high-level patient care. The complex nature of ATMPs that often target severe rare diseases with unmet medical need destines them to face a number of obstacles in their development that necessitate adaptations in the clinical design and regulatory requirements (Pizevska et al. 2022). In this chapter, we discuss the legal and regulatory framework for ATMPs in the EU, the incentives established to foster their development, challenges encountered in the clinical development and regulatory evaluation of ATMPs as well as measures taken to circumvent them, and potential issues arising in and from the regulatory decision-making.

2 The Classification of ATMPs

The classification of ATMPs is a crucial step to determine the regulatory framework applicable to the candidate product which will direct the clinical development. Thus, the European Medicines Agency (EMA) provides guidance on all relevant definitions and criteria laid out in the applicable EU legislation, i.e. Directive 2001/83/EC, amended by Commission Directive 2009/120/EC, and Regulation (EC) No 1392/2007. Since the scientific evaluation and classification of advanced therapies are often associated with challenges and require special expertise, ATMP developers have the possibility to ask the EMA for scientific recommendation on the classification of the product as an ATMP. The EMA's Committee for Advanced Therapies (CAT), a multidisciplinary body of experts, issues a scientific recommendation on ATMP classification within 60 days of receipt of the application, after consultation with the European Commission (EC). The classification procedure at the EMA is particularly important for borderline products that combine medical devices and medicinal products as other regulatory requirements might apply. In principle, a classification can be requested at any stage of the product development, even in case of a limited data package at the early stage (European Medicines Agency 2015b).

2.1 Gene Therapies

Gene therapies are being studied with great promise for use in multiple disease areas and have gained worldwide recognition, especially due to CRISPR/Cas9 systems that can be produced with greater ease (Behr et al. 2021). In order to be classified as GTMP according to Part IV of Annex I to Directive 2001/83/EC, the following criteria have to be met:

1. The active substance of the product must consist of a recombinant nucleic acid,
2. The recombinant nucleic acid must be of biologic origin irrespective of the origin of the vector system used to deliver the genetic material,
3. The recombinant nucleic acid must be used in or administered to humans with the intention to add, delete, regulate, repair, or replace a genetic sequence, and
4. The recombinant nucleic acid must be directly involved in the therapeutic, diagnostic, or prophylactic effect of the product.

Additionally, there are a number of clarifications amended to these criteria: The genetic modification does not necessarily need to occur within the human body since genetically modified cells generated ex vivo have also been classified as GTMPs. Consequently, a product that falls within the definition of a sCTMP or TEP as well as a GTMP shall be classified as GTMP, since this category poses the highest safety concerns (European Medicines Agency 2015b). Finally, genetic material aimed at the prophylaxis of infectious diseases are not considered GTMPs and are rather classified as vaccines.

2.2 Cell and Tissue Therapies

Somatic cell therapy medicinal products and tissue-engineered products are classified according to Part IV of Annex I to Directive 2001/83/EC and Article 2(1)b of Regulation (EC) No 1394/2007, respectively. Although both products are distinguished into two subcategories, they share the same criteria:

1. The product consists of cells or tissues that have been manipulated in a way that biological, physiological, or structural properties relevant for the intended clinical use have been significantly altered (sCTMPs) or
2. The product consists of cells or tissues that are not intended to be used for the same essential function as in the donor (non-homologues use) (TEP).

The purpose of use distinguishes sCTMPs and TEPs. While the first are intended to treat, prevent, or diagnose a disease through the pharmacological, immunological, or metabolic action of the active substance, TEPs are intended to regenerate, repair, or replace a human tissue. If the product exclusively consists of non-viable cells that do not exert their function via pharmacological, immunological, or metabolic means, it shall be excluded from the definition as sCTMP or TEP (European Medicines Agency 2015b).

2.3 Combined ATMPs

Combined ATMPs are defined according to Article 2(1)d of Regulation (EC) No 1394/2007. They consist of viable or non-viable cells or tissues and incorporate one or more medical devices as an integral part of the product. If cells or tissues are non-viable, they must exert the primary action of the cATMP.

3 Regulatory Framework for ATMPs

In the EU, ATMPs are governed primarily by Regulation (EC) No 1394/2007 and Directive 2001/83/EC. They not only provide definitions for the different subcategories of ATMPs but also enable and ensure a standardized marketing authorization (MA) procedure, scientific and regulatory guidance in the development of ATMPs, and set standards in quality, safety, and efficacy medicinal products have to meet. The approval of ATMPs falls under the centralized procedure described in Regulation (EC) No 726/2004 which dictates that marketing authorization applications (MAAs) are evaluated by EMA committees and authorized by the EC rather than by national regulatory agencies (European Medicines Agency 2022b). The centralized procedure guarantees that complex products such as ATMPs are evaluated by a panel of experts with relevant scientific expertise and results in a single MA valid throughout the EU/European Economic Area (EEA). The scientific evaluation of the quality, safety, and efficacy of an ATMP during the MA procedure is conducted by the CAT (European Medicines Agency 2021a). The CAT provides a draft opinion to the Committee for Medicinal Products for Human Use (CHMP) that ultimately voices a recommendation (i.e., opinion) for or against marketing authorization to the EC.

In contrast, the approval of clinical trial applications is granted by national competent authorities (NCAs) in individual EU Member States. A more harmonized approach that aims to facilitate the process will be seen in the future as a result of the application of the EU Clinical Trial Regulation EU No 536/2014 and also the possibility to submit a single clinical trial application and the simultaneous assessment by many NCAs (Salazar-Fontana 2022).

3.1 Specificities of ATMPs

ATMPs have to comply with the scientific, regulatory, and legal requirements set in the European legislation. The quality, safety, and efficacy of a medicinal product is assessed during the MA procedure based on comprehensive scientific data on the manufacturing, pre-clinical, and clinical development, which has to follow the standards of good manufacturing, laboratory, and clinical practices. However, due to the inherent complexity of ATMPs, their development bears unique challenges and these standards and requirements may need to be adapted individually. At the same time, ATMPs are at the forefront of clinical innovation in disease areas that have been neglected or challenging to treat thus far. They frequently target rare indications, address unmet medical need (i.e., conditions for which there exists no satisfactory method of diagnosis, prevention, or treatment) (European Medicines Agency 2019b), or offer a tremendous medical benefit such as curing a disease. Consequently, their successful development and authorization is of high interest for the public health. Therefore, the EMA has outlined a tailored approach with regard to ATMPs in several guidelines, taking their unique complexities and challenges into consideration (European Medicines Agency 2019a).

3.2 Incentives to Encourage Development of ATMPs

ATMPs are considered innovative treatment options due to their modality (using genetic material, cells, or tissues) and the fact that they often target diseases with unmet medical need. Originally, they were often developed by micro-, small-, and medium-sized enterprises (SMEs) or academic institutions with limited experience of the regulatory process and its requirements to obtain marketing authorization.

Moreover, the inherent complexity of ATMPs and the predominant type of targeted diseases bring along several particularities that demand a tailored approach for their development and authorization. Hence, the EMA has established comprehensive scientific and regulatory guidance (European Medicines Agency 2022a) as well as financial incentives that aim to optimize and accelerate the development and authorization of ATMPs, providing timely access to treatment for patients in need.

In its efforts to support the development of innovative treatment options as early as possible, the EMA set up the Innovation Task Force (ITF) to provide a forum for early informal dialogue with developers on innovative aspects in medicines development. It consists of experts with scientific, regulatory, and legal competences and offers briefing meetings for developers to clarify questions on the route to market for their innovative products such as ATMPs and receive advice on potential issues. These meetings are intended for the informal exchange of information between all parties and are free of charge (European Medicines Agency 2014).

The correct classification of a potential medicinal product into one of the subcategories of ATMPs is often not so trivial, but simultaneously a critical point to discern the regulatory framework that will guide the developmental plan. Especially in cases of borderline classification, the developer is strongly advised to seek guidance from the EMA. The CAT provides confirmation free of charge that the proposed product qualifies as ATMP and into which subcategory it falls (European Medicines Agency 2021b).

Furthermore, SMEs are eligible to the ATMP certification procedure of the CAT that evaluates and certifies early quality and non-clinical data (European Medicines Agency 2016b).

Developers of any medicinal product can seek scientific advice from the EMA at any given stage of a medicine's development. The aim of this guidance is to ensure that appropriate tests and studies are performed to demonstrate the safety and efficacy of a product and to minimize the number of major objections raised during a subsequent MAA. The developer raises questions on quality, non-clinical, clinical, and methodological issues and suggests proposals. The EMA, through CHMP, then gives advice on the developer's proposal.

Finally, an essential stepstone for SME and academic developers is the provision of financial incentives that EMA grants to such developers for scientific advice in the form of a 65% reduction in the fees and a 90% reduction for SME applicants or even 100% fee waiver in case the indication is a rare disease and the product has an orphan drug designation (ODD).

3.2.1 Orphan Medicinal Products

Many ATMPs are intended to treat rare diseases which imposes additional challenges on the sponsor in terms of clinical development. In order to support and to create incentives for the development of treatments for rare diseases, the EU issued the orphan medicinal products regulation (Regulation [EC] No 141/2000) which grants orphan designation to medicinal products (European Medicines Agency 2018b). To be eligible, a medicinal product needs to fulfill a number of criteria:

1. It must be intended for the treatment, prevention, or diagnosis of a disease that is life-threatening or chronically debilitating,
2. The prevalence of the disease in the EU must not be more than 5 individuals in every 10,000 or it must be unlikely that marketing of the product will generate sufficient revenue to justify the investment needed for its development, and
3. There exists no satisfactory method to diagnose, prevent, or treat the concerned condition, or if so, the proposed product must be of significant benefit to the patient population.

A significant benefit can mean that a product produces a clinically relevant advantage, is suitable for patients for whom the current treatment does not work, or is easier or more convenient to use.

EMA offers a number of financial incentives to foster the development of orphan medicinal products: Protocol assistance, a type of scientific advice specific for orphan medicinal products, and the MAA are available at reduced or waived (for SMEs) rates, and the sponsor obtains market exclusivity for the product in the authorized indication for 10 years. There is the possibility of an extension of the 10-year market exclusivity by another 2 years if the data requirements relating to administration to the pediatric population are met. This requires fulfilling the approved "Pediatric Investigation Plan," in accordance with Regulation No. 1901/2006. An example in this context is Strimvelis, which had such a pediatric study concept and thus received a total of 12 years of exclusivity (Farkas et al. 2017).

3.3 The Challenges of Development of ATMPs

Due to the complex nature of ATMPs, certain standards in manufacturing, non-clinical, and clinical studies of medicinal products are not applicable to ATMPs, thus rendering tailored development approaches to each ATMP necessary. Considering that ATMPs are a group of diverse products, it is important to state that a one-size-fits-all approach is usually not feasible. Yet, it is of utmost importance to conduct high-quality clinical trials that follow general guidelines as closely as possible to ensure the quality and safety of the product, increase chances of a successful MAA, and to nurture the trust of the general public in these innovative treatments. The diverse and complex nature of these products demands a flexible risk-based approach to define quality, non-clinical, and clinical developmental regulatory issues early in the development of ATMPs (Salazar-Fontana 2022).

3.3.1 Quality and Manufacturing

Good manufacturing practice (GMP) describes the minimum standard the production process of medicinal products must meet and has been established to guarantee the quality and safety of medicines. It covers all aspects, from starting material, equipment, manufacturing sites to staff training and hygiene standards. Compliance with GMP standards represents a major challenge for ATMPs due to their complexity in manufacturing. Furthermore, ATMPs are often personalized treatments, introducing additional challenges: Donor variability and the manufacturing of a product tailored to individual patients impede standardized manufacturing procedures and product characteristics. In an attempt to support developers of ATMPs, the EU adopted binding guidelines specifically for ATMPs that have been granted a marketing authorization or for ATMPs in clinical trials (European Commission 2017).

During development of a medicinal product, an adaptation of the manufacturing process is usually required to transition from the laboratory into the patient. This may include upscaling to provide larger quantities for clinical trials and commercialization, standardization of the procedure, and a switch to clinical grade ingredients.

The propagation of cells usually requires the use of animal- and human-derived materials like growth factors or serum which pose the risk of transmitting infectious or pathogenic agents such as viruses, bacteria, or prions. Therefore, high-quality raw materials where composition, content, and safety are controlled by the supplier need to be obtained which might be scarce or expensive, imposing a tremendous financial burden on SME or academic developers. It also often necessitates a switch to an alternative product (e.g., from bovine serum albumin to chemically-defined serum-free media) to alleviate concerns regarding safety, reproducibility, and scarcity. However, a change in raw materials can have serious effects on product characteristics, especially for sCTMPs and TEPs, and thus requires close monitoring.

Commercialization requires the production of large quantities of the product in a reproducible and robust manner. The use of expansion platforms, such as bioreactors, allows standardized manufacturing, however, it might also require a change in the previously established production protocol. Developers must ensure that the product retains key characteristics such as mode of action, purity, and safety.

To guarantee the quality and safety of the medicinal products, it is recommended to perform an in-depth characterization of the product with a range of analytical methods. For GTMPs, this may include infectivity, ratio of full/empty particles, and potency and for sCTMPs and TEPs, differentiation potential, expression of markers, biological activity, and karyotype. However, full characterization of the final product may not be feasible due to limited amounts, or test results may not be available prior to administration to patients due to the short shelf-life of the product. On this account, it is advised to establish a standardized manufacturing process with robust in-process controls to guarantee product quality without reliance on final product testing, a concept covered by the term "quality by design."

With the rising interest in ATMP-based therapies, the number of manufacturing sites that comply with GMP is increasing, making the production of the continuously increasing number of ATMPs at a high quality possible.

3.3.2 Non-clinical Development

Non-clinical studies entail in vitro and in vivo experiments in cells/tissues and animals, respectively, to demonstrate proof-of-principle, to determine the dose range, and to assess the safety of the product by characterizing its pharmacological profile. Ultimately, they give indication if it is safe to proceed with testing in humans. They are a central element in the development of all medicinal products, yet the realization of such studies in accordance with the principles of good laboratory practice (GLP) and the extrapolation of results to humans is often limited for ATMPs (Lopez-Navas et al. 2022).

In vitro studies in cells or cellular systems offer the advantage that the characteristics of the ATMP, especially in case of GTMPs, can be studied in an isolated and controlled environment and that, ideally, cells derived from patients can be used. In contrast, studies conducted in animals compared to cells and tissues have the advantage that they can assess the impact of the medicine on the body as a whole, including biodistribution and toxic effects on specific organs. However, due to ATMPs' high species-specificity, appropriate animal models that mimic humans in terms of their immune response, cellular specificity, or genome composition might not be available. To overcome this issue, either multiple animal models, genetically modified or humanized animals or homologous models with animal cells or species-specific genetic sequences are used (Agarwal et al. 2020; Ito et al. 2002). Furthermore, while the safety of conventional medicinal products is usually tested in healthy subjects, it is required to use animals with the identical genetic defect when testing GTMPs to avoid toxicity from overexpression of the gene product that would not occur in the real-world setting.

The design of non-clinical studies is as complex as ATMPs and a set of factors need to be taken into consideration (Silva Lima and Videira 2018). The assessment of the biodistribution and toxicity of ATMPs comes with unique challenges since strong pharmacological targets can often be not defined. In general, biodistribution studies should address the distribution, retention, and clearance of the ATMP itself as well as the behavior of products thereof, e.g. the expressed protein or daughter cells. Importantly, the unintended systemic distribution of sCTMPs or the non-specific transduction of viral particles and the effect of both in non-target organs need to be determined and controlled. With the use of ATMPs comes a number of risks and limitations: infections (microbial contamination of the starting material or introduced during the process); immunogenicity or rejection; tumorigenicity (off-target integration or transformation of cells); ectopic engraftment of cells into non-target tissues; loss of the active substance (silencing of the transgene or dedifferentiation of cells); integration into the germline and shedding of genetically modified organisms (GMOs) into the environment. Since many ATMPs are designed to remain in the body lifelong, the observation time of toxic effects needs to be adjusted accordingly. Ideally, these studies continue until no activity is detected anymore (transient effect intended) or until it reaches a plateau (persistent effect intended).

Although GLP-conform, non-clinical studies are not an integral part of the development of ATMPs yet, sponsors nevertheless take efforts to include them to strengthen the subsequent clinical trials and the MAA (Lopez-Navas et al. 2022).

3.3.3 Clinical Development

Non-clinical data is used for the clinical trial application at NCAs. Importantly, ATMPs that consist of or contain a GMO need to acquire a GMO authorization in addition to a clinical trial authorization that must be granted before the clinical trial commences. This is a crucial point since it is a time-consuming step that is evaluated on a national level in EU member states with different GMO regulations that can significantly delay the MA process, resulting in a call for a GMO exemption for ATMPs by the industry (Alliance for Regenerative Medicine et al. 2021). Such an exemption was granted for vaccines and ATMPs to treat or prevent COVID-19 provided that the pandemic status is given by the authorities (The European Parliament and the Council of the European Union 2020).

If the CTA is approved, the ATMP is next progressed into clinical studies. Ideally, these follow discrete steps where conclusions from smaller-scale studies support the design of subsequent larger-scale studies. In general, a new conventional medicine is first tested for safety in a small group of healthy volunteers in phase I (first-in-human) trials, then for dose-related safety and initial efficacy in about 100 patients in phase II trials, and finally for confirmation of efficacy in a large group of patients in phase III (pivotal) trials. The regulatory review then assesses if data from the clinical studies support a positive benefit–risk balance, i.e. that benefits outweigh the risks, which is mandatory for a successful MA. However, clinical studies of ATMPs usually fall short of the gold standard of controlled, randomized, double-blind trials and do not meet the same strict criteria as conventional drugs. Indeed, the most commonly identified major objections during MAA of ATMPs were raised on the clinical data package, leading to extended clock-stops and withdrawal of the MAA (Elsallab et al. 2020).

Most of the ATMPs were authorized on the basis of small, open-label, non-randomized, single-arm studies (Iglesias-Lopez et al. 2021a, b) since the complexity of ATMPs and the targeted disease limits the design of conventional studies. In general, the design of clinical studies largely depends on the target disease: An ATMP targeting a disease affecting many will face less difficulties in adhering to clinical standards in terms of patient abundance and standard of care than a rare disease with orphan status and no alternative treatment options.

Phase I trials in healthy volunteers are ethically unacceptable in the case of ATMPs, therefore the safety as well as the initial efficacy of ATMPs is usually assessed in phase I/II transitional studies that directly enroll affected patients. This is also due to the fact that most ATMPs target orphan indications and low prevalence of the targeted disease makes large cohort studies impossible (Iglesias-Lopez et al. 2021b). However, the interpretation of unexpected adverse events is complicated because symptoms may be caused by the underlying disease. Additionally, toxicities are difficult to detect in a small group size of patients and therefore, continued evaluation of safety and efficacy post-authorization and risk mitigation measures are usually mandated. These include close monitoring of treated patients and rapidly accessible treatment options (e.g. an intensive care unit and a specialized health care team). Moreover, potential risks arising from some ATMPs such as tumor formation due to mutagenesis make a longer follow-up necessary. A small number of subjects also impede statistical analysis and significance, rendering the interpretation of study results difficult. The method of administration, which is often invasive and, in some cases, even requires surgery, does not only pose additional safety concerns, but it also makes blinding and the use of controls complicated: The performance of a mock-surgery is deemed unethical, and it is nearly impossible to get CTA approval. Since often no alternative treatments options are available and many ATMPs are expected to be curative, many patients are hesitant to participate in trials with a placebo or less effective standard treatment in the control arm (Gaasterland et al. 2019). Treatment of rare diseases is often symptomatic, and the standard of care can vary from patient to patient. Therefore, the majority of trials conducted so far for ATMPs were without control arm or used historical controls, were open-labeled, and had a single-arm design (Iglesias-Lopez et al. 2021b). The efficacy of a medicine is determined by clinical endpoints, but standard clinical endpoints are often not applicable to ATMPs. The choice of study endpoints, which are often not well defined or surrogate endpoints, can severely impact the credibility of a clinical study. This may not only affect the MAA resulting in delays or refusal but also post-authorization reimbursement.

Since the authorization of ATMPs is crucial especially in disease areas with unmet medical need or major public health interest, a careful evaluation of the benefits such as treatment where there is none and risks such as uncertainties in the assessment of safety and efficacy with the so-called benefit–risk balance is of utmost importance. To this end, the EMA has introduced the risk-based approach that enables a tailor-made development program for ATMPs that can deviate from standard requirements (European Medicines Agency 2013; Kooijman et al. 2013). Thereby, the amount of data that needs to be provided at the point of the MAA depends on identified risk factors, knowledge about the product, and the sponsors' experience in development of other ATMPs. Moreover, as ATMPs are in the center of a rapidly evolving field of therapeutic innovation, methods for challenging study design and statistical evaluation are being developed that aim to overcome the caveats of traditional methods when applied to ATMPs (Iglesias-Lopez et al. 2021a).

3.4 Marketing Authorization Application

A successful clinical development culminates in the submission of an MAA to the EMA to obtain MA under the centralized procedure. The EMA established a standardized procedure to define each party's responsibilities and to enable effective and timely interaction between the applicant and the EMA (European Medicines Agency 2018a). In general, all submission steps should follow a timetable published by the EMA.

Seven to eighteen months prior to the submission of the MAA, the applicant is obligated to submit an eligibility request for review under the centralized procedure followed by a notification of the intention to submit an MAA. The MAA is submitted in the form of an electronic Common Technical Document which contains administrative content as well as the quality, safety, and efficacy data structured in several modules (European Medicines Agency 2008). Upon acceptance of the submission passing the validation, the CHMP appoints two assessment teams to evaluate the MAA based on regulatory, scientific, and procedural guidelines (European

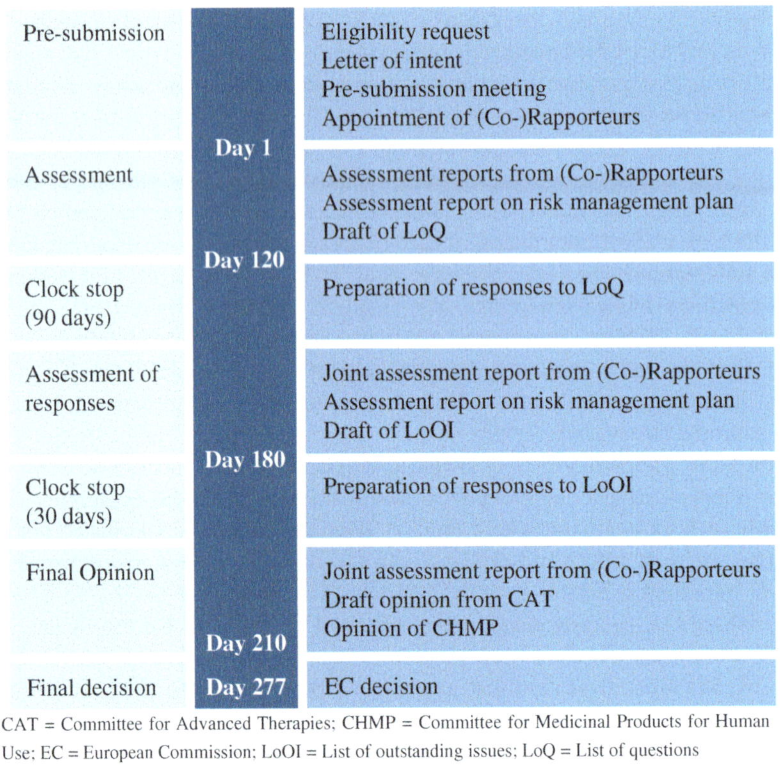
Pre-submission
Eligibility request
Letter of intent
Pre-submission meeting
Appointment of (Co-)Rapporteurs
Day 1
Assessment
Assessment reports from (Co-)Rapporteurs
Assessment report on risk management plan
Draft of LoQ
Day 120
Clock stop (90 days)
Preparation of responses to LoQ
Assessment of responses
Joint assessment report from (Co-)Rapporteurs
Assessment report on risk management plan
Draft of LoOI
Day 180
Clock stop (30 days)
Preparation of responses to LoOI
Final Opinion
Joint assessment report from (Co-)Rapporteurs
Draft opinion from CAT
Opinion of CHMP
Day 210
Final decision
Day 277
EC decision
CAT = Committee for Advanced Therapies; CHMP = Committee for Medicinal Products for Human Use; EC = European Commission; LoOI = List of outstanding issues; LoQ = List of questions

Fig. 1 Timeline of MAA evaluation. *CAT* Committee for Advanced Therapies, *CHMP* Committee for Medicinal Products for Human Use, *EC* European Commission, *LoOI* List of outstanding issues, *LoQ* List of questions

Medicines Agency 2018a). The first team consists of a rapporteur from the CAT, a coordinator from the CHMP, and a co-rapporteur from the Pharmacovigilance Risk Assessment Committee (PRAC). The second team consists of a co-rapporteur of the CAT and a corresponding CHMP member. Each team includes advisers with experience in the evaluation of quality, safety, efficacy, pharmacovigilance, and environmental risk assessment of ATMPs. Both teams are supported by a rapporteur from the PRAC.

The evaluation procedure follows a standard timetable with discrete milestones put in place by the EMA to facilitate rapid EU-wide authorization (Fig. 1) (European Medicines Agency 2018a). The CHMP opinion is provided on Day 210 (excluding clock-stops), followed by the EC decision on Day 277. The procedure starts with the electronic submission of the dossier and upon validating that the MAA includes all mandatory modules, Day 1 is initiated. From Day 1 to Day 80, the rapporteur and co-rapporteur lead the review of the application by their respective teams and subsequently each submit their assessment reports to the CAT, CHMP coordinators, CHMP, EMA, and applicant. The reports include a preliminary evaluation of the quality, safety, and efficacy of the ATMP, a provisional recommendation on the authorization of the product, and a draft list of outstanding questions. On Day 94, the PRAC rapporteur provides the risk management plan (RMP) assessment report including insights on the pharmacovigilance plan and risk minimization measures.

Based on the (co-)rapporteurs' and PRAC rapporteur's assessment reports, the CAT adopts a list of questions (LoQ) discussing objections and key scientific issues. The CHMP provides the endorsed LoQ and, based on the severity of objections, a provisional recommendation to the applicant on Day 120, which triggers a clock stop to give the applicant time to respond to the questions. The typical time frame for answering the LoQ is 90 to 180 Days.

Upon submission of the answers to the LoQ, the clock is re-initiated, and the assessment teams evaluate their suitability to address the raised concerns and issues. The (co-)rapporteurs provide their joint response assessment report to the CAT, CHMP coordinators, CHMP, PRAC rapporteur, and EMA on Day 150. It is also shared with the applicant for information only. The CAT outlines a list of outstanding issues (LoOI) which is subsequently communicated (written or oral) to the applicant by the CHMP on Day 180, which again triggers a clock stop. Submission of answers to the LoOI re-initiates the clock and is followed by the review and drafting of the joint assessment report by the (co-)rapporteurs. On Day 203, the CAT provides a draft opinion based on the joint assessment report to the CHMP and ultimately on Day 210, the CHMP adopts an opinion. In the event that the CHMP issues a positive opinion, the EC grants authorization within 67 Days given the applicant provides additional documents. In case of a negative opinion, the decision can be appealed by the applicant, resulting in a re-evaluation of the previously submitted dossier.

Regardless of the type of declared opinion, the EMA announces the outcomes of all MAAs on its website, in press releases, and in the CAT's and CHMP's monthly reports. For those products receiving MA, a European public assessment report (EPAR) is published including authorization details (i.e., details about the product and MA holder), product information (i.e., package leaflet, summary of product characteristics, therapeutic indications), and assessment history (i.e., non-commercially sensitive information from the assessment reports). A similar document including a questions and answers document is published for declined MAAs. Thus, EPARs serve as a valuable source of information for developers of new medicines.

In order to expedite the access to treatments, EMA offers accelerated assessment of MAAs, which reduces the review timeframe from 210 to 150 Days. The sponsor needs to provide sufficient justification to be eligible for this procedure, including that the medicinal product is expected to be of major public health interest (European Medicines Agency 2022f).

By September 2022, EMA authorized 20 ATMPs (12 GTMPs, 4 sCTMPs, and 4 TEPs) of which 15 hold an orphan medicinal product designation (Table 1). Six have subsequently been withdrawn due to commercial failure, the closure of manufacturing sites in the EU, safety issues, and lack of efficacy (Paul-Ehrlich Institut 2022; Iglesias-Lopez et al. 2021a; Abou-El-Enein et al. 2016). This

Table 1 Approved ATMPs in the EU (status 11 October 2022)

Name	Indication	Regulatory status	Programs
Gene therapy medicinal products			
Glybera	Hyperlipoproteinemia type I	2012 (withdrawn) MA under exceptional circumstances	Orphan drug
Imlygic	Melanoma	2015 Standard MA	
Strimvelis	Severe combined immunodeficiency	2016 Standard MA	Orphan drug
Kymriah	Precursor B-cell lymphoblastic leukemia-lymphoma, large B-cell, diffuse	2018 Standard MA	Orphan drug PRIME
Yescarta	Lymphomae, large B-cell, diffuse	2018 Standard MA	Orphan drug PRIME
Luxturna	Leber congenital amaurosis, retinitis pigmentosa	2018 Standard MA	Orphan drug
Zynteglo	β-Thalassemia	2019 (withdrawn) Conditional MA	Orphan drug PRIME
Zolgensma	Muscular atrophy, spinal	2020 Conditional MA	Orphan drug PRIME
Tecartus	Lymphoma, mantle cell	2020 Conditional MA	Orphan drug PRIME
Libmeldy	Leukodystrophy, metachromatic	2020 Standard MA	Orphan drug
Abecma	Multiple myeloma	2021 Conditional MA	Orphan drug PRIME
Somatic cell therapy medicinal products			
Provenge	Prostatic neoplasms	2013 (withdrawn) Standard MA	
Zalmoxis	Hematopoietic stem cell transplantation, graft vs. host disease	2016 (withdrawn) Conditional MA	Orphan drug
Alofisel	Rectal fistula	2018 Standard MA	Orphan drug
Carvykti	Multiple myeloma	2022 Conditional MA	Orphan drug PRIME
Tissue-engineered products			
ChondroCelect	Cartilage diseases	2009 (withdrawn) Standard MA	
MACI	Fractures, cartilage	2013 (withdrawn) Standard MA	

(continued)

Table 1 (continued)

Name	Indication	Regulatory status	Programs
Holoclar	Stem cell transplantation, corneal disease	2015 Conditional MA	Orphan drug
Spherox	Cartilage diseases	2017 Standard MA	

highlights the numerous complexities and challenges ATMP developers are facing in authorizing as well as marketing their products.

3.5 Regulatory Pathways

3.5.1 Marketing Authorization

Marketing Authorization can be granted in three ways: standard MA, conditional MA, and MA under exceptional circumstances (Detela and Lodge 2019). The type of MA largely depends on the extent of clinical data provided, the targeted indication, the size of the patient population, and the medical need. During clinical development, the applicant can obtain advice from the EMA on the most eligible route.

A standard MA is issued when a positive benefit–risk balance supported by comprehensive clinical data is provided at the time of MAA. This is the case when the efficacy and safety of the product was convincingly demonstrated in clinical trials with an adequate number of patients and a therapeutically relevant clinical endpoint. A standard MA is initially valid for 5 years, and upon renewal, for an unlimited period. The MA holder of a standard MA is usually obliged to continue monitoring safety and efficacy of the product post-authorization. Of the 20 authorized ATMPs in the EU, 12 have obtained a standard MA (Table 1).

A conditional MA is granted when comprehensive clinical data is not yet available at the time of MAA, but the medicinal product addresses an unmet medical need and the benefit of the immediate availability to patients is greater than potential safety concerns. Importantly, a conditional MAA is only granted if the benefit–risk balance is positive, and it is likely that the applicant will be able to provide comprehensive clinical data in a timely manner. A positive benefit–risk balance in the absence of comprehensive clinical data may be demonstrated through a surrogate clinical endpoint, such as a biomarker. A conditional MA is initially valid for 1 year with annual renewal and bound to specific obligations, including finishing ongoing or new clinical trials to unambiguously validate the safety and efficacy of the product and will be converted into a standard MA upon fulfillment of the obligations (European Medicines Agency 2016a). Of the 20 authorized ATMPs in the EU, 7 have obtained a conditional MA (Table 1).

An MA under exceptional circumstances is granted in the extreme case when it is not expected that comprehensive clinical data on safety and efficacy will ever be obtained, because the condition to be treated is extremely rare and the collection of sufficient data is either impossible or unethical. Therefore, it is unlikely that an MA under exceptional circumstances will ever be transformed into a standard MA. Consequently, the MAH is obliged to continuously and closely assess the safety and efficacy of the product, to report any incident related to its use and act upon it, and to allow annual re-assessment of the benefit–risk balance. An MA under exceptional circumstances is initially issued for 5 years and its extension is bound to the conclusion of the re-assessment. In the EU, MA under exceptional circumstances has so far only been issued to one ATMP, namely Glybera, a GTMP targeting the extremely rare disease hyperlipoproteinemia type I and that later on was withdrawn due to commercial failure (European Medicines Agency 2015a) (Table 1).

3.5.2 The Hospital Exemption

In Article 28(2) of Regulation 1394/2007/EC, the EU legislator gives Member States the power to authorize the use of custom-made ATMPs under extraordinary circumstances. The so-called Hospital Exemption allows, in rare cases of high unmet medical need and no treatment alternatives, an exemption from the centralized procedure, if the ATMP is used for an individual named patient on a non-commercial and non-routine basis under the exclusive responsibility of a medical practitioner in a hospital within an individual Member State of the EU. The manufacturing of the product needs to be authorized by the NCA and is regulated by national procedures. The product has to meet the same quality, traceability, and pharmacovigilance standards as an authorized product. Although the HE was originally intended to provide treatment options where none exist, experience has shown that it can be seen as a mean to circumvent a costly and time-consuming marketing authorization (European Commission 2014). The interpretation of the individual criteria of the HE within the EU is heterogenous, with regard to manufacturing and quality requirements and the extent of its use in individual Member States (Coppens et al. 2020).

3.5.3 Named Patient Use and Compassionate Use

There are other regulatory options for ATMPs, besides the HE, that are exempt from the centralized procedure pathway and allow the use of (yet) unapproved ATMPs on patients outside of clinical trials, namely the Named Patient Use and the Compassionate Use (CU) pathways. These early access pathways are not exclusive to ATMPs and allow early access to investigational medicinal products for patients in need (Coppens et al. 2020). While NPU is limited to use by individual patients, CU programs make treatments available to a specific group of patients while the product undergoes clinical trials or has entered the MAA process. In accordance with Art. 83(4) of Regulation (EC) No 726/2004, member states can make use of CU programs to help patients with life-threatening, long-lasting, or seriously debilitating illnesses, but their NCAs need to notify EMA and can optionally request an opinion from EMA regarding administration, distribution, and the use of certain medicinal products for CU.

3.6 Acceleration of Clinical Development: The PRIME Scheme

The Priority Medicines (PRIME) scheme is a program launched by EMA in 2016 to support the development of medicinal products that target an unmet medical need or offer a major therapeutic advantage over existing treatments. It builds on existing regulatory frameworks and proven tools like scientific advice and accelerated assessment to make treatments available for patients earlier by, among others, appointing rapporteurs at an early stage during clinical development and not just at the time when the intent to file an MAA is communicated. Early dialogue and enhanced interactions between the sponsor of a promising medicine and rapporteurs/EMA are intended to optimize clinical trials design to ensure that the generated data is suitable for an MAA and to increase chances of a successful MAA. Applications for PRIME need to provide evidence for eligibility in the form of early clinical data. The overall success rate is about 25%, and while ATMPs constitute only 27% of requests, they present the highest success rate of 46% of all PRIME products (European Medicines Agency 2022e).

Once a candidate medicine has been granted PRIME status, a rapporteur from the CAT is appointed to provide continuous support ahead of the MAA. Early dialogue begins with a kick-off meeting where the rapporteur and a team of multidisciplinary experts provide guidance on the overall development plan and regulatory strategy. Scientific advice is frequently offered at key developmental milestones by various stakeholders such as health-technology-assessment bodies and eligibility to accelerated assessment is confirmed at the earliest opportunity to facilitate early access to treatment.

During the first 5 years of PRIME, 18 PRIME medicines received MA and 7 of those were ATMPs (Table 1). The main therapeutic areas targeted are oncology and neurology and enrollment into PRIME reduced the evaluation time on average by about 7 months (European Medicines Agency 2022d).

4 Conclusion and Future Perspectives

Since the introduction of the regulatory framework for ATMPs in the EU 15 years ago, 20 ATMPs have been authorized with 3 more currently under evaluation (European Medicines Agency 2022c). By acknowledging the unique characteristics of these innovative medicines, numerous regulatory programs have been created to support the development of ATMPs and enable their access to the European market. Of the 20 ATMPs authorized in the EU, 15 hold an orphan drug designation, 7 were enrolled in PRIME (and 30 additional candidates are currently enrolled), and 8 have received an MA other than a standard MA (Paul-Ehrlich Institut 2022; Iglesias-Lopez et al. 2021a). Although these instruments were essential in facilitating and accelerating patients' access to treatments, the developmental and regulatory framework for ATMPs still faces numerous caveats. Flexibility on regulatory requirements allows tailored approaches for individual products, on the one hand, but also makes navigating the process complicated especially for parties unexperienced with the authorization of medicinal products like SMEs and academic institutions, on the other hand. Thus, the utilization of scientific advice greatly benefits the success of an MAA. The authorization of most ATMPs on the basis of small, open-label, uncontrolled, and single-arm pivotal trials especially for orphan diseases with low prevalence, an unmet medical need, or that are seriously debilitating may result in issues prescribing the medicine by health care providers or with reimbursement. To overcome these hurdles, the implementation of methodological improvement to clinical study design, the continued close monitoring of the safety of a product, and the integration of real-world data into the evaluation of efficacy will be essential.

ATMPs are a class of products in a fast-evolving field that demands innovation not only in scientific but also in regulatory terms. Legislative and regulatory bodies need to regularly monitor and adapt to the changing requirements of ATMP development to enable an efficient and, above all, safe entry of these innovative medicinal products to the European market.

Acknowledgment Medical writing support was provided by Marietta Hartl, SFL Regulatory Affairs & Scientific Communication, Basel, Switzerland.

References

Abou-El-Enein M, Elsanhoury A, Reinke P (2016) Overcoming challenges facing advanced therapies in the EU market. Cell Stem Cell 19(3):293–297. https://doi.org/10.1016/j.stem.2016.08.012

Agarwal Y, Beatty C, Ho S, Thurlow L, Das A, Kelly S, Castronova I, Salunke R, Biradar S, Yeshi T, Richardson A, Bility M (2020) Development of humanized mouse and rat models with full-thickness human skin and autologous immune cells. Sci Rep 10(1):14598. https://doi.org/10.1038/s41598-020-71548-z

Alliance for Regenerative Medicine, European Federation of Pharmaceutical Industries and Associations (EFPIA), European Association for Bioindustries (EuropaBio), Beattie S, Hubert A, Morrell J, Cook JA, Werner M, Ginty P, Butler G, Dahy A, Coutinho V, Roberts N, Rabbie D, Gaido M, Huh S, Olivia L, Georgieva V, Lambot N, Reimer T, de Goeij I, Romanetto J, Acha V, Tellner P (2021) Call for more effective regulation of clinical trials with advanced therapy medicinal products consisting of or containing genetically modified organisms in the European Union. Hum Gene Ther 32(19–20):997–1003. https://doi.org/10.1089/hum.2021.058

Behr M, Zhou J, Xu B, Zhang H (2021) In vivo delivery of CRISPR-Cas9 therapeutics: progress and challenges. Acta Pharm Sin B 11(8):2150–2171. https://doi.org/10.1016/j.apsb.2021.05.020

Coppens DGM, Hoekman J, De Bruin ML, Slaper-Cortenbach ICM, Leufkens HGM, Meij P, Gardarsdottir H (2020) Advanced therapy medicinal product manufacturing under the hospital exemption and other exemption pathways in seven European Union countries. Cytotherapy 22(10):592–600. https://doi.org/10.1016/j.jcyt.2020.04.092

Detela G, Lodge A (2019) EU regulatory pathways for ATMPs: standard, accelerated and adaptive pathways to marketing authorisation. Mol Ther Methods Clin Dev 13:205–232. https://doi.org/10.1016/j.omtm.2019.01.010

Elsallab M, Bravery CA, Kurtz A, Abou-El-Enein M (2020) Mitigating deficiencies in evidence during regulatory assessments of advanced therapies: a comparative study with other biologicals. Mol Ther Methods Clin Dev 18:269–279. https://doi.org/10.1016/j.omtm.2020.05.035

European Commission (2014) Report from the Commission to the European Parliament and the Council in accordance with Article 25 of Regulation (EC) No 1394/2007 of the European Parliament and of the Council on advanced therapy medicinal products and amending Directive 2001/83/EC and Regulation (EC) No 726/2004. https://eur-lex.europa.eu/legal-content/EN/TXT/PDF/?uri=CELEX:52014DC0188&from=EN. Accessed 2 Oct 2022

European Commission (2017) EudraLex, the rules governing medicinal products in the European Union (volume 4) Good Manufacturing Practice – Guidelines on Good Manufacturing Practice specific to Advances Therapy Medicinal Products. https://health.ec.europa.eu/system/files/2017-11/2017_11_22_guidelines_gmp_for_atmps_0.pdf. Accessed 12 Sept 2022

European Medicines Agency (2008) Notice to applicants – volume 2B – medicinal products for human use. Presentation and format of the dossier – Common Technical Document (CTD) https://health.ec.europa.eu/system/files/2016-11/ctd_05-2008_en_0.pdf. Accessed 7 Sept 2022

European Medicines Agency (2013) Guideline on the risk-based approach according to annex I, part IV of Directive 2001/83/EC applied to Advanced therapy medicinal products. https://www.ema.europa.eu/en/documents/scientific-guideline/guideline-risk-based-approach-according-annex-i-part-iv-directive-2001/83/ec-applied-advanced-therapy-medicinal-products_en.pdf. Accessed 12 Sept 2022

European Medicines Agency (2014) Mandate of the EMA Innovation Task Force (ITF). https://www.ema.europa.eu/en/documents/other/mandate-european-medcines-agency-innovation-task-force-itf_en.pdf. Accessed 13 Sept 2022

European Medicines Agency (2015a) Glybera EPAR. https://www.ema.europa.eu/en/documents/overview/glybera-epar-summary-public_en.pdf. Accessed 13 Sept 2022

European Medicines Agency (2015b) Reflection paper on classification of advanced therapy medicinal products. https://www.ema.europa.eu/en/documents/scientific-guideline/reflection-paper-classification-advanced-therapy-medicinal-products_en-0.pdf. Accessed 6 Sept 2022

European Medicines Agency (2016a) Guideline on the scientific application and the practical arrangements necessary to implement Commission Regulation (EC) No 507/2006 on the conditional marketing authorisation for medicinal products for human use falling within the scope of Regulation (EC) No 726/2004. https://www.ema.europa.eu/en/documents/scientific-guideline/guideline-scientific-application-practical-arrangements-necessary-implement-commission-regulation-ec/2006-conditional-marketing-authorisation-medicinal-products-human-use-falling_en.pdf. Accessed 9 Sept 2022

European Medicines Agency (2016b) Procedural advice on the certification of quality and non-clinical data for small and medium sized enterprises developing advanced therapy medicinal products. https://www.ema.europa.eu/en/documents/regulatory-procedural-guideline/procedural-advice-certification-quality-non-clinical-data-small-medium-sized-enterprises-developing_en.pdf. Accessed 6 Sept 2022

European Medicines Agency (2018a) Procedural advice on the evaluation of advanced therapy medicinal product in accordance with Article 8 of Regulation (EC) No 1394/2007. https://www.ema.europa.eu/en/documents/regulatory-procedural-guideline/procedural-advice-evaluation-advanced-therapy-medicinal-product-accordance-article-8-regulation-ec/2007_en.pdf. Accessed 7 Sept 2022

European Medicines Agency (2018b) Rare diseases, orphan medicines – getting the facts straight. https://www.ema.europa.eu/en/documents/other/rare-diseases-orphan-medicines-getting-facts-straight_en.pdf. Accessed 13 Sept 2022

European Medicines Agency (2019a) Guideline on quality, non-clinical and clinical requirements for investigantional advanced therapy medicinal products (Draft). https://www.ema.europa.eu/en/documents/scientific-guideline/draft-guideline-quality-non-clinical-clinical-requirements-investigational-advanced-therapy_en.pdf. Accessed 13 Sept 2022

European Medicines Agency (2019b) Unmet medical need: an introduction to definitions and stakeholder perceptions. https://www.ema.europa.eu/en/documents/presentation/presentation-unmet-medical-need-introduction-definitions-stakeholder-perceptions-jllinares-garcia_en.pdf. Accessed 13 Sept 2022

European Medicines Agency (2021a) Committee for Advanced Therapies (CAT). https://www.ema.europa.eu/en/documents/regulatory-procedural-guideline/cat-rules-procedure_en.pdf. Accessed 13 Sept 2022

European Medicines Agency (2021b) Procedural advice on the provision of scientific recommendation on classification of advanced therapy products in accordance with article 17 of regulation (EC) no 1394/2007. https://www.ema.europa.eu/en/documents/regulatory-procedural-guideline/procedural-advice-provision-scientific-recommendation-classification-advanced-therapy-medicinal/2007_en.pdf. Accessed 6 Sept 2022

European Medicines Agency (2022a) European Medicines Agency Guidance for Applicants seeking scientific advice and protocol assistance. https://www.ema.europa.eu/en/documents/regulatory-procedural-guideline/european-medicines-agency-guidance-applicants-seeking-scientific-advice-protocol-assistance_en.pdf. Accessed 13 Sept 2022

European Medicines Agency (2022b) European Medicines Agency pre-authorisation precedural advice for users of the centralised procedure. https://www.ema.europa.eu/en/documents/regulatory-procedural-guideline/european-medicines-agency-pre-authorisation-procedural-advice-users-centralised-procedure_en-0.pdf. Accessed 13 Sept 2022

European Medicines Agency (2022c) Medicines for human use under evaluation. https://www.ema.europa.eu/en/medicines/medicines-human-use-under-evaluation. Accessed 15 Sept 2022

European Medicines Agency (2022d) PRIME: 5 years experience. https://www.ema.europa.eu/en/documents/report/prime-5-years-experience_en.pdf. Accessed 13 Sept 2022

European Medicines Agency (2022e) PRIME: Analysis of the first 5 years' experience. https://www.ema.europa.eu/en/documents/report/prime-analysis-first-5-years-experience_en.pdf. Accessed 13 Sept 2022

European Medicines Agency (2022f) Procedural advice on the accelerated assessment of marketing authorisation applications pursuant to Article 44 (3) of Regulation (EU) No 2019/6. https://www.ema.europa.eu/en/documents/regulatory-procedural-guideline/procedural-advice-accelerated-assessment-marketing-authorisation-applications-pursuant-article-44-3/6_en.pdf. Accessed 13 Sept 2022

Farkas AM, Mariz S, Stoyanova-Beninska V, Celis P, Vamvakas S, Larsson K, Sepodes B (2017) Advanced therapy medicinal products for rare diseases: state of play of incentives supporting development in Europe. Front Med (Lausanne) 4:53. https://doi.org/10.3389/fmed.2017.00053

Gaasterland CMW, van der Weide MCJ, du Prie-Olthof MJ, Donk M, Kaatee MM, Kaczmarek R, Lavery C, Leeson-Beevers K, O'Neill N, Timmis O, van Nederveen V, Vroom E, van der Lee JH (2019) The patient's view on rare disease trial design - a qualitative study. Orphanet J Rare Dis 14(1):31. https://doi.org/10.1186/s13023-019-1002-z

Iglesias-Lopez C, Agusti A, Vallano A, Obach M (2021a) Current landscape of clinical development and approval of advanced therapies. Mol Ther Methods Clin Dev 23:606–618. https://doi.org/10.1016/j.omtm.2021.11.003

Iglesias-Lopez C, Agusti A, Vallano A, Obach M (2021b) Methodological characteristics of clinical trials supporting the marketing authorisation of advanced therapies in the European Union. Front Pharmacol 12:773712. https://doi.org/10.3389/fphar.2021.773712

Ito M, Hiramatsu H, Kobayashi K, Suzue K, Kawahata M, Hioki K, Ueyama Y, Koyanagi Y, Sugamura K, Tsuji K, Heike T, Nakahata T (2002) NOD/SCID/gamma(c)(null) mouse: an excellent recipient mouse model for engraftment of human cells. Blood 100(9):3175–3182. https://doi.org/10.1182/blood-2001-12-0207

Kooijman M, van Meer PJ, Gispen-de Wied CC, Moors EH, Hekkert MP, Schellekens H (2013) The risk-based approach to ATMP development – generally accepted by regulators but infrequently used by companies. Regul Toxicol Pharmacol 67(2):221–225. https://doi.org/10.1016/j.yrtph.2013.07.014

Lopez-Navas L, Torrents S, Sanchez-Pernaute R, Vives J (2022) Compliance in non-clinical development of cell-, gene-, and tissue-based medicines: good practice for better therapies. Stem Cells Transl Med 11(8):805–813. https://doi.org/10.1093/stcltm/szac046

Milazzo G, De Luca M, Pellegrini G (2016) Holoclar: first of its kind in more ways than one. Cell Gene Ther Insights 2(2):183–197. https://doi.org/10.18609/cgti.2016.023

Paul-Ehrlich Institut (2022) Advanced therapy medicinal products (ATMPs). https://www.pei.de/EN/medicinal-products/atmp/atmp-node.html. Accessed 9 Sept 2022

Pizevska M, Kaeda J, Fritsche E, Elazaly H, Reinke P, Amini L (2022) Advanced therapy medicinal Products' translation in Europe: a developers' perspective. Front Med (Lausanne) 9:757647. https://doi.org/10.3389/fmed.2022.757647

Salazar-Fontana LI (2022) A regulatory risk-based approach to ATMP/CGT development: integrating scientific challenges with current regulatory expectations. Front Med (Lausanne) 9:855100. https://doi.org/10.3389/fmed.2022.855100

Silva Lima B, Videira MA (2018) Toxicology and biodistribution: the clinical value of animal biodistribution studies. Mol Ther Methods Clin Dev 8:183–197. https://doi.org/10.1016/j.omtm.2018.01.003

The European Parliament and the Council of the European Union (2020) Regulation (EU) 2020/1043 of the European Parliament and of the Council on the conduct of clinical trials with and supply of medicinal products for human use containing or consisting of genetically modified organisms intended to treat or prevent coronavirus disease (COVID-19). https://eur-lex.europa.eu/legal-content/EN/TXT/PDF/?uri=CELEX:32020R1043&from=en. Accessed 7 Oct 2022

Looking to the Future: Drug Delivery and Targeting in the Prophylaxis and Therapy of Severe and Chronic Diseases

Monika Schäfer-Korting

Contents

M. Schäfer-Korting (✉)
Freie Universität Berlin, Pharmacology and Toxicology, Berlin, Germany
e-mail: monika.schaefer-korting@fu-berlin.de

M. Schäfer-Korting, U. S. Schubert (eds.), *Drug Delivery and Targeting*,
Handbook of Experimental Pharmacology 284, https://doi.org/10.1007/164_2023_696

Abstract

High molecular weight actives and cell-based therapy have the potential to revolutionize the prophylaxis and therapy of severe diseases. Yet, the size and nature of the agents – proteins, nucleic acids, cells – challenge drug delivery and thus formulation development. Moreover, off-target effects may result in severe adverse drug reactions. This makes delivery and targeting an essential component of high-end drug development. Loading to nanoparticles facilitates delivery and enables targeted mRNA vaccines and tumor therapeutics. Stem cell therapy opens up a new horizon in diabetes type 1 among other domains which may enhance the quality of life and life expectancy. Cell encapsulation protects transplants against the recipient's immune system, may ensure long-term efficacy, avoid severe adverse reactions, and simplify the management of rare and fatal diseases.

The knowledge gained so far encourages to widen the spectrum of potential indications. Co-development of the active agent and the vehicle has the potential to accelerate drug research. One recommended starting point is the use of computational approaches. Transferability of preclinical data to humans will benefit from performing studies first on validated human 3D disease models reflecting the target tissue, followed by studies on validated animal models. This makes approaching a new level in drug development a multidisciplinary but ultimately worthwhile and attainable challenge. Intense monitoring of the patients after drug approval and periodic reporting to physicians and scientists remain essential for the safe use of drugs especially in rare diseases and pave future research.

Keywords

Antitumor immunotherapy · Cell therapies · Clinical studies · Drug targeting · Gene delivery · RNA delivery · Strategic preclinical drug evaluation

Abbreviations

AAV	Adeno-associated virus
ACE-2	Angiotensin-converting enzyme 2
ADR	Adverse drug reaction(s)
AIDS	Acquired immunodeficiency syndrome
ASO	Antisense oligonucleotide(s)
ATMP	Advanced therapy medicinal products
CART	Chimeric antigen receptor T
CDN	Claudin
COVID-19	Corona virus disease 2019
CRISPR	Clustered regularly interspaced short palindromic repeat (DNA sequences)
DC	Dendritic cells
EMA	European Medicines Agency

FDA	Food and Drug Administration (USA)
GFP	Green fluorescent protein
hESC	human embryonic stem cells
i.m.	Intramuscular
i.v.	Intravenous
IDDM	Insulin-dependent diabetes mellitus
iPSCs	Induced pluripotent stem cells
LNP(s)	Lipid nanoparticle(s)
s.c.	Subcutaneous
SARS-CoV-2	Severe acute respiratory syndrome corona-virus 2
siRNA	Small interfering RNA(s)
SMA	Spinal muscular atrophy (types 1 and 2)
SMN	Genes encoding for spinal muscular atrophy (types 1 and 2)
TLR	Toll-like receptor(s)
VEGF	Vascular endothelial growth factor
VOCs	Virus variants of concern
WHO	World Health Organization

1 Introduction

Despite major successes in medical research, there are still diseases that respond either inadequately or not at all to drugs and for which surgery is not an option. Recent insights into molecular pathology indicate promising new directions which give rise to the following challenges:

- Delivery of high molecular weight drugs (proteins, gene therapeutics) and cell therapeutics
- Selective access to regions of specific interest
- The use of agents of narrow benefit/risk ratio
- Therapy of severe diseases in newborns and geriatric patients

The previous chapters outline a number of approaches opening up paths to advance in these directions. The current chapter aims to bring the various aspects together with a dual focus on safety and efficacy. An overview showcasing promising results of cooperative and efficient approaches along these lines suggests a path for future research.

The worldwide threat created by the SARS-CoV-2 virus pandemic (COVID-19) has stimulated a joint approach to drug development and approval. The close cooperation of experts from academia and industry representing virology, vaccine development, and drug delivery resulted in rapid successes. Building up new facilities for vaccine production, running intercontinental large-size clinical studies, raising significant funding – private and public – and the early involvement of drug regulatory bodies significantly slowed the spread of the disease and saved lives. Innovative, targeted mRNA-based vaccines and vector-based vaccines proved to be game changers.

The use of nucleic acids also opens up new avenues for the therapy of severe and recalcitrant diseases. In particular, tumor therapy can leverage nucleic acids targeting to enhance efficacy and reduce off-target effects. Stem cells also have the potential to prove game changers, but equally require the joint development of drugs and delivery systems. Examples and major hurdles to be overcome are presented here to envisage the future. Due to often limited predictive power of preclinical data for humans (Wong et al. 2019), the discussion preferentially focuses on data generated in human subjects.

2 Vaccines and Vaccine Delivery

2.1 SARS-CoV-2Vaccines: Entering Global Challenges

Beginning in 2019, the COVID-19 pandemic has challenged human societies. Pulmonal uptake of the virus occurs via a fusion protein anchored in the viral membrane. The inactive precursor (1,273 amino acids in size) is cleaved, releasing the receptor-binding S1 peptide and the fusion S2 peptide (Hoffmann et al. 2020). Virus binding via the S1 domain to the host cell receptor (angiotensin-converting enzyme 2; ACE-2) activates the fusion peptide S2 which enables merging of the viral envelope and host cell membrane (Shang et al. 2020).

By delivering or encoding the viral S1 protein in the prefusion conformation, vaccines induce the production of neutralizing antibodies and activate immune cells and the innate immune system (Fig. 1a, b; Mistry et al. 2022). Moreover, mRNA vaccines activate pattern-recognition receptors, resulting in self-adjuvanting effects (Linares-Fernández et al. 2020). However, vaccine activity strongly depends on the virus strain and mutations occur rapidly.

The target protein of the original virus has already undergone several mutations (Fig. 1c). Virus Variants of Concern (VOCs) are strains with several ACE-2 mutations resulting in enhanced transmissibility or severity of the disease which creates epidemiologic challenges. For instance, the Omicron variant was confirmed in 110 countries by the end of 2021 (Vitiello et al. 2022), mutations are ongoing.

Vaccination should reduce the infection rate by at least 50% in vehicle-controlled clinical trials. Drug Administrations in the EU and the USA among others have approved such vaccines. Those are

- S-protein-specific mRNA-based vaccines (*Tozinameran* or *BNT162b2*, Comirnaty® and *Elasomeran* or mRNA-1273, Spikevax®, including bivalent vaccines for the original plus Omicron variant),
- Adenovector virus-based vaccines (*AZD1222*, Vaxzevria) and (*AD26.COV2.S*, Jcovden), and
- the recombinant spike protein (Nuvaxovid®; saponin adjuvanted)

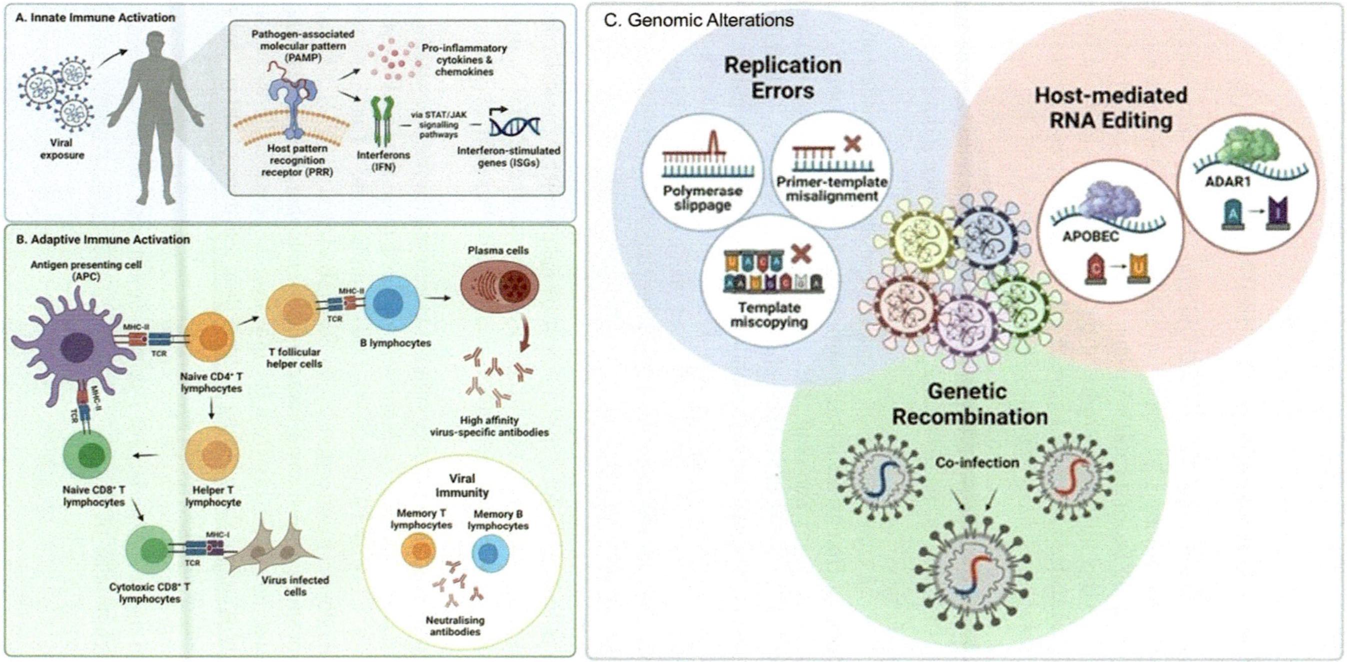

Fig. 1 Innate (**a**) and adaptive (**b**) branches of the immune system activated in viral infections and vaccines. Molecular mechanisms (**c**) introducing genomic alterations in SARS-CoV-2 (from Mistry et al. 2022, with permission from Frontiers)

Moreover, aluminum-adjuvanted vaccines containing the inactivated original (WUHAN) strain (COVID-19 Vaccine Valneva; CoronaVac) are used in the Global WHO Vaccination Strategy (Das et al. 2023).

2.1.1 mRNA Vaccines: Nanoparticle-Supported Delivery and Targeting

mRNA vaccines encoding the SARS-CoV-2 spike protein are front runners to control the COVID-19 pandemic. The rapid availability of VOC-adapted vaccines demonstrates the flexibility of the mRNA technology *and* the efficacy of joint research.

The single-stranded mRNA is produced by in vitro transcription in large scale (Cui et al. 2022). Loaded to lipid nanoparticles (LNPs) and *injected by the i.m. route*, the mRNA is *taken up by local immune cells* and transferred into the viral S-protein which induces the production and release of neutralizing antibodies.[1] Antigen-specific T helper cells, natural killer cells, and memory cells become activated (Pardi et al. 2015; Sahin et al. 2014) and T memory cells are induced (Teijaro and Farber 2021).

The LNPs (Fig. 2), around 80 nm in size, are the result of systematic optimization. They are made up of cationic ionizable phosphatidylcholine facilitating RNA encapsulation (Pardi et al. 2015; Yan et al. 2022) plus cholesterol, neutral lipid, and PEG lipid. The pro-inflammatory character enhances immunogenicity (Aliahmad et al. 2022). PEG lipids provide colloidal stability, prevent opsonin binding, and thus clearance. Moreover, PEG lipids appear to be involved in membrane fusion (Ramachandran et al. 2022). Optimization of the carrier and testing new lipid components becomes possible by robotic lipid screening. A high-throughput screening platform for fully automatic lipid handling and precise mixing generates reproducibly mRNA-loaded nanoparticles with up to 384 formulations per plate (Cui et al. 2022).

Potential alternatives include the injection of naked mRNA, mRNA loaded to cationic polymers or to dendritic cells (DCs; Ramachandran et al. 2022). In addition, the use of detachable microneedle patches is proposed (Wu et al. 2023).

Pivotal Clinical Studies Observer-blind, randomized, *vehicle-controlled Phase 3 studies* on *Elasomeran* and *Tozinameran* included more than 30,000 volunteers at high risk for COVID-19 infection or its complications. Two i.m. injections reduced the likelihood of infection by 94–95% (Baden et al. 2021; Pollack et al. 2020). The protection against severe cases was even higher. Efficacy is close to the immune response after recovery from the infection. In general, the vaccines induce minor local and systemic short lasting adverse drug reactions (ADRs). One rare but severe complication is myocarditis, predominantly in young males (≈12.6 cases per million Tozinameran vaccinations), but improvement in many cases spontaneously occurs. Due to the favorable benefit-risk assessment, vaccination is recommended for everyone ≥6 months of age.

[1] The Nobel Prize in Medicine and Physiology 2023 is awarded to Dr. Drew Weissman and Dr. Katalin Karikó because of their groundbreaking discoveries in mRNA interaction with the immune system and mRNA delivery by lipid nanoparticles.

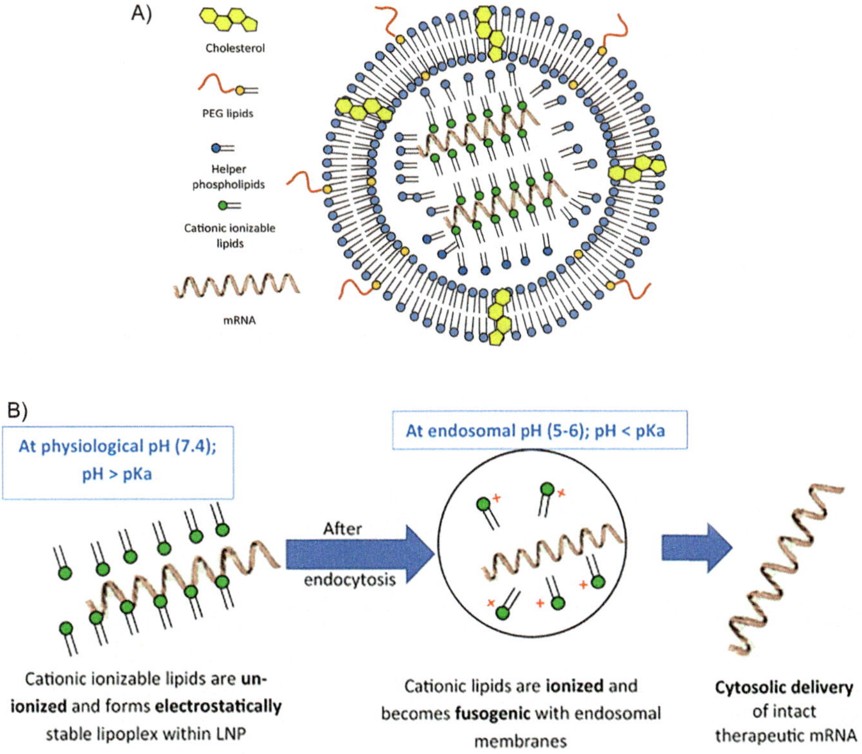

Fig. 2 Schematic depiction of liposomes transporting mRNA vaccines (**a**) and mRNA release at the site of delivery to local immune cells (**b**) (from Ramachandran et al. 2022, with permission from Springer Nature)

The rapid availability of SARS-CoV-2-vaccines, including adaptations to the Omicron variant, demonstrates the flexibility of the mRNA technology as well as the efficacy of a joint approach by the vaccine industry and academia. Moreover, the lessons learned may significantly enhance the development of other antiviral and therapeutic tumor vaccines. Lipid variations and further lipid components can induce targeting to alternate sites of interest when aiming for alternate indications. LNP compositions with specially designed lipids may enhance encapsulation efficiency, biodegradability, storage life time and reduce the formation of PEG antibodies.

2.1.2 Other SARS-CoV-2 Vaccines of Major Relevance

Adenovector-based vaccines (AZD1222 and AD26.COV2.S) deliver viral DNA which is transcribed into the S-Protein activating the immune response. Very rare (1:100,000 vaccine exposures; Sharifian-Dorche et al. 2021), yet potentially fatal intracranial venous sinus thrombosis restricts the use to less often affected persons aged 60 years and older. The severe ADR predominantly occurs in young and middle-aged females.

2.1.3 Intranasal Vaccination

In mice and *rhesus macaques* an *intranasal vaccination* by an adenovector-based vaccine induces a weaker response compared to i.m. dosing, yet macaques were protected against SARS-CoV-2 after 4 weeks (Feng et al. 2020). In mice an intranasal booster enhances IgA formation and the formation of neutralizing antibodies directed to the Omicron variant BA.5 in particular (Wang et al. 2023). The next steps will be to prove the stability of the immunogens for local degradation by proteases (Sécher and Mayor 2019) and to test the formulations for stability under storage and in use (nebulization; refer to Carneiro et al. 2022).

2.2 Immunotherapy and Cancer Vaccines

Immunotherapy in cancer addresses proteins overexpressed in transformed cells (*tumor-associated antigens*) or tumor-only expressed *neoantigens*. An ideal agent selectively addresses epitopes in tumor subtypes (or even in individual patients) and thereby improves life expectancy *and* well-being of the patient (Shemesh et al. 2021). However, the diagnostic and therapeutic approaches still are under clinical investigation (Xie et al. 2023) and related costs appear currently unforeseeable.

The front runner of cancer immunotherapy *sipuleucel-T* (Provenge®) is a fusion protein of the tumor-associated *prostatic acid phosphatase antigen* and Granulocyte-Macrophages-Colony Stimulating Factor, which is loaded to autologous mononuclear cells. Overall survival in *antiandrogen-resistant* **prostate carcinoma** is extended following 1–3 doses (Kantoff et al. 2010; Higano et al. 2019). Yet, several tumor-associated antigens in prostate cancer limit the efficacy of targeting a single one.

Gastric Cancer is among the most frequent cancers, and patients are often diagnosed in advanced stages. Current palliative chemotherapy enhances median survival by less than 1 year. The mutant tight-junction protein *claudin 18.2* is overexpressed in advanced-stage gastric cancer and limits drug access to the tumor. Binding to the mutant protein *Zolbetuximab,* a chimeric monoclonal *claudin 18.2 antibody* activates the complement system and induces antibody-dependent cytotoxicity. Added to the established first-line therapy zolbetuximab improves progression-free survival and overall survival without an increase in ADR (Sahin et al. 2021).

2.2.1 mRNA Vaccines for Immunotherapy in Oncology

mRNA technology can also be used to generate "tumor vaccines": Encoded antibodies target tumor-specific mutations in unresectable gastric cancer, melanoma, non-small cell bronchial tumor, pancreas carcinoma, glioblastoma. In principle, even *individual mRNA tumor vaccines* addressing up to 20 neoantigens per patient can be produced and delivered "on demand."

In an uncontrolled study, mRNA encoding five tumor-specific antigens (RNActive®) plus local irradiation were applied in locally advanced or metastatic **non-small cell lung cancer** (26 patients) *after the standard therapy*. Tumor-specific T cells and antibody formation increased in 84% and 40% of the patients, respectively. Adverse effects were mild or moderate reactions at the injection site and flu-like symptoms (Papachristofilou et al. 2019).

A Phase I study indicated the formation of neoantigen-specific T cells in 8 out of 16 patients with **pancreatic ductal adenocarcinoma** and increased recurrence-free survival in responders (Rojas et al. 2023). mRNA adaptations appear possible in case of mutation-associated regrowth of a tumor. Whether this leads to tumor control for a relevant period of time is still open. Combinations with a potent vaccine adjuvant and/or a "classical" anticancer drug may further enhance activity.

In **unresectable melanoma**, liposomal mRNA encoding four antigens including melanoma-associated antigen A3 (*Melanoma FixVac*) induced $CD4^+$ and $CD8^+$ responses and partial regression of tumor lesions including checkpoint-inhibitor pre-treated patients ($n = 89$; Sahin et al. 2020). Effects were also seen in *murine models* when applying iontophoresis for mRNA delivery (Husseini et al. 2023).

A Major Challenge: Glioblastoma Overcoming the blood–brain barrier (BBB) and the rapid mutation of target proteins, however, are major obstacles in treating glioblastoma. Transient BBB opening of localized brain regions by Magnetic-Resonance-Imaging-guided ultrasound in animals may allow for a noninvasive, regional, and transient drug exposure to the tumor while limiting exposure of the healthy brain. However, transferability is challenged by the thickness and variability of human skulls (Burgess and Hynynen 2013). Whether the loss of claudin-3 and altered expression of other tight-junction proteins enables access of personalized vaccines and/or CART immunotherapies (Yu and Quail 2021) remains an open question, too. Long-term glioblastoma survivors often exhibit favorable prognostic factors such as small tumors and young age (Armocida et al. 2019).

2.2.2 Outlook

The success of mRNA-based tumor vaccines might be further enhanced by the use of synthetic self-replicating mRNA (srRNA) vaccines generating higher amounts of proteins for an extended time. Delivery occurs by lipid nanoparticles and polymers (Aliahmad et al. 2022) as described.

3 RNA Interference and Gene Therapy

The heterogenous group of Advanced Therapeutic Medicinal Products (ATMPs) encompasses gene therapeutics, products for somatic cell therapy, and tissue-engineered products. ATMPs are approved for orphan diseases and unmet clinical needs. The active component is recombinant nucleic acid aimed to regulate, repair, replace, add, or remove a nucleotide sequence in humans. Effects should be organ specific and long lasting in chronic diseases. A single-dose therapy is the final goal in gene therapy.

Potent and specific delivery systems offer therapeutic options in previously untreatable diseases and those poorly responding to drugs. Defenses keeping invading nucleic acids out of the cells can be overcome by *cationic nanoparticles* close to those of mRNA vaccines (Zhang et al. 2009; Chen et al. 2023). Binding of *GalNac drug conjugates* to asialoglycoprotein receptors on *hepatocytes* induces liver targeting (Nair et al. 2014). Moreover, human non-pathogenic *adeno-associated viruses* (AAV) can be used for targeted delivery. AAV5 is used to target the liver, AAV9 and AAV2 are used for delivery to the brain. Yet, the first-generation AAVs appear to be suboptimal for human use. Potentially low efficacy in human asks for relatively large vector doses inducing immune responses in human and tropism in animal models may not translate to human (Srivasta 2023).

Moreover, detailed insights into particle–cell interactions enable tissue-specific delivery by systematic modifications of nanoparticle surfaces, so-called selective organ targeting *(SORT)*. The inclusion of quaternary ammonium headgroups ($pK_A > 9$) favors pulmonal delivery and anionic lipids (pK_A 2–6) induce spleen targeting (Dilliard et al. 2021).

Clinical development and drug approval, however, are challenged by often low numbers of patients to be enrolled in clinical studies. Pivotal clinical trials are often small, open-labeled, single-arm studies. In addition, since efficacy is often compared to historical controls, the standard of care may not reflect current therapy. Unmet clinical needs as well as the complexity of these agents can justify approval of an innovative agent despite limited clinical data availability. Thus, ongoing intense monitoring of benefits and risks is essential (Iglesias-Lopez et al. 2021).

3.1 Antisense Oligonucleotides (ASOs) and Small Interfering RNAs (siRNAs)

By binding to complementary mRNA segments, single-stranded ASOs and double-stranded siRNAs inhibit protein synthesis. To improve drugability, ASOs are chemically modified to improve stability against cleavage by RNases and hydrolases. The modifications also enhance cellular uptake as size (often >12 kDa), strong anionic charge (>40 phosphodiester linkages), and hydrophilicity ($\log P < 1$) impair the diffusion of cell membranes. siRNAs, however, are delivered by lipid nanoparticles close to those used for mRNA vaccines (for further information on delivery, refer to chapter Reichel and Träger 2023).

Transthyretin Amyloidosis Transthyretin gene mutation results in protein misfolding and the accumulation of protein fragments with amyloid deposits in heart and peripheral nerves. Cardiomyopathy and neuropathy limit life expectancy after diagnosis to 2–6 and 4–17 years, respectively. In particular, the cardiac function appears to improve following the therapy. The ASO *Inotersen* (Tegsedi®) and the siRNAs *Patisiran* (Onpattro™) and *Vutrisiran* inhibit the formation of disturbed transthyretin (Aimo et al. 2022). The slow elimination of the *Vutrisiran* allows for an extended dosing interval (3 months) and this siRNA appears to be better tolerated (Adams et al. 2023), too. For CRISPR-cas9 therapy, see Sect. 3.4.

Hypercholesterolemia GalNac conjugated siRNAs target hepatocytes. *Inclisiran* (Leqvio) induces the breakdown of the mRNA strand of the PCSK9 gene, thereby reducing hepatic cholesterol and LDL-C formation by about 50% (Frampton 2023). The very slowly eliminated drug (McDougall et al. 2022) is applied by s.c. injections on day 1, 90, and every 6 months thereafter for statin-intolerant *hypercholesterolemia* and – in combination with statins – in patients failing to normalize on statin monotherapy. First-line therapy of hypercholesterolemia should be considered based on the benefits and risks associated with statins and inclisiran in the long run. This is currently unknown for the new drug.

For *Nusinersen,* see Sect. 3.3.

3.2 Gene Therapies

Ideally, application of a single dose should lead to ongoing improvement under gene therapy. Yet, gene delivery to the target organ is a challenge. With respect to the eye, however, subretinal injection enables direct access to the retina (see also Sect. 4.2.1).

Voretigene neparvovec (Luxturna®) is a copy of the all-trans retinyl isomerase gene. Subretinal injection improves loss of vision in *inherited retinal dystrophy due to the RPE65 mutation.* However, only the minority of **retinitis pigmentosa** patients have this genetic defect. Moreover, for a relevant stabilization of vison, the retina must still contain a sufficient number of functional cells. In contrast to gene therapy, cell therapies replacing deficient receptors might also be effective in advanced retinitis pigmentosa (Russel et al. 2017).

The outcome of voretigene neparvovec therapy, however, could have a major impact on research: because of the *nonreplicating target cell,* a single dose should induce a permanent improvement. Unfortunately, this does not apply to the majority of genetic diseases (Chiu et al. 2021).

In addition, gene therapy is becoming available for rare inborn genetic diseases including **hemophilia A**. The need for factor VIII infusions in severe bleeding decreases by 98.6% following AAV5-delivered factor VIII (1 year study period; Ozelo et al. 2022). Long-term larger size studies will show if a single-dose therapy will be suitable for hemophilia A therapy.

3.3 Spinal Muscular Atrophies: Gene and ASO Therapies

The lack of functional Survival Motor Neuron (SMN) proteins results in spinal muscular atrophy (SMA). SMA1 is a neurodegenerative disease caused by biallelic mutations in the SMN1 gene – the SMN2 gene produces only a minor SMN protein amount. SMA1 manifests in neonates and results in motor neuron degeneration, progressive muscle atrophy, weakness, and early death. Before the emergence of disease-modifying therapies, children did not achieve the ability to sit independently and less than 10% survived beyond 20 months of age without permanent ventilator support (Reilly et al. 2023).

In *SMA1,* the SMN1 gene *Onasemnogene abeparvovec* (Zolgensma®) is AAV9 delivered to the brain. Following a *single-dose therapy*, patients can sit or stand. Efficacy is best with early treatment (Mendell et al. 2021). Among 18-month-olds, all children studied (14) survived without ventilation and could sit independently. The normal development of 11 children demonstrates the efficacy of the drug and of newborn screening (Strauss et al. 2022). The future will show whether the single-dose therapy maintains the anticipated ongoing efficacy.

The **ASO** *Nusinersen* (Spinraza®) is indicated for *SMA2* in newborns, children, and adults. The 2′-methyl-O-ethylether substituent of ribose modifies *SMN2* pre-mRNA splicing, resulting in the formation of an SMN2 protein of higher activity. Event-free and overall survival time increase if therapy starts before the end of month 3 (Crooke et al. 2021). Nusinersen is incapable of crossing the BBB, intrathecally applied ASOs distribute into spinal cord and brain with a maximum uptake of about 4%. Elimination occurs by slow redistribution (Monine et al. 2021). ADRs are linked to the essential *repeated intrathecal injections*.

Oral therapy becomes possible using the **small molecule** *Risdiplam* (Evrysdi), surmounting the BBB and modifying *SMN2* pre-mRNA splicing. In *SMA1,* however, Risdiplam appears less potent than Onasemnogen abeparovec (Reilly et al. 2023).

Complex genetics challenge drug development. Thus, in *amyotrophic lateral sclerosis* and *Alzheimer's disease* (among other diseases) improved understanding of the various causative genes appears essential (Suzuki et al. 2023; Imbimbo et al. 2023).

3.4 CRISPR-cas9 Therapy

Alterations of short DNA nucleotide sequences are targeted by Clustered Regularly Interspaced Short Palindromic Repeat (CRISPR) RNA. The flexible system can be used ex vivo (genome editing of hematopoietic progenitor cells in *sickle cell anemia*; Doudna 2020) and in vivo. However, the sophisticated synthesis of RNA oligonucleotides, the need for optimized genome editing enzymes, and the lack of vehicles for delivery which avoid off-target effects challenge research and the application to humans (van Haasteren et al. 2020; Rees et al. 2021). Delivery is possible by AAVs, yet safety appears to be superior with lipid- and polymer-based nanoparticles (Wang et al. 2022).

A Phase 1 study in 6 *transthyretin amyloidosis* patients indicates that CRISPR-cas9 therapy (using lipid nanoparticles for delivery) interferes with the ongoing accumulation of the misfolded protein in nerves and heart (87% following a single 0.3 mg/kg dose; Gillmore et al. 2021).

4 Cell Therapies

Modified autologous T cells significantly add to the armamentarium for tumor therapy. Stem cell therapy is at the horizon for ocular diseases and insufficiently controlled *insulin-dependent diabetes mellitus* (IDDM) among others. Delivery systems protecting the actives on their path to the target are frequently included into the initial research strategy, as exemplified here.

4.1 Chimeric Antigen Receptor T (CART) Cell Immunotherapies

CART cells comprise an extracellular antigen-recognition domain joint to an intracellular T cell activation domain. Ex vivo genetic modification of autologous T cells – typically by *lentiviral transduction* – results in the expression of chimeric receptors targeting antigens highly expressed in tumors. CART immunotherapy is effective even for advanced hematological tumors poorly responding to other drugs. In lymphoma, remissions over 2 years following *ciltacabtagene autoleucel* have been reported (Martin et al. 2023). Yet, CART cell production and therapy come at significant costs. An economic evaluation of CART cell therapy as with ATMP therapy in general is unreliable as long as life extension and quality of life are unknown (Lloyd-Williams and Hughes 2021).

4.2 Approaching Stem Cell Therapy

4.2.1 Ocular Diseases

Retinal neovascularization and local edema induce major *macular degeneration* which becomes obvious by blurred vision. Due to the small anatomical size of the macula a low number of induced pluripotent stem cells (iPSC) appear sufficient to improve the vision in **age-related macular degeneration** and in **retinitis pigmentosa** which already occurs at a younger age. Applied into the subretinal space iPSC can halt disease progression by integration into the outer retinal layers. Application of cell suspensions appears to be less prone to complications while cell sheets keep cells properly oriented. Major needs are standardized cell sources and procedures, clinical trials are ongoing. Lessons learned are summarized (Fortress et al. 2023).

4.2.2 Diabetes Mellitus Type 1

Insulin therapy (+/– additional antidiabetic drugs) by 1–2 injections a day or using an implantable insulin pump enables a significant reduction of blood glucose levels and a relevant, though not full, extension of life expectancy in insulin-dependent diabetes mellitus (IDDM). 1,665 patients using *fully-automated insulin delivery systems* did not report major adverse drug reactions, in particular no life-threatening changes in blood glucose. Treatment burdens were linked to the size and appearance of the devices (Munoz-Velandia et al. 2019). On this will be results of further attempts to improve the therapy of type-1 diabetics to be measured.

Transplantation of stem cells differentiated to β-cells might further improve life expectancy and quality of life. Yet, allogenic islet transplantation is investigational and available only very rarely – in particular, if kidney transplantation is needed, too. Donors of human pancreatic islets are scarce and the islet isolation process is not yet optimized. Implementation of CRISPR/cas9 for genome engineering may facilitate knocking-out Human Leukocyte Antigen (HLA) surface molecules implicated in autoimmunity. Yet, immune and non-immune stressors induce islets attrition (Triolo and Bellin 2021).

Thus "safe-space" delivery systems (Fig. 3; Melton 2021) are aimed for to protect implants against the host's immune system and were already *studied in animals*. For example, a nanofibrous device prevents the evasion of β-cells while maintaining maximum insulin transfer. Normoglycemia is rapidly restored and lasts for up to 60 days in immunocompetent and 120 days in immunodeficient animals, respectively (Wang et al. 2021). The use of materials impeding cellular overgrowth (Liu et al. 2021) and oxygen-generating microbeads may overcome hypoxia-induced destruction of transplants in the critical phase shortly after implantation (Liang et al. 2021).

Long-term studies in humans have to demonstrate ongoing efficiency and safety of stem cell transplantation with and without safe-space delivery. This may also pave the path for personalized regenerative therapies beyond diabetes mellitus.

INCLUDEPICTURE "D:\crvar\crfolders\cr82 \cr_ln_926d1wd1n0zwy00xf6s80000gn\crT\crcom.microsoft.Word \crWebArchiveCopyPasteTempFiles\crpage1image50911952" * MERGEFORMAT

4.2.3 Disorders of the Brain

Drug delivery to the brain is extremely challenged by the blood–brain barrier (BBB). This particularly holds true for the delivery of hydrophilic and high molar mass drugs and with cells. Several noninvasive measures have been developed. In particular,

- increasing lipophilicity by prodrug formation,
- AAV9 supported gene delivery,
- loading drugs to nanocarriers, and
- transient BBB opening in localized brain regions by guided ultrasound (Burgess and Hynynen 2013; for use in human, see Sect. 2.2.1).

Stem cells delivered to the brain by co-developed innovative devices may become game changers for major neurological diseases in the aging population (in particular Parkinson's disease and Huntington's disease; Berlet et al. 2022; Barker et al. 2021).

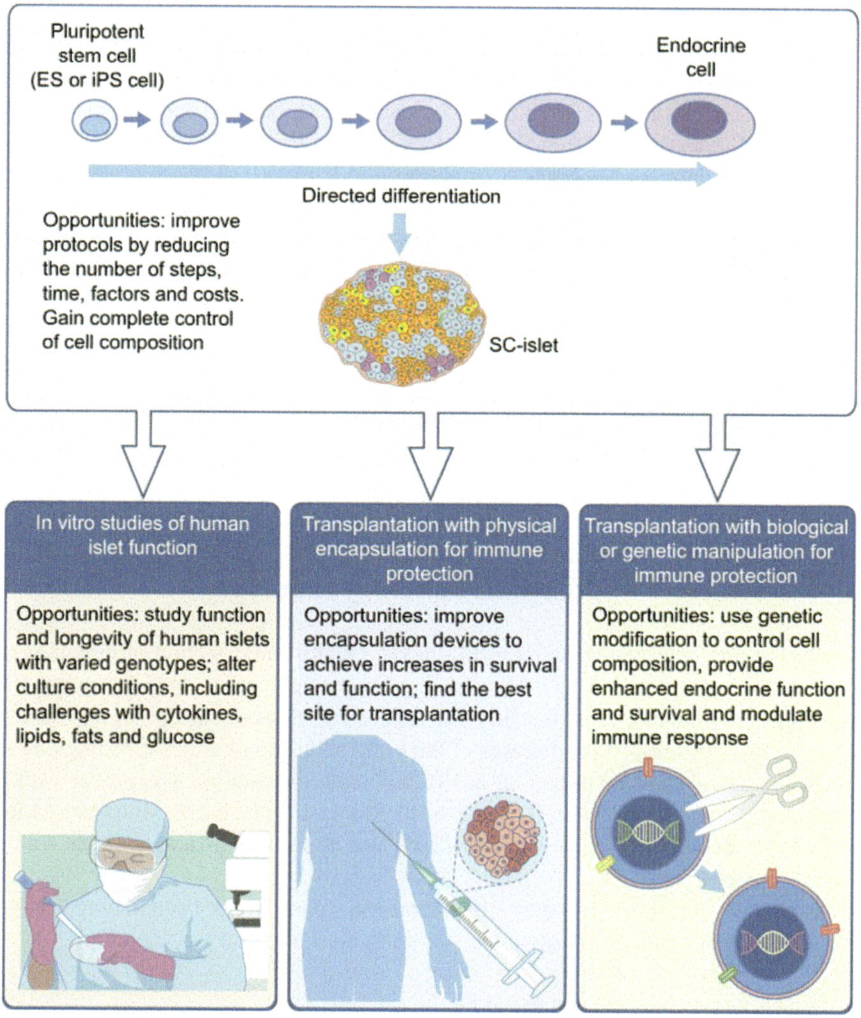

Fig. 3 Approaching improved therapy of severe type-1 diabetes mellitus (from Melton 2021, with permission from Springer Nature)

The neurorestorative approach may enable more people to live independently in old age.

Parkinson's Disease (PD) results from the ongoing degeneration of dopaminergic neurons in the substantia nigra, which leads to a decline in dopamine production and storage. Consequently, current long-term therapy using dopaminergic (+/– anticholinergic) drugs loses efficiency over time and fluctuating motility occurs. Grafting dopamine-producing stem cells from bone marrow or transfecting gene-encoding enzymes involved in dopamine synthesis may restore the dopamine loss in resident cells and retard the fading of the improved motility, on-off-target effects should decline. This is indicated by a Phase I/II clinical study on early-stage Parkinson patients *intraputaminally* exposed to dopamine neurotrophic factor (infusions via implanted catheters). For larger clinical trials and an introduction to therapy, a less burdensome application is requested (Lindholm and Saarma 2022), suitable delivery systems need to be developed. Long-term studies will have to prove ongoing efficacy and tolerability.

Ischemic stroke, the second leading cause of death globally, arises from thrombic or embolic events disrupting the blood supply in the brain resulting in irreversible neuronal damage. Reperfusion by tissue plasminogen activators is possible, but prone to severe ADRs. Transplanted stem-cell-derived progenitor cells, while efficacious and safe in animal models, fail in humans (Borlongan 2019). Therefore, rigorous stem cell characterization and standardized clinical application in future studies have been requested (Brooks et al. 2022). Whether improved delivery may be an answer remains open. Facing the current limited transferability of results in animals to human, this topic has to be taken up early in drug research as outlined below.

5 Strategic Approaches: Bundling Expertise

Understanding diseases at the molecular level enables the detection of new targets and the design of new drugs. However, overcoming barriers to the targets still challenges drug therapy, particularly for cancer and diseases in the brain. In fact, 85% of drugs developed for diseases of the brain and 96% of anticancer drugs have failed in clinical trials (Wong et al. 2019) indicating the need for preclinical testing based on *qualified methods*. It is better to fail fast and cheap. Moreover, drug delivery and targeting must be considered by multidisciplinary research teams from the outset.

Essential questions in drug development, particularly concerning drugs addressing new or incompletely understood targets and pathways, include:

- Which targets must be addressed by the actives?
- Which off-targets are likely addressed and what about the related risks?
- Will efficacy and safety benefit from drug targeting and which delivery system appears most suitable?
- Is ongoing efficacy expected, if long-term therapy is needed?
- What is the anticipated benefit of the new therapy compared to established treatments? Is the scientific basis sound?
- What measures are necessary to protect first-time and early-stage users of new drugs?
- Can validated methods address these questions and allow to determine the benefit–risk ratio?

Framing a benefit–risk analysis is essential at the start of a project and again when preparing for the next major steps of a research program.

5.1 Predictive Preclinical Approaches

In Silico/In Vitro/Ex Vivo Studies Early stages of drug development for human use should explicitly *engage with the complexity of human biology* combining respective computational (molecular modeling) and experimental knowledge in a conceptual framework, thereby bridging the gap between molecular entities and the cellular phenotype (Wray and Whitmore 2022). To be close to the patient, the test matrix should be the diseased target organ (Frombach et al. 2019) or a rigorously characterized human cell-based organotypic disease model. Testing on juvenile cells is preferred because of the higher proliferation rate, but its predictability is often poor for diseases in the aged.

Significant progress has been made in this area. Preclinical testing increasingly uses qualified *human cell-based 3D disease models* (Schäfer-Korting and Zoschke 2021). Combined with the human on-the-chip technology significantly enhancing tissue viability, a first insight into effects over time and following repeated exposure (Ma et al. 2021) will become possible.

Human genetic variants can be studied on material from cell banks (Carss et al. 2023) and engineered cells, models generated from genetic variant cells can provide an early insight into the efficacy and safety in a broader population. The results will improve the predictability of preclinical data for human.

For example, organoids generated from human-induced pluripotent stem cells are developed for screening the transduction efficacy of engineered AAV vectors to be used in retinal gene therapy. GFP signaling in the organoids reveals differences in the potency of vector candidates (Pavlou et al. 2021). An independent, small size study (9 patients) in CNGA3-gene associated achromatopsia indicates safety and some improvement following AAV8 gene delivery (Fischer et al. 2020). The future will show if preclinical approaches as suggested here meet the expectation, and gene therapies for currently untreatable ocular diseases can be realized.

Drug metabolism in human is foreseeable from results generated in in vitro studies. Low clearance drugs should be tested in liver microsomes or primary hepatocytes in microfluidic systems because of a rather stable enzyme activity. In vitro models of liver and kidney diseases as well as cerebral organoids and brain-on-a-chip models are established including those generated from human cells (Youhanna et al. 2022). In fact, respective research appears to be almost exploding.

Animal experiments, however, remain essential in order to further minimize the exposure of humans to inefficient or unsafe drugs. For transferability of results to humans, the relative age of the animals has to be aligned with the life stage of the target population. For example, preclinical studies on stroke therapy often fail to be predictive because of testing in young animals, neglecting to incorporate co-morbidities or using doses not applicable to human (Nilles et al. 2022). Animal care and stress reduction are essential for predictive and reproducible results, too.

Novel therapeutics that lack relevant animal models to reveal their intrinsic safety profile will benefit from the application of human genetics. Assessing potential on- and off-target events as well as carcinogenicity risks should be subject of translational safety studies and surveillance strategies to decide to continue or discontinue a program (Carss et al. 2023). For gene therapeutics in particular adequate models are a major challenge and in fact, since December 2022, animal testing is no longer an essential prerequisite for drug approval according to US law.

5.2 High-End Analytics

The quantification of drug levels is needed both in preclinical and clinical studies. Low doses of potent actives ask for high-end analytics (MS/MS spectroscopy in particular) to quantify drug access to the target site (Yamamoto et al. 2016). Modeling drug concentrations over time reveals short-term and long-run drug exposure (Saeidpour et al. 2017; Schulz et al. 2017), which facilitates the planning of clinical studies. Sample collection, handling, and analytics of mRNA drugs deviate from those applicable to small molecules and proteins (Guelman et al. 2022). Results of those studies will allow to focus clinical studies of mRNA agents.

5.3 Drug Delivery: New Approaches in Carrier Development

In particular in chronic diseases, *adherence to therapy* is another hurdle to success, requiring well-tolerated and easy-to-use medication to promote compliance. Thus, drug delivery and targeting must be considered by multidisciplinary research teams from the outset as they envision the "product drug."

Computer modeling of carriers can complement experimental approaches. Its relevance will increase with a detailed understanding of the influences of particle structure and aggregation, stability, size and surface, interactions with proteins and cell surfaces on cargo delivery (Ramezanpour et al. 2016). Machine learning and artificial intelligence, which facilitate insights into nanoparticle delivery in tumors (Lin et al. 2022), may allow for an a priori selection of promising systems (Tomé et al. 2021) in the future. Similarly, robotic processes for head-to-head comparisons of vehicles (Cui et al. 2022) should gain relevance.

5.4 Clinical Studies

Ultimately, clinical studies must prove the efficacy and safety of the therapy. Control groups have to receive the currently established therapy. Gordon Gyatt has outlined important standards for clinical research and has been awarded the Individual Award 2022 by the Einstein Foundation Berlin for his research in evidence-based medicine (einsteinfoundation.de).

5.5 Enhancing Knowledge Acquisition and Risk Assessment

Following drug approval, strong networks are of outmost importance collecting, evaluating, and reporting on efficacy and safety. Most challenging are drugs approved for rare and severe disorders. International committees of outstanding experts including those not involved in the development of a respective drug should take-over data analysis and activate alarm systems, if needed.

5.6 Ethical Aspects and Conclusions

As outlined, several paths have the potential to generate novel prophylaxes and therapies of recalcitrant diseases including those in late and very early stages of life. Gene and cell therapy hold major promise in this regard and often are expected to result in healing. As currently ongoing efficacy is not assured, the promises and associated challenges of genome editing require responsible use (Doudna 2020). The preferences of informed patients and their families must be included in the decision making. This is of particular importance when deciding on gene therapy in children and prenatally. Intense monitoring of the patients and detailed reporting will enhance understanding of benefits and risks. Finally, access to the most advanced and costly therapies already challenges the health systems. Societies and parliaments must discuss rules for how to proceed.

Acknowledgment I would like to thank Prof. Dr. Burkhard Kleuser and PD Dr. Christian Zoschke for their collegial and critical approach to this chapter.

References

Adams D, Tournev IL, Taylor MS et al (2023) Efficacy and safety of vutrisiran for patients with hereditary transthyrethrin-mediated amyloidosis with polyneuropathy: a randomized clinical trial. Amyloid 30:1–9

Aimo A, Castiglione V, Rapezzi C et al (2022) RNA-targeting and gene editing therapies for transthyretin amyloidosis. Nat Rev Cardiol 19:655–667

Aliahmad P, Miyake-Stoner SJ, Geall AJ et al (2022) Next generation self-replicating RNA vectors for vaccines and immunotherapies. Cancer Gene Ther 30:785–793

Armocida D, Pesce A, Di Giammarco F et al (2019) Long term survival in patients suffering from glioblastoma multiforme: a single-centre observational cohort study. Diagnostics 9:209

Baden LR, El Sahli HM, Essink B et al (2021) Efficacy and safety of the mRNA-1273 SARS-CoV-2 vaccine. N Engl J Med 384:403–416

Barker RA, Cutting EV, Daft DM (2021) Bringing advanced therapy medicinal products (ATMPs) for Parkinson's disease to the clinic: the investigator's perspective. J Parkinsons Dis 11(Suppl 2):S129–S134

Berlet R, Galang Cabantan DA, Gonzales-Portillo D (2022) Enriched environment and exercise enhance stem cell therapy for stroke, Parkinson's disease and Huntington's disease. Front Cell Dev Biol 10:798826

Borlongan CV (2019) Concise review: stem cell therapy for stroke patients: are we there yet? Stem Cells Transl Med 8:983–988

Brooks B, Ebedes D, Usmani A et al (2022) Mesenchymal stromal cells in brain injury. Cell 11: 1013
Burgess A, Hynynen K (2013) Noninvasive and targeted drug delivery to the brain using focused ultrasound. ACS Chem Neurosci 4:519–526
Carneiro W, Müller JT, Merkel OM (2022) Molecular therapeutics for pulmonary diseases. In: Schäfer-Korting et al (ed) Drug delivery and targeting, handbook of experimental pharmacology
Carss KJ, Deaton AM, Del Rio-Espinola A (2023) Using human genetics to improve safety assessment of therapeutics. Nat Rev Drug Discov 22:145–162
Chen T, Xu J, Zhu L et al (2023) Cancer-cell-membrane-camouflaged supramolecular self-assembly of antisense oligonucleotide and chemodrug for targeted combination therapy. Nanoscale 15:1914–1924
Chiu W, Lin T-Y, Chang Y-C et al (2021) An update on gene therapy for inherited retinal dystrophy: experience in Leber congenital amaurosis clinical trials. Int J Mol Sci 22:4534
Crooke ST, Baker BF, Crooke RM et al (2021) Antisense technology: an overview and prospectus. Nat Rev Drug Discov 20:427–453
Cui L, Pereira S, van Pelt SS et al (2022) Development of a high-throughput platform for screening lipid nanoparticles for mRNA delivery. Nanoscale 14:1480–1491
Das R, Hyer RN, Burton P et al (2023) Emerging heterologous mRNA-based booster strategies within the COVID-19 vaccine landscape. Hum Vaccin Immunother 19:2153532
Dilliard SA, Cheng Q, Siegwart DJ (2021) On the mechanism of tissue-specific mRNA delivery by selective organ targeting nanoparticles. Proc Natl Acad Sci U S A 118:e2109256118
Doudna JA (2020) The promise and challenge of therapeutic genome editing. Nature 578:229–236
Feng L, Wang Q, Shan C et al (2020) An adenovirus-vectored COVID-19 vaccine confers protection from SARS-COV-2 challenge in rhesus macaques. Nat Commun 11:4207
Fischer DM, Michalakis S, Wilhelm B et al (2020) Safety and vision outcomes of subretinal gene therapy targeting cone photoreceptors in achromatopsia: a nonrandomized controlled trial. JAMA Ophthalmol 138:643–651
Fortress AM, Miyagishima KI, Reed AA et al (2023) Stem cell sources and characterization in the development of cell-based products for treating retinal disease: an NEI town hall report. Stem Cell Res Ther 14:53
Frampton JE (2023) Inclisiran: a review in hypercholesterolemia. Am J Cardiovasc Drugs 23:219–230
Frombach J, Unbehauen M, Kurniashi IN et al (2019) Core-multishell nanocarriers enhance drug penetration and reach keratinocytes and antigen-presenting cells in intact human skin. J Control Release 299:138–148
Gillmore JD, Gane E, Taubel J et al (2021) CRISPR-Cas9 in vivo gene editing for transthyretin amyloidosis. New Engl J Med 385:493–502
Guelman S, Zhou Y, Brady A et al (2022) A fit-fur-purpose method to measure circulating levels of the mRNA component of a liposomal-formulated individualized neoantigen-specific therapy for cancer. AAPS J 24:64
Higano CS, Armstrong AJ, Sartor AO et al (2019) Real-world outcomes of sipuleucel-T treatment in PROCEED, a prospective registry of men with metastatic castration-resistant prostate cancer. Cancer 125:4172–4180
Hoffmann M, Kleine-Weber H, Pöhlmann S (2020) A multibasic cleavage site in the spike protein of SARS-CoV-2 is essential for infection of human lung cells. Mol Cell 78:779–784
Husseini RA, Abe N, Hara T et al (2023) The use of iontophoresis technology for transdermal delivery of a minimal mRNA vaccine as a potential melanoma therapeutic. Biol Pharm Bull 46: 301–308
Iglesias-Lopez C, Agusti A, Vallano A et al (2021) Current landscape of clinical development and approval of advanced therapies. Mol Ther Methods Clin Dev 23:606–618
Imbimbo BP, Triaca V, Imbimbo C et al (2023) Investigational treatments for neurodegenerative diseases caused by inheritance of gene mutations: lessons learned from recent clinical studies. Neural Regen Res 18:1679–1683

Kantoff PW, Higano CS, Shore ND et al (2010) Sipuleucel-T immunotherapy for castration-resistant prostate cancer. New Engl J Med 363:411–422

Liang JP, Accola RP, Soundirajan M et al (2021) Engineering a microporous oxygen-generating scaffold for enhancing islet cell transplantation within an extrahepatic site. Acta Biomater 130: 268–280

Lin Z, Chou WC, Cheng YH et al (2022) Predicting nanoparticle delivery to tumors using machine learning and artificial intelligence approaches. Int J Nanomed 17:1365–1379

Linares-Fernández S, Lacroix C, Exposito J-Y et al (2020) Tailoring mRNA vaccine to balance innate/adaptive immune response. Trends Mol Med 26:311–23

Lindholm P, Saarma M (2022) Cerebral dopamine neurotrophic factor protects and repairs dopamine neurons by novel mechanism. Mol Psychiatry 27:1310–1321

Liu Q, Wang X, Chiu A et al (2021) A zwitterionic polyurethan nanoporous device with low foreign-body response for islet encapsulation. Adv Mater 33:e2102852

Lloyd-Williams H, Hughes DA (2021) A systematic review of economic evaluations of advanced therapy medicinal products. Br J Clin Pharmacol 87:2428–2443

Ma C, Peng Y, Li H (2021) Organ-on-a-chip: a new paradigm for drug development. Trends Pharmacol Sci 42:119–133

Martin T, Usmani SZ, Berdeja JG et al (2023) Ciltacabtagene autoleucel, an anti-B-cell maturation antigen chimeric antigen receptor T-cell therapy, for relapsed/refractory multiple myeloma: CARTITUDE-1 2-year follow-up. J Clin Oncol 41:1265–1274

McDougall R, Ramsden D, Agarwal S et al (2022) The nonclinical disposition and pharmacokinetic/pharmacodynamic properties of N-acetylgalactosamine-conjugated small interfering RNA are highly predictable and build confidence in translation to human. Drug Metab Dispos 50: 781–797

Melton D (2021) The promise of stem cell-derived islet replacement therapy. Diabetologica 64: 1030–1036

Mendell JR, Al-Zaidy SA, Lehman KJ et al (2021) Five-year extension results of the phase 1 START trial of onasemnogene abeparvovec in spinal muscular atrophy. JAMA Neurol 78: 834–841

Mistry P, Barmania F, Mellet J et al (2022) SARS-CoV-2 variants, vaccines and host immunity. Front Immunol 12:809244

Monine M, Norris D, Wang Y et al (2021) A physiologically-based pharmacokinetic model to describe antisense oligonucleotide distribution after intrathecal administration. J Pharmacokinet Pharmacodyn 48:639–654

Munoz-Velandia O, Guyatt G, Devji T et al (2019) Patient values and preference regarding continuous subcutaneous insulin infusion and artificial pancreas in adults with type 1 diabetes: a systematic review of quantitative and qualitative data. Diabetes Technol Ther 21:183–200

Nair JK, Willoughby JL, Chan A et al (2014) Multivalent N-acetylgalactosamine-conjugated siRNA localizes in hepatocytes and elicits robust RNAi-mediated gene silencing. J Am Chem Soc 136:16958–16961

Nilles KL, Williams EI, Betterton RD et al (2022) Blood-brain barrier transporters: opportunities for therapeutic development in ischemic stroke. Int J Mol Sci 23:1898

Ozelo MC, Mahlangu J, Pasi KJ et al (2022) Valoctogene roxaparvovec gene therapy for hemophilia A. New Engl J Med 386:1013–1025

Papachristofilou A, Hipp MM, Klinkhardt U et al (2019) Phase Ib evaluation of a self-adjuvanted protamine formulated mRNA-based active cancer immunotherapy, BI1361849 (CV9202), combined with local radiation treatment in patients with stage IV non-small cell lung cancer. J Immunotherapy Cancer 7:38

Pardi N, Tuyishime S, Muramatsu H et al (2015) Expression kinetics of nucleoside-modified mRNA delivered in lipid nanoparticles to mice by various routes. J Control Release 217:345–351

Pavlou M, Schön C, Occelli LM et al (2021) Novel AAV capsids for intravitreal gene therapy of photoreceptor disorders. EMBO Mol Med 13:e13392

Pollack FP, Thomas SJ, Kitchin N et al (2020) Safety and efficacy of the BNT162b2 mRNA Covid-19 vaccine. N Engl J Med 383:2603–2615
Ramachandran S, Satapathy SR, Dutta T (2022) Delivery strategy for mRNA vaccines. Pharmaceut Med 36:11–20
Ramezanpour M, Leung SSW, Delgado-Magnero KH et al (2016) Computational and experimental approaches for investigating nanoparticle-based drug delivery systems. Biochim Biophys Acta 1858:1688–1709
Rees HA, Minella AC, Burnett CA et al (2021) CRISPR-derived genome editing therapies: progress from bench to bedside. Mol Ther 29:3125–3139
Reichel LS, Träger A (2023) Stimuli-responsive non-viral nanoparticles for gene delivery. In: Schäfer-Korting M, Schubert U (eds) Handbook of experimental pharmacology drug delivery and targeting
Reilly A, Chehade L, Kothary R (2023) Curing SMA: are we there yet? Gene Ther 30:8–17
Rojas LA, Sethna Z, Soares KC (2023) Personalized RNA neoantigen vaccines stimulate T cells in pancreatic cancer. Nature 618:144–150
Russel S, Bennett J, Wellman JA et al (2017) Efficacy and safety of voretigene neparvovec (AAV2-hRPE65v2) in patients with RPE-65-mediated inherited retinal dystrophy: a randomized, controlled, open-label, phase 3 trial. Lancet 390:849–860
Saeidpour S, Lohan SB, Anske M et al (2017) Localization of dexamethasone within dendritic core-multishell (CMS) nanoparticles and skin penetration properties studied by multi-frequency electron paramagnetic resonance (EPR) spectroscopy. Eur J Pharm Biopharm 116:94–101
Sahin U, Karikó K, Türeci Ö (2014) mRNA-based therapeutics – developing a new class of drugs. Nat Rev Drug Discov 13:759–780
Sahin U, Oehm P, Derhovanessian E et al (2020) An mRNA vaccine drives immunity in checkpoint-inhibitor-treated melanoma. Nature 585:107–126
Sahin U, Türeci O, Manikhas G et al (2021) FAST: a randomised phase II study of zolbetuximab (IMAB362) plus EOX versus EOX alone for first-line treatment of advanced CLDN18.2-positive gastric and gastro-esophageal adenocarcinoma. Ann Oncol 32:609–619
Schäfer-Korting M, Zoschke C (2021) How qualification of 3D disease models cuts the Gordian knot in preclinical drug development. In: Schäfer-Korting M, Maria-Engler SS, Landsiedel R (eds) Organotypic models in drug development. Handbook of experimental pharmacology, vol 265, Springer, Heidelberg, pp 29–58
Schulz R, Yamamoto K, Klossek A et al (2017) Data-based modeling of drug penetration relates human skin barrier function to the interplay of diffusivity and free-energy profiles. Proc Nat Acad Sci 114:3631–3636
Sécher T, Mayor A, Heuzé-Vourc'h N (2019) Inhalation of immuno-therapeutics/-prophylactics to fight respiratory tract infections: an appropriate drug at the right place! Front Immunol 10:2760
Shang J, Wan Y, Luo C et al (2020) Cell entry mechanism of SARS-CoV-2. Proc Natl Acad Sci U S A 117:11727–11734
Sharifian-Dorche M, Bahmanyar M, Sharifian-Dorche A (2021) Vaccine-induced immune thrombocytopenia and cerebral venous sinus thrombosis post COVID-19 vaccination; a systematic review. J Neurol Sci 428:117607
Shemesh CS, Hsu JC, Hosseini I et al (2021) Personalized cancer vaccines: clinical landscape, challenges, and opportunities. Mol Ther 29:555–570
Srivasta A (2023) Rationale and strategies for the development of safe and effective optimized AAV vectors for human gene therapy. Mol Ther Nucleid Acids 32:949–959
Strauss KA, Farrar MA, Muntoni F et al (2022) Onasemnogen abeparvovec for presyptomatic infants with two copies of *SMN2* at risk for spinal muscular atrophy type 1: the phase III SP1INT trial. Nat Med 28:1381–1389
Suzuki N, Nishiyama A, Warita H et al (2023) Genetics of amyotrophic lateral sclerosis: seeking therapeutic targets in the era of gene therapy. J Hum Genet 68:131–153
Teijaro JR, Farber DL (2021) COVID-19 vaccines: modes of immune vaccination and future challenges. Nat Rev Immunol 21:195–197

Tomé I, Francisco V, Fernandes H et al (2021) High throughput screening of nanoparticles in drug delivery. APL Bioeng 5:031511

Triolo TM, Bellin MD (2021) Lessons learned from human islet transplantation inform stem cell-based approaches in the treatment of diabetes. Front Endocrinol 12:636824

van Haasteren J, Li J, Scheideler OJ et al (2020) The delivery challenge: fulfilling the promise of therapeutic genome editing. Nat Biotechnol 38:845–855

Vitiello A, Ferrara F, Auti AM et al (2022) Advances in the omicron variant development. J Intern Med 292:81–90

Wang X, Maxwell KG, Wang K et al (2021) A nanofibrous encapsulation device for safe delivery of insulin producing cells to treat type 1 diabetes. Sci Transl Med 13(596):eabb4601. https://doi.org/10.1126/scitranslmed.abb4601

Wang SW, Gao C, Zheng Y-M et al (2022) Current applications and future perspective of CRISPR/Cas9 gene editing in cancer. Mol Cancer 21:57. https://doi.org/10.1186/s12943-022-01518-8

Wang Q, Yang C, Lin L et al (2023) Intranasal booster using an omicron vaccine confers broad mucosal and systemic immunity against SARS-CoV-2 variants. Signal Transduct Target Ther 8:167

Wong CH, Siah KW, Lo AW (2019) Estimation of clinical trial success rates and related parameters. Biostatistics 20:273–286

Wray J, Whitmore A (2022) Network-driven drug discovery. Methods Mol Biol 2390:177–190

Wu Y, Hutton A, Pandya A et al (2023) Microneedle and polymeric films – delivery of proteins, peptides and nucleic acids. In: Schäfer-Korting M, Schubert U (eds) Handbook of experimental pharmacology drug delivery and targeting

Xie N, Shen G, Gao W et al (2023) Neoantigens: promising targets for cancer therapy. Sign Transduct Target Ther 8:9

Yamamoto K, Klossek A, Flesch R et al (2016) Core-multishell nanocarriers: transport and release of dexamethasone probed by soft X-ray spectromicroscopy. J Control Release 242:64–70

Yan Y, Liu X-Y, Lu A et al (2022) Non-viral vectors for RNA delivery. J Control Release 342:241–279

Youhanna S, Kemas AM, Preiss L et al (2022) Organotypic and microphysiological human tissue models for drug discovery and development – current state-of-the-art and future perspectives. Pharmacol Rev 74:141–206

Yu MW, Quail DF (2021) Immunotherapy for glioblastoma: current progress and challenges. Front Immunol 12:676301

Zhang C, Newsome JT, Mewani R et al (2009) Systemic delivery and pre-clinical evaluation of nanoparticles containing antisense oligonucleotides and siRNAs. Methods Mol Biol 480:65–83